Handbook of Chronic Kidney Disease

Handbook of Chronic Kidney Disease

Edited by Felicity Darko

hayle medical
New York

Hayle Medical,
750 Third Avenue, 9th Floor,
New York, NY 10017, USA

Visit us on the World Wide Web at:
www.haylemedical.com

ISBN: 978-1-63241-928-6

Cataloging-in-Publication Data

Handbook of chronic kidney disease / edited by Felicity Darko.
p. cm.
Includes bibliographical references and index.
ISBN 978-1-63241-928-6
1. Kidneys--Diseases. 2. Chronic diseases. 3. Kidneys--Diseases--Diagnosis.
4. Kidneys--Diseases--Treatment. I. Darko, Felicity.
RC903 .H36 2020
616.61--dc23

Table of Contents

Preface

Every book is a source of knowledge and this one is no exception. The idea that led to the conceptualization of this book was the fact that the world is advancing rapidly; which makes it crucial to document the progress in every field. I am aware that a lot of data is already available, yet, there is a lot more to learn. Hence, I accepted the responsibility of editing this book and contributing my knowledge to the community.

Chronic kidney disease (CKD) is a disease of the kidneys whereby they lose their function gradually over time. It also increases the risk of developing cardiovascular disease. The cause of mortality in individuals with CKD is cardiovascular disease. CKD progresses over a number of stages in increasing order of kidney damage. Kidney damage with glomerular filtration rate (GFR) greater than 90 ml/min and persistent albuminuria qualifies for stage 1. As it advances, GFR reduces progressively. Finally when GFR becomes less than 15 ml/min (stage 5), kidney failure sets in and the disease enters its end-stage. At this stage, a permanent renal replacement therapy is required for survival of the patient. Although renal replacement therapies can sustain people indefinitely, the quality of life is severely compromised. For individuals with hypertension, diabetes or obesity, above 60 years of age, or with a history of cardiovascular disease or kidney disease in family, screening is recommended. Research in CKD is aimed at the development of effective compounds for treating the disease. The efficacy of sulodexide and olmesartan medoxomil in the management of CKD is currently under investigation. This book provides comprehensive insights into chronic kidney disease. It presents researches and studies performed by experts across the globe. Those in search of information to further their knowledge will be greatly assisted by this book.

While editing this book, I had multiple visions for it. Then I finally narrowed down to make every chapter a sole standing text explaining a particular topic, so that they can be used independently. However, the umbrella subject sinews them into a common theme. This makes the book a unique platform of knowledge.

I would like to give the major credit of this book to the experts from every corner of the world, who took the time to share their expertise with us. Also, I owe the completion of this book to the never-ending support of my family, who supported me throughout the project.

Editor

1

Ergocalciferol and Microcirculatory Function in Chronic Kidney Disease and Concomitant Vitamin D Deficiency

Gavin Dreyer[1,3], Arthur T. Tucker[4], Steven M. Harwood[3], Rupert M. Pearse[2], Martin J. Raftery[1], Muhammad M. Yaqoob[1,3]*

1 Department of Renal Medicine, Barts Health NHS Trust, London, United Kingdom, **2** Department of Critical Care Medicine, Barts Health NHS Trust, London, United Kingdom, **3** Department of Translational Medicine and Therapeutics, Queen Mary University of London, London, United Kingdom, **4** Ernest Cooke Microvascular Unit, Barts Health NHS Trust, London, United Kingdom

Abstract

Background and Objectives: Vitamin D deficiency and endothelial dysfunction are non-traditional risk factors for cardiovascular events in chronic kidney disease. Previous studies in chronic kidney disease have failed to demonstrate a beneficial effect of vitamin D on arterial stiffness, left ventricular mass and inflammation but none have assessed the effect of vitamin D on microcirculatory endothelial function.

Study Design: We conducted a randomised controlled trial of 38 patients with non diabetic chronic kidney disease stage 3–4 and concomitant vitamin D deficiency (<16 ng/dl) who received oral ergocalciferol (50,000 IU weekly for one month followed by 50,000 IU monthly) or placebo over 6 months. The primary outcome was change in microcirculatory function measured by laser Doppler flowmetry after iontophoresis of acetylcholine. Secondary endpoints were tissue advanced glycation end products, sublingual functional capillary density and flow index as well as macrovascular parameters. Parallel *in vitro* experiments were conducted to determine the effect of ergocalciferol on cultured human endothelial cells.

Results: Twenty patients received ergocalciferol and 18 patients received placebo. After 6 months, there was a significant improvement in the ergocalciferol group in both endothelium dependent microcirculatory vasodilatation after iontophoresis of acetylcholine ($p = 0.03$) and a reduction in tissue advanced glycation end products ($p = 0.03$). There were no changes in sublingual microcirculatory parameters. Pulse pressure ($p = 0.01$) but not aortic pulse wave velocity was reduced. There were no significant changes in bone mineral parameters, blood pressure or left ventricular mass index suggesting that ergocalciferol improved endothelial function independently of these parameters. In parallel experiments, expression of endothelial nitric oxide synthase and activity were increased in human endothelial cells in a dose dependent manner.

Conclusions: Ergocalciferol improved microcirculatory endothelial function in patients with chronic kidney disease and concomitant vitamin D deficiency. This process may be mediated through enhanced expression and activity of endothelial nitric oxide synthase.

Trial Registration: Clinical trials.gov NCT00882401

Editor: Giuseppe Danilo, University of Milan, Italy

Funding: This study was funded by grants from the British Renal Society (www.britishrenal.org) (Grant number BRS 09/010) and the Barts and the London charitable Trust (Barts and the London charitable Trust). The funders had no role in study design, data collection and analysis, decision to publish, or preparation of the manuscript.

Competing Interests: The authors have declared that no competing interests exist.

* Email: m.m.yaqoob@qmul.ac.uk

Introduction

Patients with chronic kidney disease (CKD) are far more likely to die of cardiovascular disease (CVD) than progress to end stage kidney disease (ESKD) [1]. Traditional risk factors including age, hypertension, smoking and diabetes mellitus do not entirely account for the excess of CVD mortality in patients with CKD. Vitamin D deficiency, a non-traditional CVD risk factor in patients with all stages of kidney disease [2,3,4], is highly prevalent in patients with CKD [5,6] and is associated with elevated cardiovascular (CV) morbidity and mortality [7,8,9].

Vitamin D deficiency in patients with CKD has been shown to correlate with impairment in endothelial function [10,11]. In pre-clinical [12] and clinical studies [13], endothelial dysfunction has been identified as a non-traditional risk factor for CVD in CKD with improvements in endothelial function reflecting improved global vascular health and a reduced risk of CVD [14].

Observational studies [15,16,17,18,19,20] have provided support for the protective role of vitamin D therapy in reducing the risk of CVD in patients with CKD and ESKD. However, these studies were heterogeneous in design, therapeutic intervention and patient populations (CKD vs ESKD) and have not elucidated the mechanism by which vitamin D reduces CV risk in this patient group. Several *in vitro*, pre-clinical and clinical studies have demonstrated that endothelial and therefore microcirculatory function can be ameliorated after treatment with both activated and nutritional forms of vitamin D [21,22,23,24,25]. However, none of these studies have included patients with CKD. Two previous studies in patients with non-dialysis and CKD and ESKD evaluating the effect of nutritional vitamin D compounds on endothelial biomarkers and conduit artery function have provided conflicting results [26,27].

The microcirculation, defined as blood vessels <150 μm in diameter [28] located within tissue parenchyma, is intricately linked to endothelial function and predicts the function of the microcirculatory beds in renal and cardiac tissue [29,30,31,32,33]. A review of cardiovascular assessment in patients with CKD [34] has highlighted the need for further assessments of microcirculatory dysfunction in patients with CKD as a method for predicting adverse CV outcomes. To date, there have been no prospective, randomized controlled studies investigating the effect of vitamin D on microcirculatory endothelial function or CV endpoints in patients with CKD [35].

We therefore conducted an exploratory, double blind, randomised, controlled trial to determine if therapy with ergocalciferol compared to placebo improves microcirculatory endothelial function in patients with CKD and concomitant vitamin D deficiency. We also conducted parallel *in vitro* experiments to elucidate the mechanistic pathway of ergocalciferol in cultured human endothelial cells.

Methods

Study design

The protocol for this trial and supporting CONSORT checklist are available as supporting information; see Checklist S1 and Protocol S1. This was a single centre, double blind, exploratory randomised controlled trial comparing oral ergocalciferol to placebo in patients with CKD stage 3–4 (estimated glomerular filtration rate (eGFR) 60–15 ml/min/1.73 m^2) and concomitant vitamin D deficiency (defined as a serum 25 hydroxy vitamin D (25 (OH) D) level of <16 ng/ml). The study was conducted at the Royal London Hospital, UK, between 1/5/2009 and 1/9/2010. All patients provided written informed consent and ethical approval was obtained from the East London Research Ethics Committee. The trial was registered at clinicaltrials.gov (Clinical trials number- NCT00882401, http://clinicaltrials.gov/ct2/show/NCT00882401) and conducted in accordance with the Declaration of Helsinki.

Inclusion/exclusion criteria

The principle inclusion criteria were an eGFR between 15 and 60 ml/min/1.73 m^2 with evidence of 2 consecutive measures of eGFR <60 ml/min/1.73 m^2 by the 4 variable MDRD equation [36] at least 3 months apart, serum 25 (OH) D levels <16 ng/ml, age >18 and <80 years, no evidence of diabetes mellitus (fasting blood sugar <128 mg/dl, not taking any diabetic medication), not receiving nor having had renal replacement therapy in the preceding three months

The principle exclusion criteria were current vitamin D therapy of any type, serum calcium above 10.4 mg/dl (based on the upper limit of the laboratory reference range [37]), pregnant or lactating women, presence of conditions which predispose to hypercalcaemia, renal calculi and presence of a disease other than CKD associated with microcirculatory dysfunction.

Intervention and randomization

Patients were randomised to either ergocalciferol (Sanofi Aventis, New Jersey, USA) or a matching placebo. The dose of ergocalciferol was 50,000 IU weekly for one month followed by 50,000 IU monthly for 5 months resulting in a total dose of 450,000 IU over 6 months. This was in line with existing K/DOQI guidelines for the replacement of vitamin D in patients with CKD at the time the study was designed [37]. The dose of ergocalciferol was standardized for all patients to ensure equal dosing of ergocalciferol over the duration of the study to avoid the potentially confounding effect of varying doses of ergocalciferol based on initial serum concentrations of 25 (OH) D. The control arm received a matching placebo given at the same dose schedule as ergocalciferol. All patients received dietary advice appropriate to their stage of CKD from specialist renal dietitians which included advice on dietary intake of calcium, phosphate, sodium, potassium and protein. Patients were reviewed monthly for 6 months. A 2 week washout period for any vitamin D containing drugs or over the counter supplements was included before randomization, however no subjects required vitamin D washout. The randomization schedule was developed by an independent accountant. Sequentially numbered, sealed envelopes were used to achieve allocation concealment. Envelopes were stored and sequentially dispensed to study patients by the hospital clinical trial pharmacy who were blinded to the intervention and allocation as were the remainder of the study team.

Study endpoints

The primary outcome measure was microcirculatory endothelial function assessed by laser Doppler flowmetry (LDF) over forearm skin after iontophoresis of acetylcholine (ACh). Secondary outcome measures were microvascular parameters including skin autofluorescence (AF) and side stream dark field imaging (SDF) of the sub lingual microcirculation as well as macrovascular parameters including blood pressure, pulse pressure, aortic pulse wave velocity (aPWV), left ventricular mass index (LVMI) and bone mineral parameters (see File S1 for details of all techniques).

Clinical assessments

All patients were reviewed at the Royal London Hospital kidney unit. Patients were instructed to wear loose clothing, avoid caffeine and nicotine for 12 hours prior to assessments and rested for 15 minutes in a temperature and humidity controlled room before microcirculatory assessments.

Iontophoresis and laser Doppler flowmetry

Iontophoresis involves the delivery of charged particles to the local microcirculation, through the skin, using electrically repulsive forces. Laser Doppler flowmetry is a non-invasive technique which uses the Doppler principle to measure flux of erythrocytes in sub dermal capillaries. Increasing red cell flux after iontophoresis reflects microcirculatory vasodilatation as a consequence of improved endothelial function. The combination of these techniques is a validated method for studying endothelial function in the microcirculation in various pathologies including CKD. [38,39,40] A 1% solution of both ACh and sodium nitroprusside (SNP) were iontophoresed on the volar aspect of the non-dominant forearm using a low current protocol to reduce galvanic effect [41] with a maximum achieved dose of 75 μA after 7.5 minutes. To eliminate baseline variability, relative percentage change from baseline flux after the maximum iontophoretic dose is the primary outcome measure (see Figure S1 and Table S1 in File S1) [38].

Skin autofluorescence

Tissue advanced glycation end (AGE) product levels are an independent risk predictor of microcirculatory complications and are predictors of CVD in renal failure [42]. The technique utilises the AGE reader (Diagnoptics, Netherlands) which provides a non-invasive measure of AGE in the skin. AGE products correlate with measures of skin AF provided by the output from the AGE reader device [42].

Side stream dark field imaging of the sublingual microcirculation

This is a non-invasive, real time, imaging tool to assess intra-vital capillary blood flow. An analysis of the moving cells in the recorded video images permits the quantitative measurement of red blood cell flow in the capillaries. SDF images were scored and interpreted according to standard guidelines [43].

Macrocirculatory parameters

Aortic pulse wave velocity (Vicorder device, Skidmore Medical, UK) was measured to determine if changes in microcirculatory function occurred independently of changes in large conduit vessels. LVMI was measured by cardiac magnetic resonance imaging (cMRI) to determine if the hypothesized improved microcirculatory function resulted in reduced peripheral resistance leading to reduced cardiac workload and subsequent reductions in LVMI.

Biochemical analysis

All biochemical tests were performed in our hospital laboratory by a Roche modular unit analyser (F. Hoffmann-La Roche Ltd, Switzerland). Serum vitamin D levels were assessed by UPLC-MS/MS, which is a quantitative ultra-performance liquid chromatography tandem mass spectrometry assay. Parathyroid hormone (PTH) levels were assessed by the Roche E170 intact PTH assay (Roche Diagnostics, Mannheim)

Experimental work

Human aortic endothelial cells (HAEC, Promocell, UK) were cultured and incubated for 24 h using either low (12 ng/dl) or high (120 ng/dl) concentrations of ergocalciferol. Real time polymerase chain reaction (RT-PCR) was used to evaluate the effect of ergocalciferol on the expression of endothelial nitric oxide synthase (eNOS). Nitrite levels in cell supernatant, to evaluate the downstream effect of changes in eNOS expression in cells, were measured by a chemiluminescent technique [44] (see File S1 and figures S1-5 for full description of all techniques).

Statistical analysis

At the time of designing the study, there was insufficient available evidence of the effect of ergocalciferol therapy on microcirculatory parameters to undertake a standard power calculation. Our hypothesis was that ergocalciferol would significantly improve the function of the endothelium in patients with CKD and concomitant vitamin D deficiency. Given the profoundly low levels of 25 (OH) D in this patient group, the expected rise in serum 25 (OH) D levels with ergocalciferol and predicted lack of change of 25 (OH) D levels in the placebo group, we estimated that 30% of patients in the placebo group and 80% of the patients in the ergocalciferol group would have an improvement in peripheral LDF measured by relative change from baseline flux after 6 months of therapy. At 80% power and with a significance level of 0.05, this required 19 patients per arm. An intention to treat analysis was performed.

Clinical trial subjects

The two groups were compared for similarity at baseline and after 6 months of therapy using the Student's t test for normally distributed variables, Mann Whitney tests for non-parametric data and Chi squared tests or Fisher's exact test for proportions. Differences in 25 (OH) D levels and change from baseline flux measured by LDF after iontophoresis were analysed using a two way repeated measures ANOVA test followed by Bonferroni post tests for comparisons at pre determined time points (1, 3 and 6 months). We confirmed our findings using a mixed effects model. Forearm laser Doppler flowmetry is expressed as the percentage increase in flux from baseline after iontophoresis of ACh [38]. Four patients in the ergocalciferol group and 1 in the placebo group completed an initial 3 months on therapy before the end of the predetermined study period and this data was included in the analysis. The analysis of data at 6 months includes data from all remaining patients who completed the full follow up period. SDF imaging of the sublingual microcirculation was expressed as functional capillary density (mm^{-1}) and microvascular flow index as described previously [43]. LVMI, SDF imaging, skin AF and bone mineral parameters were analysed using t tests and Mann Whitney tests based on the distribution of the data. A p value of $<$ 0.05 was considered statistically significant. Analysis was conducted on Stata version 10 (www.stata.com) and GraphPad Prism software version 5 (see File S1 and figures S2–S5 for sub-group analysis).

Cell experiments

RT-PCR data were analyzed with ABI 7900HT Prism sequence detector software (SDS Version 2.3, Applied Biosystems) to determine differential gene expression for eNOS compared to β actin. Differences in nitrite levels were assessed using the Student t-test. Ethanol is included since this was used to dilute the ergocalciferol. Statistical analysis was performed using GraphPad Prism software (version 5).

Results

Patient screening, enrolment and randomization are shown in figure 1. The treatment and placebo groups were similar with respect to demographic, clinical (table 1) and laboratory parameters (table 2). Two patients were lost to follow up in the ergocalciferol arm and 1 in the placebo arm. All patients self reported complete compliance and this was confirmed by manual inspection of study medication bottles at each visit. No patients were taking nitrate containing medications that may have acted as vasodilators through the donation of nitric oxide. After 6 months of treatment with ergocalciferol, 25 hydroxy vitamin D (25 (OH) D) levels increased significantly in the treatment group ($p<0.0001$) (figure 2) but there were no significant changes in other biochemical parameters (table 3).

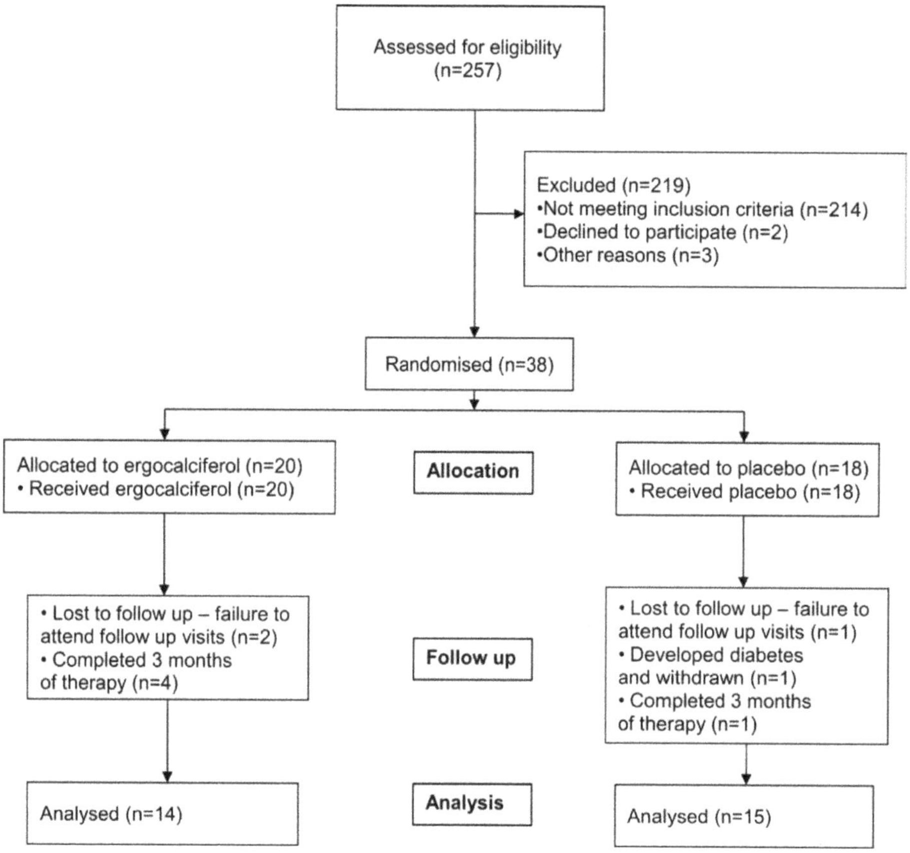

Figure 1. Recruitment schedule for study patients.

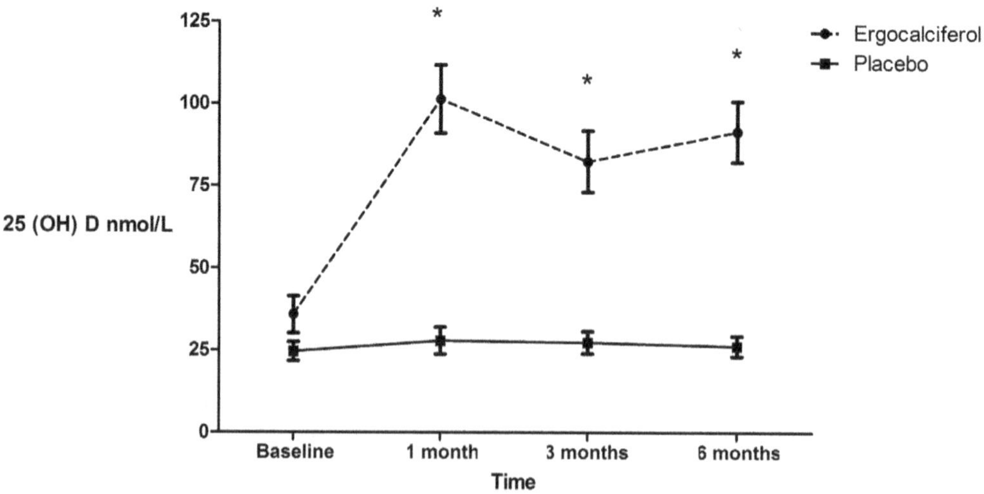

Number at risk

	Baseline	1 month	3 months	6 months
Ergocalciferol	20	19	18	14
Placebo	18	18	16	15

Figure 2. 25 (OH) D levels in patients treated with ergocalciferol and placebo. Bonferroni post tests following two way repeated measures ANOVA at 1,3 and 6 months $p<0.0001$. (* = statistically significant).

Table 1. Baseline demographic and clinical data for patients.

	Ergocalciferol (n = 20)	Placebo (n = 18)	p value
Age years	45.8 (10.0)	48.8 (12.2)	0.39
Sex (% male)	14 (60.9%)	14 (73.7%)	0.22
Body mass index	30.4 (7.1)	29.2 (3.4)	0.51
Ethnicity			0.57
Caucasian	5 (21.8%)	6 (31.6%)	
Non-Caucasian	15 (78.2%)	12 (68.4%)	
Cause of CKD			0.74
Hypertension	5 (25%)	7 (38.9%)	
Glomerulonephritis	8 (40%)	5 (27.8%)	
ADPKD	2 (10%)	1 (5.6%)	
Other~	5 (25%)	5 (27.7%)	
Smoking status			0.59
Current smoker	1 (5%)	2 (11.1%)	
Never/Ex-smoker	19 (95%)	16 (88.9%)	
Presence of endovascular stent devices	0 (0%)	1 (5.6%)	0.47
ACE-I/ARB	16 (80%)	12 (66.7%)	0.33
β Blocker	7 (35%)	6 (33.3%)	0.57
Statin use	9 (45%)	7 (38.9%)	0.84
Anti platelet therapy	2 (10%)	3 (16.7%)	0.48
Folic acid	1 (5.0%)	1 (5.6%)	1.00
Nitrate containing medications#	0 (0%)	0 (0%)	1.00
Medications containing Vitamin D	0 (0%)	0 (0%)	1.00
BP in past history	15 (65.2%)	11 (57.9%)	0.63
Systolic BP (mmHg)	114 (10)	119 (10)	0.11
Diastolic BP (mmHg)	70 (8)	71 (7)	0.57
MAP (mmHg)	84 (8)	87 (8)	0.29
Pulse pressure (mmHg)	45 (7)	48 (6)	0.08
aPWV (m/s)	8.5 (1.1)	8.5 (1.5)	0.66
LVMI (g/m2)	96.1 (36.3)	87.5 (174)	0.55
Skin AF (AU)	2.8 (0.9)	3.1 (0.9)	0.26
FCD (mm-1)	5.2 (0.5)	5.0 (0.5)	0.78
MFI (AU)	2.5 (0.1)	2.4 (0.1)	0.54

Figures in brackets are standard deviation of the mean or % of total in treatment group. ADPKD – autosomal dominant polycystic kidney disease. BP = blood pressure, ACE-I angiotensin converting enzyme inhibitor, ARB – angiotensin receptor blocker, MAP = mean arterial pressure, aPWV = aortic pulse wave velocity, LVMI – left ventricular mass index, AF – auto fluorescence, FCD – functional capillary density, MFI – microvascular flow index. AU – arbitrary units

#- any form of glyceryl trinitrate, isosorbide mononitrate, isosorbide dinitrate or other esters of nitric acid

~- Additional causes of CKD in ergocalciferol group: tubulo-interstitial nephritis (n = 1), reflux nephropathy (n = 2), unknown (n = 2). Placebo group: reflux nephropathy (n = 2), ischaemic nephropathy presumed due to reno-vascular disease (n = 1), unknown (n = 2).

The effect of ergocalciferol on microcirculatory parameters

Treatment with ergocalciferol compared to placebo was associated with a significant increase in change from baseline flux measured by LDF after iontophoresis of ACh (repeated measures 2 way ANOVA $p = 0.03$) with a significant difference between treatment groups observed at 6 months (Bonferroni post test $p = 0.012$) (figure 3). There were no significant differences in change from baseline flux after the iontophoresis of SNP between treatment groups at 6 months (repeated measures 2 way ANOVA $p = 0.18$) (figure 4). The use of a mixed effects model did not change the significance of these findings (change from baseline after iontophoresis at 6 months follow up: ACh $p = 0.03$, SNP $p = 0.36$).

Skin AF was significantly lower in patients treated with ergocalciferol after 6 months, reflecting reduced levels of tissue oxidative stress ($p = 0.03$). At the end of the follow up period, there were no differences in parameters of functional capillary density (FCD) or microvascular flow index (MFI) assessed by SDF imaging of the sublingual microcirculation (table 4).

The effect of ergocalciferol on macrocirculatory parameters

Pulse pressure was significantly lower in patients treated with ergocalciferol after 6 months ($p = 0.01$) but systolic, diastolic and

Table 2. Baseline laboratory data for CKD patients randomised to either ergocalciferol or placebo.

	Ergocalciferol (n = 20)	Placebo (n = 18)	p value
Creatinine (mg/dl)	2.3 (0.8)	2.0 (1.0)	0.60
eGFR (ml/min/1.73 m^2)	33.0 (13.5)	38.7 (15)	0.39
Stage of CKD			0.33
Stage 3	9 (45%)	13 (72.2%)	
Stage 4	11 (55%)	5 (27.8%)	
Hb (g/dl)	12.8 (1.8)	12.6 (1.4)	0.63
Calcium (mg/dl)	8.8 (0.8)	8.8 (0.8)	0.74
Phosphate (mg/dl)	3.8 (0.6)	3.5 (0.6)	0.16
Calcium phosphate product (mg^2/dl^2)	33.0 (4.2)	31.2 (5.1)	0.25
PTH (pg/L)	102.8 (76.4)	118.9 (103.8)	0.60
CRP (mg/L)	7.6 (17.2)	5.9 (9.8)	0.71
Urine P:CR	190.8 (276.4)	102.7 (147.0)	0.32
Total cholesterol (mg/dl)	201 (53)	185 (39)	0.36
High density lipoprotein cholesterol (mg/dl)	57.5 (24.0)	46.7 (15.9)	0.20

Figures in brackets are standard deviation of the mean. eGFR = estimated glomerular filtration rate, 25 (OH) D = 25 hydroxy vitamin D, Hb = haemaglobin, PTH = parathyroid hormone, CRP = C reactive protein, P:CR = protein:creatinine ratio.

mean arterial pressures were similar between treatment groups. There were no differences between the study groups in aPWV or LVMI after 6 months of therapy (table 4).

Safety data

There were no serious adverse events reported. Three patients in each group experienced episodes of gout that resolved with analgesia. The highest 25 (OH) D level recorded was 68.5 ng/ml. There were no recorded episodes of hypercalcaemia (defined as a serum calcium >10.4 mg/dl).

The effect of ergocalciferol on eNOS expression and nitrite levels in cultured human aortic endothelial cells

RT-PCR analysis for the fold-increase of eNOS compared to β-actin as a control gene demonstrated a dose dependent increase in expression with a 2.4-fold increase in eNOS expression after 24 h of incubation with high concentration ergocalciferol (120 ng/dl) compared to a 1.6 fold increase with low dose ergocalciferol (12 ng/dl) ($p = 0.002$). Only high concentration ergocalciferol resulted in a statistically significant increase in fold expression of eNOS compared to the control experiment ($p < 0.001$) (figure 5). There was no significant difference in nitrite levels between control and low dose ergocalciferol treated cells at 24 h. However, high dose ergocalciferol treatment produced a significant rise in nitrite compared to both low dose ($p = 0.007$) and vehicle control ($p = 0.003$) (figure 6).

Discussion

In this study, ergocalciferol therapy over 6 months in patients with CKD and concomitant vitamin D deficiency was associated with improved endothelium dependent microcirculatory function and a reduction in measures of tissue oxidative stress. The increase

Table 3. Laboratory results in both groups after 6 months of therapy.

	Ergocalciferol (n = 14)	Placebo (n = 15)	p value
Creatinine (mg/dl)	2.4 (0.9)	2.3 (1.1)	0.80
eGFR (ml/min/1.73 m^2)	31.4 (10.6)	35.0 (14.5)	0.44
Hb (g/dl)	12.6 (2.1)	12.4 (1.3)	0.73
Calcium (mg/dl)	9.1 (0.7)	8.9 (0.6)	0.43
Phosphate (mg/dl)	3.7 (0.74)	3.7 (1.2)	0.98
Calcium phosphate product (mg^2/dl^2)	33.6 (8.2)	32.6 (3.5)	0.66
PTH (pg/L)	97.2 (74.5)	135.8 (96.2)	0.26
CRP (mg/L)	7.5 (15.0)	9.7 (19.8)	0.76
Urine P:CR	154.0 (210.3)	117.5 (126.3)	0.62
Total cholesterol (mg/dl)	193 (38)	174 (35)	0.21
High density lipoprotein cholesterol (mg/dl)	54.2 (25.2)	50.8 (15.3)	0.67

Figures in brackets are standard deviation of the mean. eGFR = estimated glomerular filtration rate, 25 (OH) D = 25 hydroxy vitamin D, Hb = haemaglobin, PTH = parathyroid hormone, CRP = C reactive protein, P:CR = protein:creatinine ratio.

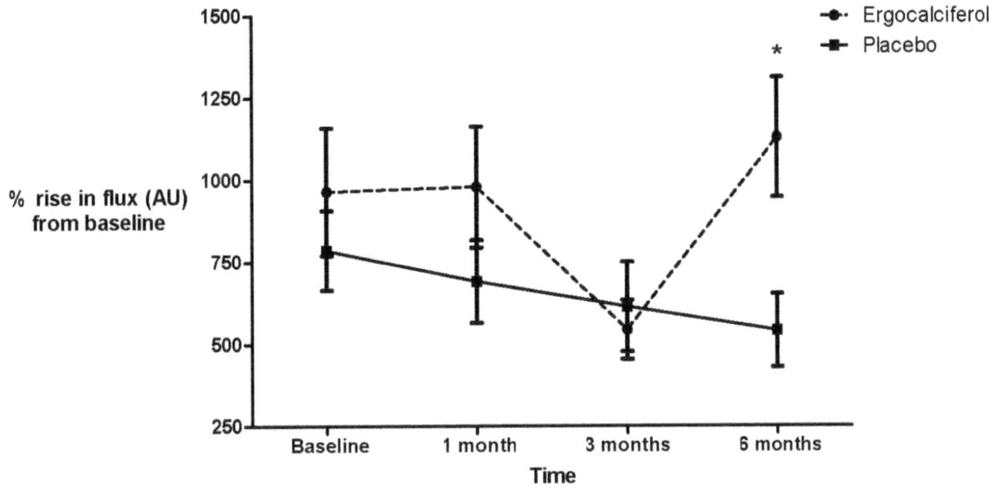

Number at risk

	Baseline	1 month	3 months	6 months
Ergocalciferol	20	19	18	14
Placebo	18	18	16	15

Figure 3. Percentage rise from baseline flux in arbitrary units (AU) after iontophoresis of ACh. Absolute values of percentage change in flux (AU): baseline - ergocalciferol 964.8, placebo 785.9 (p = NS). 1 month - ergocalciferol 979.5, placebo 690.9 (p = NS). 3 months – ergocalciferol 543.7, placebo 613.5 (p = NS). 6 months – ergocalciferol 1130.0, placebo 540.6 (p = 0.012). p values are Bonferroni post test following two way repeated measures ANOVA. (* = statistically significant).

in relative change of flux from baseline after iontophoresis with ACh but not SNP in subjects treated with ergocalciferol indicates improved microcirculatory function occurred through an endothelium dependent mechanism. Reduction in measures of skin AF in the ergocalciferol group correlates with reduced oxidative stress in these patients which will contribute to improved endothelial function and a reduced risk of future CV events [42]. This is in line with previous experimental work that demonstrated the protective effect of calcitriol in human endothelial cells cultured with AGE products [21].

In our study, bone mineral parameters, kidney function, C reactive protein, blood pressure and aPWV were similar at 6

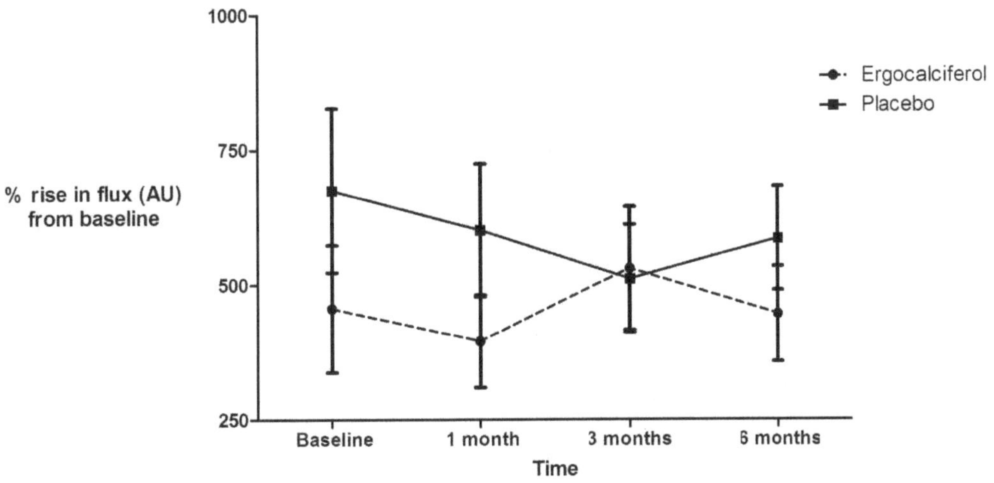

Number at risk

	Baseline	1 month	3 months	6 months
Ergocalciferol	20	19	18	14
Placebo	18	18	16	15

Figure 4. Percentage rise from baseline flux in arbitrary units (AU) after iontophoresis of SNP. Absolute values of percentage change in flux (AU): baseline - ergocalciferol 455.8, placebo 670.1 (p = NS). 1 month - ergocalciferol 395.5, placebo 601.3 (p = NS). 3 months – ergocalciferol 530.2, placebo 511.2 (p = NS). 6 months – ergocalciferol 445.7, placebo 585.9 (p = NS). p values are Bonferroni post test following two way repeated measures ANOVA.

Table 4. Measures of macrovascular parameters in both groups after 6 months of therapy.

	Ergocalciferol (n = 14)	Placebo (n = 15)	p value
Systolic BP (mmHg)	118 (10)	123 (15)	0.26
Diastolic BP (mmHg)	74 (6)	70 (9)	0.15
MAP (mmHg)	89 (7)	88 (10)	0.77
Pulse pressure (mmHg)	44 (8)	53 (12)	0.01
aPWV (m/s)	8.4 (1.3)	8.5 (1.2)	0.78
LVMI (g/m²)	94.7 (28.4)	110 (54.3)	0.44
Skin AF (AU)	2.8 (0.6)	3.5 (0.9)	0.03
FCD (mm⁻¹)	5.3 (0.7)	5.4 (0.8)	0.90
MFI (AU)	2.4 (0.2)	2.4 (0.2)	0.81

Figures in brackets are standard deviation of the mean. BP = blood pressure, MAP = mean arterial pressure, aPWV = aortic pulse wave velocity, LVMI - left ventricular mass index, AF - auto fluorescence, FCD - functional capillary density, MFI - microvascular flow index. AU - arbitrary units.

month follow up suggesting that functional changes to the microcirculation occurred independently of these parameters, adding strength to the argument that ergocalciferol may have a specific mechanism of action within the microcirculation. In contrast to other studies [45,46], proteinuria was unaffected in the ergocalciferol group although the differences in vitamin D compounds, dose schedule, study duration and populations between those studies and ours may explain this difference. aPWV did not decrease in line with the reduction in pulse pressure and this finding may reflect the short duration of the study. Studies with a longer follow up duration are more likely to demonstrate a fall in pulse wave velocity which may occur after a reduction in pulse pressure

After 6 months of therapy with ergocalciferol, there was no increase in the functional capillary density or flow within the microcirculation. This implies that the observed improvements in endothelium dependent microcirculatory function did not involve the recruitment of extra functionally relevant capillaries or changes in blood flow but rather that the endothelium dependent function of the existing microcirculatory network was improved by the direct effect of ergocalciferol.

This hypothesis is supported by the results of parallel *in vitro* experiments in which ergocalciferol, in a dose dependent manner, upregulated eNOS expression measured by RT-PCR. Nitric oxide generation compared to vehicle was numerically but not statistically significantly increased with low dose ergocalciferol but was significantly increased with high dose ergocalciferol. This suggests that higher doses of ergocalciferol are required to increase the functional effect of ergocalciferol on the endothelium and therefore that there may be a threshold 25 (OH) D concentration

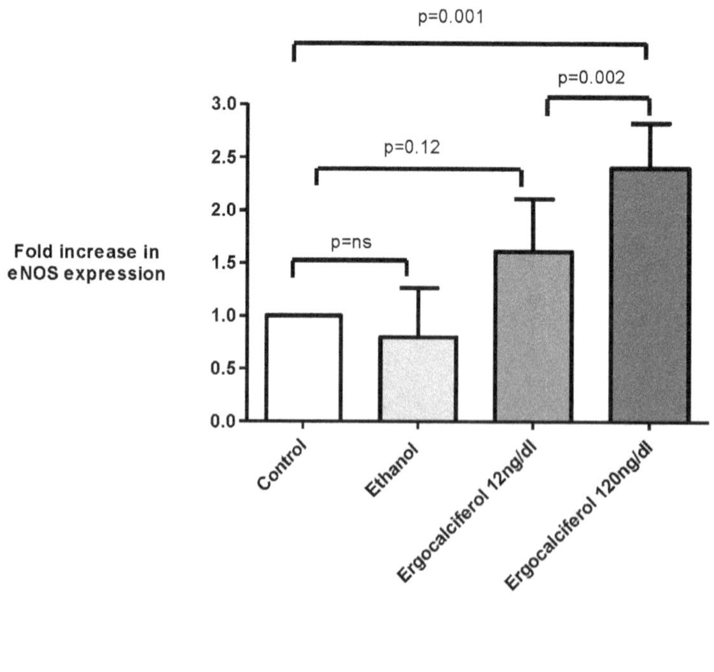

eNOS – endothelial nitric oxide synthase

Figure 5. Fold increase in eNOS expression by RT-PCR in cultured HAEC.

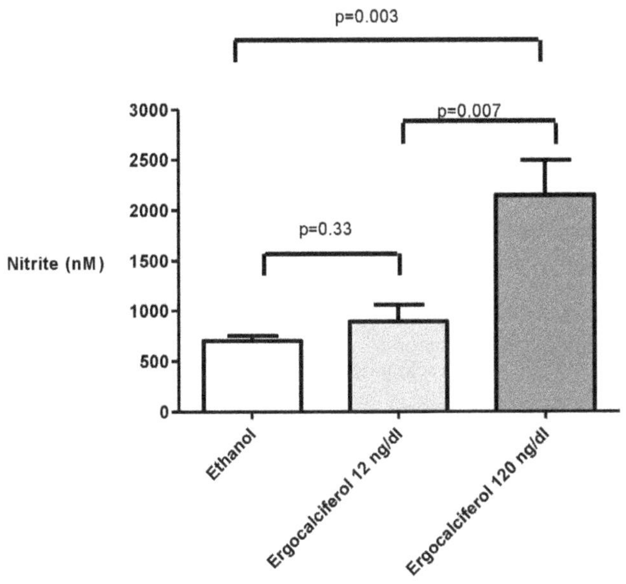

Figure 6. Nitrite levels in supernatants of HAEC. Cultured in low dose (12 ng/dl) and high dose (120 ng/dl) ergocalciferol after 24 h incubation.

above which the maximum effects of ergocalciferol on the microcirculation are achieved.

The present study is the first of its kind to explore the effect of vitamin D on microcirculatory function in patients with CKD and concomitant vitamin D deficiency. The exclusion of patients with diabetes mellitus allowed us to evaluate the effect of ergocalciferol on the microcirculation in CKD without the potentially confounding effect of diabetes on endothelial function.

Prospective studies of the effect of vitamin D therapy in patients with CKD have so far failed to show a beneficial effect of vitamin D on endpoints including LVMI, aPWV, blood pressure and inflammatory biomarkers. [27,47] The effect of nutritional vitamin D compounds on endothelial biomarkers and conduit artery endothelial function in kidney disease has been evaluated in two studies which have produced conflicting results. Marckmann *et al.* [27] compared the effect of 8 weeks of 40,000 IU of weekly cholecalciferol compared to a placebo in patients with both CKD and ESKD treated with haemodialysis. Patients in the control and intervention group were similar at baseline including cause of kidney disease, dialysis status and serum 25 (OH) D, 1,25 $(OH)_2$ D_3 and bone mineral parameters (PTH, Ca, PO_4) levels. There was a significant increase in 25 (OH) D levels in the treatment compared to control group (154.7 nmol/L vs 23.5 nmol/L) and a significant increase in 1,25 $(OH)_2$ D_3 levels although the increase in 1,25 $(OH)_2$ D_3 levels was higher in non-dialysis compared to dialysis requiring CKD (median increase in the CKD group 49 pmol/L ($p<0.01$) compared to 14 pmol/L in the dialysis group ($p>0.05$)). After 8 weeks of treatment, PTH fell significantly in non-dialysis CKD patients but not in dialysis requiring CKD patients. Despite the significant increase in vitamin D levels in the cholecalciferol group, there was no reduction in markers of endothelial dysfunction including D-dimer, von Willebrand factor, fibrinogen and interleukin (IL) 8 or C reactive protein. Additionally, blood pressure, aPWV and aortic augmentation index did not change between the two groups. Specifically, there were no significant differential effects on these parameters when comparing cholecalciferol treated and untreated patients in the dialysis and non-dialysis groups.

Assimon *et al.* [26] have evaluated the effect of ergocalciferol (n = 20 on ergocalciferol for a mean of 39.2 weeks and n = 20 not receiving ergocalciferol) on markers of vascular endothelial adhesion in a case control study of 40 patients undergoing maintenance haemodialysis. There were no significant differences in baseline parameters including dialysis vintage and both groups were receiving an equivalent dose of doxercalciferol. Serum 25 (OH) D levels were higher in the ergocalciferol group (90.8 nmol/L compared to 60.2 nmol/L, $p = 0.03$). In the ergocalciferol group, there was reduction in levels of vascular adhesion molecules sVCAM-1, sICAM-1, P-selectin and in all patients there was a significant negative correlation between serum 25 (OH) D levels and P-selectin and E-selectin. There was no difference in inflammatory biomarkers including IL-6 and TNF-α. However, the functional response of the endothelium was not evaluated and the case control design of this study means that the causal relationship between endothelial adhesion molecules and ergocalciferol cannot be established.

Despite the prompt and sustained rise in 25 (OH) D levels in our patients, significant differences in key microcirculatory end points were only observed after 6 months of therapy with ergocalciferol even though 25 (OH) D levels were similar at 1,3 and 6 months. Previous clinical studies using high dose ergocalciferol or cholecalciferol in healthy and diabetic patients without significant kidney disease demonstrated improved microcirculatory function between 8–12 weeks [24,25,48]. The delay in attainment of significantly improved microvascular function in the current study and lack of improvement over 8 weeks in Marckmann *et al.* study [27] may be a consequence of the uraemic milieu reducing the response of the microcirculation both to the upregulation of eNOS [49] and its downstream effects [50] in increasing availability of vasodilator moieties.

The findings from our study suggest that treatment with high dose ergocalciferol over an extended period of time is required before there is an improvement in microcirculatory endothelial function. This concept will have important implications for determining both the optimum duration of therapy of ergocalciferol and the optimum serum 25 (OH) D level to ensure a maximally beneficial effect on the microcirculation.

The strengths of our study are its double blind randomised placebo control design, replacement of vitamin D in line with international guidelines [37] that was standardised for all patients and commensurate with baseline serum concentrations of 25 (OH) D as well as the use of techniques that specifically assessed both conduit artery and microcirculatory endothelial function. At the time of designing this study, microcirculatory endothelial function had not previously been evaluated in patients with CKD and concomitant VDD in a clinical trial setting. Iontophoresis has been used in the setting of clinical trials to evaluate endothelial function. [51,52,53,54] The experimental conditions and iontophoretic protocol in the present study were standardised and changes in endothelial function were compared with baseline prior to treatment with ergocalciferol. The use of a low current iontophoresis protocol will have reduced the direct galvanic effect from the iontophoretic process on the endothelium seen when a higher current is used. [41] Therefore, any change seen in LDF after iontophoresis must be due to the direct effect of ergocalciferol itself on microvascular endothelial function.

Limitations of this study include the short follow up time and small sample size. The study duration is insufficient to detect significant differences between treatment groups in key outcome measures including CV events. Excluding patients with diabetes mellitus has limited the external validity but improved the internal validity and precision of the present study. Human aortic endothelial cells were not cultured in media consistent with the degree of CKD in the clinical trial subjects due to the complexity of establishing a culture medium that accurately reflects the earlier rather than more advanced stages of CKD. Consequently, the results from the *in vitro* experiments cannot be directly generalised to the uraemic milieu associated with CKD stage 3–4. The current study did not assess the effect of ergocalciferol on endothelial progenitor cells which are important mediators of endothelial repair and function and are reduced in patients at high risk of CVD [55]. Additional studies are required to address the effect of ergocalciferol on endothelial cells cultured in a medium more representative of the earlier stages of CKD as well as the effect of ergocalciferol on EPC number and function in CKD stage 3–4.

Conclusions

High dose ergocalciferol therapy over 6 months improved microcirculatory function and reduced tissue oxidative stress in patients with CKD stage 3–4 and concomitant vitamin D deficiency. *In vitro* studies suggest this effect is mediated through increased expression of eNOS and greater generation of nitric oxide. The primary endpoint of the study reflects global vascular health [14] and it is therefore logical to consider that the observed improvements in microcirculatory function will translate into improved clinical outcomes including a reduction in CV events.

To test this hypothesis, studies in patients with CKD and concomitant vitamin D deficiency with longer follow up and adequately powered to detect CV end points are now required to determine both if improved microcirculatory endothelial function through ergocalciferol therapy subsequently reduces CV endpoints and to determine the optimum serum level of 25 (OH) D to maximize microvascular endothelial function.

Supporting Information

Figure S1 Examples of iontophoresis dose response curves after 6 months of treatment for 2 patients after delivery of ACh demonstrating greater relative increase from baseline in flux in the ergocalciferol compared to placebo treated patient. Flux measured in arbitrary units (AU). Epoch reflects sequential dose increments of the iontophoretic protocol.

Figure S2 Percentage rise in flux from baseline after iontophoresis of ACh in patients with hypertension. Absolute values of percentage change in flux (AU): baseline - ergocalciferol 505.9, placebo 889.2 (p = NS). 1 month - ergocalciferol 853.5, placebo 1051.0 (p = NS). 3 months – ergocalciferol 519.2, placebo 1103.0 (p = NS). 6 months – ergocalciferol 671.6, placebo 1024.0 (p = NS). p values are Bonferroni post test following two way repeated measures ANOVA.

Figure S3 Percentage rise in flux from baseline after iontophoresis of SNP in patients with hypertension. Absolute values of percentage change in flux (AU): baseline - ergocalciferol 339.7, placebo 675.1 (p = NS). 1 month - ergocalciferol 866.9, placebo 724.0 (p = NS). 3 months – ergocalciferol 573.2, placebo 735.0 (p = NS). 6 months – ergocalciferol 682.2, placebo 579.0 (p = NS). p values are Bonferroni post test following two way repeated measures ANOVA.

Figure S4 Percentage rise in flux from baseline after iontophoresis of ACh in patients with glomerulonephritis. Absolute values of percentage change in flux (AU): baseline - ergocalciferol 762.9, placebo 1220.0 (p = NS). 1 month - ergocalciferol 1141.0, placebo 483.8 (p = NS). 3 months – ergocalciferol 647.7, placebo 1023.0 (p = NS). 6 months – ergocalciferol 1086, placebo 661.8 (p = NS). p values are Bonferroni post test following two way repeated measures ANOVA.

Figure S5 Percentage rise in flux from baseline after iontophoresis of SNP in patients with glomerulonephritis. Absolute values of percentage change in flux (AU): baseline - ergocalciferol 794.2, placebo 637.4 (p = NS). 1 month - ergocalciferol 690.6, placebo 708.8 (p = NS). 3 months – ergocalciferol 455.6, placebo 830.8 (p = NS). 6 months – ergocalciferol 387.3, placebo 504.1 (p = NS). p values are Bonferroni post test following two way repeated measures ANOVA.

Protocol S1 Full study protocol.

Checklist S1 Study CONSORT check list.

File S1 Full methodology. Contains Table S1, full iontophoresis protocol.

Acknowledgments

We are grateful to Amanda Smith for helpful advice on scoring SDF videos, Mawdsley Brooks UK for assistance with importing of the ergocalciferol, Alex Farrel and Jeanette Hansen for advice about dispensing the study drug, Dr Mark Westwood for advice about cMRI imaging and Dr Alex Milsom for her assistance with measuring nitrite levels. We are grateful to Dr Mavuto Mukaka for statistical advice.

Author Contributions

Conceived and designed the experiments: GD AT SH RP MJR MMY. Performed the experiments: GD SH. Analyzed the data: GD MJR MMY. Contributed reagents/materials/analysis tools: ATT SH RP MMY. Wrote the paper: GD SH MJR MMY. Conceived the original hypothesis: GD MMY Designed and executed the study: GD MJR MMY Provided scientific advice and equipment for microvascular studies: ATT RP Contributed to and have reviewed the final manuscript: GD ATT SH RP MJR MMY.

References

1. Feehally J, Griffith KE, Lamb EJ, O'Donoghue DJ, Tomson CR (2008) Early detection of chronic kidney disease. BMJ 337: a1618.
2. Li YC, Kong J, Wei M, Chen ZF, Liu SQ, et al. (2002) 1,25-Dihydroxyvitamin D(3) is a negative endocrine regulator of the renin-angiotensin system. J Clin Invest 110: 229–238.
3. Muller K, Haahr PM, Diamant M, Rieneck K, Kharazmi A, et al. (1992) 1,25-Dihydroxyvitamin D3 inhibits cytokine production by human blood monocytes at the post-transcriptional level. Cytokine 4: 506–512.
4. de Boer IH, Ioannou GN, Kestenbaum B, Brunzell JD, Weiss NS (2007) 25-Hydroxyvitamin D levels and albuminuria in the Third National Health and Nutrition Examination Survey (NHANES III). Am J Kidney Dis 50: 69–77.
5. Blair D, Byham-Gray L, Lewis E, McCaffrey S (2008) Prevalence of vitamin D [25(OH)D] deficiency and effects of supplementation with ergocalciferol (vitamin D2) in stage 5 chronic kidney disease patients. J Ren Nutr 18: 375–382.
6. LaClair RE, Hellman RN, Karp SL, Kraus M, Ofner S, et al. (2005) Prevalence of calcidiol deficiency in CKD: a cross-sectional study across latitudes in the United States. Am J Kidney Dis 45: 1026–1033.
7. Pilz S, Iodice S, Zittermann A, Grant WB, Gandini S (2011) Vitamin D status and mortality risk in CKD: a meta-analysis of prospective studies. Am J Kidney Dis 58: 374–382.

8. de Boer IH, Katz R, Chonchol M, Ix JH, Sarnak MJ, et al. (2011) Serum 25-hydroxyvitamin D and change in estimated glomerular filtration rate. Clin J Am Soc Nephrol 6: 2141–2149.
9. de Boer IH, Kestenbaum B, Shoben AB, Michos ED, Sarnak MJ, et al. (2009) 25-hydroxyvitamin D levels inversely associate with risk for developing coronary artery calcification. J Am Soc Nephrol 20: 1805–1812.
10. Chitalia N, Recio-Mayoral A, Kaski JC, Banerjee D (2012) Vitamin D deficiency and endothelial dysfunction in non-dialysis chronic kidney disease patients. Atherosclerosis 220: 265–268.
11. Recio-Mayoral A, Banerjee D, Streather C, Kaski JC (2011) Endothelial dysfunction, inflammation and atherosclerosis in chronic kidney disease—a cross-sectional study of predialysis, dialysis and kidney-transplantation patients. Atherosclerosis 216: 446–451.
12. Tatematsu S, Wakino S, Kanda T, Homma K, Yoshioka K, et al. (2007) Role of nitric oxide-producing and -degrading pathways in coronary endothelial dysfunction in chronic kidney disease. J Am Soc Nephrol 18: 741–749.
13. Pannier B, Guerin AP, Marchais SJ, Metivier F, Safar ME, et al. (2000) Postischemic vasodilation, endothelial activation, and cardiovascular remodeling in end-stage renal disease. Kidney Int 57: 1091–1099.
14. Cohn JN, Quyyumi AA, Hollenberg NK, Jamerson KA (2004) Surrogate markers for cardiovascular disease: functional markers. Circulation 109: IV31–46.
15. Teng M, Wolf M, Ofsthun MN, Lazarus JM, Hernan MA, et al. (2005) Activated injectable vitamin D and hemodialysis survival: a historical cohort study. J Am Soc Nephrol 16: 1115–1125.
16. Andress DL (2006) Vitamin D in chronic kidney disease: a systemic role for selective vitamin D receptor activation. Kidney Int 69: 33–43.
17. Shoben AB, Rudser KD, de Boer IH, Young B, Kestenbaum B (2008) Association of oral calcitriol with improved survival in nondialyzed CKD. J Am Soc Nephrol 19: 1613–1619.
18. Tentori F, Hunt WC, Stidley CA, Rohrscheib MR, Bedrick EJ, et al. (2006) Mortality risk among hemodialysis patients receiving different vitamin D analogs. Kidney Int 70: 1858–1865.
19. Wolf M, Thadhani R (2007) Vitamin D in patients with renal failure: a summary of observational mortality studies and steps moving forward. J Steroid Biochem Mol Biol 103: 487–490.
20. Santoro D, Gitto L, Ferraro A, Satta E, Savica V, et al. (2011) Vitamin D status and mortality risk in patients with chronic kidney disease. Ren Fail 33: 184–191.
21. Talmor Y, Golan E, Benchetrit S, Bernheim J, Klein O, et al. (2008) Calcitriol blunts the deleterious impact of advanced glycation end products on endothelial cells. Am J Physiol Renal Physiol 294: F1059–1064.
22. Borges AC, Feres T, Vianna LM, Paiva TB (1999) Effect of cholecalciferol treatment on the relaxant responses of spontaneously hypertensive rat arteries to acetylcholine. Hypertension 34: 897–901.
23. Wong MS, Delansorne R, Man RY, Vanhoutte PM (2008) Vitamin D derivatives acutely reduce endothelium-dependent contractions in the aorta of the spontaneously hypertensive rat. Am J Physiol Heart Circ Physiol 295: H289–296.
24. Shab-Bidar S, Neyestani TR, Djazayery A, Eshraghian MR, Houshiarrad A, et al. (2011) Regular consumption of vitamin D-fortified yogurt drink (Doogh) improved endothelial biomarkers in subjects with type 2 diabetes: a randomized double-blind clinical trial. BMC Med 9: 125.
25. Sugden J DJ, Witham M, Morris A, Struthers A (2007) Vitamin D improves endothelial function in patients with Type 2 diabetes mellitus and low vitamin D levels. Diabetic Medicine 25: 320–325.
26. Assimon MM, Salenger PV, El-Fawal HA, Mason DL (2012) Nutritional vitamin D supplementation in haemodialysis: A potential vascular benefit? Nephrology (Carlton) 17: 237–242.
27. Marckmann P, Agerskov H, Thineshkumar S, Bladbjerg EM, Sidelmann JJ, et al. (2012) Randomized controlled trial of cholecalciferol supplementation in chronic kidney disease patients with hypovitaminosis D. Nephrol Dial Transplant.
28. Clough G, Cracowski JL (2012) Spotlight issue: Microcirculation-from a clinical perspective. Microcirculation 19: 1–4.
29. Pignocchino P, Conte MR, Scarnato S, Grande A (1994) [Study of cutaneous microcirculation using the laser-Doppler method in syndrome X]. Cardiologia 39: 193–197.
30. Economides PA, Caselli A, Zuo CS, Sparks C, Khaodhiar L, et al. (2004) Kidney oxygenation during water diuresis and endothelial function in patients with type 2 diabetes and subjects at risk to develop diabetes. Metabolism 53: 222–227.
31. Tur E, Yosipovitch G, Bar-On Y (1991) Skin reactive hyperemia in diabetic patients. A study by laser Doppler flowmetry. Diabetes Care 14: 958–962.
32. Jung F, Mrowietz C, Labarrere C, Schuler S, Park JW (2001) Primary cutaneous microangiopathy in heart recipients. Microvasc Res 62: 154–163.
33. Shamim-Uzzaman QA, Pfenninger D, Kehrer C, Chakrabarti A, Kacirotti N, et al. (2002) Altered cutaneous microvascular responses to reactive hyperaemia in coronary artery disease: a comparative study with conduit vessel responses. Clin Sci (Lond) 103: 267–273.
34. McIntyre C JS, Jefferies H (2008) Advances in the cardiovascular assessment of patients with chronic kidney disease. NDT Plus 6: 383–391.
35. de Boer IH, Kestenbaum B (2008) Vitamin D in chronic kidney disease: is the jury in? Kidney Int 74: 985–987.
36. Levey AS, Bosch JP, Lewis JB, Greene T, Rogers N, et al. (1999) A more accurate method to estimate glomerular filtration rate from serum creatinine: a new prediction equation. Modification of Diet in Renal Disease Study Group. Ann Intern Med 130: 461–470.
37. (2003) K/DOQI Clinical Practice Guidelines for Bone Metabolism and Disease in Chronic Kidney Disease. Am J Kidney Dis 42: S1–S201.
38. Cupisti A, Rossi M, Placidi S, Caprioli R, Morelli E, et al. (2000) Responses of the skin microcirculation to acetylcholine and to sodium nitroprusside in chronic uremic patients. Int J Clin Lab Res 30: 157–162.
39. Cupisti A, Rossi M, Placidi S, Fabbri A, Morelli E, et al. (2000) Responses of the skin microcirculation to acetylcholine in patients with essential hypertension and in normotensive patients with chronic renal failure. Nephron 85: 114–119.
40. Morris SJ, Shore AC, Tooke JE (1995) Responses of the skin microcirculation to acetylcholine and sodium nitroprusside in patients with NIDDM. Diabetologia 38: 1337–1344.
41. Droog EJ, Henricson J, Nilsson GE, Sjoberg F (2004) A protocol for iontophoresis of acetylcholine and sodium nitroprusside that minimises nonspecific vasodilatory effects. Microvasc Res 67: 197–202.
42. Gerrits EG, Smit AJ, Bilo HJ (2009) AGEs, autofluorescence and renal function. Nephrol Dial Transplant 24: 710–713.
43. De Backer D, Hollenberg S, Boerma C, Goedhart P, Buchele G, et al. (2007) How to evaluate the microcirculation: report of a round table conference. Crit Care 11: R101.
44. Ignarro LJ, Fukuto JM, Griscavage JM, Rogers NE, Byrns RE (1993) Oxidation of nitric oxide in aqueous solution to nitrite but not nitrate: comparison with enzymatically formed nitric oxide from L-arginine. Proc Natl Acad Sci U S A 90: 8103–8107.
45. de Zeeuw D, Agarwal R, Amdahl M, Audhya P, Coyne D, et al. (2010) Selective vitamin D receptor activation with paricalcitol for reduction of albuminuria in patients with type 2 diabetes (VITAL study): a randomised controlled trial. Lancet 376: 1543–1551.
46. Molina P, Gorriz JL, Molina MD, Peris A, Beltran S, et al. (2013) The effect of cholecalciferol for lowering albuminuria in chronic kidney disease: a prospective controlled study. Nephrol Dial Transplant.
47. Thadhani R, Appelbaum E, Pritchett Y, Chang Y, Wenger J, et al. (2012) Vitamin D therapy and cardiac structure and function in patients with chronic kidney disease: the PRIMO randomized controlled trial. JAMA 307: 674–684.
48. Tarcin O, Yavuz DG, Ozben B, Telli A, Ogunc AV, et al. (2009) Effect of vitamin D deficiency and replacement on endothelial function in asymptomatic subjects. J Clin Endocrinol Metab 94: 4023–4030.
49. Rashid G, Benchetrit S, Fishman D, Bernheim J (2004) Effect of advanced glycation end-products on gene expression and synthesis of TNF-alpha and endothelial nitric oxide synthase by endothelial cells. Kidney Int 66: 1099–1106.
50. Arese M, Strasly M, Ruva C, Costamagna C, Ghigo D, et al. (1995) Regulation of nitric oxide synthesis in uraemia. Nephrol Dial Transplant 10: 1386–1397.
51. Witham MD, Adams F, Kabir G, Kennedy G, Belch JJ, et al. (2013) Effect of short-term vitamin D supplementation on markers of vascular health in South Asian women living in the UK - A randomised controlled trial. Atherosclerosis 230: 293–299.
52. Hobbs DA, Goulding MG, Nguyen A, Malaver T, Walker CF, et al. (2013) Acute ingestion of beetroot bread increases endothelium-independent vasodilation and lowers diastolic blood pressure in healthy men: a randomized controlled trial. J Nutr 143: 1399–1405.
53. Tehrani S, Mobarrez F, Lins PE, Adamson U, Wallen HN, et al. (2013) Impaired endothelium-dependent skin microvascular function during high-dose atorvastatin treatment in patients with type 1 diabetes. Diab Vasc Dis Res 10: 483–488.
54. Kaiser SE, Sanjuliani AF, Estato V, Gomes MB, Tibirica E (2013) Anti-Hypertensive Treatment Improves Microvascular Rarefaction and Reactivity in Low-Risk Hypertensive Individuals. Microcirculation.
55. Pellegatta F, Bragheri M, Grigore L, Raselli S, Maggi FM, et al. (2006) In vitro isolation of circulating endothelial progenitor cells is related to the high density lipoprotein plasma levels. Int J Mol Med 17: 203–208.

2

Estimated Glomerular Filtration Rate is a Poor Predictor of the Concentration of Middle Molecular Weight Uremic Solutes in Chronic Kidney Disease

Nathalie Neirynck[1*], Sunny Eloot[1], Griet Glorieux[1], Daniela V. Barreto[2,3], Fellype C. Barreto[2,3], Sophie Liabeuf[2,3], Aurélie Lenglet[2,4], Horst D. Lemke[5], Ziad A. Massy[2,3,4], Raymond Vanholder[1]

1 Nephrology Section, Department of Internal Medicine, Ghent University Hospital, Gent, Belgium, **2** INSERM U-1088, Amiens, France, **3** Clinical Research Centre, Division of Clinical Pharmacology, Amiens University Hospital, Amiens, France, and the Jules Verne University of Picardy, Amiens, France, **4** Division of Nephrology, Amiens University Hospital, Amiens, France, **5** EXcorLab GmbH, Obernburg, Germany

Abstract

Background: Uremic solute concentration increases as Glomerular Filtration Rate (GFR) declines. Weak associations were demonstrated between estimated GFR (eGFR) and the concentrations of several small water-soluble and protein-bound uremic solutes (MW<500Da). Since also middle molecular weight proteins have been associated with mortality and cardiovascular damage in Chronic Kidney Disease (CKD), we investigated the association between several eGFR formulae and the concentration of Low Molecular Weight Proteins (LMWP) (MW>500Da).

Materials and Methods: In 95 CKD-patients (CKD-stage 2–5 not on dialysis), associations between different eGFR-formulae (creatinine, CystatinC-based or both) and the natural logarithm of the concentration of several LMWP's were analyzed: i.e. parathyroid hormone (PTH), Cystatin C (CystC), interleukin-6 (IL-6), tumor necrosis factor-alpha (TNF-α), leptin, retinol binding protein (RbP), immunoglobin light chains kappa and lambda (Ig-κ and Ig-λ), beta-2-microglobulin (β_2M), myoglobin and fibroblast growth factor-23 (FGF-23)).

Results: The regression coefficients (R^2) between eGFR, based on the CKD-EPI-Crea-CystC-formula as reference, and the examined LMWP's could be divided into three groups. Most of the LMWP's associated weakly (R^2 <0.2) (FGF-23, leptin, IL-6, TNF-α, Ig-κ, Ig-λ) or intermediately (R^2 0.2–0.7) (RbP, myoglobin, PTH). Only β_2M and CystC showed a strong association (R^2 >0.7). Almost identical R^2-values were found per LMWP for all eGFR-formulae, with exception of CystC and β_2M which showed weaker associations with creatinine-based than with CystC-based eGFR.

Conclusion: The association between eGFR and the concentration of several LMWP's is inconsistent, with in general low R^2-values. Thus, the use of eGFR to evaluate kidney function does not reflect the concentration of several LMWP's with proven toxic impact in CKD.

Editor: Emmanuel A. Burdmann, University of Sao Paulo Medical School, Brazil

Funding: This study was funded by a Grant of the Amiens University hospital [PHRC: 2006/0100 (27/03/2006)] and a Grant from European Uremic Toxin Workgroup (EUTox). SE received post-doctoral grant of the Belgian Fund for research Flanders (FWO Vlaanderen). DVB and FCB received postdoctoral grants from the Picardy Regional Council/Jules Verne University of Picardy and postdoctoral scolarships from the National Council of Technological and Scientific Development (CNPq), Brazil. The funders had no role in the study design, data collection and analysis, decision to publish, or preparation of the manuscript.

Competing Interests: DHL is employer at EXcorLab GmbH. This does not alter the authors' adherence to all PLoS ONE policies on sharing data and materials.

* E-mail: n.neirynck@ugent.be

These authors contributed equally to this work.

Introduction

Chronic Kidney Disease (CKD) is an independent risk factor for mortality and cardiovascular disease (CVD) [1]. As Framingham risk calculation cannot correctly predict this risk [2,3], other than traditional risk factors are at play. When kidney function declines, retention of uremic solutes with potential to cause vessel damage and other toxic effects, conceivably plays a role in this [4,5].

Glomerular Filtration Rate (GFR) is used to express kidney function and this can accurately be measured by time-consuming and labor-intensive methods [6]. In clinical practice, serum creatinine (Crea) based formulae are used to calculate estimated GFR (eGFR), which offer an acceptable estimate of measured GFR (mGFR) [6–9]. However, if possible, mGFR is to be preferred as it may differ from eGRF especially in the lower GFR range in a CKD population or in patients with a body constitution that deviates from the average [6,10]. On the other hand, measuring GFR by one of these techniques is more costly and labor-intensive than to determine eGFR. Also, current guidelines classify CKD based on the Modification of Diet in Renal Disease study (MDRD) formula [11,12]. More recently, the CKD-EPI-Crea formula [13] has been proposed as a valid alternative, especially if eGFR is >60 ml/min/1.73 m^2 [9], so that it possibly will be incorporated into the upcoming KDIGO guideline [14].

Since concentrations of uremic solutes rise when GFR deteriorates, it has been thought that GFR reflects the retention state of the patient and that the elevation of individual solute concentration of uremic toxins is closely related to the gradual deterioration of GFR. However, Eloot *et al.* [15] found very low regression coefficients between eGFR and several low molecular weight retention solutes in a CKD population.

The low molecular weight proteins (LMWP) are among the main representatives of the middle molecules, the third family of uremic retention solutes [16], and are interesting to study for their relationship with eGFR as with normal kidney function they are freely filtered through the glomerular basement membrane (GBM) and then mainly degraded into amino acids by the proximal tubules [17]. Furthermore the concentrations of several of the investigated LMWP's, such as inflammatory parameters and FGF-23, are already elevated in patients with a moderate reduction in GFR [18–21] or in more advanced CKD [22]. As a consequence, associations between these solutes and eGFR are often assumed. Assessing the predictive value of eGFR for their concentration is furthermore also relevant, because several LMWP's, such as interleukin-6 (IL-6) [23–26], tumor necrosis factor-alpha (TNF-α) [27,28], beta-2-microglobulin (β_2M) [29,30], and fibroblast growth factor-23 (FGF-23) [31–33], have been linked to mortality or surrogate outcomes like vascular damage or progression of kidney failure. In addition, active removal of middle molecules by dialysis has been associated with better outcome [34].

Therefore, we investigated in a CKD population whether the concentration of several LMWP's would associate with eGFR, calculated by several eGFR formulae.

Materials and Methods

Ethics Statement

The study was approved by the local ethical committee (Comité Consultatif de Protection des Personnes dans la Recherche Biomédicale (CCPPRB) de Picardie, CHU Amiens, Amiens, France) and performed in accordance to the Declaration of Helsinki. Written informed consent was obtained from all patients.

Study Population

This evaluation is a planned sub-analysis of a study undertaken over an 18-month period (January '06- June '07), which screened 150 Caucasian patients with prevalent CKD stage 2–5D from the Nephrology Department at Amiens University Hospital, in which uremic retention solutes in relation to clinical outcomes were analyzed [23,35–37].

All patients were over 40 years old and had a confirmed diagnosis of CKD (two previous eGFR measures of <90 ml/min, calculated by the Cockcroft-Gault formula with an interval of 6–9 months) [38]. Exclusion criteria were chronic inflammatory disease, atrial fibrillation, complete heart block, abdominal aorta aneurysm, an aortic and/or femoral artery prosthesis, primary hyperparathyroidism, kidney transplantation, and any acute cardiovascular event in a 3 month period prior to screening for inclusion.

From the 140 patients who met the inclusion criteria, 45 were excluded from the current study because of hemodialysis treatment, which has an impact on solute concentration and on eGFR. The 95 patients, included in this study, were classified in CKD stages according to the CKD-EPI-Crea-CystC formula for further analysis [8].

Sampling and Laboratory Methods

Blood samples of all patients were collected in the morning from 9 a.m. on, centrifuged, aliquoted, frozen and stored at −80°C. Cystatin C (CystC) (MW: 13.3 kDa) concentration was determined by immune-nephelometry (N latex Cystatin C®, Siemens Healthcare, Dade Behring, Marburg, Germany) and that of intact parathyroid hormone (PTH) (MW: 9.5kDa) with a chemiluminometric immunoassay (Liaison N-tact PTH CLIA®, Diasorin, Stillwater, MN, USA). The determination of retinol binding protein (RbP) (MW: 21kDa), beta-2-microglobulin (β_2M) (MW: 11.8kDa), myoglobin (MW: 17kDa) and total immunoglobulin light chains kappa (Ig-κ) and lambda (Ig-λ) (MW: 23kDa) was performed by laser nephelometry (BNProSpec®, Siemens Healthcare, Dade Behring, Marburg, Germany). ELISA's were used to determine the levels of interleukin-6 (IL-6) (MW: 23kDa), tumor necrosis factor-alpha (TNF-α) (MW: 17kDa) (R&D Systems, Wiesbaden, Germany), and leptin (MW: 16kDa) (DRG diagnostics, Marburg, Germany). Intact fibroblast growth factor-23 (FGF-23) (MW: 32kDa), was measured by a two-site (N-terminal and C-terminal) ELISA (Immunotopics, San Clemente, CA, USA). Serum creatinine (Crea) (MW: 113Da) was measured colorimetrically by standard laboratory methods.

eGFR- Calculation

Six different formulae were used to estimate GFR: the CKD-EPI formula, based on Crea and CystC (CKD-EPI-Crea-CystC) $eGFR = 177.6 \cdot Crea^{-0.65} \cdot CystC^{-0.57} \cdot age^{-0.20} \cdot 0.82$ (if female) [8]; two formulae based on Crea alone: the MDRD $eGFR = 175 \cdot Crea^{-1.154} \cdot age^{-0.203} \cdot (0.742 \text{ if female}) \cdot (1.21 \text{ if black})$ [7] and the CKD-EPI creatinine (CKD-EPI-Crea) $eGFR = 141 . \min(Crea/\kappa, 1)^{\alpha} \cdot \max(Crea/\kappa, 1)^{-1.209} \cdot 0.993^{Age} \cdot 1.018 \text{ (if female)} \cdot 1.159 \text{ (if black)}$ (κ: 0.7 if female, 0.9 if male; α: −0.329 if female, −0.411 if male) [13]; and three formulae based on CystC alone: Stevens $eGFR = 127.7 \cdot CystC^{-1.17} \cdot age^{-0.13} \cdot 0.91 \text{ (if female)} \cdot 1.06 \text{ (if black)}$ [8], Le Bricon $eGFR = [78 \cdot (1/CystC)] + 4$ [39] and Rule $eGFR = 66.8 \cdot (CystC)^{-1.3}$ [40].

Statistical Analysis

The data are expressed as mean ± standard deviation and analysed by ANOVA if they were normally distributed. For data that were not normally distributed, median with interquartile range and Kruskall-Wallis test were used. Linear regressions and Pearson correlations were calculated on semi-logarithmic (LN) concentrations as a function of eGFR. Multifactorial analysis was performed to correct for well-known influencing factors for the concentration of several solutes. The regression model of CystC, β_2M, IL-6, TNF-α, Ig-κ and Ig-λ was adjusted for C-reactive protein (CRP), the one of FGF-23 and PTH for calcium, phosphorus and vitamin D-supplementation, the one of leptin for body mass index (BMI) and gender, and the one of RbP for BMI, 1/CRP and diabetes mellitus. A $P<0.05$ was considered as statistically significant. All statistical analyses were performed using SPSS Statistics 19 (SPSS Inc, Chicago, IL) for Windows (Microsoft Corp, Redmond, WA).

Results

Ninety-five patients at different stages of CKD were included: 11.5% CKD stage 2, 39.0% CKD stage 3, 39.0% CKD stage 4, and 10.5% CKD stage 5 not on dialysis. Table 1 summarizes the demographic and clinical characteristics of the study population.

The concentrations of the studied LMWP's, except for the immunoglobulin light chains, increased progressively with declining kidney function (Table 2).

Table 1. Main demographic and clinical characteristics of the study population (n = 95).

	CKD stage					P
	Stage 2–5	stage 2	stage 3	stage 4	stage 5	
Number n (%)	95 (100)	11 (11.5)	37 (39.0)	37 (39.0)	10 (10.5)	
eGFR (ml/min/1.73m^2)	35±18	69±8	43±9	22±4	11±3	<0.001
Age (years)	68±12	65±8	69±12	65±13	66±15	0.07
Male gender n (%)	59 (62)	9 (82)	24 (65)	22 (60)	4 (40)	0.39
Diabetes Mellitus n (%)	45 (47)	4 (36)	19 (51)	18 (49)	4 (40)	0.50
BMI (kg/m^2)	29±7	26±5	29±6	31±7	28±7	0.28
Cholesterol (mmol/l)	5.0±1.1	5.4±0.7	4.6±1.1	5.3±1.1	4.6±0.5	0.02
Triglycerides (mmol/l)	1.9±1.4	1.7±0.9	1.6±0.7	2.4±1.9	2.2±1.2	0.06
CRP (mg/l)	3.11 [1.1–6.7]	2.3 [0.7–4.9]	2.8 [1.4–5.0]	3.7 [0.8–8.5]	4.1 [0.4–15.6]	0.696
Albumin (g/l)	38.9±6.4	40.6±8.8	38.4±5.7	39.9±5.8	33.8±6.7	0.07
Hemoglobin (g/l)	12.5±1.7	14.0±1.2	12.7±1.5	12.0±1.6	10.9±1.4	<0.001
Calcium (mmol/l)	2.3±0.1	2.3±0.1	2.3±0.1	2.3±0.2	2.3±0.2	0.96
Phosphate (mmol/l)	1.2±0.3	0.9±0.3	1.1±0.2	1.4±0.3	1.5±0.5	<0.001
Vit D supplement n (%)	17 (18)	1 (9)	5 (13)	6 (16)	5 (50)	0.06

CKD stages according to the CKD-EPI-Crea-CystC formula. Data are expressed as mean ± SD, median with interquartile range between square brackets or number for binary variables, with percentages between brackets per CKD class. CKD, chronic kidney disease; eGFR, estimated glomerular filtration rate; BMI, body mass index; Statistical analysis: ANOVA or Kruskall-Wallis; P-values comparing all stages.

Our analysis primarily focused on the linear regression analysis with the natural logarithm (LN) of the concentration of each studied uremic retention solute concentration as dependent variable and the CKD-EPI-Crea-CystC eGFR as independent variable. This formula was chosen as reference because it is considered as one of the most accurate ones at this time while it incorporates both Crea and CystC, in contrast to all other studied formulae which are based on either Crea or CystC [8]. Associations between eGFR and LMWP's were expressed as regression coefficients (R^2) and are summarized in table 3 and figure 1.

The R^2-values per individual solute were divergent; according to these, associations could be arbitrarily divided into three groups: strong (R^2 >0.7), moderate (R^2 0.2–0.7) and weak (R^2 <0.2) (Figure 1). As expected, CystC ($R^2 = 0.828$) was strongly associated as it is one of the used parameters in the formula. Only β_2M showed a similar association ($R^2 = 0.770$). Retinol binding protein (RbP), myoglobin and parathyroid hormone (PTH) were moderately associated to eGFR with R^2-values of 0.423, 0.303 and 0.231, respectively. The association with eGFR was only weak for IL-6 ($R^2 = 0.117$), leptin ($R^2 = 0.084$), FGF-23 ($R^2 = 0.058$) and TNF-α ($R^2 = 0.056$). There was even no association for immuno-

Table 2. Concentrations of uremic solutes ± standard deviation according to CKD-stage (CKD-EPI-Crea-CystC).

	CKD stage					P- value
	stage 2–5	stage 2	stage 3	stage 4	stage 5	
CystC (mg/l)	1.9±0.9	0.9±0.2	1.4±0.5	2.4±0.7	3.5±0.7	<0.001
β_2M (mg/l)	6.1 [3.2–9.3]	2.6 [2.1–4.6]	3.8 [3.0–5.3]	8.2 [6.7–10.4]	13.9 [12.8–16.4]	<0.001
PTH (pg/ml)	77.0 [42.5–135.5]	39.5 [25.5–44.0]	62.0 [42.0–83.5]	124.0 [74.0–196.0]	111.5 [22.0–173.0]	<0.001
RbP (mg/l)	82.0±32.8	52.9±15.2	67.0±21.8	102.6±32.2	95.9±31.5	<0.001
Myoglobin (mg/l)	82.7 [54.9–115.0]	49.9 [32.4–57.4]	72.3 [49.7–104.8]	98.8 [75.4–125.5]	170.5 [62.8–244.0]	<0.001
IL-6 (pg/ml)	2.6 [1.3–5.1]	1.1 [0.4–1.9]	2.2 [1.3–4.0]	3.0 [1.3–5.2]	7.0 [2.2–14.0]	0.001
TNF-α (pg/ml)	3.4 [2.2–4.6]	1.1 [1.1–2.5]	4.1 [2.2–4.6]	2.6 [2.2–5.1]	4.1 [3.1–7.2]	0.016
Leptin (ng/ml)	12.8 [2.0–43.5]	0.56 [<0.48–5.3]	8.5 [2.5–33.4]	21.4 [4.3–59.2]	26.3 [0.7–>105]	0.012
FGF-23 (pg/ml)	30.6 [26.8–34.4]	26.6 [25.8–27.3]	31.5 [27.6–34.5]	30.6 [27.6–34.9]	34.4 [33.1–35.0]	0.007
Ig-κ (g/l)	2.6 [2.2–3.0]	2.4 [2.3–2.8]	2.4 [2.1–4.8]	2.8 [2.4–3.0]	2.5 [2.1–3.1]	0.330
Ig-λ (g/l)	1.5 [1.3–1.8]	1.5 [1.3–1.7]	1.5 [1.3–1.7]	1.6 [1.4–1.8]	1.2 [1.2–1.8]	0.280

Concentrations are expressed as mean ± SD or median with interquartile range (between square brackets) as appropriate. CKD: chronic kidney disease, CystC: cystatin C, β_2M: beta-2-microglobulin, PTH: parathyroid hormone, RbP: retinol binding protein, IL-6: interleukin-6, TNF-α: tumor necrosis factor-alpha, Ig-κ: immunoglobulin light chain kappa, Ig-λ: immunoglobulin light chain lambda, FGF-23: fibroblast growth factor-23. Statistical analysis: ANOVA or Kruskall-Wallis; P comparing all stages.

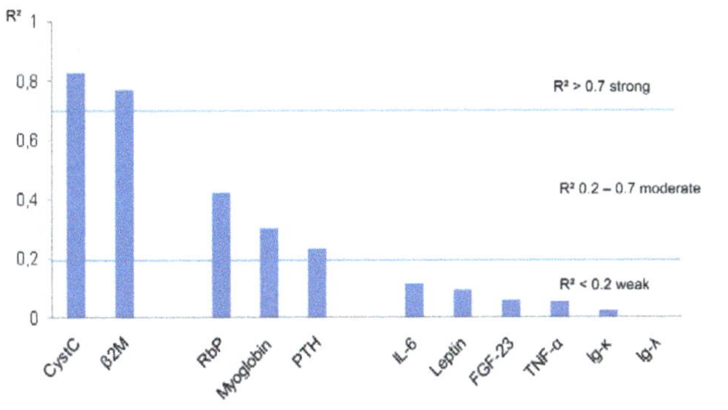

Figure 1. Regression coefficients between LN of studies LMWP's and eGFR. The coefficients of the linear regression analysis between the natural logarithm of the studied low molecular weight protein concentrations and estimated Glomerular Filtration Rate, according to CKD-EPI-Crea-CystC, can be divided into 3 groups: strong (R^2 >0.7), moderate (R^2 0.2–0.7) and weak (R^2 <0.2). The dashed lines indicate $R^2 = 0.2$ and 0.7. All correlations were significant except for Ig-κ and Ig-λ. LN: natural logarithm, LMWP: low molecular weight protein, eGFR estimated glomerular filtration rate, R^2: regression coefficient, Cyst C: Cystatin C, β_2M: beta-2-microglobulin, RbP: retinol binding protein, PTH: parathyroid hormone, IL-6: interleukin-6, FGF-23: fibroblast growth factor-23, TNF-α: tumor necrosis factor-alpha, Ig-κ: immunoglobulin light chain kappa, Ig-λ: immunoglobulin light chain lambda.

globulin light chain kappa (Ig-κ) ($R^2 = 0.021$) and immunoglobulin light chain lambda (Ig-λ) ($R^2 = 0$) (P = N.S.).

Figure 2 shows the dot plots of solute concentrations as a function of eGFR. Whereas the relation is strong with little scatter around the linear regression line for β_2M (Panel A), the scatter is much larger for solutes with moderate to weak R^2-values, as illustrated for myoglobin (Panel B), IL-6 (Panel C) and especially Ig-λ (Panel D) for which there is no association at all. The large standard deviations or wide interquartile ranges of the individual solute concentrations per CKD-stage also illustrate the large inter-individual variability of LMWP concentration within the same eGFR-range (Table 2).

In addition we analyzed the correlation coefficients between the concentrations of the different LMWP and eGFR (CKD-EPI-Crea-CystC) in the group CKD stage 2–3 versus CKD stage 4–5. The correlation between RbP, PTH, myoglobin, FGF-23 and eGFR was significant in CKD-stage 2–3 while not in CKD stage 4–5. For the other investigated solutes, the R^2-values in CKD stage 2–3 and CKD stage 4–5 were more confirm to each other. The respective R^2-values are summarized in table 4.

In a second step, the same analysis was performed with the other formulae under evaluation and compared to the results with the CKD-EPI-Crea-CystC-formula. The R^2-values between all eGFR formula and individual solutes were strikingly similar with only one exception (Table 3). β_2M was only moderately associated to Crea-based eGFR, with R^2-values of approximately 0.55, as compared to CystC-based eGFR (R^2 >0.8). In this way β_2M followed the same pattern as CystC, for which this discrepancy could be attributed to whether CystC was included as a factor in the formula or not. Considering the other studied LMWP's, only PTH showed a moderately similar trend, with R^2 approximately 0.27 compared to R^2 approximately 0.13, with CystC- or Crea-based eGFR-formulae, respectively.

Finally, we performed multifactorial regression analysis for the different LMWP's with adjustment for several relevant variables. However, only two models induced a marked increase in R^2-value: for leptin the association rose from weak to moderate when BMI

Table 3. Regression coefficients of LMWP's and different eGFR formulae.

R^2	CKD-EPI-Cr-CystC	MDRD	CKD-EPI-Cr	Stevens	Le Bricon	Rule
	R^2 >0.7					
Cyst C	0.828	0.572	0.569	0.920	0.939	0.902
β_2M	0.770	0.559	0.549	0.838	0.855	0.820
	R^2 0.2–0.7					
RbP	0.423	0.348	0.343	0.383	0.397	0.390
Myoglobin	0.303	0.246	0.262	0.287	0.297	0.293
PTH	0.231	0.130	0.132	0.279	0.274	0.276
	R^2 <0.2					
IL-6	0.117	0.090	0.097	0.126	0.127	0.123
Leptin	0.084	0.056	0.059	0.092	0.065	0.065
FGF-23	0.058	0.008	0.008	0.095	0.101	0.094
TNF-α	0.056	0.043	0.044	0.066	0.058	0.061
Ig-κ	0.021	0.021	0.020	0.016	0.015	0.011
Ig-λ	0.000	0.000	0.000	0.001	0.001	0.001

LMWP: Low Molecular Weight Protein, R^2: regression coefficient, eGFR: estimated glomerular filtration rate, CKD-EPI-Crea-CystC: CKD-EPI formula based on creatinine and cystatin C, MDRD: Modification of Diet in Renal Disease formula, CKD-EPI-Crea: CKD-EPI formula based on creatinine. CystC: cystatin C, β_2M: beta-2-microglobulin, RbP: retinol binding protein, PTH: parathyroid hormone, IL-6: interleukin-6, FGF-23: fibroblast growth factor-23, TNF-α: tumor necrosis factor-alpha, Ig-κ: immunoglobulin light chain kappa, Ig-λ: immunoglobulin light chain lambda.

was added to the regression model (R^2 from 0.084 to 0.346), with BMI as an independent predictor for the leptin concentration. Likewise, after adjustment for CRP, IL-6 became moderately associated with eGFR (R^2 from 0.117 to 0.305 after adjustment). For all other solutes there was no change in R^2. (Data not shown).

Discussion

We analyzed the linear regression coefficients between the concentrations of several LMWP's retained in CKD and different eGFR-formulae in a CKD population, stage 2–5 not on dialysis. As a main finding, the R^2-values diverged considerably, ranging from high, R^2 >0.7, to low, R^2 <0.2. The majority of the evaluated LMWP's associated weakly (R^2 <0.2 for IL-6, TNF-α, FGF-23 and leptin) or moderately (R^2: 0.2–0.7 for RbP, myoglobin and PTH). There was no correlation at all for the immunoglobulin light chains. Only CystC and β_2M showed a strong association with eGFR (R^2 >0.7) (Figure 1, Table 3). Although in some studies a correlation was sought for individual LMWP's and eGFR of mGFR, this present study seeked out the association of the concentration of several LMWP's and eGFR formulae together allowing their comparison.

The R^2-values for the weakly and moderately associating LMWP's did not differ substantially whether eGFR was calculated with the CKD-EPI-Crea-CystC-formula [8], the Crea-based formulae (MDRD [7] and CKD-EPI-Crea [13]), or the three different CystC-based formulae, (Stevens [8], Rule [40] and Le Bricon [39]) (Table 3). These low regression coefficients can partially be attributed to the known limitations of eGFR, as an index of mGFR [6,41]. However in at least four other studies, almost identical low regression coefficients were found between mGFR, assessed with different techniques, and the concentration

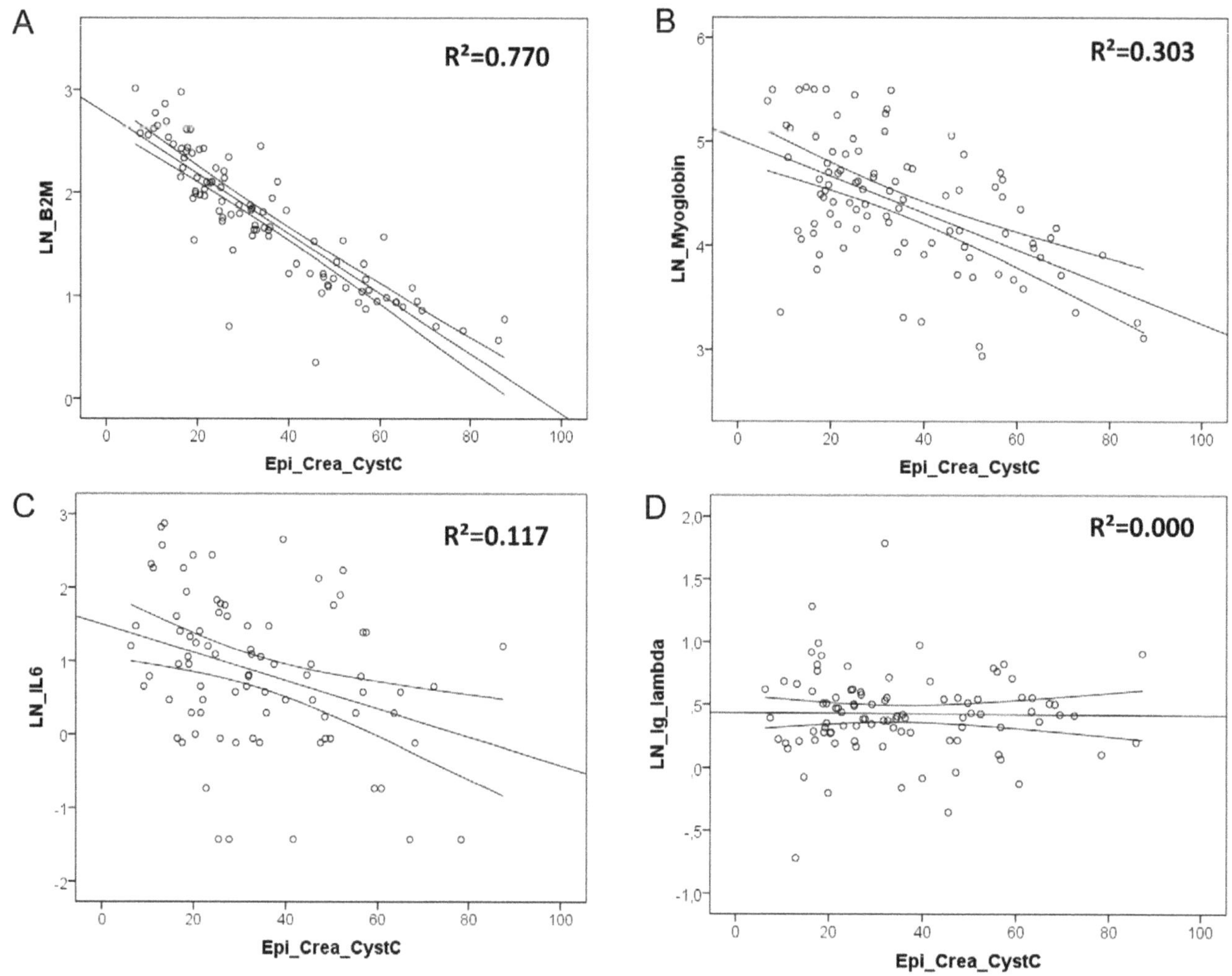

Figure 2. Dot plots with best fit linear regression lines for LN of LMWP's in function of eGFR. Dot plots with best fit linear regression lines for natural logarithms of β_2M, myoglobin, IL-6 and Ig-λ, as examples of strongly, moderately and weakly correlating low molecular weight proteins, in function of estimated Glomerular Filtration Rate, calculated by CKD-EPI-Crea-CystC. The dots represent the individual concentrations and the lines the best fit linear regression line with the 95% confidence interval. LN: natural logarithm, LMWP: low molecular weight protein, β_2M : beta-2-microglobulin, IL-6: Interleukin-6, Ig-λ: immunoglobulin light chain lambda, EPI-Crea-CystC: CKD-EPI formula based on serum creatinine and Cystatin C, R^2: regression coefficient, LN: natural logarithm.

of RbP (R^2 0.16) [42], myoglobin (R^2 0.38) [43], leptin (R^2 0.0004) [44] and FGF-23 (R^2 0.09) [45] as in our study, be it that transformation of the concentrations varied from study to study. In addition, the imperfect reflection of true GFR by eGFR can explain that regression coefficients are substantially lower than 1, but not that the range in between individual molecules is so discordant, whereas per molecule they are almost identical (Table 3, Figure 1). There was also an unpredictable and large variability in concentrations of different solutes within each eGFR stratum (Table 2). These data suggest another reason for the sometimes deceiving associations than a discrepancy among mGFR and eGFR, namely that uremic solute concentration depends on other factors than GFR as well. In this way, our study corroborates findings in an earlier study with small water-soluble and protein-bound compounds [15,46].

These results are somewhat unexpected from a physiological point of view as the renal clearance of these LMWP's depends to a large extent on GFR alone. All these LMWP's are freely filtered through the GBM, followed, at normal physiological concentrations, by an almost entire uptake by the proximal tubules via a receptor-mediated process to be degraded subsequently into amino acids in the tubular lysosomes [17,47]. In this way, the proximal tubulus plays an important role in LMWP metabolism but without a direct contribution to their renal clearance; regarding the latter, GFR is the rate limiting step. This probably explains why we did not find any association between eGFR and the total (free plus bound) immunoglobulin light chains, in contrast to Hutchison et al who evaluated only free light chains for their association to eGFR (free Ig-κ: R^2: 0.52; free Ig-λ: R^2: 0.44) [48], as only the free fraction passes the GBM. This is also in contrast to the small water-soluble and protein-bound uremic toxins, for which tubular secretion and/or reabsorption play an important role in renal clearance [15,46].

However, the concentration of small water-soluble and protein-bound solutes may be further influenced by many other factors as well, such as enzymatic metabolism, intestinal secretion/absorption, generation by intestinal flora, diet and changes in distribution volume [15,46]. It is conceivable that also the concentration of the

Table 4. Regression coefficients (R^2) of the concentration of LMWP's and eGFR (CKD-EPI-Crea-CystC) comparing CKD stage 2–3 versus CKD stage 4–5.

R^2	CKD stage 2-3 (n = 48)	CKD stage 4-5 (n = 47)
Cyst C	0.782	0.555
β_2M	0.619	0.549
RbP*	0.254	0.001
PTH*	0.195	0.000
Myoglobin*	0.257	0.059
IL-6	0.074	0.117
TNF-α	0.107	0.087
Leptin	0.060	0.001
FGF-23*	0.120	0.033
Ig-κ	0.013	0.016
Ig-λ	0.001	0.006

LMWP: Low Molecular Weight Protein, eGFR: estimated glomerular filtration rate, CKD-EPI-Crea-CystC: CKD-EPI formula based on creatinine and cystatin C. CystC: cystatin C, β_2M: beta-2-microglobulin, RbP: retinol binding protein, PTH: parathyroid hormone, IL-6: interleukin-6, TNF-α: tumor necrosis factor-alpha, FGF-23: fibroblast growth factor-23, Ig-κ: immunoglobulin light chain kappa, Ig-λ: immunoglobulin light chain lambda. *: LMWP's with a significant correlation in CKD stage 2–3, but no significant correlation in CKD stage 4–5.

weakly and moderately correlating LMWP's depends on other mechanisms than GFR, which even seem to have more important weight than GFR. Some known influencing factors such as changes in generation, homeostatic mechanisms and extra-renal clearance are summarized in table 5. Multifactorial regression analysis for the respective LMWP's including some of these parameters, increased the R^2-value as expected. E.g. for leptin, R^2 rose from 0.084 to 0.346 when corrected for BMI,which was an independent covariate for leptin concentration in a model with eGFR and BMI. The R^2-value between IL-6 and eGFR became 0.305 instead of 0.117, when adjusted for CRP, which, in contrast to BMI for leptin concentration, did however not independently predict IL-6 concentration in a model with eGFR and CRP. The majority of potentially influencing factors did however not importantly affect the R^2-values. This suggests that other than well known mediators may influence these LMWP concentrations as well. In more advanced CKD, the influence of confounders, for example bone metabolism, is probably more important, which could explain partially that no significant associations were observed between PTH or FGF-23 and eGFR in CKD stage 4–5, while they were present in CKD stage 2–3 (table 4). Another contributing factor to this discrepancy in associations between CKD stage 2–3 versus CKD stage 4–5 might be purely mathematical, as the GFR-range in CKD 2–3 (30–90 ml/min/ 1.73 m^2) is much larger than CKD 4–5 (±10–30 ml/min/ 1.73 m^2).

This study demonstrates that eGFR is not a reliable predictor of the concentration of most of the evaluated LMWP's, although several of them such as IL-6 [23–26], TNF-α [27,28] and FGF-23 [31–33,49] have been associated with mortality or with intermediate endpoints, such as vascular dysfunction or progression to end stage renal disease (ESRD) in CKD- or hemodialysis patients. Presumably, some of these solutes, especially if they would be representative for a cluster of other solutes, might by themselves become useful predictors of morbidity or mortality in CKD independently from eGFR. Based on the data collected in the present study, we investigated the mutual correlations between the concentrations of the different LMWP's; however, we could not identify such a marker, correlating strongly to other LMWP's without correlating to eGFR, among the investigated solutes (data not shown). This question, however, would be worthwhile to be investigated in larger populations.

In contrast to these weakly and moderately correlating LMWP's, there is a remarkable similarity in regression coefficients between CystC and β_2M. First, these molecules are the sole LMWP's studied that result in acceptably high associations with eGFR (Table 3). Second, they associate better with CystC-based eGFR formulae [8,39,40] than with Crea-based ones [7,13], the CKD-EPI-Crea-CystC [8] which contains both factors being intermediate (Table 3). Whereas this is no surprise for CystC which is included in some formulae and not in others, the pattern for β_2M seems to be identical. This suggests that the kinetics of both molecules during progression of CKD depend on similar factors or at least factors with a similar impact on solute concentration. Of note, some of the non-renal elements with impact on both concentrations [50,51], like chronic inflammatory disease or malignancy were among the exclusion criteria of this study. CystC was a superior marker of the association of GFR with outcome in a study by Peralta *et al.*, who showed that the predictive value for mortality or CVD of eGFR <60 ml/min/ 1.73 m^2, based on a CystC-based eGFR, was better than eGFR based on the CKD-EPI-Crea-formula [45]. Recently, in a general population, CystC and β_2M were stronger predictors of mortality, CVD and evolution to ESRD than eGFR based on the CKD-EPI-Crea [52].

The present study has some shortcomings. First, the study population was rather small, with even smaller subgroups per CKD-stage. Second, we used eGFR which gives only an approximate value for glomerular filtration in comparison to more exact methods such as EDTA-clearance. We preferred to use methods which are applied on a day to day basis. As the differences in correlations are so striking, it is very likely that these findings can be extrapolated to GFR in general. The strengths of this study lie in the fact that several LMWP's are evaluated together in the same population for different eGFR formulae based on Crea, CystC or both.

Our present data, together with the previous ones [15], showing extremely variable associations between uremic retention solutes and a surrogate of GFR, suggests that eGFR per se is an inadequate indicator of the uremic status. This is also suggested by other studies. In a CKD population, Lilitkarntakul *et al.* [53] demonstrated that renal function did not independently predict arterial stiffness or endothelial dysfunction while the uremic retention solutes asymmetric dimethylarginine (ADMA), isoprostanes or endothelin-A did. In the Initiating Dialysis Early and Late (IDEAL) trial [54], approximately 75% of the patients randomized to start dialysis at low eGFR (5–7 ml/min/1.73 m^2), initiated dialysis earlier, mainly because of uremic symptoms.

In this study, the regression coefficients of different LMWP's in relation to eGFR are diverse and in general low. This shows that other factors than GFR are important for the development of the 'uremic status'. Further research is needed to evaluate whether these uremic toxins can be used as biomarkers for the risk stratification associated to uremic toxicity within the different CKD-stages and beyond eGFR.

Table 5. Main factors influencing the concentrations of the studied LMWP's, other than GFR.

	Extra renal handling	Generation
CystC	–	Gender, age, hyperthyroidism, corticosteroid intake, malignancy, inflammation
β_2M	+ (~5%)	Inflammation, malignancy
RbP	?	Insulin resistance, obesity, DM, Zn-deficiency, liver dysfunction, infection
PTH	+	Hypocalcemia, hyperphosphatemia, hypo-VitD
Myoglobin	+ (in uremia?)	Different generation in uremia (?)
Leptin	+	Obesity, gender, low energy expenditure, insulin resistance
IL-6	+	Inflammation
TNF-α	+	Inflammation
FGF-23	+ ?	Hyperphosphatemia, regulation mineral metabolism
Ig-κ	+ ?	B-cell lymphoproliferative disorders, inflammation
Ig-λ	+ ?	B-cell lymphoproliferative disorders, inflammation

CystC: Cystatin C, β_2M: beta-2-microglobulin, RbP: retinol binding protein, PTH: parathyroid hormone, IL-6: interleukin-6, TNF-α: tumor necrosis factor-alpha, FGF-23: fibroblast growth factor-23, Ig-κ: immunoglobulin light chain kappa, Ig-λ: immunoglobulin light chain lambda, Zn: Zinc, DM: diabetes mellitus, Ca: Calcium, P: Phosphorus, VitD: Vitamin-D. For references: see Table S1.

Author Contributions

Conceived and designed the experiments: ZAM RV. Performed the experiments: DVB FCB SL AL ZAM. Analyzed the data: SE NN GG. Contributed reagents/materials/analysis tools: HDL ZAM SL. Wrote the paper: NN RV.

References

1. Weiner DE, Tighiouart H, Amin MG, Stark PC, MacLeod B, et al. (2004) Chronic Kidney Disease as a Risk Factor for Cardiovascular Disease and All-Cause Mortality: A Pooled Analysis of Community-Based Studies. J Am Soc Nephrol 15: 1307–1315.
2. Weiner DE, Tighiouart H, Elsayed EF, Griffith JL, Salem DN, et al. (2007) The Framingham predictive instrument in chronic kidney disease. J Am Coll Cardiol 50: 217–224.
3. Sciarretta S, Valenti V, Tocci G, Pontremoli R, Rosei EA, et al. (2010) Association of renal damage with cardiovascular diseases is independent of individual cardiovascular risk profile in hypertension: data from the Italy - Developing Education and awareness on MicroAlbuminuria in patients with hypertensive Disease study. J Hypertens 28: 251–258.
4. Vanholder R, De Smet R (1999) Pathophysiologic effects of uremic retention solutes. J Am Soc Nephrol 10: 1815–1823.
5. Vanholder R, Baurmeister U, Brunet P, Cohen G, Glorieux G, et al. (2008) A bench to bedside view of uremic toxins. J Am Soc Nephrol 19: 863–870.
6. Stevens LA, Levey AS (2009) Measured GFR as a Confirmatory Test for Estimated GFR. J Am Soc Nephrol 20: 2305–2313.
7. Levey AS, Coresh J, Greene T, Stevens LA, Zhang YL, et al. (2006) Using standardized serum creatinine values in the modification of diet in renal disease study equation for estimating glomerular filtration rate. Ann Intern Med 145: 247–254.
8. Stevens LA, Coresh J, Schmid CH, Feldman HI (2008) Estimating GFR using Cystatin C alone or in combination with creatinine: a pooled analysis of 3418 individuals with CKD. Am J Kidney Dis 51: 395–406.
9. Stevens LA, Schmid CH, Greene T, Zhang YP, Beck GJ, et al. (2010) Comparative Performance of the CKD Epidemiology Collaboration (CKD-EPI) and the Modification of Diet in Renal Disease (MDRD) Study Equations for Estimating GFR Levels Above 60 mL/min/1.73 m(2). Am J Kidney Dis 56: 486–495.
10. Kuan Y, Hossain M, Surman J, El Nahas AM, Haylor J (2005) GFR prediction using the MDRD and Cockcroft and Gault equations in patients with end-stage renal disease. Nephrol Dial Transplant 20: 2394–2401.
11. National Kidney Foundation (2002) K/DOQI clinical practice guidelines for chronic kidney disease: evaluation, classification, and stratification. Am J Kidney Dis 39: S1–266.
12. Levey AS, Eckardt KU, Tsukamoto Y, Levin A, Coresh J, et al. (2005) Definition and classification of chronic kidney disease: a position statement from Kidney Disease: Improving Global Outcomes (KDIGO). Kidney Int 67: 2089–2100.
13. Levey AS, Stevens LA, Schmid CH, Zhang YP, Castro AF, et al. (2009) A New Equation to Estimate Glomerular Filtration Rate. Ann Intern Med 150: 604–607.
14. Levey AS, de Jong PE, Coresh J, El Nahas M, Astor BC, et al. (2011) The definition, classification, and prognosis of chronic kidney disease: a KDIGO Controversies Conference report. Kidney Int 80: 17–28.
15. Eloot S, Schepers E, Barreto DV, Barreto FC, Liabeuf S, et al. (2011) Estimated glomerular filtration rate is a poor predictor of concentration for a broad range of uremic toxins. Clin J Am Soc Nephrol 6: 1266–1273.
16. Vanholder R, De Smet R, Glorieux G, Argiles A, Baurmeister U, et al. (2003) Review on uremic toxins: Classification, concentration, and interindividual variability. Kidney Int 63: 1934–1943.
17. Maack T, Johnson V, Kau ST, Fugueiredo J, Sigulem D (1979) Renal filtration, transport, and metabolism of low-molecular- weight proteins: A review. Kidney Int 16: 251–270.
18. Ix JH, Shlipak MG, Wassel CL, Whooley MA (2010) Fibroblast growth factor-23 and early decrements in kidney function: the Heart and Soul Study. Nephrol Dial Transplant 25: 993–997.
19. Isakova T, Wahl P, Vargas GS, Gutierrez OM, Scialla J, et al. (2011) Fibroblast growth factor 23 is elevated before parathyroid hormone and phosphate in chronic kidney disease. Kidney Int 79: 1370–1378.
20. Keller C, Katz R, Cushman M, Fried LF, Shlipak M (2008) Association of kidney function with inflammatory and procoagulant markers in a diverse cohort: a cross-sectional analysis from the Multi-Ethnic Study of Atherosclerosis (MESA). BMC Nephrol 9: 9doi:10.1186/1471-2369-9-9.
21. Upadhyay A, Larson MG, Guo CY, Vasan RS, Lipinska I, et al. (2011) Inflammation, kidney function and albuminuria in the Framingham Offspring cohort. Nephrol Dial Transplant 26: 920–926.
22. Pecoits R, Heimburger O, Barany P, Suliman M, Fehrman-Ekholm I, et al. (2003) Associations between circulating inflammatory markers and residual renal function in CRF patients. Am J Kidney Dis 41: 1212–1218.
23. Barreto DV, Barreto FC, Liabeuf S, Temmar M, Lemke HD, et al. (2010) Plasma interleukin-6 is independently associated with mortality in both hemodialysis and pre-dialysis patients with chronic kidney disease. Kidney Int 77: 550–556.
24. Tripepi G, Mallamaci F, Zoccali C (2005) Inflammation markers, adhesion molecules, and all-cause and cardiovascular mortality in patients with ESRD: searching for the best risk marker by multivariate modeling. J Am Soc Nephrol 16 Suppl 1: S83–S88.
25. Panichi V, Maggiore U, Taccola D, Migliori M, Rizza GM, et al. (2004) Interleukin-6 is a stronger predictor of total and cardiovascular mortality than C-reactive protein in haemodialysis patients. Nephrol Dial Transplant 19: 1154–1160.
26. Pecoits-Filho R, Barany P, Lindholm B, Heimburger O, Stenvinkel P (2002) Interleukin-6 is an independent predictor of mortality in patients starting dialysis treatment. Nephrol Dial Transplant 17: 1684–1688.

27. Kimmel PL, Phillips TM, Simmens SJ, Peterson RA, Weihs KL, et al. (1998) Immunologic function and survival in hemodialysis patients. Kidney Int 54: 236–244.
28. Futh R, Herder C, Forster S, Muller-Scholze S, Kruse N, et al. (2004) Evaluation of diagnostic relevance of mRNA levels in peripheral blood: predictive value for mortality in hemodialysis patients. Cytokine 27: 166–172.
29. Okuno S, Ishimura E, Kohno K, Fujino-Katoh Y, Maeno Y, et al. (2009) Serum beta(2)-microglobulin level is a significant predictor of mortality in maintenance haemodialysis patients. Nephrol Dial Transplant 24: 571–577.
30. Cheung AK, Rocco MV, Yan GF, Leypoldt JK, Levin NW, et al. (2006) Serum beta-2 microglobulin levels predict mortality in dialysis patients: Results of the HEMO study. J Am Soc Nephrol 17: 546–555.
31. Isakova T, Xie HL, Yang W, Xie DW, Anderson AH, et al. (2011) Fibroblast Growth Factor 23 and Risks of Mortality and End-Stage Renal Disease in Patients With Chronic Kidney Disease. J Am Med Assoc 305: 2432–2439.
32. Jean G, Terrat JC, Vanel T, Hurot JM, Lorriaux C, et al. (2009) High levels of serum fibroblast growth factor (FGF)-23 are associated with increased mortality in long haemodialysis patients. Nephrol Dial Transplant 24: 2792–2796.
33. Yilmaz MI, Sonmez A, Saglam M, Yaman H, Kilic S, et al. (2010) FGF-23 and vascular dysfunction in patients with stage 3 and 4 chronic kidney disease. Kidney Int 78: 679–685.
34. Locatelli F, Martin-Malo A, Hannedouche T, Loureiro A, Papadimitriou M, et al., for the Membrane Permeability Outcome (MPO) Study Group (2009) Effect of Membrane Permeability on Survival of Hemodialysis Patients. J Am Soc Nephrol 20: 645–654.
35. Barreto FC, Barreto DV, Liabeuf S, Meert N, Glorieux G, et al. (2009) Serum indoxyl sulfate is associated with vascular disease and mortality in chronic kidney disease patients. Clin J Am Soc Nephrol 4: 1551–1558.
36. Liabeuf S, Barreto DV, Barreto FC, Meert N, Glorieux G, et al. (2010) Free p-cresylsulphate is a predictor of mortality in patients at different stages of chronic kidney disease. Nephrol Dial Transplant 25: 1183–1191.
37. Schepers E, Barreto DV, Liabeuf S, Glorieux G, Eloot S, et al., On behalf of the European Uremic Toxin Work Group (EUTox) (2011) Symmetric Dimethylarginine as a Proinflammatory Agent in Chronic Kidney Disease. Clin J Am Soc Nephrol 6: 2374–2383.
38. Cockcroft DW, Gault MH (1976) Prediction of creatinine clearance from serum creatinine. Nephron 16: 31–41.
39. Le Bricon T, Thervet E, Froissart M, Benlakehal M, Bousquet B, et al. (2000) Plasma cystatin C is superior to 24-h creatinine clearance and plasma creatinine for estimation of glomerular filtration rate 3 months after kidney transplantation. Clin Chem 46: 1206–1207.
40. Rule AD, Bergstralh EJ, Slezak JM, Bergert J, Larson TS (2006) Glomerular filtration rate estimated by cystatin C among different clinical presentations. Kidney Int 69: 399–405.
41. Stevens LA, Coresh J, Greene T, Levey AS (2006) Assessing kidney function–measured and estimated glomerular filtration rate. N Engl J Med 354: 2473–2483.
42. Donadio C, Lucchesi A, Ardini M, Giordani R (2001) Cystatin C, beta 2-microglobulin, and retinol-binding protein as indicators of glomerular filtration rate: comparison with plasma creatinine. J Pharm Biomed Anal 24: 835–842.
43. Hallgren R, Karlsson FA, Roxin LE, Venge P (1978) Myoglobin Turnover - Influence of Renal and Extra-Renal Factors. J Lab Clin Med 91: 246–254.
44. Menon V, Wang X, Greene I, Beck GJ, Kusek JW, et al. (2004) Factors associated with serum leptin in patients with chronic kidney disease. Clin Nephrol 61: 163–169.
45. Bacchetta J, Dubourg L, Harambat J, Ranchin B, bou-Jaoude P, et al. (2010) The Influence of Glomerular Filtration Rate and Age on Fibroblast Growth Factor 23 Serum Levels in Pediatric Chronic Kidney Disease. J Clin Endocrinol Metabol 95: 1741–1748.
46. Vanholder R, Eloot S, Schepers E, Neirynck N, Glorieux G, et al. (2012) An Obituary for GFR as the Main Marker for Kidney Function? Semin Dial 25: 9–14.
47. Christensen EI, Birn H (2001) Megalin and cubilin: synergistic endocytic receptors in renal proximal tubule. Am J Physiol - Renal Physiol 280: F562–F573.
48. Hutchison CA, Harding S, Hewins P, Mead GP, Townsend J, et al. (2008) Quantitative Assessment of Serum and Urinary Polyclonal Free Light Chains in Patients with Chronic Kidney Disease. Clin J Am Soc Nephrol 3: 1684–1690.
49. Gutierrez OM, Mannstadt M, Isakova T, Rauh-Hain JA, Tamez H, et al. (2008) Fibroblast growth factor 23 and mortality among patients undergoing hemodialysis. N Engl J Med 359: 584–592.
50. Drueke TB, Massy ZA (2009) Beta2-microglobulin. Semin Dial 22: 378–380.
51. Seronie-Vivien S, Delanaye P, Pieroni L, Mariat C, Froissart M,et al. (2008) Cystatin C: current position and future prospects. Clin Chem Lab Med 46: 1664–1686.
52. Astor BC, Shafi T, Hoogeveen RC, Matsushita K, Ballantyne CM, et al.(2012) Novel Markers of Kidney Function as Predictors of ESRD, Cardiovascular Disease, and Mortality in the General Population. Am J Kidney Dis 653–662.
53. Lilitkarntakul P, Dhaun N, Melville V, Blackwell S, Talwar DK, et al. (2011) Blood pressure and not uraemia is the major determinant of arterial stiffness and endothelial dysfunction in patients with chronic kidney disease and minimal co-morbidity. Atherosclerosis 216: 217–225.
54. Cooper BA, Branley P, Bulfone L, Collins JF, Craig JC, et al.(2010) A randomized, controlled trial of early versus late initiation of dialysis. N Engl J Med 363: 609–619.

Bone Biomarkers Help Grading Severity of Coronary Calcifications in Non Dialysis Chronic Kidney Disease Patients

Marion Morena[1,2,3], Isabelle Jaussent[4], Aurore Halkovich[1], Anne-Marie Dupuy[1], Anne-Sophie Bargnoux[1,3], Leila Chenine[5], Hélène Leray-Moragues[5], Kada Klouche[3,6], Hélène Vernhet[7], Bernard Canaud[2,3,5], Jean-Paul Cristol[1,3]*

1 Laboratoire de Biochimie, CHRU de Montpellier, Montpellier, France, **2** Institut de Recherche et de Formation en Dialyse, Montpellier, France, **3** UMR 204, Nutripass, Université Montpellier I, Montpellier, France, **4** INSERM, U1061, and Université Montpellier I, Montpellier, France, **5** Service de Néphrologie-Hémodialyse et Soins Intensifs, CHRU de Montpellier, Montpellier, France, **6** Service de Réanimation Métabolique, CHRU de Montpellier, Montpellier, France, **7** Service de Radiologie, CHRU de Montpellier, Montpellier, France

Abstract

Background: Osteoprotegerin (OPG) and fibroblast growth factor-23 (FGF23) are recognized as strong risk factors of vascular calcifications in non dialysis chronic kidney disease (ND-CKD) patients. The aim of this study was to investigate the relationships between FGF23, OPG, and coronary artery calcifications (CAC) in this population and to attempt identification of the most powerful biomarker of CAC: FGF23? OPG?

Methodology/Principal Findings: 195 ND-CKD patients (112 males/83 females, 70.8 [27.4–94.6] years) were enrolled in this cross-sectional study. All underwent chest multidetector computed tomography for CAC scoring. Vascular risk markers including FGF23 and OPG were measured. Logistic regression analyses were used to study the potential relationships between CAC and these markers. The fully adjusted-univariate analysis clearly showed high OPG (≥10.71 pmol/L) as the only variable significantly associated with moderate CAC ([100–400[) (OR = 2.73 [1.03;7.26]; p = 0.04). Such association failed to persist for CAC scoring higher than 400. Indeed, severe CAC was only associated with high phosphate fractional excretion ($FEPO_4$) (≥38.71%) (OR = 5.47 [1.76;17.0]; p = 0.003) and high FGF23 (≥173.30 RU/mL) (OR = 5.40 [1.91;15.3]; p = 0.002). In addition, the risk to present severe CAC when FGF23 level was high was not significantly different when OPG was normal or high. Conversely, the risk to present moderate CAC when OPG level was high was not significantly different when FGF23 was normal or high.

Conclusions: Our results strongly suggest that OPG is associated to moderate CAC while FGF23 rather represents a biomarker of severe CAC in ND-CKD patients.

Editor: Olivier Kocher, Harvard Medical School, United States of America

Funding: This work was partly supported by a grant from Ministère de la Santé (PHRC-UF 7853). No additional external funding was received for this study. The funders had no role in study design, data collection and analysis, decision to publish, or preparation of the manuscript.

Competing Interests: The authors have declared that no competing interests exist.

* E-mail: jp-cristol@chu-montpellier.fr

Introduction

Coronary artery calcifications (CAC) are recognized as a strong predictor of all-cause and cardiovascular mortality in hemodialysis (HD) patients [1]. Recent studies now provide strong evidence for the risk of death with a high CAC score in chronic kidney disease (CKD) patients before onset of dialysis [2,3]. Presence of CAC has been associated with numerous traditional risk factors including aging, hypertension and diabetes as well as with non traditional risk factors including mineral metabolism disorders, hyperparathyroidism, inflammation, osteoprotegerin (OPG) and more recently fibroblast growth factor 23 (FGF23) [4].

OPG is a bone regulating protein belonging to the TNF receptor superfamily. With its ligand, the receptor activator of nuclear factor kB ligand (RANKL), it regulates important aspects of osteoclast/osteoblast formation [5]. RANKL increases the pool of active osteoclasts by activating its specific receptor RANK located partly on osteoclastic cells, thus increasing bone resorption, whereas OPG, which neutralizes RANKL, has opposite effects. RANKL and OPG are produced by bone marrow derived stromal cells and osteoblasts and are regulated by various calcitropic cytokines, hormones, and drugs. The actions of OPG and RANKL in the vasculature and heart are still unclear but no doubt exists about the strong association of OPG with the prevalence of vascular calcifications in predialysis [6] and HD patients [7].

FGF23 is the main regulator of phosphate homeostasis. It is produced by osteocytes in response to hyperphosphatemia and exerts its effects on its receptor, the Klotho-FGFR1c heterodimer, in the kidney where it inhibits the expression of Na-Pi cotransporters resulting in hyperphosphaturia. Literature data are more controversial regarding FGF23 association with vascular calcifications according to the stage of CKD. Relationships between FGF23 and aortic calcifications [8] or peripheral vascular calcifications [9,10] are well documented in HD patients. By contrast, studies in non dialysis CKD (ND-CKD) patients could not evidence any association after multivariable adjustment [11] but rather relationships to atherosclerosis [12] and left ventricular hypertrophy [11,13].

We therefore investigated in this cross-sectional study the relationships between FGF23, OPG and CAC prevalence in a population of ND-CKD patients and attempted to identify the most powerful biomarker(s) of CAC: FGF23? OPG?

Methods

Ethics Statement

The study was conducted according to the principles of the Declaration of Helsinki and in compliance with International Conference on Harmonization/Good Clinical Practice regulations. According to the French Law, the study has been registered at "Ministère de la Santé et des Solidarités" after approval by the Montpellier University Hospital's ethics committee (Comité de Protection des Personnes Sud Méditerranée IV) with the following number 2006-A00416-45. All patients gave their written informed consent.

Subjects

One hundred and ninety five ND-CKD patients at various stages of kidney disease, issued from the outpatient general nephrology consultation of the Montpellier Lapeyronie university hospital, were enrolled in this cross-sectional study. Inclusion criteria were age≥18 years and presence of CKD defined by glomerular filtration rate (GFR) in agreement with the National Kidney Foundation [14].

Causes of CKD were glomerulonephritis (n = 25), cystic renal disease (n = 14), diabetic nephropathy (n = 21), diabetic and hypertensive nephropathy (n = 21), angiosclerosis and hypertensive nephropathy (n = 79), infectious/obstructive interstitial nephropathy (n = 4), renal neoplasia (n = 1), genetic/congenital cause (n = 1), necrotizing angiitis (n = 3), unknown cause (n = 9), other cause (n = 17).

Detailed medical history including age, gender, weight, height, diabetes mellitus, hypertension, past or current smoking, presence of atherosclerotic cardiovascular disease was recorded.

Existence of hypertension was defined by brachial blood pressure higher or equal to 130/80 mmHg and/or by a current antihypertensive treatment.

Presence of atherosclerotic cardiovascular disease was defined by the presence of at least one of the three following manifestations: coronary heart disease (CHD), cerebrovascular disease (CVD) or peripheral vascular disease (PVD). *CHD* was defined as documented angina pectoris or history of myocardial infarction. Angina pectoris was described as chest pain arising at exertion and disappearing with nitroglycerine or rest. The diagnosis may also have been made by a positive evaluation in nuclear medicine or a coronary stenosis >75% of luminal diameter evidenced by angiography. Myocardial infarction was defined as clinical symptoms, such as chest pain or dyspnea, associated with abnormal electrocardiogram and elevated troponins. *CVD* was defined as previous clinical cerebral disease (transient ischemic attack or stroke) or the presence of atheromatous plaques on internal carotid arteries. *PVD* included clinical symptoms such as intermittent claudication, abolished peripheral pulses or diminished arterial pulses or signs of atheromatous involvement of the lower limb diagnosticated by doppler ultrasound.

Procedures

Laboratory measurements. Blood samples were collected as part of our regular CKD patient follow-up, centrifuged and supernatant was stored at −80°C for processing of creatinine, calcium, PO_4, 25(OH) vitamin D, 1.25$(OH)_2$ vitamin D, intact parathyroid hormone (PTH), albumin, high sensitive C reactive protein (hs CRP), fibrinogen, FGF23 and OPG. All measurements were sequentially done with less than one year intervals after freezing.

Creatinine was measured by enzymatic method (Olympus, Rungis, France) using reagents from Randox (Randox, Mauguio, France). Calcium and PO_4 were assessed by colorimetric method (Olympus, Rungis, France). 25(OH) vitamin D and 1.25$(OH)_2$ vitamin D were measured by radioimmunoassay (Immunodiagnostic Systems, Boldon, UK). Intact PTH and insulin were measured by immunoradiometric assay (N-Tact PTH SP IRMA Kit, DiaSorin, Stillwater, MN, USA; Bi Ins IRMA, Cisbio International, Bagnols sur Cèze, France). Albumin was measured by immunonephelometry (Immage Beckman Coulter, Villepinte, France). hs CRP was determined by immunoturbidimetry (Olympus, Rungis, France). Fibrinogen was measured by Von Clauss method (STA Fibrinogen, Diagnostica Stago, Asnières, France). FGF23 was measured with an enzyme linked immunosorbent assay (ELISA) detecting both intact FGF23 and C-terminal fragments (Immutopics International Inc, San Clemente; CA, USA). OPG was determined by ELISA (Biovendor Laboratory Medicine, Brno, Czech Republic) [15,16].

GFR was estimated using the reexpressed 4-variable Modification of Diet in Renal Disease (MDRD) study equation [17].

Urinary PO_4 excretion was expressed as Fractional excretion of PO_4 ($FEPO_4$) calculated as follows: $FEPO_4$ (%) = urine[PO_4] × plasma[Creat] × 100/urine[Creat] ×plasma[PO_4].

Coronary artery calcification imaging. All patients underwent multidetector computed tomography (MDCT).

Regarding data acquisition, all MDCT scans derived from a multidetector-row spiral CT (Lightspeed VCT, General Electric Medical System, Milwaukee, WI, USA). Prospective ECG-triggered step-scan was performed using with 2.5-mm collimation width ×64 detectors so that the center of the temporal window corresponded to 70% of the R-R interval. The scanning parameters were a gantry rotation speed of 0.35 s/rotation, 120 kV and 300 mA 8×2.5 collimation, and 20 mm table feed per rotation. The matrix size was 512×512 pixels and the display field of view was 25 cm. The reconstruction kernel was standard. The temporal resolution was 250 ms.

Regarding image evaluation, calcium score was calculated using a semi-automatically software (Smartscore version 3.5, Advantage Window 4.4 workstation, General Electric, Milwaukee, WI, USA). Coronary calcification was defined as a plaque of > = 4 pixels (area = 1.37 mm^2) with a density of greater than or equal to 130 Hounsfield units. Quantitative calcium scores were calculated according to the method described by Agatston et al. [18]. Coronary calcium scoring was performed by either a physician or computed tomography technician with specific training for the methodology described above.

Statistical Methods

Characteristics of the population were described by using proportions for categorical variables and median and range for quantitative variables since their distributions were tested with the Shapiro-Wilk statistic and were mostly skewed.

Associations between the extent of CAC divided into three groups (<100, [100–400[, ≥400) and patient characteristics, vascular risk biomarkers, biological parameters were quantified with odds-ratio (OR) and their 95% confidence intervals (CI). Clinical and sociodemographic variables associated with CAC (at $p<0.15$) were included in multinomial logistic regression models to estimate adjusted OR for biological parameters (especially OPG and FGF23). The cut-off used for CAC has been chosen by respect to CAC scoring: those with CAC<100 (considered as patients with insignificant or mild CAC), those with CAC in the range [100–400[(presence of moderate CAC) and those with CAC≥400 (presence of severe CAC) [19,20]. Biological parameters were divided into tertiles. In the case of FGF23 and OPG, patients were divided into two categories, those with a low level (<173.30 RU/mL for FGF23; <10.71 pmol/L for OPG, corresponding to the 1st and 2nd tertiles) and those with a high level (≥173.30 RU/mL for FGF23; ≥10.71 pmol/L for OPG, corresponding to the 3rd tertile).

Spearman correlation coefficient (rho) was used to determine the relationships between quantitative variables.

Significance was set at $p<0.05$. All analyses were carried out with SAS software, version 9.2 (SAS Institute, Cary, NC, USA).

Results

Clinical characteristics for the 195 CKD patients are summarized in **Table 1**.

Sex ratio of the patients was 112/83 (male/female), median age was 70.8 with a range of 27.4–94.6 years and median BMI was 26.7 [14.3–47.7] kg/m^2.

Ninety five (49.0%) patients had ever smoked. Diabetes and hypertension were found in 63 (32.3%) and 180 (92.3%) patients respectively. History of CHD was present in 39 patients (20.0%), 14 (7.2%) patients had history of CVD and 34 (17.4%) had history of PVD.

One hundred and twenty four (63.6%) patients were receiving vitamin D supplements, 64 (37.2%) patients were receiving statins, 12 (7.0%) patients were receiving sevelamer HCl, none of them were receiving cinacalcet. Erythropoiesis stimulating agents were administered to 37 (18.97%) patients.

Median eGFR using MDRD was 33.2 [6.5–91.9] mL/min/1.73 m^2. Median hs CRP was 2.2 [0.1;56.1] mg/L, median intact PTH was 47.0 [4.0–493.0] pg/mL, median 1.25(OH)$_2$ vitamin D was 30 [5–80] pg/mL, median 25(OH) vitamin D was 19.5 [6.6–76.4] ng/mL, median FGF23 was 126.4 [42.9–3415.0] RU/mL and median OPG level was 9.1 [2.7–37.6] pmol/L.

Median CAC was 188 [0–3942].

Stratification of FGF23 and OPG median values (quartiles) according to CKD stages are presented in **Figure 1**.

Table 1. Characteristics of the chronic kidney disease patients.

Parameter	Total
No. of patients	195
Gender, male	112 (57.4%)
Age *years*	70.8 [27.4–94.6]
BMI *kg/m²*	26.7 [14.3–47.7]
Smoking habits	95 (49.0%)
Diabetes mellitus	63 (32.3%)
Hypertension	180 (92.3%)
Coronary heart disease	39 (20.0%)
Cerebrovascular disease	14 (7.2%)
Peripheral vascular disease	34 (17.4%)
Vitamin D supplements	
Alfacalcidol	99 (50.8%)
Cholecalciferol	21 (10.8%)
Calcifediol	4 (2.1%)
Statins	64 (37.2%)
Sevelamer hydrochloride	12 (7%)
Erythropoiesis stimulating agents	37 (18.97%)
eGFR (MDRD study equation) (mL/min/1.73 m^2)	33.2 [6.5–91.9]
>60 mL/min/1.73 m^2	19 (9.7%)
60-30 mL/min/1.73 m^2	91 (46.7%)
<30 mL/min/1.73 m^2	85 (43.6%)
Triglycerides (mmol/L)	1.65 [0.36–4.93]
HDL cholesterol (mmol/L)	1.49 [0.64–3.37]
LDL cholesterol (mmol/L)	2.90 [1.12–6.46]
hs C reactive protein (mg/L)	2.2 [0.1–56.1]
Calcium (mmol/L)	2.38 [1.68–2.73]
Phosphate (mmol/L)	1.07 [0.58–2.34]
Parathyroid hormone (pg/mL)	47.0 [4.0–493.0]
1.25(OH)$_2$ vitamin D (pg/mL)	30 [5–80]
25(OH) vitamin D (ng/mL)	19.5 [6.6–76.4]
Hemoglobin (g/dL)	13 [8.9–16.9]
FGF23 (RU/mL)	126.4 [42.9–3415.0]
OPG (pmol/L)	9.1 [2.7–37.6]
CAC	188 [0–3942]

Values were described by using proportions for categorical variables and median [range] for quantitative variables.

Characteristics of the patients according to the level of CAC

Among the 195 patients studied, 79 (40.5%) had insignificant or mild CAC (score below 100), 50 (25.6%) patients had moderate CAC (score in the range [100–400[) and 66 (33.9%) presented severe CAC (score greater than or equal to 400).

The univariate analysis revealed that presence of moderate CAC (score in the range [100–400[) was significantly associated with male gender (OR = 3.17 [1.51;6.65]); age (OR = 2.75 [1.83;4.13] for 10 years increased) and diabetes (OR = 4.48 [1.91;10.5]). Presence of severe CAC (score greater or equal to 400) was significantly associated with the same parameters (male gender: OR = 4.71 [2.30;9.62]; age: OR = 3.04 [2.04;4.51] for 10 years increased; diabetes: OR = 6.08 [2.64;14.0]) including smoking (OR = 3.11 [1.57;6.16]). No significant relationship between therapeutic interventions and moderate or severe CAC was evidenced (**Table 2**).

Relationships between biological markers of vascular risk and the extent of CAC

Among the biological markers of vascular risk studied, the logistic regression analysis clearly showed high OPG (≥10.71 pmol/L) as the only one variable to be significantly associated with moderate CAC ([100–400[) (OR = 2.73 [1.03;7.26]; p = 0.04) after adjustment for age, gender, diabetes

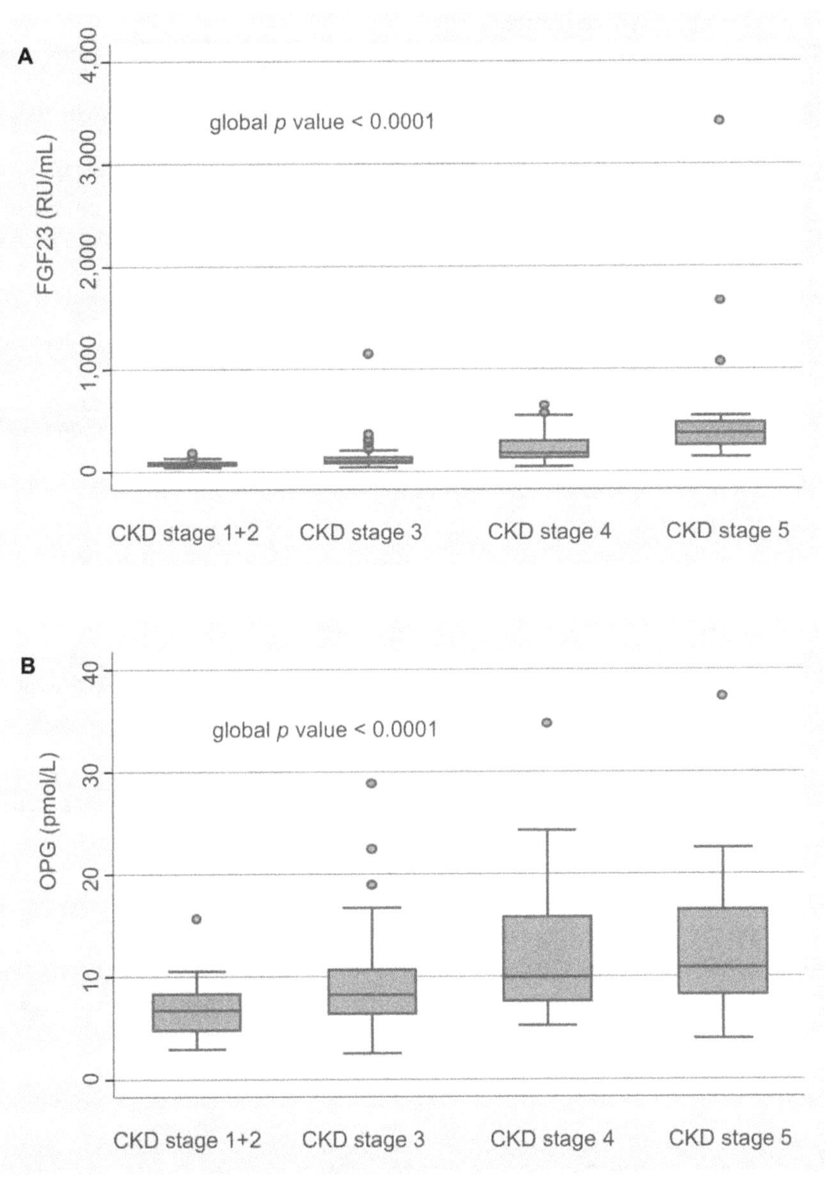

Figure 1. Stratification of bone biomarkers according to CKD stages. FGF23 (A) and OPG (B) median values (quartiles) are depicted according to CKD stages (with a glomerular filtration rate estimated using the reexpressed 4-variable Modification of Diet in Renal Disease (MDRD) 175 study equation).

and smoking. Such association failed to persist for CAC scoring higher than 400 (OR = 2.41 [0.91;6.39]). Indeed, severe CAC score was only associated with high $FEPO_4$ (≥38.71%) (OR = 5.47 [1.76;17.0]; p = 0.003) and high FGF23 (≥173.30 RU/mL) (OR = 5.40 [1.91;15.3]; p = 0.002) (**Table 3**). Besides, a strong positive correlation was observed between $FEPO_4$ and FGF23 whatever the CAC score was (all CAC: rho = 0.53, p<0.0001; CAC<100: rho = 0.45, p<0.0001; CAC [100–400[: rho = 0.51, p = 0.0003; CAC≥400: rho = 0.61, p<0.0001).

Prevalence of high OPG and FGF-23 levels according to the extent of CAC

To further compare the relative prevalence of abnormally high (greater than the lower bound of third tertile) OPG versus FGF23 levels across the spectrum of CAC, the proportions of participants with normal or high OPG and FGF23 values within each category of CAC were determined. (**Figure 2A**). As expected, the predominant pattern in the range of insignificant or mild CAC (<100) was normal FGF23/normal OPG (63.3%). In the range of moderate CAC, an isolated increase in OPG (46.0%) was the most common pattern and was more likely than an isolated increase in FGF23 (28.0%). By contrast, at the level of severe CAC, the most common pattern was characterized by an isolated increase in FGF23 (47.0%).

Relationships between OPG/FGF23 (as a composite criterium) and the extent of CAC

Logistic regression model clearly showed that, in these patients, the risk to present severe CAC when FGF23 level was high (≥173.30 RU/mL) was not significantly different when OPG was normal (OR = 7.33 [2.02;26.60]) or high (OR = 7.34

Table 2. Clinical markers associated to increased coronary artery calcifications.

	Coronary artery calcifications							*Coronary artery calcifications*	
	<100 (n = 79)		*[100–400[(n = 50)*		*≥400 (n = 66)*			*[100–400[vs <100*	*≥400 vs <100*
Variable	*n*	*%*	*n*	*%*	*n*	*%*	*P-value**	*OR [CI 95%]*	*OR [CI 95%]*
Gender									
Female	49	62.03	17	34.00	17	25.76	<.0001	1	1
Male	30	37.97	33	66.00	49	74.24		**3.17 [1.51;6.65]**	**4.71 [2.30;9.62]**
Median Age [min-max]									
OR For 10 Years increased	61.2 [27.4–85.1]		73.4 [45.7–94.6]		75.9 [49.7–86.7]		<.0001	**2.75 [1.83;4.13]**	**3.04 [2.04;4.51]**
Body mass index									
<25	39	49.37	16	32.00	22	33.33	0.20	1	1
[25–30[	28	35.44	21	42.00	30	45.45		1.83 [0.81;4.12]	1.90 [0.91;3.96]
≥30	12	15.19	13	26.00	14	21.21		2.64 [0.99;7.01]	2.07 [0.81;5.25]
Smoking									
No	51	64.56	24	48.00	24	36.92	0.004	1	1
Yes	28	35.44	26	52.00	41	63.08		1.97 [0.96;4.06]	**3.11 [1.57;6.16]**
Diabetes mellitus									
No	68	86.08	29	58.00	35	53.03	<0.0001	1	1
Yes	11	13.92	21	42.00	31	46.97		**4.48 [1.91;10.5]**	**5.48 [2.46;12.2]**
Hypertension									
No	8	10.13	5	10.00	2	3.03	0.26	1	1
Yes	71	89.87	45	90.00	64	96.97		1.01 [0.31;3.29]	3.60 [0.74;17.6]
Dyslipidemia									
No	13	16.67	10	20.00	7	10.77	0.38	1	1
Yes (LDL ≥ 2.62 mmol/L or statin use)	65	83.33	40	80.00	58	89.23		0.80 [0.32;2.00]	1.66 [0.62;4.43]
Vitamin D supplements									
No	27	34.18	18	36.00	25	37.88	0.90	1	1
Yes	52	65.82	32	64.00	41	62.12		0.92 [0.44;1.94]	0.85 [0.43;1.68]
Sevelamer HCl									
No	76	96.20	47	94.00	60	90.91	0.44	1	1
Yes	3	3.80	3	6.00	6	9.09		1.62 [0.31;8.35]	2.53 [0.61;10.6]
Erythropoiesis stimulating agents									
No	66	83.54	43	86.00	49	74.24	0.22	1	1
Yes	13	16.46	7	14.00	17	25.76		0.83 [0.31;2.24]	1.76 [0.78;3.96]
Calcium-based phosphate binders									
No	63	79.75	41	82.00	58	87.88	0.42	1	1
Yes	16	20.25	9	18.00	8	12.12		0.86 [0.35;2.14]	0.54 [0.22;1.36]
Non-calcium-based phosphate binders									
No	77	97.47	47	94.00	61	92.42	0.40	1	1
Yes	2	2.53	3	6.00	5	7.58		2.46 [0.40;15.3]	3.16 [0.59;16.8]

*p-value (for variables with more than two categories, the p-value of the test for trend is given).

[1.63;33.00]). Conversely, even though only a tendancy exists, the risk to present moderate CAC when OPG level was high (≥10.71 pmol/L) was not significantly different when FGF23 was normal (OR = 3.27 [0.99;10.80]) or high (OR = 3.53 [0.77;16.30]) (**Figure 2B**).

Discussion

In this study, clinical variables such as age, diabetes mellitus and smoking habits were associated with CAC in our population of ND-CKD patients. Among biomarkers of vascular calcifications, our results clearly confirmed that both high OPG and FGF23

Table 3. Biological markers associated to increased coronary artery calcifications after adjustment for age, gender, diabetes mellitus and smoking (the p-value of the test for trend is given).

	Coronary artery calcifications							*Coronary artery calcifications*	
	<100 (n = 79)		*[100–400[(n = 50)*		*≥400 (n = 66)*			*[100–400[vs <100*	*≥400 vs <100*
Variable	*n*	*%*	*n*	*%*	*n*	*%*	*Global P-value*	*OR [CI 95%]*	*OR [CI 95%]*
Hemoglobin (g/dL)									
<12.5	23	29.11	16	32.65	22	33.85	0.49	1	1
[12.5–13.8[	27	34.18	18	36.73	20	30.77		0.53 [0.17;1.61]	0.37 [0.12;1.16]
≥13.8	29	36.71	15	30.61	23	35.38		0.50 [0.16;1.61]	0.52 [0.17;1.62]
Serum creatinine (μmol/L)									
<137	32	40.51	18	36.00	14	21.21	0.25	1	1
[137–190[	26	32.91	14	28.00	24	36.36		0.77 [0.27;2.22]	1.59 [0.55;4.55]
≥190	21	26.58	18	36.00	28	42.42		1.76 [0.61;5.13]	**3.17 [1.07;9.37]**
Calcium (mmol/L)									
<2.32	25	31.65	22	44.00	20	30.30	0.34	1	1
[2.32–2.44[	32	40.51	11	22.00	19	28.79		0.53 [0.18;1.53]	1.04 [0.36;2.97]
≥2.44	22	27.85	17	34.00	27	40.91		1.16 [0.41;3.32]	2.08 [0.72;6.04]
Phosphate (mmol/L)									
<0.97	23	29.11	21	42.00	19	28.79	0.46	1	1
[0.97–1.16[	28	35.44	18	36.00	23	34.85		0.95 [0.35;2.58]	1.30 [0.47;3.64]
≥1.16	28	35.44	11	22.00	24	36.36		0.54 [0.17;1.74]	1.44 [0.46;4.45]
$FEPO_4$ (%)									
<25.86	33	43.42	14	31.11	13	22.03	0.01	1	1
[25.86–38.71[	24	31.58	19	42.22	17	28.81		**2.95 [1.01;8.64]**	2.66 [0.86;8.21]
≥38.71	19	25.00	12	26.67	29	49.15		2.15 [0.67;6.95]	**5.47 [1.76;17.0]**
1.25 $(OH)_2$ vitamin D (pg/mL)									
<23	23	29.11	18	36.00	18	27.27	0.20	1	1
[23–38[	27	34.18	15	30.00	23	34.85		**0.23 [0.07;0.79]**	0.30 [0.09;1.03]
≥38	29	36.71	17	34.00	25	37.88		0.33 [0.10;1.05]	0.45 [0.14;1.44]
25(OH) vitamin D (ng/mL)									
<15.7	24	32.00	19	38.00	20	30.77	0.94	1	1
[15.7–25.0[	23	30.67	15	30.00	24	36.92		1.13 [0.39;3.26]	1.53 [0.54;4.40]
≥25.0	28	37.33	16	32.00	21	32.31		1.01 [0.36;2.89]	1.22 [0.42;3.49]
Intact PTH (pg/mL)									
<36	32	40.51	15	30.00	16	24.24	0.35	1	1
[36–75[	26	32.91	20	40.00	20	30.30		1.40 [0.50;3.94]	1.11 [0.38;3.24]
≥75	21	26.58	15	30.00	30	45.45		1.15 [0.39;3.36]	2.10 [0.74;5.97]
FGF 23 (RU/mL)									
<173.30	58	73.42	36	72.00	35	53.03	0.003	1	1
≥173.30	21	26.58	14	28.00	31	46.97		2.05 [0.71;5.92]	**5.40 [1.91;15.3]**
Osteoprotegerin (pmol/L)									
<10.71	65	82.28	27	54.00	37	56.06	0.11	1	1
≥10.71	14	17.72	23	46.00	29	43.94		**2.73 [1.03;7.26]**	2.41 [0.91;6.39]

levels were associated with CAC in this population. Original findings of our study are that association of both markers with CAC depends on the severity of CAC extension: OPG is associated to moderate CAC while FGF23 rather represents a biomarker of severe CAC in these patients.

Previous studies have reported an association between high OPG levels and CAC in CKD (in particular one from our group) [6], HD [7,10,21] and diabetic patients [22,23]. Here, we demonstrated for the first time that high OPG is only associated to moderate rather than severe coronary calcifications. These interesting results are in total agreement with a previous study from Morony et al. [24] in a model of atherogenic diet-fed *ldlr* $^{(-/-)}$ mice. Indeed, the authors clearly showed that plasma OPG level increased with initiation of the atherogenic diet, reached a maximum value after one month of diet and did not increase further during the four following months while aortic atherosclerosis lesions were still progressing. In our

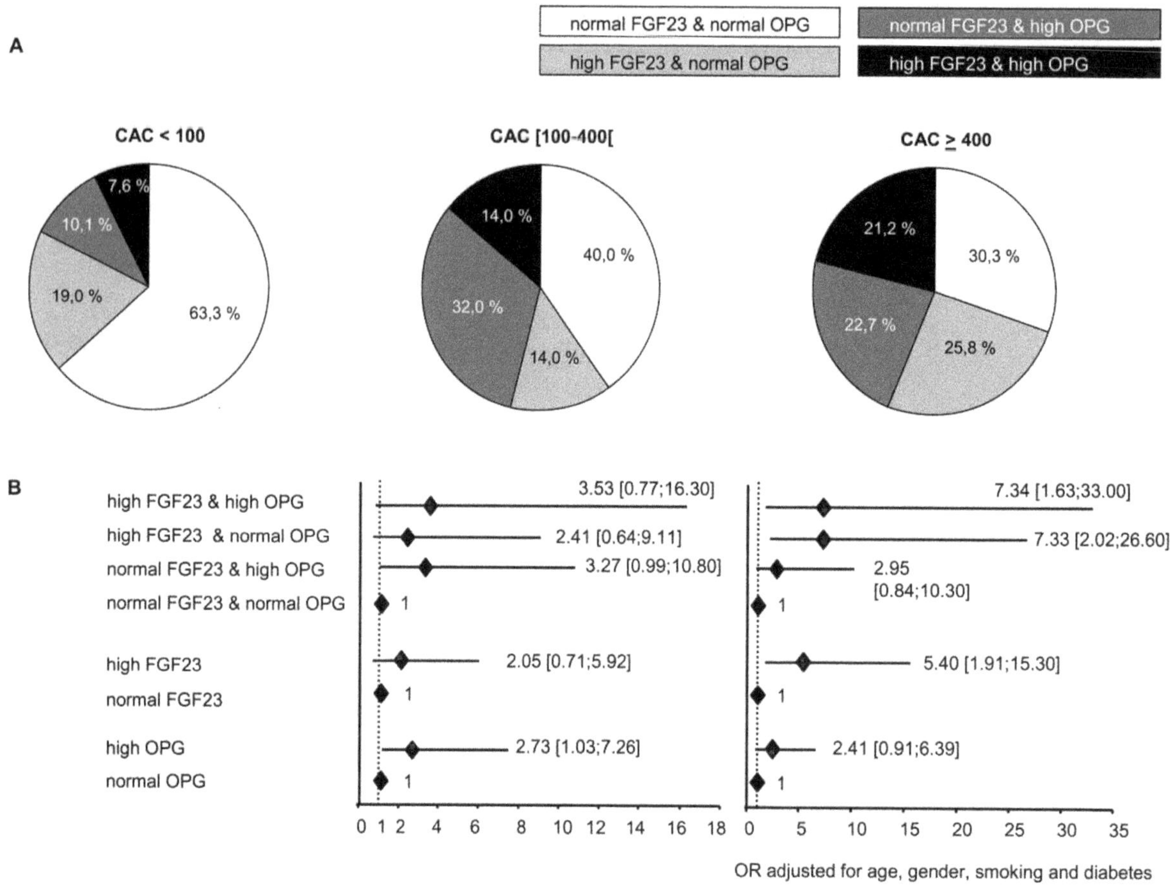

Figure 2. Fibroblast growth factor 23 and Osteoprotegerin are differently associated to the severity of CAC. (A) Proportions of patients with normal (<173.30 RU/mL) or high (≥173.30 RU/mL) fibroblast growth factor 23 (FGF23) and normal (<10.71 pmol/L) or high (≥10.71 pmol/L) osteoprotegerin (OPG) levels within each coronary artery calcification (CAC) category. Sections of pie charts indicate proportions of patients with FGF23 and/or OPG levels by CAC category. (B) Prevalence rate ratio of CAC associated with increased levels of FGF23 and/or OPG levels.

study, the same pattern is observed. OPG values are significantly increased in patients with moderate ([100–400[) compared with mild (<100) CAC, this increased level being comparable with that of patients presenting severe (>400) CAC. This clearly suggests that OPG appears as a marker of atherosclerosis/vascular calcification onset rather than its severity or progression. Considerable controversy exists regarding the role of OPG in the development and progression of vascular calcifications. However, the only theory we can speculate on is that OPG is increased in response to vascular insult as the component of a complex compensatory mechanism, probably secondary to inflammatory processes. Indeed, proinflammatory mediators, particularly TNF-alpha, which participate to the development of vascular calcification through induction of alkaline phosphatase can also stimulate OPG synthesis in vascular smooth muscle cells and endothelial cells [25–27] in an attempt to possibly counteract osteogenic or pro-apoptotic calcification mechanisms. However, further in vitro and in vivo studies need to be conducted in order to elucidate the exact implication of such molecule in the early progression of vascular calcifications.

Regarding FGF23, although its association with CAC was evidenced in HD [8,9], this relationship was not clear in all studies related to ND-CKD patients. In their analysis, Gutierrez et al. [11] could describe an association between FGF23 and CAC. However, this association was no longer significant after multivariable adjustment or when examined on a continuous scale. The recent study from Desjardins et al. [28] clearly demonstrated in 142 ND-CKD patients an association between high FGF23 and aortic calcifications and to a lesser extent an association with CAC in a subgroup of 93 patients. As previously observed by Gutierrez et al., FGF23 was also no longer associated to CAC in their multivariate analysis. The authors speculated that, contrary to aortic calcifications, the lack of association between CAC and FGF23 may be explained by the different type of calcifications observed (intimal for coronaries and medial in the case of aorta): FGF23 being more related to mineral metabolism disturbances, would favor medial rather than intimal atheromatous calcifications. Actually, the persisting association between CAC and FGF23 after full adjustment, observed here, in more than twice the number of patients, may probably reflect a power limitation of their study. Desjardins et al. also depicted correlations between aortic as well as coronary calcifications and FGF23. In the present study, we were not able to evidence any correlation, as our results clearly demonstrated an association between FGF23 and severe rather than moderate CAC. Interestingly, these latter findings were also described in the study from Jean et al. in HD patients [10].

The potential evidence of high FGF23 as a biomarker of severe CAC in our study cannot lead to the conclusion of a real role of FGF23 in the pathogenesis of CAC. Indeed, it was initially postulated that FGF23, due to its phosphaturic and hypophosphatemic actions [29], may be considered as a protective molecule against vascular calcifications. During decline in renal function, the commonly observed rise in FGF23 should probably reflect an increased production by osteocytes to help maintening normophosphatemia rather than a lack of removal by the kidney [30]. However, a previous work in this population could report a preponderance of C-terminal fragments (secondary to proteolytic cleavage of intact FGF23) suggesting that less than one-quarter of the circulating FGF23 was bioactive in these patients [31]. In addition, the original work from Goetz et al. [32] could provide evidence that proteolytic cleavage of this molecule abrogated its activity by removing FGF23's binding site for the FGF receptor-Klotho complex and also by generating an endogenous inhibitor of FGF23. Therefore, taken into account all these findings, it could be postulated that the high levels of FGF-23 (both intact and C-terminal fragments) measured in our population might reflect a lack of efficiency rather than an excess activity of this phosphatonin. However, importantly we observed a significant association between high levels of $FEPO_4$, the first target of FGF23, and CAC. Finally, as no association was reported between phosphatemia and CAC in our study, we may also assume that such association between FGF23 and CAC involves phosphate-independent mechanismes. Indeed, the recent report of Faul et al. [33] in an animal model strongly suggests that FGF-23 *per se* is able to induce an impairment in cardiac function. Besides, the lack of association observed here between serum phosphate and CAC is surprising but not unexpected as previous studies also reported similar findings in predialysis patients [2,34]. Russo et al. suggested that a single measurement of serum phosphate could not reflect the lifetime exposure due to rapidly changes over time for compensatory mechanisms that are mostly active early in the course of CKD [35].

Our study acknowledged some limitations. Both intact FGF23 and C-terminal fragments have been measured here. Even though several studies reported strong correlations ($r = 0.97$; $p<0.0001$) existing with the active intact FGF23 [36], this assay does not exactly reflect the biologically active form of FGF23. However, it is to note that a strong positive correlation ($rho = 0.52731$; $p<0.0001$) was observed here between C-terminal fragments and $FEPO_4$, the intact FGF23 first target. Circulating klotho levels are missing due to the lack of availability of assays in plasma or urine. The relatively small sample size of this study may have prevented some of the detected associations from being statistically significant. Finally, the cross-sectional nature of this study can not clearly evidence the kinetic of OPG and FGF23 over the progression of coronary calcifications, a prospective study being strongly required.

In conclusion, even though both OPG and FGF23 constitute strong predictors of mortality in HD patients, their relationships to vascular calcifications are different, especially in ND-CKD population. Our results clearly showed that both high OPG and FGF23 levels were associated with CAC in this population of ND-CKD patients, OPG being nevertheless a stronger associated factor of moderate CAC while FGF23 rather represents a biomarker of severe CAC.

Acknowledgments

The authors would like to acknowledge the nurses from Policlinique at Lapeyronie Hospital especially Anne Bebengut and Hélène Lebihan for patient appointment scheduling and blood withdrawals.

Author Contributions

Conceived and designed the experiments: MM AMD KK HV BC JPC. Performed the experiments: MM AH AMD ASB LC HLM KK HV BC JPC. Analyzed the data: MM IJ AMD BC JPC . Wrote the paper: MM IJ BC JPC . Reviewed, revised and approved the final paper: MM IJ AH AMD ASB LC HLM KK HV BC JPC.

References

1. London GM, Guerin AP, Marchais SJ, Metivier F, Pannier B, et al. (2003) Arterial media calcification in end-stage renal disease: impact on all-cause and cardiovascular mortality. Nephrol Dial Transplant 18: 1731–40.
2. Chiu YW, Adler SG, Budoff MJ, Takasu J, Ashai J, et al. (2010) Coronary artery calcification and mortality in diabetic patients with proteinuria. Kidney Int 77: 1107–14.
3. Haas MH (2010) The risk of death in patients with a high coronary calcification score: does it include predialysis patients? Kidney Int 77: 1057–9.
4. Moe SM, Chen NX (2008) Mechanisms of vascular calcification in chronic kidney disease. J Am Soc Nephrol 19: 213–6.
5. Trouvin A, Goëb V (2010) Receptor activator of nuclear factor-kappa B ligand and osteoprotegerin: maintaining the balance to prevent bone loss. Clin Interv Aging 19: 345–354.
6. Morena M, Dupuy AM, Jaussent I, Vernhet H, Gahide G, et al. (2009) A cut-off value of plasma osteoprotegerin level may predict the presence of coronary artery calcifications in chronic kidney disease patients. Nephrol Dial Transplant 24: 3389–97.
7. Nitta K, Akiba T, Uchida K, Otsubo S, Takei T, et al. (2004) Serum osteoprotegerin levels and the extent of vascular calcification in haemodialysis patients. Nephrol Dial Transplant 19: 1886–9.
8. Nasrallah MM, El-Shehaby AR, Salem MM, Osman NA, El Sheikh E, et al. (2010) Fibroblast growth factor-23 (FGF-23) is independently correlated to aortic calcification in haemodialysis patients. Nephrol Dial Transplant 25: 2679–85.
9. Inaba M, Okuno S, Imanishi Y, Yamada S, Shioi A, et al. (2006) Role of fibroblast growth factor-23 in peripheral vascular calcification in non-diabetic and diabetic hemodialysis patients. Osteoporos Int 17: 1506–13.
10. Jean G, Bresson E, Terrat JC, Vanel T, Hurot JM, et al. (2009) Peripheral vascular calcification in long-haemodialysis patients: associated factors and survival consequences. Nephrol Dial Transplant 24: 948–955.
11. Gutierrez OM, Januzzi JL, Isakova T, Laliberte K, Smith K, et al. (2009) Fibroblast growth factor 23 and left ventricular hypertrophy in chronic kidney disease. Circulation 119: 2545–52.
12. Mirza MA, Hansen T, Johansson L, Ahlstrom H, Larsson A, et al. (2009) Relationship between circulating FGF23 and total body atherosclerosis in the community. Nephrol Dial Transplant 24: 3125–31.
13. Mirza MA, Larsson A, Lind L, Larsson TE (2009) Circulating fibroblast growth factor-23 is associated with vascular dysfunction in the community. Atherosclerosis 205: 385–90.
14. Goolsby MJ (2002) National Kidney Foundation Guidelines for chronic kidney disease: evaluation, classification, and stratification. J Am Acad Nurse Pract 14: 238–42.
15. Avignon A, Sultan A, Piot C, Elaerts S, Cristol JP, et al. (2005) Osteoprotegerin is associated with silent coronary artery disease in high-risk but asymptomatic type-2 diabetic patients. Diabetes Care 28: 2176–2180.
16. Maïmoun L, Couret I, Mariano-Goulart D, Dupuy AM, Cristol JP, et al. (2005) Changes in osteoprotegerin/RANKL system, bone mineral density and bone biochemical markers in patients with recent spinal cord injury. Calcified Tissue International 76: 404–411.
17. Levey AS, Coresh J, Greene T, Stevens LA, Zhang YL, et al. (2006) Using standardized serum creatinine values in the modification of diet in renal disease study equation for estimating glomerular filtration rate. Ann Intern Med 145: 247–54.
18. Agatston AS, Janowitz WR, Hildner FJ, Zusmer NR, Viamonte M, Jr., et al. (1990) Quantification of coronary artery calcium using ultrafast computed tomography. J Am Coll Cardiol 15: 827–32.
19. Brindis RG, Douglas PS, Hendel RC, Peterson ED, Wolk MJ, et al. (2005) ACCF/ASNC appropriateness criteria for single-photon emission computed tomography myocardial perfusion imaging (SPECT MPI): a report of the American College of Cardiology Foundation Quality Strategic Directions Committee Appropriateness Criteria Working Group and the American Society of Nuclear Cardiology endorsed by the American Heart Association. J Am Coll Cardiol 46: 1587–605.
20. Greenland P, Bonow RO, Brundage BH, Budoff MJ, Eisenberg MJ, et al. (2007) ACCF/AHA 2007 clinical expert consensus document on coronary artery calcium scoring by computed tomography in global cardiovascular risk assessment and in evaluation of patients with chest pain: a report of the American College of Cardiology Foundation Clinical Expert Consensus Task Force (ACCF/AHA Writing Committee to Update the 2000 Expert Consensus Document on Electron Beam Computed Tomography) developed in collaboration with the Society of Atherosclerosis Imaging and Prevention and the Society of Cardiovascular Computed Tomography. J Am Coll Cardiol 49: 378–402.

21. Nitta K, Akiba T, Uchida K, Kawashima A, Yumura W, et al. (2003) The progression of vascular calcification and serum osteoprotegerin levels in patients on long-term hemodialysis. Am J Kidney Dis 42: 303–9.
22. Anand DV, Lahiri A, Lim E, Hopkins D Corder R (2006) The relationship between plasma osteoprotegerin levels and coronary artery calcification in uncomplicated type 2 diabetic subjects. J Am Coll Cardiol 47: 1850–7.
23. Mikami S, Hamano T, Fujii N, Nagasawa Y, Isaka Y, et al. (2008) Serum osteoprotegerin as a screening tool for coronary artery calcification score in diabetic pre-dialysis patients. Hypertens Res 31: 1163–70.
24. Morony S, Tintut Y, Zhang Z, Cattley R, Van G, et al. (2008) Osteoprotegerin inhibits vascular calcification without affecting atherosclerosis in ldlr(−/−) mice. Circulation 117: 411–20.
25. Collin-Osdoby P (2004) Regulation of vascular calcification by osteoclast regulatory factors RANKL and osteoprotegerin. Circ Res 95: 1046–57.
26. Collin-Osdoby P, Rothe L, Anderson F, Nelson M, Maloney W, et al. (2001) Receptor activator of NF-kappa B and osteoprotegerin expression by human microvascular endothelial cells, regulation by inflammatory cytokines, and role in human osteoclastogenesis. J Biol Chem 276: 20659–72.
27. Shioi A, Katagi M, Okuno Y, Mori K, Jono S, et al. (2002) Induction of bone-type alkaline phosphatase in human vascular smooth muscle cells: roles of tumor necrosis factor-alpha and oncostatin M derived from macrophages. Circ Res 91: 9–16.
28. Desjardins L, Liabeuf S, Renard C, Lenglet A, Lemke H, et al. (2011) FGF23 is independently associated with vascular calcification but not bone mineral density in patients at various CKD stages. Osteoporos Int doi: 10.1007/s00198-011-1838-0.
29. Strewler GJ (2001) FGF23, hypophosphatemia, and rickets: has phosphatonin been found? Proc Natl Acad Sci U S A 98: 5945–6.
30. Gutierrez O, Isakova T, Rhee E, Shah A, Holmes J, et al. (2005) Fibroblast growth factor-23 mitigates hyperphosphatemia but accentuates calcitriol deficiency in chronic kidney disease. J Am Soc Nephrol 16: 2205–15.
31. Weber TJ, Liu S, Indridason OS, Quarles LD (2003) Serum FGF23 levels in normal and disordered phosphorus homeostasis. J Bone Miner Res 18: 1227–34.
32. Goetz R, Nakada Y, Hu MC, Kurosu H, Wang L, et al. (2010) Isolated C-terminal tail of FGF23 alleviates hypophosphatemia by inhibiting FGF23-FGFR-Klotho complex formation. Proc Natl Acad Sci U S A 107: 407–12.
33. Faul C, Amaral AP, Oskouei B, Hu MC, Sloan A, et al. (2011) FGF23 induces left ventricular hypertrophy. J Clin Invest 121: 4393–408.
34. Russo D, Palmiero G, De Blasio AP, Balletta MM, Andreucci VE (2004) Coronary artery calcification in patients with CRF not undergoing dialysis. Am J Kidney Dis 44: 1024–30.
35. Russo D, Battaglia Y, Buonanno E (2010) Phosphorus and coronary calcification in predialysis patients. Kidney Int 78: 818; author reply 18.
36. Olauson H, Qureshi AR, Miyamoto T, Barany P, Heimburger O, et al. (2010) Relation between serum fibroblast growth factor-23 level and mortality in incident dialysis patients: are gender and cardiovascular disease confounding the relationship? Nephrol Dial Transplant 25: 3033–8.

4

Human Embryonic Mesenchymal Stem Cell-Derived Conditioned Medium Rescues Kidney Function in Rats with Established Chronic Kidney Disease

Arianne van Koppen[1], Jaap A. Joles[1], Bas W. M. van Balkom[1], Sai Kiang Lim[2], Dominique de Kleijn[3], Rachel H. Giles[1], Marianne C. Verhaar[1]*

1 Department of Nephrology and Hypertension, University Medical Center Utrecht, Utrecht, the Netherlands, **2** Institute of Medical Biology, A*STAR, Singapore, Republic of Singapore, **3** Department of Experimental Cardiology, University Medical Center Utrecht, Utrecht, the Netherlands

Abstract

Chronic kidney disease (CKD) is a major health care problem, affecting more than 35% of the elderly population worldwide. New interventions to slow or prevent disease progression are urgently needed. Beneficial effects of mesenchymal stem cells (MSC) have been described, however it is unclear whether the MSCs themselves or their secretome is required. We hypothesized that MSC-derived conditioned medium (CM) reduces progression of CKD and studied functional and structural effects in a rat model of established CKD. CKD was induced by 5/6 nephrectomy (SNX) combined with L-NNA and 6% NaCl diet in Lewis rats. Six weeks after SNX, CKD rats received either 50 µg CM or 50 µg non-CM (NCM) twice daily intravenously for four consecutive days. Six weeks after treatment CM administration was functionally effective: glomerular filtration rate (inulin clearance) and effective renal plasma flow (PAH clearance) were significantly higher in CM vs. NCM-treatment. Systolic blood pressure was lower in CM compared to NCM. Proteinuria tended to be lower after CM. Tubular and glomerular damage were reduced and more glomerular endothelial cells were found after CM. DNA damage repair was increased after CM. MSC-CM derived exosomes, tested in the same experimental setting, showed no protective effect on the kidney. In a rat model of established CKD, we demonstrated that administration of MSC-CM has a long-lasting therapeutic rescue function shown by decreased progression of CKD and reduced hypertension and glomerular injury.

Editor: Jean-Claude Dussaule, INSERM, France

Funding: This study was financially supported by the Dutch Kidney foundation, grant C06.2174 and foundation "De Drie Lichten" in The Netherlands (grant 28/08), and a Utrecht University Focus and Massa grant (DIGD-DGK-DHL). MCV is supported by the Netherlands organisation for Scientific Research (NWO) Vidi-grant 016.096.359. The funders had no role in study design, data collection and analysis, decision to publish, or preparation of the manuscript.

Competing Interests: I have read the journal's policy and have the following conflicts: Sai Kiang Lim has a patent application in progress on the use of MSC-derived CM. This does not alter the authors' adherence to all the PLoS ONE policies on sharing data and materials.

* E-mail: m.c.verhaar@umcutrecht.nl

Introduction

The number of patients with chronic kidney disease (CKD) is rising to epidemic proportions [1]. In 2008, the median prevalence of CKD was 7% in persons aged 30 years or older. In persons aged 64 years or older prevalence of CKD varied from 23% to 36% and is still increasing [2]. The ensuing end-stage kidney disease, as well as the associated increase in cardiovascular risk, has significant socio-economic and major public health implications [3]. Nowadays, renal replacement therapy consists of either dialysis or, preferably, kidney transplantation, which is severely limited due to donor shortage. Both renal replacement strategies are associated with increased morbidity and mortality [4]. Consequently, new interventions to slow or prevent CKD progression are being actively pursued. Mesenchymal stem cell (MSC)-based therapies have been proposed as potential new treatment modality.

Administration of MSCs has been shown to offer protection in several models of acute kidney injury [5]. Some data demonstrate a positive effect of MSC treatment on the loss of renal function in early stage CKD models as well [6]. In these studies, however, incorporation and trans-differentiation of injected MSCs were rare events, suggesting that MSCs primarily have a supportive function, probably by secreting growth factors and cytokines [7]. Such a paracrine mode of action has the therapeutic potential for cell-free treatment strategies using MSC-secreted factors. Importantly, if administration of MSC-derived secreted factors can reduce CKD progression, this may have major clinical relevance as such therapy could overcome problems associated with (allogenic) MSC administration such as immune incompatibility, MSC maldifferentiation [8,9] and tumorgenicity [10,11]. Thus far, the *in vivo* effects of MSC-secreted factors have only been studied in acute kidney disease. Bi et al. demonstrated that administration of conditioned medium (CM) from bone marrow-derived MSCs in a model of acute kidney injury (AKI) increased survival and limited renal injury, assessed as decreased blood urea nitrogen (BUN) concentrations [12]. Geishara et al., however, could not confirm such beneficial effects of MSC-CM in experimental AKI [13].

The relevance of these observations in AKI to CKD is unclear. To our knowledge, the effect of MSC secreted factors has not been investigated in a model of established CKD.

The paracrine factors secreted by MSC that are responsible for the (reno) protective effects have not been fully elucidated. Next to immunomodulatory and anti-inflammatory properties of MSC, important roles were suggested for proangiogenic factors like vascular endothelial growth factor (VEGF), hepatocyte growth factor (HGF) and insulin-like growth factor (IGF) [14–17]. Recent reports support a central role for microvesicles [18,19] or exosomes [20] in MSC-mediated tissue repair. In experimental myocardial infarction the cardio-protective effects of human embryonic MSC-CM were attributed to exosomes [21,22].

We hypothesized that MSC-secreted factors have a therapeutic rescue function by supporting renal repair and hence renal function and thus reduce progression of established CKD. Therefore, in the setting of established CKD induced by subtotal nephrectomy, the effects of repeated intravenous delivery of human embryonic MSC-derived CM on renal hemodynamics and injury were studied.

Results

CM Treatment Reduces CKD Progression

Six weeks after SNX, CKD was established and rats received treatment with CM or NCM. At 6 weeks after treatment (12 weeks after SNX), treatment with CM resulted in significantly higher GFR and ERPF compared to treatment with NCM (both $p<0.05$) at t = 12 weeks (figure 1). No differences were observed in hematocrit, mean arterial pressure (MAP), renal vascular resistance (RVR), filtration fraction (FF) and fractional excretion of sodium and potassium between CM and NCM (table 1). We observed no significant differences in GFR and ERPF in healthy controls between CM and NCM treatment. Exosome treatment had no effect on CKD progression (table S1).

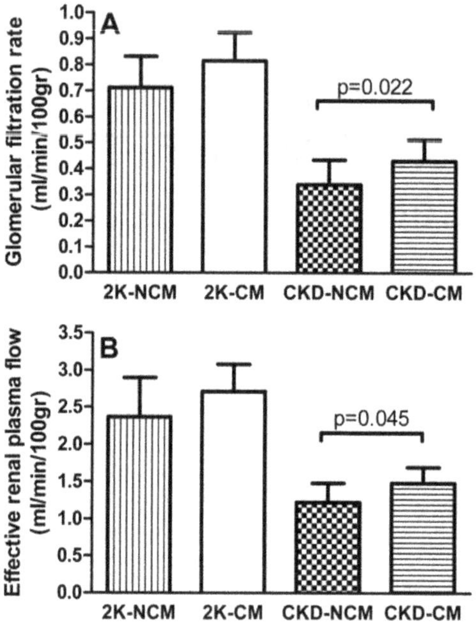

Figure 1. CM treatment increases kidney function. CM treatment increased glomerular filtration rate (GFR) (A) and effective renal plasma flow (ERPF) (B) in CKD. 2K-NCM (n = 6); 2K-CM (n = 6); CKD-CM (n = 13); CKD-NCM (n = 13). Post-hoc test p-value is shown.

CM Treatment Reduces the Increase of Systolic Blood Pressure (SBP) in CKD Rats

CKD animals showed significant hypertension compared to healthy controls (figure 2a). SBP was significantly lower in CKD-CM treated rats compared to CKD-NCM treated rats at week 11 (146±17 vs. 163±21 mm Hg; $p<0.05$, figure 2a). CKD rats showed more proteinuria compared to healthy controls. Protein excretion tended to be lower in CKD-CM-treated compared to CKD-NCM-treated rats (figure 2b; $p = 0.071$). No differences were observed in urea and creatinine clearance between CKD-CM and CKD-NCM rats at wk 11 (table 2). Plasma creatinine was increased in CKD-NCM compared to CKD-CM ($p = 0.05$). Importantly, CM or NCM administration did not influence SBP, proteinuria or creatinine clearance in healthy control rats. Exosome treatment had no effect of SBP (table S2).

CM Increases the Number of Glomerular Endothelial Cells and Reduces Glomerulosclerosis and Tubular Damage in CKD Rats

The percentage of glomerular endothelial cells, (JG12 positive), was significantly higher in CKD-CM compared to CKD-NCM-treated rats ($p<0.05$, fig. 3). Both CKD-CM and CKD-NCM-treated rats showed marked glomerulosclerosis as compared to healthy rats with respectively 31% and 26% normal, non-sclerotic glomeruli as compared to more than 85% normal glomeruli in healthy controls. Comparing the number of partly and totally sclerotic glomeruli between the CKD groups reveals a favourable shift with significantly more partly sclerotic glomeruli and less totally sclerotic glomeruli in CKD-CM compared to CKD-NCM-treated rats (figure 4). DNA damage and repair was measured by induction of cellular γ-H2AX; γ-H2AX expression has been

Table 1. Terminal kidney function measurements.

	2K-NCM n = 6	2K-CM n = 6	CKD-NCM n = 13	CKD-CM n = 13
Body weight (g)	442±43	432±23	364±22*	355±16*
MAP (mm Hg)	99±9	93±13	122±22*	135±19*
RBF (ml/min/100 g)	4.64±1.37	5.22±0.66	2.10±0.49*	2.56±0.43*
RVR (mm Hg/ml/min)	4.9±1.1	4.1±0.6	17±9*	15±4*
Hematocrit	50±1	49±2	45±2*	46±2*
FF	0.32±0.03	0.30±0.05	0.28±0.05	0.29±0.05
FeNa (%)	0.44±0.24	0.38±0.24	1.59±1.79*	1.55±0.77*
FeK (%)	13±6	14±6	38±11*	45±13*

Mean±SD *P<0.05: 2K vs. CKD.
MAP = mean arterial pressure. RBF = renal blood flow. RVR = renal vascular resistance. FF = filtration fraction. FeNa = fractional excretion of sodium. FeK = fractional excretion of potassium.

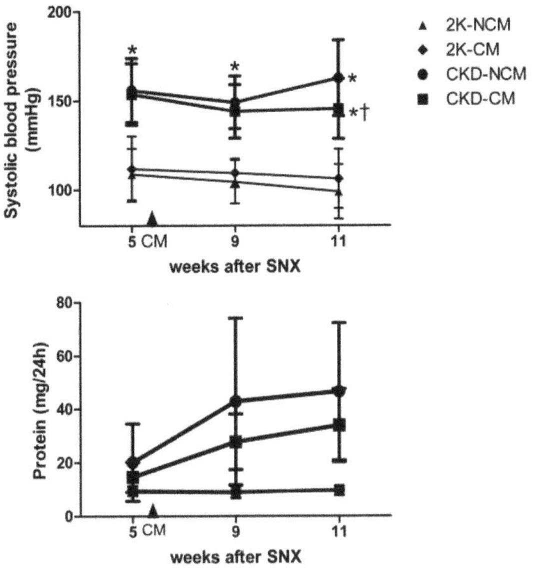

Figure 2. CM treatment decreased systolic blood pressure (A) and proteinuria (B) in CKD. 2K-NCM (n = 6); ◆ 2K-CM (n = 6); ■ CKD-CM (n = 13); ● CKD-NCM (n = 13). *$P<0.05$: CKD vs. 2K, † $P<0.05$: CKD-CM vs. CKD-NCM.

established as a sensitive indicator of clonogenic survival after tissue damage and induction of DNA damage repair [23,24]. We noted with interest that CM significantly increased glomerular γ-H2AX induction in CKD rats compared to healthy rats whereas CKD-NCM rats were not different compared to healthy rats (figure 5). The numbers of glomerular proliferating cells as determined by Ki67 and glomerular inflammatory $CD3^+$ and $ED\text{-}1^+$ cells were not different between the CKD-CM and CKD-NCM -treated rats (table 3).

Compared to healthy rats, both CKD-NCM and CKD-CM-treated rats demonstrated enhanced tubulo-interstitial damage. However, tubular atrophy and interstitial fibrosis were significantly lower after CM treatment in CKD rats (figure 6). Tubular deposition of collagen I and III was decreased in CKD-CM rats compared to CKD-NCM rats (figure 7).

The number of endothelial cells per tubular field was not different between CKD-NCM and CKD-CM treatment, neither were the numbers of tubular $ED\text{-}1^+$ and $CD3^+$ cells. The number of apoptotic cells was not different in glomeruli and tubulo-interstitium of CM and NCM as determined by TUNEL staining (table 3). Exosome treatment had no effect of renal damage (figure S1).

Cytokine Profile in Remnant Kidney is Altered after CM Treatment

To screen whether CM affected local production of inflammatory cytokines by kidney cells in healthy and CKD kidneys, a cytokine array was performed on kidney homogenates (figure 8a). Seven inflammatory cytokines, Monokine Induced by Gamma-Interferon (MIG); Macrophage Inflammatory Protein-1 alpha (MIP1α); Macrophage Inflammatory Protein-3 alpha (MIP3α); thymus chemokine, Tissue Inhibitor of Metalloproteinase-1 (TIMP-1); VEGF and Interleukin 1 Receptor Antagonist (IL1-RA) were only detected in CKD and not in healthy kidneys.

Fractalkine and Regulated upon Activation, Normal T-cell Expressed, and Secreted (RANTES) were lower in CKD kidneys, whereas L-selectin was higher in CKD kidneys compared to healthy kidneys. In healthy kidneys CM had no significant effects on cytokines, whereas in CKD kidneys CM increased the expression of both Fractalkine and IL-1Ra. Gene expression of Fractalkine was decreased in CKD compared to healthy controls and increased by CM in CKD (figure 8b).

CM Effectively Induces Angiogenesis and Wound Closure

To evaluate the effectiveness of CM *in vitro*, an angiogenesis assay and wound closure assay were performed. CM was able to significantly induce angiogenesis compared to NCM (figure 9a). Exosome treatment showed also increased angiogenesis (figure S2). We also analysed the effect of CM on wound closure in an *in vitro* scratch wound assay. As PBS induces cell death in the scratch wound assay, PBS could not be used as vehicle or control. We therefore used CM and NCM diluted in DMEM. CM-treated HMECs showed increased wound closure compared to NCM treatment (figure 9b).

Table 2. Longitudinal measurements after CM treatment at week 6 after SNX.

	2K-NCM n = 6	2K-CM n = 6	CKD-NCM n = 13	CKD-CM n = 13	P (CKD-CM vs. CKD-NCM)
Urea (mmol/L)					
wk 5	5.7±0.9	6.2±1.0	10.3±2.4*	10.2±2.5*	0.854
wk 9	5.9±0.5	5.9±1.1	10.8±2.2*	12.2±1.9*	0.058
wk 11	6.5±0.8	6.9±1.5	9.7±1.9*	9.9±1.8*	0.701
Plasma creatinine (μmol/L)					
wk 5	20.1±3.3	20.8±1.1	49.7±8.8*	48.6±9.9*	0.948
wk9	21.8±6.6	25.6±4.5	44.9±11.4*	42.9±6.6*	0.558
wk11	28.9±7.5	22.7±3.1	51.0±14.2*	42.8±6.9*	0.050
Creatinine clearance (ml/min)					
wk 5	4.18±0.52	4.13±1.31	1.18±0.22*	1.13±0.25*	0.795
wk 9	3.84±1.27	3.00±0.44*	1.48±0.36*	1.43±0.21*	0.801
wk 11	2.84±0.74	3.27±0.93	1.32±0.35*	1.50±0.28*	0.386

Week numbers indicate the week after SNX. Week 5 represents the week before treatment.
*$P<0.05$ vs. respective 2K controls. Posthoc p-value is shown.

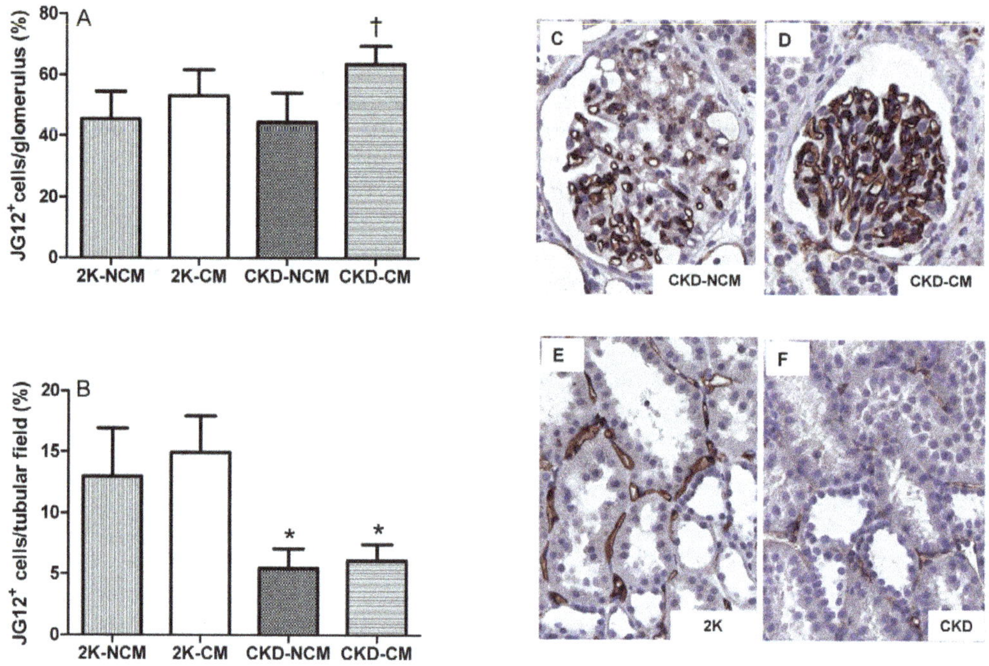

Figure 3. CM treatment increased the number of glomerular endothelial cells (A, C-D), but did not increase tubular endothelial cell number (B, E-F) shown by a JG12 staining. 2K-NCM (n = 6); 2K-CM (n = 6); CKD-NCM (n = 13); CKD-CM (n = 13). *P<0.05: CKD vs. 2K, †P<0.05: CKD-CM vs. CKD-NCM.

Discussion

Our study demonstrates for the first time that repeated IV administration of human embryonic MSC derived CM as a 'rescue intervention'– i.e. 6 weeks after CKD induction - can markedly attenuate the reduction of both GFR and ERPF as assessed by classical "gold standard" inulin and PAH clearance methodology and that this effect is detectable at 6 weeks after administration indicating long-term protection. Furthermore, histology showed a reduction in renal injury.

Previous studies showed beneficial effects of MSC administration in models of AKI (reviewed in [5,7]) and have even led to phase I clinical trials on allogenic MSC administration in AKI (clinicaltrial.gov Identifier: NCT00733876 and NCT01275612).

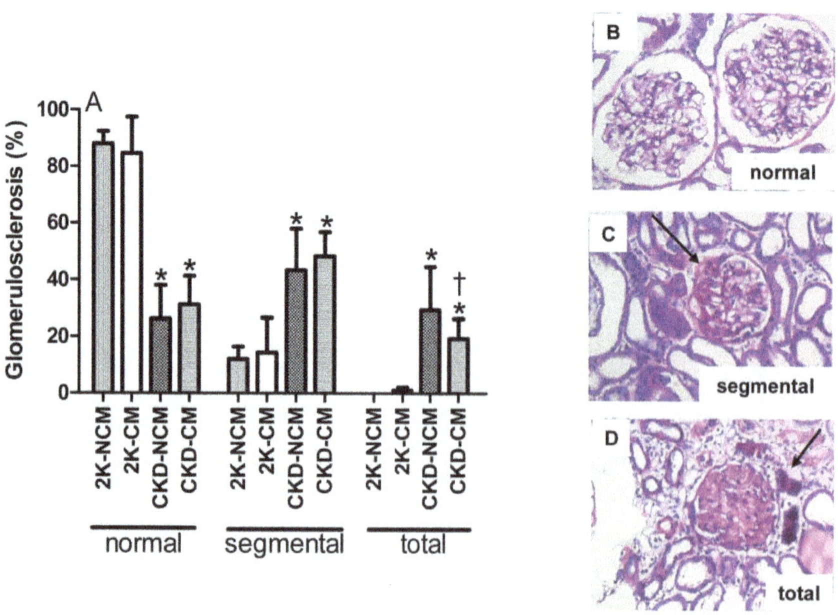

Figure 4. Glomerulosclerosis was reduced by CM treatment. On PAS-stained sections, glomeurosclerosis was reduced after CM treatment (A). Normal (B), segmental (C) and totally sclerotic are shown (D). Black arrows indicate sclerotic areas. 2K-NCM (n = 6); 2K-CM (n = 6); CKD-NCM (n = 13); CKD-CM (n = 13). *P<0.05: CKD vs. 2K, †P<0.05: CKD-CM vs. CKD-NCM.

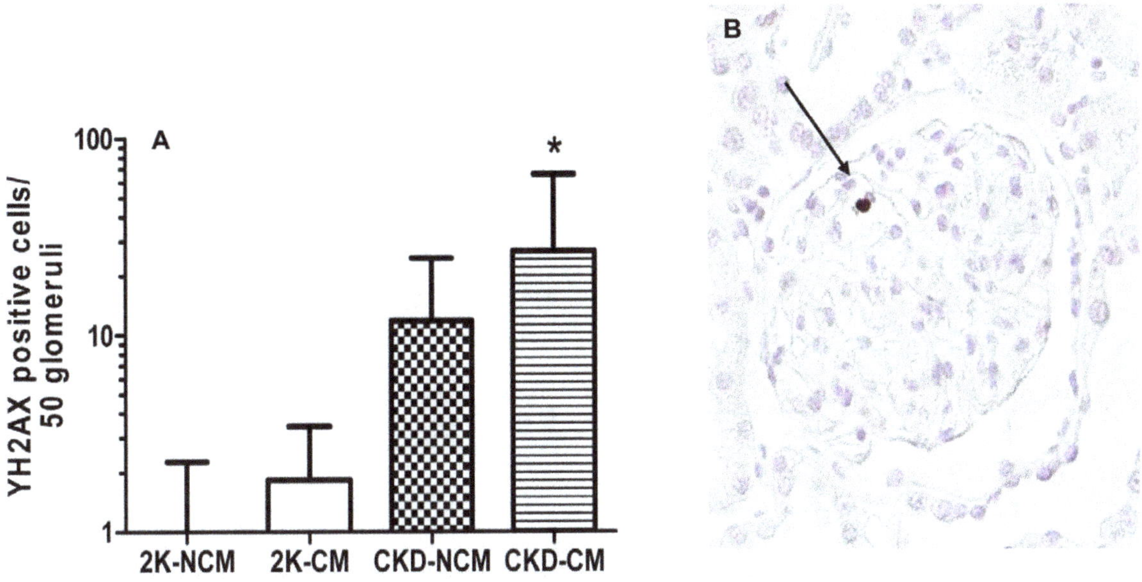

Figure 5. CM treatment increased DNA damage repair. After logarithmic transformation, more γ-H2AX positive cells, indicating glomerular nuclei undergoing DNA damage repair, were found after CM treatment in CKD (A). Black arrow indicates positive nucleus (B). 2K-NCM (n = 6); 2K-CM (n = 6); CKD-NCM (n = 13); CKD-CM (n = 13). *P<0.05: CKD vs. 2K.

However, the relevance of these observations in AKI to CKD is unclear and data on MSC administration in CKD are sparse. In a few studies, administration of MSC was shown to prevent development of CKD if administered directly after induction of the disease [6,25–28] or at early stages of CKD [29]. However, studies aiming at therapeutic 'rescue' in established CKD have not been reported. Furthermore, although most of the reports on beneficial effects suggest that the therapeutic effect is at least in part mediated by paracrine factors secreted by the cells [30], only two studies have applied MSC-CM as therapeutic strategy, and both were performed in AKI models and report conflicting results [12,13]. More recently, two studies reported beneficial effects of microvesicles derived from human adult MSC-CM in experimental AKI [18,19].

We intravenously administered human embryonic MSC-CM that was harvested using a clinically compliant protocol. We used the $5/6^{th}$ nephrectomy ablation model, a known experimental model of progressive renal disease, associated with systemic and glomerular hypertension, capillary loss, renal inflammation and gradual development of glomerulosclerosis, resembling human CKD [31,32]. Creatinine clearance tends to underestimate the decline in GFR due to extensive tubular creatinine secretion in rats [33], underlining the importance of the gold standard method to determine renal function by inulin and PAH clearance [34]. We previously showed a marked reduction of GFR and ERPF in this model using classic clearance technology, while this was less apparent from changes in plasma creatinine, plasma urea, or creatinine clearance [35]. Injection of CM IV at 6 weeks after induction of CKD, a time point at which kidney failure is established, resulted in a long-term beneficial effect on GFR and ERPF as well as a marked reduction in SBP of up to 27 mmHg, lasting up to at least six weeks post-injection between groups. Besides these functional effects, glomerulosclerosis was reduced and glomerular DNA damage repair increased. Our findings of a beneficial effect of human embryonic MSC secretions on progression of experimental established CKD may have relevance for treatment of human CKD. Clinical use of cell-free MSC secretions may have important advantages over MSC administration, for example with regard to risks of malignant [10,11] or non-malignant transdifferentiation [8,9].

Table 3. Renal morphology.

	2K-NCM n = 6	2K-CM n = 6	CKD-NCM n = 13	CKD-CM n = 13
Glomerular measurements				
Ki 67⁺ cells/glomerulus	3.85±1.01	4.17±1.38	5.11±1.52	5.99±1.60*
ED1⁺ cells/glomerulus	1.33±0.51	1.33±0.51	2.70±1.34*	2.59±0.84*
CD3⁺ cells/glomerulus	0.14±0.08	0.09±0.07	0.46±0.36*	0.34±0.13
Tubular measurements				
ED1⁺ cells/tubular field	12.7±0.8	13.5±3.5	32.9±10.2*	34.3±3.9*
CD3⁺ cells/20 tubular fields	2.2±0.9	1.4±0.7	49.3±23.7*	48.8±8.0*
TUNEL⁺cells/tubular field	0.65±0.68	0.23±0.14	1.75±1.12	1.30±0.77*

Mean±SD. *P<0.05: 2K vs. CKD;

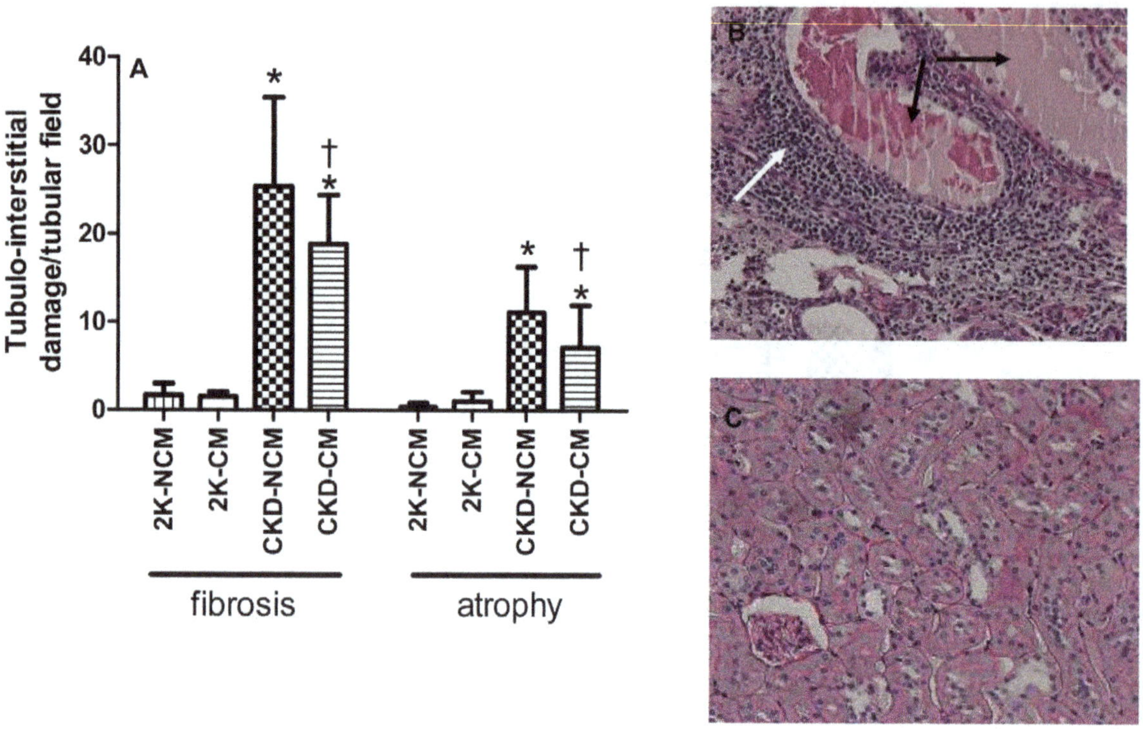

Figure 6. Tubulo-interstitial damage on PAS-stained sections was reduced after CM treatment in CKD rats. CM treatment decreased tubular fibrosis and atrophy (A). Differences between CKD (B) and healthy (C) tubular kidney tissue are shown. White arrow indicates infitration, black arrows showing proteincasts. 2K-NCM (n = 6); 2K-CM (n = 6); CKD-NCM (n = 13); CKD-CM (n = 13). *P<0.05: CKD vs. 2K, †P<0.05: CKD-CM vs. CKD-NCM.

Several mechanisms have been proposed for the beneficial effects of paracrine factors secreted by MSC on the injured kidney: immunosuppressive and inflammatory actions, proangiogenic, antifibrotic and anti-apoptotic effects. Our data points at enhanced glomerular endothelial regeneration and genome integrity preservation through active DNA damage signaling. Such enhancement of glomerular endothelial repair has previously been shown to provide protection against glomerulosclerosis progression [36]. We observed a favorable shift in glomerulosclerosis after CM as compared to NCM treatment, which was associated with higher glomerular endothelial cell numbers after CM, whereas glomerular size was not different. Approximately 10% fewer glomeruli were totally sclerotic hence non-functional in CKD-CM rats which match the increase of GFR compared to CKD-NCM rats. The constant filtration fraction points at increased preglomerular and intraglomerular vascular capacity, possibly by preserved endothelial function.

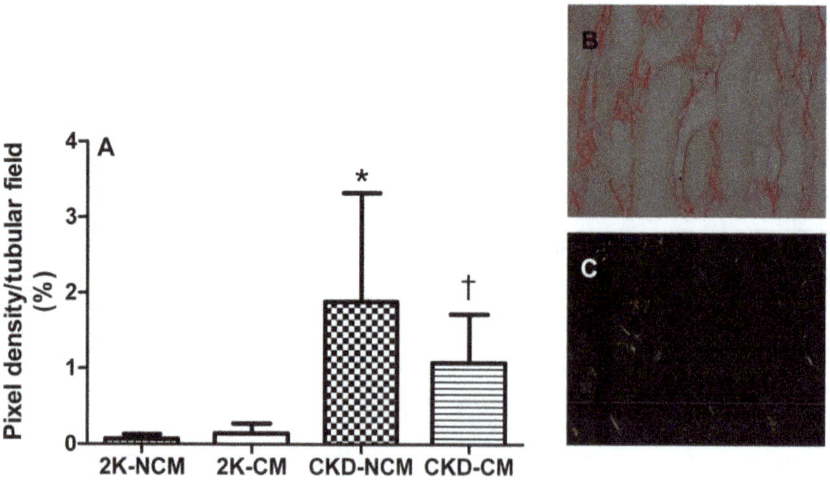

Figure 7. Tubular collagen I and III deposition was reduced after CM treatment in CKD rats. CM treatment reduced sirius red staining (A). Raw (B) and polarized (C) pictures are shown. 2K-NCM (n = 6); 2K-CM (n = 6); CKD-NCM (n = 13); CKD-CM (n = 13). *P<0.05: CKD vs. 2K, †P<0.05: CKD-CM vs. CKD-NCM.

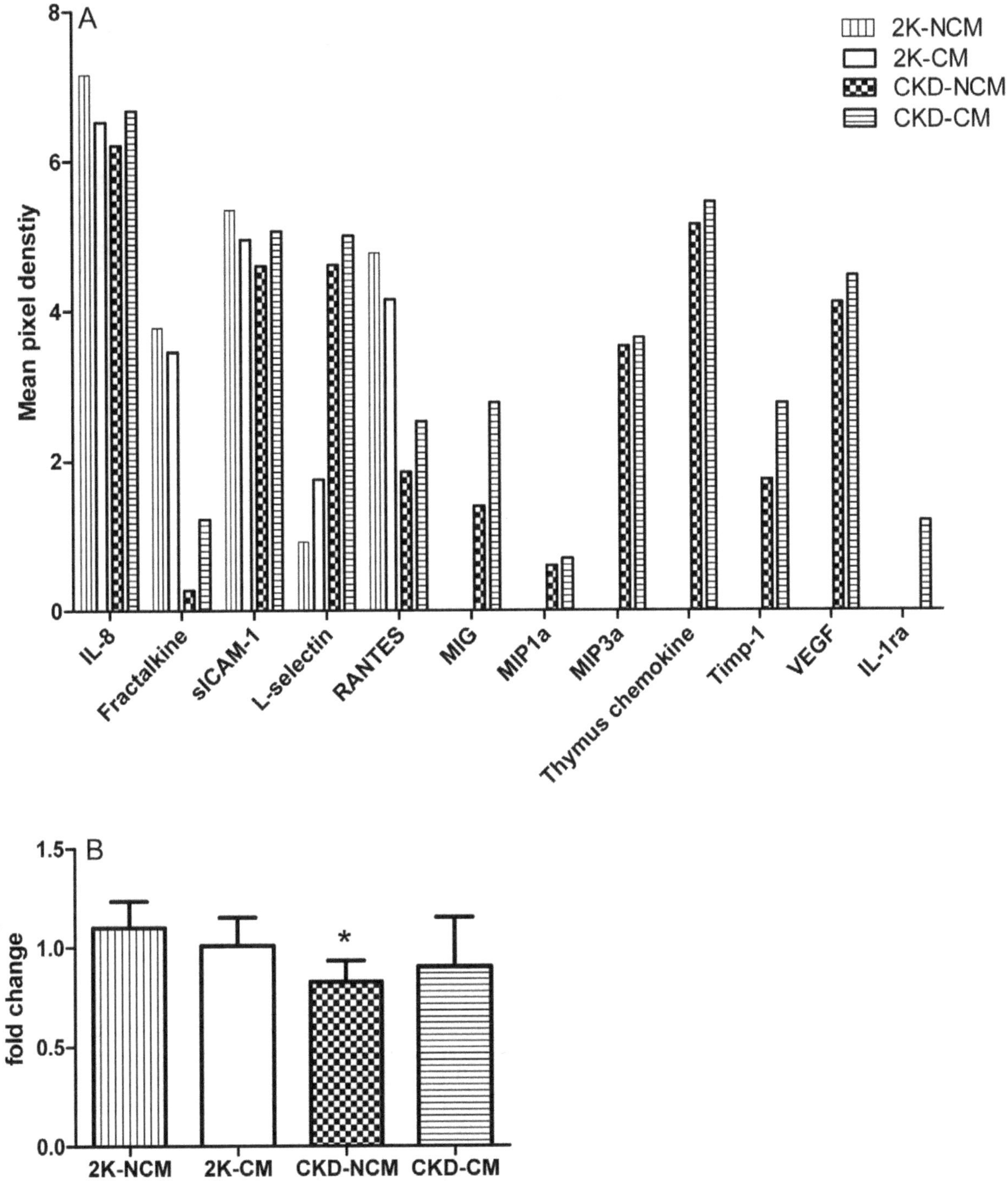

Figure 8. Inflammatory cytokine expression in healthy and CKD kidneys. A: Cytokine array in array. Striped bars = 2K-CM (n = 6); dotted bars = 2K-NCM (n = 6); black bars = CKD-NCM (n = 7); white bars = CKD-CM (n = 4). IL-8 = interleukin 8; sICAM = soluble Inter-Cellular Adhesion Molecule; L-selectin = leucocyte cell-adhesion molecule; RANTES = Regulated upon Activation, Normal T-cell Expressed, and Secreted; MIG = Monokine Induced by Gamma-Interferon; MIP1α = Macrophage Inflammatory Protein-1 alpha; MIP3α = Macrophage Inflammatory Protein-3 alpha; Timp-1 = Tissue Inhibitor of Metalloproteinase 1; VEGF = Vascular Endothelial Growth Factor; IL-1RA = Interleukin 1 Receptor Antagonist. **B: Fractalkine mRNA in healthy and CKD kidneys.** Striped bars = 2K-CM (n = 6); dotted bars = 2K-NCM (n = 6); black bars = CKD-NCM (n = 7); white bars = CKD-CM (n = 4). *$P<0.05$: CKD vs. 2K.

Furthermore, we show that human embryonic MSC CM enhanced endothelial cell migration and angiogenesis *in vitro*. These observations are in line with a report by Togel et al demonstrating *in vitro* vasculotropic effects of adult rat MSC CM [15]. Recently, our human embryonic MSC-CM was also shown to increase capillary density and improve cardiac function after acute myocardial infarction in a pig model [22]. In our CKD model, at 6 weeks after injection of MSC-CM or MSC-NCM we found no differences in the numbers of apoptotic and proliferating cells, nor in the presence of VEGF in the kidney, however, we

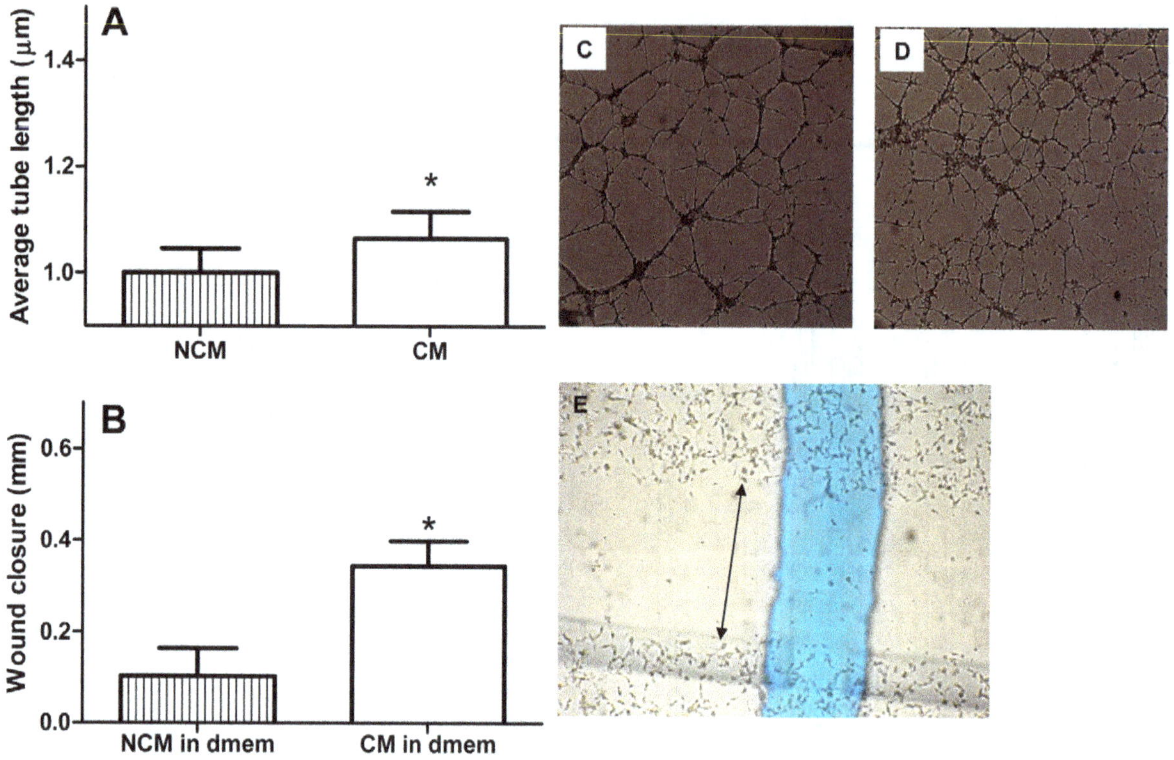

Figure 9. CM stimulates in vitro angiogenesis (A) and wound closure (B). Average tube length was increased after CM treatment compared to NCM (C+D). In a scratch wound assay, CM treatment increased wound (indicated by black arrow in E) closure compared to NCM treatment. *P<0.05 CM vs. NCM.

cannot exclude that anti-apoptotic, mitogenic or VEGF effects have occurred in an earlier stage. We did observe a reduction in tubular inflammation and fibrosis as well as increased expression of fractalkine and Il-1RA, two cytokines that are involved in recruitment of inflammatory response [37,38] after CM as compared to NCM treatment, suggesting a role for paracrine anti-inflammatory and anti-fibrotic effects, consistent with findings in other disease models [39,40].

Recent studies on the effects of MSC-derived microvesicles in acute kidney injury models support a potential exosome-mediated renoprotective effect. Bruno et al. reported that human adult MSC-derived microvesicles, which include exosomes, mimicked the protection against AKI as provided by intravenously administered MSC [18]. Gatti et al showed that single administration of human MSC-derived microvesicles immediately after ischemia-reperfusion injury protected against the development of both acute and chronic kidney injury [19]. Furthermore, in a mouse myocardial infarction model it was recently shown that cardioprotection by human embryonic MSC was mediated by exosomes [21]. Based on the above reports we proposed exosomes to be the CM components that provide protection against CKD progression. However, repeated IV administration of human embryonic MSC derived exosomes in our model of established CKD did not affect progression of CKD (text S1).

We used exosome concentrations in CKD rats that were approximately fourfold the concentration of exosomes present in CM, similar to the exosome concentrations previously shown to improve cardiac function after myocardial infarction [21]. Moreover, *in vitro* both human embryonic MSC derived exosomes and CM effectively induced wound closure and angiogenesis. Lack of a significant therapeutic effect of exosomes in this model of chronic renal injury may be due to tissue specific requirements regarding exosome content and/or dose. Our results suggest that the beneficial effect in our model of CKD was mediated by soluble factors and cytokines. Whether rat exosomes would be more effective in the damaged kidney is unknown.

In line with an effect via soluble factors and cytokine, Togel et al. demonstrated that adult rat MSC-CM contains VEGF, HGF and IGF [15] which mediate renoprotection. Previous analysis on the secretory product of human embryonic MSC showed the presence of several gene products that play a role in angiogenesis; kinase insert domain receptor, VEGF, interleukin 8, angiopoietin and fibroblast growth factor [41]. Studies showing that MSC with knockdown of IGF-1 or VEGF failed to protect rats from AKI [14,16] support a role for proangiogenic factors. Semedo et al. found higher levels of anti-inflammatory cytokines in kidney extracts of MSC-treated animals after ischemia reperfusion injury [29], which is consistent with our observations 6 weeks after CM administration in CKD.

A limitation of our study is that we did not administer CM depleted of exosomes in our CKD model. Therefore we cannot exclude that exosomes mediate the beneficial effect in CKD but need an immunomodulatory or anti-inflammatory factor that is present in the CM. In this respect a recent study may be of interest which reported that porcine MSC have limited immune-modulating activity which abolishes their protective efficacy in AKI [42].

In conclusion, our study demonstrates a marked renoprotective effect of human embryonic MSC derived CM in a rat model with established CKD, as shown by a higher GFR and considerably less glomerular damage after a CM administration. This is probably due to increased endothelial cell regeneration through active DNA damage repair, proliferation and angiogenesis. These findings provide a basis for further research towards potential clinical application of CM-based therapies in human CKD.

Materials and Methods

Animals

Ethics Statement. The protocol was approved by the Utrecht University committee of Animal Experiments (DEC nr 2007.II.050.131).

Animal model. Male inbred Lewis rats (Charles River, Sulzfeld, Germany) were housed under standard conditions in a light-, temperature- and humidity-controlled environment.

CKD was induced in 8-week-old inbred male Lewis rats by two-stage subtotal nephrectomy (SNX) as described (t = 0) [43]. Briefly, the right kidney was removed (wk –1) and one week later (wk 0) the poles of the left kidney were cut off, equalling approximately 66+/−4% of the weight of the previously removed kidney. Progression of CKD was accelerated with L-N^G-Nitroarginine (L-NNA), a nitric oxide (NO)-synthase inhibitor (20 mg/L) in drinking water for 8 wk, (wk −4 to wk 4), and after wk 0, animals were fed standard powdered chow (CRM-FG; Special Diet Services Ltd., Witham, Essex, UK) supplemented with 6% NaCl.

MSC-CM Preparation

The protocols for MSC generation and CM preparation have been described previously [41]. In short, a chemically defined serum free culture medium (Dulbecco's modified eagle medium (DMEM), supplemented with insulin, transferrin, and selenoprotein, fibroblast growth factor 2, platelet derived growth factor AB, glutamine-penicillin-streptomycin, and ß-mercapto-ethanol) was conditioned by MSCs derived from human embryonic stem cells (hESCs) using a clinically compliant protocol. Three polyclonal, karyotypically stable and phenotypically MSC-like cultures that did not express pluripotency-associated markers but displayed MSC-like surface antigens ($CD29^+$, $CD44^+$, $CD49a^+/e^+$, $CD105^+$, $CD166^+$, $CD34^-$, $CD45^-$) and gene expression profile, were generated by trypsinization and propagation of hESCs from either HuES9 hESC line or H1 hESC line in feeder- and serum-free selection media [44]. One of these cultures, HuES9.E1 could be stably expanded for at least 80 population doublings. To harvest MSC secretions, hESC-derived MSC cultures were transferred to a chemically defined, serum free culture medium to condition the medium for three days before the media containing MSC secretions were collected, clarified by centrifugation, concentrated 25 times using 10 kDa MW cut-off ultra-filtration membranes and sterilized by filtration through a 220 nm filter. After these steps, the protein concentration was 0.50 mg/ml. As a negative control, the above-mentioned serum free culture medium was processed equally (non-conditioned medium, NCM). To study the effect of MSC-specific proteins, CM and NCM were diluted in sterile PBS in parallel before administration to reach a protein concentration of 50 µg/250 µl. For MSC-derived exosomes preparation, see text S1.

Effects of Administration of MSC-derived Conditioned Medium in CKD Rats

At week 5 rats with confirmed CKD were stratified based on plasma urea (>9 mmol/L) and systolic blood pressure (SBP) to receive CM or NCM via tail vein injections (twice daily for 4 consecutive days) at week 6 when stable CKD has developed, as follows: **healthy-NCM** (n = 6), healthy rats received 250 µl NCM per injection; **healthy-CM** (n = 6), healthy rats received 250 µl CM per injection; **CKD-NCM** (n = 13), rats with CKD received 250 µl NCM per injection; **CKD-CM** (n = 13), rats with CKD received 250 µl NCM per injection.

At week 12 terminal kidney function was measured under barbiturate anesthesia (see below). Directly thereafter, rats were sacrificed and tissues were collected and either frozen in liquid nitrogen or fixed in 4% paraformaldehyde (PFA) for embedding in paraffin. For detailed time-line, see figure 10. MSC-derived exosomes were studied in the same experimental set-up (text S1).

Longitudinal Chronic Kidney Disease Evaluation

Rats were weighed weekly. In week 5, 9 and 11, 24 h urine, blood samples were collected and SBP was measured by tail cuff sphygmomanometry [45]. To collect 24 h urine, rats were placed in metabolism cages without food for 24 h, but with free access to water with 2% glucose. Urine was collected on antibiotic/antimycotic solution (Sigma, St. Louis, MO; A5955) and stored at –80°C. Blood samples were collected from the tail vein. Urine protein was measured with Coomassie blue. Sodium and potassium were determined by flame photometry.

Terminal Kidney Function

Kidney function was assessed by inulin clearance to determine glomerular filtration rate (GFR) and para-ammino hippuric acid (PAH) clearance to determine the effective renal plasma flow (ERPF) as described [45]. Briefly, rats were anesthetized with intraperitoneal pentobarbital sodium (60 mg/kg) and placed on a servo-controlled surgical table that maintained body temperature at 37°C. The trachea was cannulated with a PE-10 cathether. A PE-50 catheter was placed in the left jugular vein for infusion of solutions and a PE-10 catheter was introduced in this PE-50 cathether for supplemental anesthetic. The left femoral artery was cannulated with PE-50 tubing for measurement of mean arterial pressure (MAP) and blood sampling. A PE-50 catheter was placed in the bladder for urine collection. During surgery, animals received an intravenous infusion of a 150 mM NaCl solution containing 6% bovine serum albumin (BSA). Following surgery, the infusion was switched to a 150 mM NaCl solution with 1% BSA at the same infusion rate. This infusion was maintained throughout the experiment. The solution also contained inulin and para-amino hippurate (PAH) for clearance measurements. A 60-min equilibration period was observed before the start of the 60-min clearance measurements. During this clearance measurement urine was sampled for 15 minute periods and before and after the clearance measurement blood was sampled. Clearances and fractional excretions were calculated by standard formulae. Renal blood flow was calculated from ERPF and hematocrit.

Renal Morphology

Glomerulosclerosis and tubular interstitial damage were scored on 3 µm periodic acid Schiff (PAS)-stained paraffin-embedded slides [46]. Collagen I and III contents was stained with Sirius red, visualized with circular polarized light and digitally analyzed using ImageJ software [46]. The percentage of collagen area was calculated by dividing the Sirius red stained area by the total image area. Monocytes/macrophages (ED-1 stain) and leucocytes (CD3 stain) were counted in glomeruli and tubulo-interstitum [47]. Terminal deoxynucleotidyl transferase-mediated dUTP-biotin nick end labeling (TUNEL) staining (Apoptag Plus in situ Peroxidase kit, Millipore, Temecula, CA, USA) was performed according to manufacturer guidelines. The number of apoptotic cells was determined as the number of

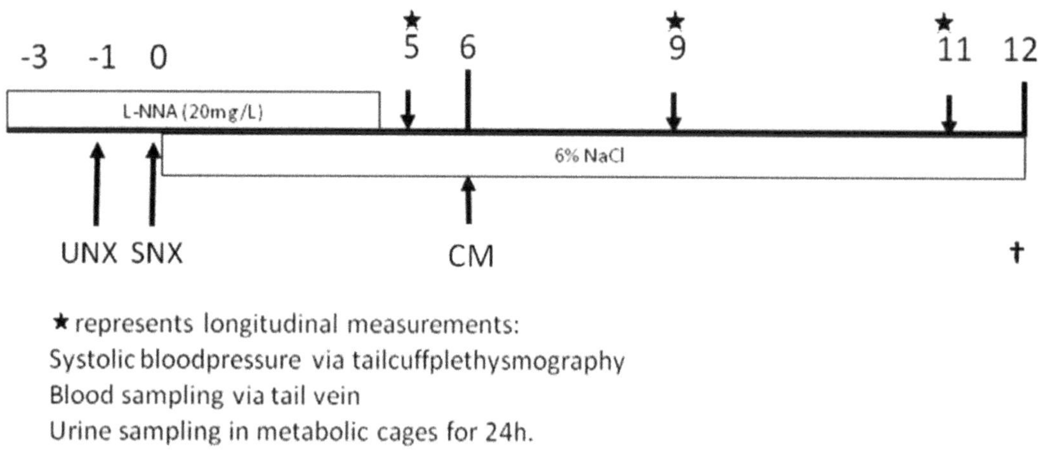

Figure 10. Representation of experimental set up. UNX = uninephrectomy; SNX = subtotal nephrectomy; CM = conditioned medium administration. Stars indicate longitudinal measurements.

TUNEL-positive cells in the images of 50 randomly selected fields (x200 magnification) per section. Endothelial cells were stained with JG12 (Bender Medsystems GmbH, Vienne, Austria) after heat antigen retrieval in citrate buffer (pH 6.0) [48]. JG12 positive cells were determined in the glomeruli (calculated in at least 100 glomeruli per animal) and in peritubular areas (calculated in 20 peritubular fields per animals) using Adobe Photoshop software, version 8.0.1 (Adobe Systems; San Jose, CA) and ImageJ software, version 1.42q (National Institutes of Health; Bethesda, MD). To score nuclei repairing DNA damage, paraffin-embedded kidney sections were deparafinized and treated with PO block for 15 minutes and incubated at 100°C in Citrate/HCL buffer for 20 minutes. The sections were stained with mouse anti-γH2AX (ser139) (Millipore, 1:200) overnight at 4°C. Polyclonal rabbit anti-mouse HRP (Dako, 1:100) was incubated 30 minutes at RT. Finally, BrightVision Poly HRP-Anti Rabbit IgG (Immunologic) was incubated for 1 hour RT. Nova RED substrate kit for Peroxidase (Vector, SK-4800) was used and counterstained with hematoxyline. Analysis was performed using the Aperio ImageScope software.

Cytokine Array and Gene Expression in Renal Tissue

Kidney samples were collected at termination (6 weeks after CM or NCM administration) and quickly frozen in liquid nitrogen. A rat cytokine array (R&D systems) was performed on kidney homogenates according to manufacturer's instructions to screen whether CM treatment stimulated local secretion of specific inflammatory cytokines by the host kidney cells. Samples were pooled per treatment group and equal amounts of protein were loaded on the blots. From all pooled samples blots were performed in duplicate and averages of these two pixel densities were used to calculate the average density with Image J software. Background staining and spot size were analysed as recommended by the manufacturer. Briefly, pictures were converted to 8-bit inverted jpeg files and spots were encircled. Per blot, equal spot sizes were analysed.

To determine whether a local production of cytokines could be confirmed on mRNA level, cDNA was isolated from frozen remnant kidney tissue and expression of fractalkine was determined using quantitative real-time RT-PCR (ABi PRiSM 790Sequence Detection SYStem, applied Biosystems, Foster City, CA). The following TaqMan® Gene Expression Assays (Applied Biosystems) were used: (fractalkine (CX3CL1): Rn00593186_m1), (ß-actin: Rn00667869_m1) and (calnexin: Rn00596877_m1). Reactions were carried out in duplicate. Cycle time (Ct) values for fractalkine were normalized for mean Ct-values of Calnexin and β-actin, which we previously determined to be the two most stable housekeeping genes across all groups using the geNorm-program (http://medgen.ugent.be/~jvdesomp/genorm/), and expressed relative to a calibrator (the sample with the lowest expression: the 2K controls), using the ΔΔCt-method. Hence, steady state mRNA levels were expressed as *n*-fold difference relative to the calibrator.

In vitro Angiogenesis Assay

The potential of CM to stimulate angiogenic tube formation was assessed *in vitro*. For this, 10 µl matrigel (Millipore, Temecula, CA, USA) was added in the inner compartment of an ibidi µ-angiogenesis slide (Ibidi, Munchen, Germany). After the matrigel had solidified, 50 µl of tests-suspension was added, containing respectively 10 µg CM or 10 µg NCM. Subsequently, 10 µl unsupplemented MCDB medium containing 10.000 trypsinized human microvascular endothelial cells (HMEC-1) cells (HMECs; Centers for Disease Control and Prevention, Atlanta, USA) was added. The angiogenesis area was photographed using light microscopy after 18 hours incubation at 37°C, 5% CO_2 and the mean tubule length, used as a measure of angiogenesis, was determined using Angioquant software [49]. Each sample was assayed in triplicate. The angiogenic potential of MSC-derived exomes was also studied (see text S1).

In vitro Scratch Wound Assay

The potential of CM to stimulate endothelial cell migration was assessed by *in vitro* scratch wound assay. A mechanical scratch was created with a pipet tip in a confluent monolayer of HMECs. After washing with PBS, 200 µl DMEM medium containing respectively 40 µg CM or 40 µg NCM was placed on the cells. DMEM without supplementation served as control. Reference lines were made on the bottom of the wells to obtain exactly the same field during image acquisition. The scratched area was photographed using light microscopy at start and after 6 hours incubation (37°). The extent of closure after 6 hours was determined relative to the starting width of the scratch (Image-Pro plus software, Media Cybernetics 3.0). Each sample was measured in two wells and two picture-fields per well were examined. Results were averaged for analysis.

Statistical Analyses

Data are presented as mean ± standard deviation and analyzed by analysis of variance (One-way ANOVA with a Newman-Keuls post-test, Two-way ANOVA with a Newman-Keuls post-test) or Student's T-test, where appropriate. $P<0.05$ was considered significant.

Supporting Information

Figure S1 Glomerulosclerosis and tubulo-interstitial damage after exosome treatment. A: Segmental (segm) and total (tot) glomerulosclerosis (GS); B: Tubulo-interstitial damage. Exosomes (n = 8); PBS (n = 7). There were no significant differences.

Figure S2 Exosomes stimulates in vitro angiogenesis. Average tube length was increased after exosome treatment compared to PBS. *$P<0.05$: exosomes vs. PBS

Table S1 Terminal kidney function measurements in the exosome and PBS groups. There were no significant differences.

Table S2 Longitudinal measurements after exosome treatment at week 6 after SNX. Week numbers indicate the week after SNX. Week 5 represents the week before treatment. There were no significant differences.

Text S1 Supporting text including materials and methods, results and references.

Acknowledgments

We thank Krista den Ouden, Nel Willekes, Chantal Tilburgs, Frits Meeuwsen, Paula Martens and Nicole van Vliet for their expert technical assistance.

Author Contributions

Conceived and designed the experiments: AvK JAJ BWMvB MCV. Performed the experiments: AvK. Analyzed the data: AvK JAJ MCV. Contributed reagents/materials/analysis tools: SKL DdK RHG BWMvB. Wrote the paper: AvK JAJ MCV.

References

1. Vinhas J, Gardete-Correia L, Boavida JM, Raposo JF, Mesquita A, et al. (2011) Prevalence of Chronic Kidney Disease and Associated Risk Factors, and Risk of End-Stage Renal Disease: Data from the PREVADIAB Study. Nephron Clin Pract 119: c35-c40.
2. Zhang QL, Rothenbacher D (2008) Prevalence of chronic kidney disease in population-based studies: systematic review. BMC Public Health 8: 117.
3. Levin A, Stevens PE (2011) Early detection of CKD: the benefits, limitations and effects on prognosis. Nat Rev Nephrol 7: 446–457.
4. McDonald SP, Tong B (2011) Morbidity burden of end-stage kidney disease in Australia: Hospital separation rates among people receiving kidney replacement therapy. Nephrology (Carlton) 16: 758–766.
5. Imai N, Kaur T, Rosenberg ME, Gupta S (2009) Cellular therapy of kidney diseases. Semin Dial 22: 629–635.
6. Choi SJ, Kim JK, Hwang SD (2010) Mesenchymal stem cell therapy for chronic renal failure. Expert Opin Biol Ther 10: 1217–1226.
7. Humphreys BD, Bonventre JV (2008) Mesenchymal stem cells in acute kidney injury. Annu Rev Med 59: 311–325.
8. Kunter U, Rong S, Boor P, Eitner F, Muller-Newen G, et al. (2007) Mesenchymal stem cells prevent progressive experimental renal failure but maldifferentiate into glomerular adipocytes. J Am Soc Nephrol 18: 1754–1764.
9. Breitbach M, Bostani T, Roell W, Xia Y, Dewald O, et al. (2007) Potential risks of bone marrow cell transplantation into infarcted hearts. Blood 110: 1362–1369.
10. Foudah D, Redaelli S, Donzelli E, Bentivegna A, Miloso M, et al. (2009) Monitoring the genomic stability of in vitro cultured rat bone-marrow-derived mesenchymal stem cells. Chromosome Res 17: 1025–1039.
11. Jeong JO, Han JW, Kim JM, Cho HJ, Park C, et al. (2011) Malignant tumor formation after transplantation of short-term cultured bone marrow mesenchymal stem cells in experimental myocardial infarction and diabetic neuropathy. Circ Res 108: 1340–1347.
12. Bi B, Schmitt R, Israilova M, Nishio H, Cantley LG (2007) Stromal cells protect against acute tubular injury via an endocrine effect. J Am Soc Nephrol 18: 2486–2496.
13. Gheisari Y, Ahmadbeigi N, Naderi M, Nassiri SM, Nadri S, et al. (2011) Stem cell-conditioned medium does not protect against kidney failure. Cell Biol Int 35: 209–213.
14. Imberti B, Morigi M, Tomasoni S, Rota C, Corna D, et al. (2007) Insulin-like growth factor-1 sustains stem cell mediated renal repair. J Am Soc Nephrol 18: 2921–2928.
15. Togel F, Weiss K, Yang Y, Hu Z, Zhang P, et al. (2007) Vasculotropic, paracrine actions of infused mesenchymal stem cells are important to the recovery from acute kidney injury. Am J Physiol Renal Physiol 292: F1626–F1635.
16. Togel F, Zhang P, Hu Z, Westenfelder C (2009) VEGF is a mediator of the renoprotective effects of multipotent marrow stromal cells in acute kidney injury. J Cell Mol Med 13: 2109–2114.
17. Zarjou A, Kim J, Traylor AM, Sanders PW, Balla J, et al. (2011) Paracrine effects of mesenchymal stem cells in cisplatin-induced renal injury require heme oxygenase-1. Am J Physiol Renal Physiol 300: F254–F262.
18. Bruno S, Grange C, Deregibus MC, Calogero RA, Saviozzi S, et al. (2009) Mesenchymal stem cell-derived microvesicles protect against acute tubular injury. J Am Soc Nephrol 20: 1053–1067.
19. Gatti S, Bruno S, Deregibus MC, Sordi A, Cantaluppi V, et al. (2011) Microvesicles derived from human adult mesenchymal stem cells protect against ischaemia-reperfusion-induced acute and chronic kidney injury. Nephrol Dial Transplant 26: 1474–1483.
20. Camussi G, Deregibus MC, Bruno S, Cantaluppi V, Biancone L (2010) Exosomes/microvesicles as a mechanism of cell-to-cell communication. Kidney Int 78: 838–848.
21. Lai RC, Arslan F, Lee MM, Sze NS, Choo A, et al.(2010) Exosome secreted by MSC reduces myocardial ischemia/reperfusion injury. Stem Cell Res 4: 214–222.
22. Timmers L, Lim SK, Hoefer IE, Arslan F, Lai RC, et al. (2011) Human mesenchymal stem cell-conditioned medium improves cardiac function following myocardial infarction. Stem Cell Res 6: 206–214.
23. MacPhail SH, Banath JP, Yu Y, Chu E, Olive PL (2003) Cell cycle-dependent expression of phosphorylated histone H2AX: reduced expression in unirradiated but not X-irradiated G1-phase cells. Radiat Res 159: 759–767.
24. MacPhail SH, Banath JP, Yu TY, Chu EH, Lambur H, et al. (2003) Expression of phosphorylated histone H2AX in cultured cell lines following exposure to X-rays. Int J Radiat Biol 79: 351–358.
25. Caldas HC, Fernandes IM, Gerbi F, Souza AC, Baptista MA, et al. (2008) Effect of whole bone marrow cell infusion in the progression of experimental chronic renal failure. Transplant Proc 40: 853–855.
26. Cavaglieri RC, Martini D, Sogayar MC, Noronha IL (2009) Mesenchymal stem cells delivered at the subcapsule of the kidney ameliorate renal disease in the rat remnant kidney model. Transplant Proc 41: 947–951.
27. Lee SR, Lee SH, Moon JY, Park JY, Lee D, et al. (2010) Repeated administration of bone marrow-derived mesenchymal stem cells improved the protective effects on a remnant kidney model. Ren Fail 32: 840–848.
28. Villanueva S, Ewertz E, Carrion F, Tapia A, Vergara C, et al. (2011) Mesenchymal stem cell injection ameliorates chronic renal failure in a rat model. Clin Sci (Lond) 121: 489–499.
29. Semedo P, Correa-Costa M, Antonio CM, Maria Avancini Costa MD, Antonia dos RM, et al. (2009) Mesenchymal stem cells attenuate renal fibrosis through immune modulation and remodeling properties in a rat remnant kidney model. Stem Cells 27: 3063–3073.
30. La Manna G, Bianchi F, Cappuccilli M, Cenacchi G, Tarantino L, et al. (2010) Mesenchymal stem cells in renal function recovery after acute kidney injury. Use of a differentiating agent in a rat model. Cell Transplant.
31. Fleck C, Appenroth D, Jonas P, Koch M, Kundt G, et al. (2006) Suitability of 5/6 nephrectomy (5/6NX) for the induction of interstitial renal fibrosis in rats–influence of sex, strain, and surgical procedure. Exp Toxicol Pathol 57: 195–205.
32. Griffin KA, Picken MM, Churchill M, Churchill P, Bidani AK (2000) Functional and structural correlates of glomerulosclerosis after renal mass reduction in the rat. J Am Soc Nephrol 11: 497–506.
33. Darling IM, Morris ME (1991) Evaluation of "true" creatinine clearance in rats reveals extensive renal secretion. Pharm Res 8: 1318–1322.

34. Hostetter TH, Meyer TW (2004) The development of clearance methods for measurement of glomerular filtration and tubular reabsorption. Am J Physiol Renal Physiol 287: F868–F870.
35. van Koppen A, Joles JA, Bongartz LG, van den Brandt J, Reichardt HM, et al. (2012) Healthy bone marrow cells reduce progression of kidney failure better than CKD bone marrow cells in rats with established chronic kidney disease. Cell Transplant in press.
36. Rookmaaker MB, Smits AM, Tolboom H, Van't Woud K, Martens AC, et al. (2003) Bone-marrow-derived cells contribute to glomerular endothelial repair in experimental glomerulonephritis. Am J Pathol 163: 553–562.
37. Mizutani N, Sakurai T, Shibata T, Uchida K, Fujita J, et al. (2007) Dose-dependent differential regulation of cytokine secretion from macrophages by fractalkine. J Immunol 179: 7478–7487.
38. Arend WP, Malyak M, Guthridge CJ, Gabay C (1998) Interleukin-1 receptor antagonist: role in biology. Annu Rev Immunol 16: 27–55.
39. Katsha AM, Ohkouchi S, Xin H, Kanehira M, Sun R, et al. (2011) Paracrine factors of multipotent stromal cells ameliorate lung injury in an elastase-induced emphysema model. Mol Ther 19: 196–203.
40. Yew TL, Hung YT, Li HY, Chen HW, Chen LL, et al. (2011) Enhancement of Wound Healing by Human Multipotent Stromal Cell Conditioned Medium: The Paracrine Factors and p38 MAPK Activation. Cell Transplant 20: 693–706.
41. Sze SK, de Kleijn DP, Lai RC, Khia Way TE, Zhao H, et al. (2007) Elucidating the secretion proteome of human embryonic stem cell-derived mesenchymal stem cells. Mol Cell Proteomics 6: 1680–1689.
42. Brunswig-Spickenheier B, Boche J, Westenfelder C, Peimann F, Gruber AD, et al. (2010) Limited immune-modulating activity of porcine mesenchymal stromal cells abolishes their protective efficacy in acute kidney injury. Stem Cells Dev 19: 719–729.
43. Tornig J, Amann K, Ritz E, Nichols C, Zeier M, et al. (1996) Arteriolar wall thickening, capillary rarefaction and interstitial fibrosis in the heart of rats with renal failure:the effects of ramipril, nifedipine and moxonidine. J Am Soc Nephrol 7: 667–675.
44. Lian Q, Lye E, Suan YK, Khia Way TE, Salto-Tellez M, et al. (2007) Derivation of clinically compliant MSCs from CD105+. Stem Cells 25: 425–436.
45. Koeners MP, Racasan S, Koomans HA, Joles JA, Braam B (2007) Nitric oxide, superoxide and renal blood flow autoregulation in SHR after perinatal L-arginine and antioxidants. Acta Physiol (Oxf) 190: 329–338.
46. Bongartz LG, Braam B, Verhaar MC, Cramer MJ, Goldschmeding R, et al. (2010) The nitric oxide donor molsidomine rescues cardiac function in rats with chronic kidney disease and cardiac dysfunction. Am J Physiol Heart Circ Physiol 299: H2037–H2045.
47. Attia DM, Verhagen AM, Stroes ES, van Faassen EE, Grone HJ, et al. (2001) Vitamin E alleviates renal injury, but not hypertension, during chronic nitric oxide synthase inhibition in rats. J Am Soc Nephrol 12: 2585–2593.
48. Kunter U, Rong S, Djuric Z, Boor P, Muller-Newen G, et al. (2006) Transplanted mesenchymal stem cells accelerate glomerular healing in experimental glomerulonephritis. J Am Soc Nephrol 17: 2202–2212.
49. Niemisto A, Dunmire V, Yli-Harja O, Zhang W, Shmulevich I (2005) Robust quantification of in vitro angiogenesis through image analysis. IEEE Trans Med Imaging 24: 549–553.

5

Prevalence of Chronic Kidney Disease and Progression of Disease Over Time among Patients Enrolled in the Houston West Nile Virus Cohort

Melissa S. Nolan[1], Amber S. Podoll[2], Anne M. Hause[3], Katherine M. Akers[2], Kevin W. Finkel[2], Kristy O. Murray[1]*

1 Department of Pediatrics, Baylor College of Medicine, Houston, Texas, United States of America, **2** Department of Internal Medicine, Medical School, University of Texas Health Science Center at Houston, Houston, Texas, United States of America, **3** Department of Epidemiology, School of Public Health, University of Texas Health Science Center at Houston, Houston, Texas, United States of America

Abstract

Introduction: In experimental models of West Nile virus (WNV) infection, animals develop chronic kidney infection with histopathological changes in the kidney up to 8-months post-infection. However, the long term pathologic effects of acute infection in humans are largely unknown. The purpose of this study was to assess renal outcomes following WNV infection, specifically the development of chronic kidney disease (CKD).

Methods: In a cohort of 139 study participants with a previous diagnosis of WNV infection, we investigated the prevalence of CKD using the Kidney Disease Outcomes Quality Initiative (KDOQI) criteria based on the Modification of Diet in Renal Disease (MDRD) formula and urinary abnormalities, and assessed various risk factors and biomarkers.

Results: Study participants were primarily male (60%) and non-Hispanic white (86%) with a mean age of 57 years. Most (83%) were four to nine years post-infection at the time of this study. Based on the KDOQI definition, 40% of participants had evidence of CKD, with 10% having Stage III or greater and 30% having Stage I–II. By urinary dipstick testing, 26% of patients had proteinuria and 23% had hematuria. Plasma NGAL levels were elevated in 14% of participants while MCP-1 levels were increased in 12%. Over 1.5 years, the average change in eGFR was -3.71 mL/min/1.73 m^2. Only a history of Neuroinvasive WNV disease was independently associated with CKD following multivariate analysis.

Discussion: We found a high prevalence of CKD after long term follow-up in a cohort of participants previously infected with WNV. The majority of those with CKD are in Stage I-II indicating early stages of renal disease. Traditional risk factors were not associated with the presence of CKD in this population. Therefore, clinicians should regularly evaluate all patients with a history of WNV for evidence of CKD.

Editor: Tian Wang, University of Texas Medical Branch, United States of America

Funding: This project was generously funded by the Gillson Longenbaugh Foundation and the NIH/NIAID (5R01AI091816-01, K23AI057341, N01 AI 50027-03, and U19AI089992-01). The funders had no role in study design, data collection and analysis, decision to publish, or preparation of the manuscript.

Competing Interests: The authors have declared that no competing interests exist.

* E-mail: KMurray@bcm.edu

Introduction

West Nile virus (WNV), a member of the Flaviviridae family, has become endemic in the United States, with more than 1.7 million persons estimated to have been infected [1]. The long-term effects of acute infection with this disease are largely unknown. Several animal models have been developed to understand the chronic pathologic effects of WNV infection. One model indicates that renal disease can result from acute experimental infection with WNV [2]. Importantly, after clinical recovery from WNV infection, animals develop chronic kidney infection with histopathological changes in renal tissue and viuria detectable for up to 8 months after acute infection.

Similar to the animal models, three studies have found evidence of virus in the urine of human WNV patients; however, these studies did not assess the renal impact of WNV infection [3,4,5]. In Houston, we previously reported that 9% of hospitalized WNV patients developed acute renal failure at the time of initial infection [6]. In this same cohort, only 8% of patients had a history of renal insufficiency prior to infection [7]. In Colorado a recent study assessing delayed mortality several years post infection, found that 21% of deceased WNV patients had documented renal failure as a contributory cause or underlying condition [8].

Thus far, the relationship between WNV infection and possible development of CKD in humans has not been thoroughly examined. We performed an observational study to determine the prevalence of CKD and examine biomarkers for renal dysfunction in a cohort of WNV study participants years past their initial infection.

Methods

In 2003, a cohort of WNV patients was established in Houston, Texas and followed prospectively from the time of acute infection to up to nine years post-infection. To date, 217 patients have been enrolled into the study. Over time, 45 participants were withdrawn from the study either due to death, lost-to-follow-up, or voluntary withdrawal. Of the remaining eligible study participants, 139 had complete information to analyze for CKD prevalence. All study activities were approved by the University's Institutional Review Board (HSC-SPH-03-039) prior to subject enrollment.

For the purposes of this study, participants were assessed during April 2010-November 2011 and were evaluated every six months from the initial start date. Evaluation included a questionnaire and sample collections, including blood and urine. The questionnaire obtained the following demographic data: age, race, ethnicity, and height and weight for body mass index calculation. In addition subjects self-reported a diagnosis of diabetes mellitus, hypertension, or a family history of CKD, which are known risk factors for CKD.

Blood was analyzed by Quest Diagnostic Laboratories Inc. for complete metabolic profiles and complete blood counts [9]. Serum creatinine levels were obtained and estimated glomerular filtration rate (eGFR) was calculated using the Modification of Diet in Renal Disease (MDRD) study formula [10]. Chronic kidney disease was defined according to Kidney Disease Outcomes Quality Initiative (KDOQI) criteria for stages of CKD [11]. Participants were considered to have proteinuria and hematuria if urinalysis indicated greater than trace levels. Urinalysis was performed using Siemens Multistix® 10 SG reagent strips. Two potential biomarkers for renal dysfunction were also analyzed on a sub-set of fifty randomly selected participants. Neutrophil gelatinase associated lipocalin (NGAL) and monocyte chemotactic protein-1 (MCP-1) were measured in both plasma and urine using Quantikine Immunoassays (R&D Systems: Minneapolis, MN). We recorded the presence of common complications of CKD including anemia, elevated serum blood urea nitrogen (BUN), and hyperkalemia.

Descriptive statistics were used to describe the cohort and CKD risk factors, indicators and biomarkers. Univariate logistic regression analysis was performed to assess potential associations between stages of CKD with CKD risk factors. A cumulative grouping of all stages of CKD with CKD risk factors was subjected to multivariate logistic regression analysis to identify independent risk factors and test for potential confounding. All risk factors on univariate analysis with $p \leq 0.25$ were included in multivariate analysis. A backwards step elimination of the highest non-significant value method was used. Only those factors with $p \leq 0.10$ were considered significant in the multivariate analysis. All calculations were run using STATA® v12.0 software (College Station, TX).

Results

A descriptive summary of the 139 participants is provided in Table 1. Timing of WNV infection in study participants ranged from recent (within the year) to up to 9 years, with the majority (83%) being more than four years post-infection. The population was predominately composed of non-Hispanic white males with a mean age of 57. Approximately one-half of the patients presented with an initial WNV diagnosis of acute Neuroinvasive WNV disease (meningitis and/or encephalitis). Mild (febrile) and asymptomatic infection comprised the other half of the population. Hypertension and advanced age were prevalent among the population.

We found 40% of study participants met the KDOQI definition of CKD with 10% having Stage III or greater and 30% having Stage I–II. The prevalence of proteinuria and hematuria was 26% and 23%, respectively. Plasma NGAL levels were elevated in 14% of participants while MCP-1 levels were increased in 12%. Urinary levels NGAL and MCP-1 were elevated in 0% and 10%, respectively. The prevalence of anemia, elevated BUN, and hyperkalemia were 60%, 33%, and 12%, respectively.

We analyzed the eGFR values and their change over the course of the study period (Figure 1). Follow-up data for analyzing the change in eGFR was available for 112 participants. The average change in eGFR was -3.71 mL/min/1.73 m^2 over the 1.5 year study period. After adjusting for a leading cause of eGFR decline, non-diabetics had a significantly ($p \leq 0.00$) different decline in eGFR values than diabetics [12].

Results of the univariate logistic regression are provided in Table 2. Univariate analysis found Stage III or greater CKD was significantly associated with being age 65 or older ($p \leq 0.01$) and having hypertension ($p = 0.01$) at time of evaluation. No significant associations were found between Stage I–II CKD and CKD risk factors. Multivariate logistic regression was performed on the cumulative category of all stages of CKD with CKD risk factors. Based on univariate analysis, the following risk factors were included in the multivariate model: African American race ($p = 0.10$, $OR = 3.31$) and history of Neuroinvasive WNV disease ($p = 0.06$, $OR = 1.95$). After multivariate analysis, only Neuroinvasive WNV disease ($p = 0.058$, $OR = 1.95$) was found to be significantly associated with any stage of CKD.

Discussion

The goal of this study was to assess the long-term renal outcomes among a cohort of study participants with a history of WNV infection. In a previous study of WNV patients in Houston, we found 8% of participants had a history of renal insufficiency at the time of initial infection [7], and an additional 9% developed acute renal failure as a result of their illness [6]. In this follow-up study, we found 40% of our study population met the KDOQI definition for CKD when assessed up to nine years post-WNV infection. The majority of patients had CKD Stages I–II (30%) with CKD Stages III or greater being less frequent (10%). In multivariate analysis, traditional risk factors for CKD including age, and the presence of hypertension or diabetes mellitus were not associated with the presence of CKD. In fact, the analysis found history of Neuroinvasive WNV disease as the only significant risk factor associated with CKD. We cannot exclude severe infection with WNV as a factor in the development of CKD, especially considering the data from animal studies and the presence of persistent viuria in some human subjects.

Since CKD is a slowly progressive disease, we looked for any potential associations between years post-acute infection (PAI) and CKD. Due to sample size restraints, we grouped years into categories. We found an overall trend of increasing odds of CKD Stage progression as the years PAI increased. Those participants who were nine to seven years PAI had 1.61 greater odds than those with zero to six years PAI of having CKD Stages III–V, while those zero to three years PAI were more likely to have CKD Stages I–II. While a larger sample size is needed to confirm this finding, our data suggests that CKD progresses in the years following acute WNV infection. Chronic renal decline is also supported by findings of extended IgM titers several years post-

Table 1. Descriptive summary of cohort demographics, CKD risk factors, CKD indicators, and CKD biomarkers.

	All WNV participants n = 139 (%)	Neuroinvasive WNV n = 67 (%)	Mild WNV n = 44 (%)	Asymptomatic WNV n = 28 (%)
Years Post-Acute WNV Infection				
Zero to Three	23 (17)	8 (12)	7 (16)	8 (33)
Four to Six	56 (40)	19 (28)	22 (50)	15 (26)
Seven to Nine	60 (43)	40 (60)	15 (34)	5 (8)
Demographics				
Male	84(60)	45(67)	22(50)	17(61)
Anglo	119(86)	52(78)	43(98)	24(86)
Black	9(6)	6(9)	1(2)	2(7)
Asian	2(1)	1(1)	0(0)	1(4)
Hispanic	9(6)	8(12)	0(0)	1(4)
CKD Risk Factors				
Aged 65 and older	42(30)	30(45)	9(20)	3(11)
Obesity	32(25)	18(28)	7(17)	7(25)
Diabetes mellitus	17(13)	14(22)	3(7)	0(0)
Hypertension	47(35)	29(44)	14(33)	4(14)
Family History of CKD	2(2)	1(2)	1(3)	0(0)
CKD Prevalence				
CKD, All Stages	55 (40)	32 (48)	12 (27)	11 (39)
CKD Stages 3–5	13 (10)	9 (13)	3 (7)	1 (4)
CKD Stage 1–2	42 (30)	23 (34)	9 (20)	10 (36)
CKD Indicators				
Proteinuria	36(26)	21(31)	9(20)	6(21)
Hematuria	32(23)	18(27)	7(16)	7(24)
Anemia	80(60)	40(60)	23(58)	17(63)
Elevated serum BUN	46(33)	30(45)	12(27)	5(18)
Hyperkalemia	16(12)	8(12)	7(16)	1(4)
Elevated plasma NGAL	7/50 (14)	5/24 (21)	2/16 (13)	0/10 (0)
Elevated plasma MCP-1	6/50 (12)	3/24 (13)	1/16 (6)	2/10 (20)

infection in a substantial percent of WNV infected persons, including up to eight years post-infection [3,13–15].

A previous study within this cohort found 20% (5/25) positive for viuria [19]. Viuria testing was not a main focus of this article since the authors are in the process of optimizing the viuria detection technique, and not all participants were tested for viuria due to logistic challenges. However, preliminary data does infer viuria testing as a possible diagnostic tool for WNV-related CKD. Of those who met the clinical definition for CKD, 50% (25/50) tested positive for viral RNA in the urine. In fact, more pronounced kidney decline was even more associated with viruira, with 83% (10/12) of those with moderate to severe CKD testing positive for viuria. While these findings are preliminary, we do intend to further investigate the possibility of viuria serving as a diagnostic marker for WNV-related renal disease.

Our data also suggest that WNV patients who are hypertensive or are 65 years or older are more likely to progress into stage III–V advanced renal disease. Since hypertension and older age are significant risk factors for severe WNV disease, it is unclear what their direct association is with the progression of CKD in this particular population. It is possible that these comorbidities serve a surrogate indicator of neuroinvasive disease's effect on renal decline. Current studies are underway aiming to evaluate long-term neurologic effects of WNV years post-infection and any correlation to renal decline among this population.

Evaluation of renal tubular injury biomarkers, NGAL and MCP-1, were not prevalent among our cohort. Increased NGAL levels have been demonstrated in several studies of kidney injury and we were not able to reproduce those findings [16–19]. MCP-1 is an indicator of interstitial inflammation among lupus patients [16]. Its low prevalence and lack of statistical significance suggests that MCP-1 is not relevant among our cohort and interstitial inflammation is not a dominant factor among our cohort. A larger sample size is needed to validate our findings.

We found a significant decline of eGFR values in our study population. Healthy populations have an average eGFR value decline of -1 mL/min/1.73 m^2 per year [9,10]. Our study population had an average eGFR value decline of -3.71 mL/min/1.73 m^2 over 1.5 years. Even after adjusting for diabetes a known cause of eGFR decline [12], we still found the decline to be greater than expected. Additionally we found 15% of the study population had eGFR declines consistent with progression of CKD from milder to more severe stages over the 1.5 year period of observation. The lack of diabetes as an associated risk factor for

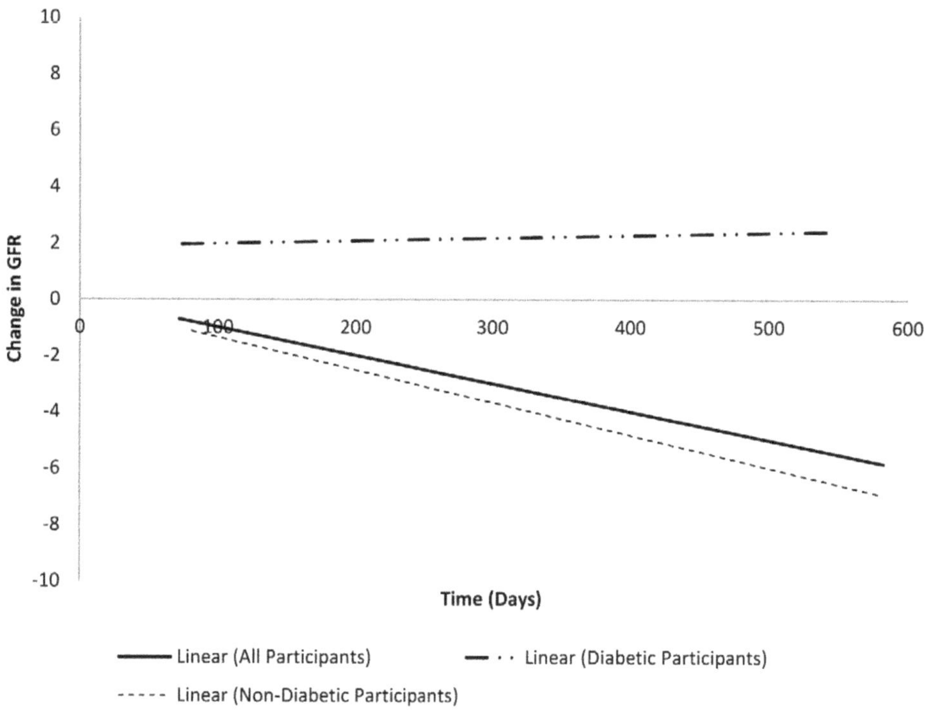

Figure 1. Change in eGFR values over time among 112 study participants, April 2010 to November 2011.

eGFR decline suggests an alternate cause of progression. Therefore WNV may play a role in chronic renal dysfunction as noted by declining eGFR values.

We found a high prevalence of CKD among the cohort. While an alternative equation has been indicated as a more accurate estimator of eGFR values in the <90 range [20], we used the standard discipline for calculating our eGFR values. It is possible that using the standard equation could lead to inaccuracy and thereby misclassification. We ultimately decided to use the MDRD equation since it is believed to be the most commonly used equation by clinicians at this time. Additionally, since we used the KDOQI definition for stages of CKD which incorporates both eGFR values and evidence of kidney damage, we feel the specific equation used has minimal influence on the overall rates of CKD. When calculating the stages of CKD, we defined kidney damage as having proteinuria and/or hematuria. Proteinuria is known to be accurately measured by dipstick, although studies are inconclusive regarding the accuracy of dipstick measurement of hematuria [21]. Due to the observational nature of this study, we found dipstick measurements to be appropriate. Based on all the measurements we used to define CKD, we feel confident that our estimation that 40% of participants with CKD is accurate.

Based on our observational findings, it is evident that more extensive research is needed to understand the exact association between WNV and the development of CKD. We are in the process of developing an age-, gender-, and race/ethnicity-matched case control study with two control populations (CKD non-WNV patients and general medicine patients) to better understand the potential role of WNV infection and development of CKD. The main goals of this case-control study are to first

Table 2. Univariate logistic regression analysis between presence of CKD and CKD risk factors and indicators.

	CKD, All Stages No. (%) p-value; OR (95%CI)	**CKD, Stages 3–5 No. (%) p-value; OR (95%CI)**	**CKD, Stages 1–2 No. (%) p-value; OR (95%CI)**
CKD Risk Factors			
African American Race	6/55 (11%) 0.101 3.31 (0.79–13.82)	1/13 (8%) 0.852 1.23 (0.14–10.68)	5/42 (12%) 0.086 3.31 (0.84–13.00)
Hispanic Ethnicity	4/55 (7%) 0.757 1.24 (0.32–4.83)	1/13 (8%) 0.852 1.23 (0.14–10.68)	3/42 (7%) 0.952 1.04 (0.26–4.25)
Aged 65 and older	18/55 (33%) 0.602 1.22 (0.58–2.54)	9/13 (69%) 0.004 6.34 (1.83–21.97)	9/42 (21%) 0.131 0.52 (0.22–1.21)
Obesity	12/54 (22%) 0.594 0.80 (0.35–1.82)	5/12 (42%) 0.160 2.41 (0.71–8.20)	7/42 (17%) 0.153 0.51 (0.20–1.29)
Diabetes mellitus	6/54 (11%) 0.672 0.80 (0.28–2.30)	2/13 (15%) 0.750 1.30 (0.26–6.43)	4/41 (10%) 0.579 0.72 (0.22–2.34)
Hypertension	22/55 (40%) 0.273 1.49 (0.73–3.06)	9/13 (69%) 0.011 5.03 (1.46–17.36)	13/42 (31%) 0.402 0.72 (0.33–1.55)
Neuroinvasive WNV Disease	32/55 (58%) 0.058 1.95 (0.98–3.88)	9/13 (69%) 0.122 2.64 (0.77–9.01)	23/42 (55%) 0.401 1.36 (0.66–2.80)

Family History of Chronic Kidney Disease was excluded from the table since there were insufficient numbers to calculate statistical values. OR = Odds Ratio, CI = Confidence Interval.

identify if neuroinvasive WNV is serving as a surrogate marker for immunosuppression leading to renal decline. While our data does not suggest this is the case, we cannot rule it out without a proper control group. We anticipate to find that WNV is indeed a factor in renal decline, at which point we aim to then differentiate between factors associated with persistent WNV related renal decline and other causes of renal decline.

We found a high prevalence of CKD in long term follow-up of patients with a history of acute WNV infection. Over 1.5 years of follow-up, the average decline in eGFR was −3.71 mL/min/1.73 m^2. The majority of those with CKD were found to be classified as Stage I–II, indicating mild disease. Those in this range are likely to be unaware that they are in the early stages of CKD and therefore at higher risk for disease progression. Traditional risk factors, such as diabetes, hypertension, obesity, and family history of CKD, were not found to be significantly associated with CKD among this population. However, there was an association with Neuroinvasive WNV infection at initial presentation. In light of our findings, we cannot rule out the influence of WNV with declining renal functioning. Physicians should monitor the kidney health of patients with a history of WNV infection.

Acknowledgments

We would like to thank Charuta Kale and Kyle McCauley for their assistance with data collection. We would also like to thank the participants of the cohort for their continued support.

Author Contributions

Conceived and designed the experiments: MSN ASP AMH KMA KOM. Analyzed the data: MSN AMH. Contributed reagents/materials/analysis tools: KWF KOM. Wrote the paper: MSN KWF KOM.

References

1. Lindsey NP, Staples JE, Lehman JA, Fischer M (2010) Surveillance for human West Nile virus disease–United States, 1999–2008. *Morb Mort Weekly Report* 59:1–17.
2. Tesh RB, Siirin M, Guzman H, Travassos da Rosa APA, Wu X, et al. (2010) Persistent west nile virus infection in the gold hamster: Studies on its mechanism and possible implications for other flavivirus infections. *J Infect Dis.* 192:287–295.
3. Murray K, Walker C, Herrington E, Lewis JA, McCormick J, et al. (2010) Persistent infection with West Nile virus years after initial infection. *J Infect Dis.* 201(1):2–4.
4. Tonry JH, Brown CB, Cropp CB, Co JK, Bennett SN, et al (2005) West Nile virus detection in urine. *Emerg Infect Dis.* 11(8):1294–1296.
5. Baty SA, Gibney KB, Staples JE, Patterson AB, Levy C, et al. (2012) Evaluation for West Nile Virus (WNV) RNA in Urine of Patients Within 5 Months of WNV Infection. *J Infect* Dis205(9):1476–1477.
6. Murray KO, Baraniuk S, Resnick M, Arafat R, Kilborn C, et al. (2008) Clinical Investigation of Hospitalized West Nile Virus Cases in Houston, 2002–2004. *Vector Borne Zoonotic Dis* 8:167–174.
7. Murray K, Baraniuk S, Resnick M, Arafat R, Kilborn C, et al. (2006) Risk factors for encephalitis and death from west nile virus infection. *Epidemiol Infect.* 12;134(6):1325–1332.
8. Lindsey NP, Sejvar JJ, Bode AV, Pape WJ, Campbell GL (2012) Delayed mortality in a cohort of persons hospitalized with West Nile virus disease in Colorado in 2003. *VectorBorne Zoonotic* Dis12(3): 230–235.
9. directory of services. Quest Diagnostics Incorporated; 2010.
10. Levey AS, Bosch JP, Lewis JB, Greene T, Rogers N, et al. (1999) A more accurate method to estimate glomerular filtration rate from serum creatinine: A new prediction equation. *Ann Inter Med* 130(6):461–470.
11. KDOQI clinical practice guidelines for chronic kidney disease: Evaluation, classification, and stratification [Internet].: Kidney Disease Outcomes Quality Initiative; 2002. Available: http://www.kidney.org/professionals/KDOQI/guidelines_ckd/toc.htm.
12. Altemtam N, Russell J, El Nahas M (2012) A study of the natural history of diabetic kidney disease (DKD). *Nephrol Dial* Transpl27(5):1847–1854.
13. Murray KO, Nolan MS, Yan C Persistence of Immunoglobulin-M antibodies up to 8 years following infection with West Nile virus. Clin Vaccine Immunol Submitted.
14. Prince HE, Tobler LH, Lape-Nixon M, Foster GA, Stramer SL, et al. (2005) Development and persistence of West Nile virus-specific immunoglobulin M (IgM), IgA, and IgG in viremic blood donors. J Clin Microbiol. 43(9):4316–4320.
15. Papa A, Danis K, Athanasiasdou A, Delianidou M, Panagiotopoulos T (2011) Persistence of West Nile virus immunoglobulin M antibodies, Greece. J Med Virol. 83(10):1857–1860.
16. Zhang X, Nagaraja HN, Nadasdy T, Song H, McKinley A, et al. (2012) A composite urine biomarker reflects interstitial inflammation in lupus nephritis kidney biopsies. Kidney Int 81(4):401–406.
17. Damman K, van Veldhuisen DJ, Navis G, Voors AA, Hillege HL (2008) Urinary neutrophil gelatinase associated lipocalin (NGAL), a marker of tubular damage, is increased in patients with chronic heart failure. *Eur J Heart Fail* 10:997–1000.
18. Devarajan P(2010) Review: Neutrophil gelatinase-associated lipocalin: A troponin-like biomarker for human acute kidney injury. J *Nephrol* 15:419–428.
19. Haase-Fielitz A, Bellomo R, Devarajan P, Bennett M, Story D, et al. (2009) The predictive performance of plasma neutrophil gelatinase-associated lipocalin (NGAL) increases with grade of acute kidney injury. *Nephrol Dial* Transpl24:3349–3354.
20. Levey AS, Stevens LA, Schmid CH, Zhang Y, Castro AF, et al. (2009) A new equation to estimate glomerular filtration rate. *Ann Inter Med* 150(9): 604–612.
21. Clark WF, Macnab JJ, Sontrop JM, Jain AK, Moist L, et al. (2011) Dipstick proteinuria as a screening strategy to identify rapid renal decline. *Clin JAm SoNephro.* 22(9):1729–1736.

6

Culture-Modified Bone Marrow Cells Attenuate Cardiac and Renal Injury in a Chronic Kidney Disease Rat Model via a Novel Antifibrotic Mechanism

Darren A. Yuen[1]¶, Kim A. Connelly[1]¶, Andrew Advani[1], Christine Liao[1], Michael A. Kuliszewski[1], Judy Trogadis[1], Kerri Thai[1], Suzanne L. Advani[1], Yuan Zhang[2], Darren J. Kelly[2], Howard Leong-Poi[1], Armand Keating[3], Philip A. Marsden[1], Duncan J. Stewart[4], Richard E. Gilbert[1]*

1 Keenan Research Centre of the Li Ka Shing Knowledge Institute, St. Michael's Hospital, Department of Medicine, University of Toronto, Toronto, Ontario, Canada, **2** Department of Medicine, St. Vincent's Hospital, University of Melbourne, Melbourne, Victoria, Australia, **3** Department of Medicine, Princess Margaret Hospital, University of Toronto, Toronto, Ontario, Canada, **4** Ottawa Health Research Institute, University of Ottawa, Ottawa, Ontario, Canada

Abstract

Background: Most forms of chronic kidney disease are characterized by progressive renal and cardiac fibrosis leading to dysfunction. Preliminary evidence suggests that various bone marrow-derived cell populations have antifibrotic effects. In exploring the therapeutic potential of bone marrow derived cells in chronic cardio-renal disease, we examined the anti-fibrotic effects of bone marrow-derived culture modified cells (CMCs) and stromal cells (SCs).

Methodology/Principal Findings: *In vitro*, CMC-conditioned medium, but not SC-conditioned medium, inhibited fibroblast collagen production and cell signalling in response to transforming growth factor-ß. The antifibrotic effects of CMCs and SCs were then evaluated in the 5/6 nephrectomy model of chronic cardio-renal disease. While intravascular infusion of 10^6 SCs had no effect, 10^6 CMCs reduced renal fibrosis compared to saline in the glomeruli (glomerulosclerosis index: 0.8 ± 0.1 *v* 1.9 ± 0.2 arbitrary units) and the tubulointersitium (% area type IV collagen: 1.2 ± 0.3 *v* 8.4 ± 2.0, $p<0.05$ for both). Similarly, 10^6 CMCs reduced cardiac fibrosis compared to saline (% area stained with picrosirius red: 3.2 ± 0.3 *v* 5.1 ± 0.4, $p<0.05$), whereas 10^6 SCs had no effect. Structural changes induced by CMC therapy were accompanied by improved function, as reflected by reductions in plasma creatinine (58 ± 3 *v* 81 ± 11 µmol/L), urinary protein excretion ($9\times/\div1$ *v* $64\times/\div1$ mg/day), and diastolic cardiac stiffness (left ventricular end-diastolic pressure-volume relationship: 0.030 ± 0.003 *v* 0.058 ± 0.011 mm Hg/µL, $p<0.05$ for all). Despite substantial improvements in structure and function, only rare CMCs were present in the kidney and heart, whereas abundant CMCs were detected in the liver and spleen.

Conclusions/Significance: Together, these findings provide the first evidence suggesting that CMCs, but not SCs, exert a protective action in cardio-renal disease and that these effects may be mediated by the secretion of diffusible anti-fibrotic factor(s).

Editor: Arnold Schwartz, University of Cincinnati, United States of America

Funding: This work was supported by grants from the Canadian Institutes of Health Research (CIHR) and the Physicians' Services Incorporated Foundation of Ontario. Dr. Yuen is supported by a KRESCENT postdoctoral fellowship. Dr. Gilbert is supported by a generous donation from George and Diane Mara. Dr. Connelly is supported by a Clinician Scientist award from the Heart and Stroke Foundation of Ontario. Dr. Advani is supported by a Clinician Scientist award from the Canadian Diabetes Association. Dr. Leong-Poi is supported by a Phase II Clinician Scientist Award from the Heart and Stroke Foundation of Ontario and an Early Researcher Award from the Ministry of Research and Innovation, Ontario, Canada. Dr. Keating holds the Gloria and Seymour Epstein Chair in Cell Therapy and Transplantation at the University Health Network and the University of Toronto. The funders had no role in study design, data collection and analysis, decision to publish, or preparation of the manuscript.

Competing Interests: The authors have declared that no competing interests exist.

* E-mail: richard.gilbert@utoronto.ca

¶ These authors contributed equally to this work.

Introduction

Repair by connective tissue formation is a fundamental response to acute injury. If unchecked, however, the resulting fibrotic response leads to parenchymal replacement and organ dysfunction, estimated to account for nearly 45% of all deaths in the industrialized world [1]. Chronic kidney disease (CKD), for instance, now estimated to affect almost 20 million adults in the United States alone, is characterized by progressive renal fibrosis with attendant reduction in glomerular filtration that ultimately results in the need for dialysis or transplantation to preserve life [2]. Moreover, in CKD, the fibrotic pathology is not confined to the kidney but is also present in the heart [3], where even mild degrees of renal impairment are associated with ventricular stiffening, impaired relaxation and diastolic dysfunction that increase as kidney function worsens [4]. Importantly, diastolic dysfunction is a primary contributor to cardiovascular morbidity and mortality in CKD patients, where its presence portends a particularly poor prognosis [5].

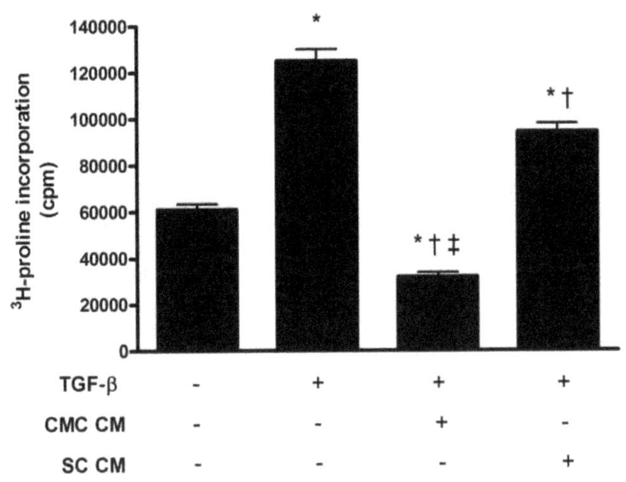

Figure 1. ***In vitro*** **conditioned medium ^{3}H-proline incorporation assays (n = 3 independent experiments).** * $p<0.05$ vs. control (no TGF-β, serum-free EBM-2 medium). † $p<0.05$ vs. serum-free EBM-2 medium + TGF-β. ‡ $p<0.05$ vs. SC-CM + TGF-β. Abbreviations: CMC CM: CMC conditioned medium. SC CM: SC conditioned medium. TGF-β: transforming growth factor-β. cpm = counts per minute.

Studies conducted over almost two decades have consistently implicated transforming growth factor-ß (TGF-ß) as a key mediator of pathological fibrosis [6]. Moreover, in addition to its profibrotic effects, TGF-ß has also been implicated in microvascular loss [7], cardiomyocyte hypertrophy [8], and podocyte dysfunction [9] that characterize cardio-renal disease. Indeed, inhibition of TGF-ß has been a major target for drug discovery with several small molecules, antibodies and nucleic acid-based strategies in development [10].

While most experimental and clinical studies of bone marrow derived cell (BMDC) therapy have been undertaken for the treatment of large vessel angio-occlusive disease [11,12,13], others have demonstrated that various BMDC populations may exert beneficial effects in other settings also, including fibrosis in the liver [14], an organ in which a dual blood supply renders it ischemia-resistant. With this in mind, we speculated as to whether this effect might be common to the two types of BMDCs that are currently under investigation as potential therapeutic agents: bone marrow-derived culture-modified cells (CMCs) and stromal cells (SCs).

Here we show that CMCs reduce collagen formation, inhibit TGF-ß signaling and also effectively reduce renal and cardiac fibrosis in a rodent model of chronic cardio-renal disease that mimics human disease. Importantly, these effects were associated with improvements in kidney and heart function, an effect not seen with current clinically available therapies.

Results

Conditioned Medium from CMCs Inhibits Fibroblast Collagen Production

Progenitor cells have been shown to secrete factors with pro-angiogenic activity that might contribute to their beneficial effects. We therefore considered whether such cells might also secrete factor(s) with anti-fibrotic activity. Accordingly, we incubated CMCs and marrow stromal cells (SCs) in serum-free medium for 24 hours. The effects of these conditioned media on TGF-ß induced collagen production were then compared with serum-free medium (SFM) in a fibroblast assay system. While conditioned medium from SCs had minimal effect, CMC-CM dramatically reduced TGF-ß-induced fibroblast ^{3}H-proline incorporation, a robust marker of collagen production (Fig. 1).

Conditioned Medium from CMCs but Not SCs Inhibits TGF-β Signalling

To further explore the effects of the conditioned media on TGF-ß induced collagen production, we considered whether medium derived from CMCs might inhibit the early stages of the TGF-ß signalling cascade by examining phosphorylation of Smad2. As expected, TGF-β stimulated robust phosphorylation of intracellular Smad2 in cultured fibroblasts. While conditioned medium from SCs had minimal effect, CMC-CM significantly reduced TGF-β-induced Smad2 phosphorylation (Fig. 2a–b).

CMC Infusion Attenuates Renal Dysfunction in the SNX Rat

Given the potent antifibrotic effects of CMCs *in vitro*, we next examined the effects of CMC infusion *in vivo* using the 5/6 subtotally nephrectomized (SNX) rat as a model of progressive, non-immune-

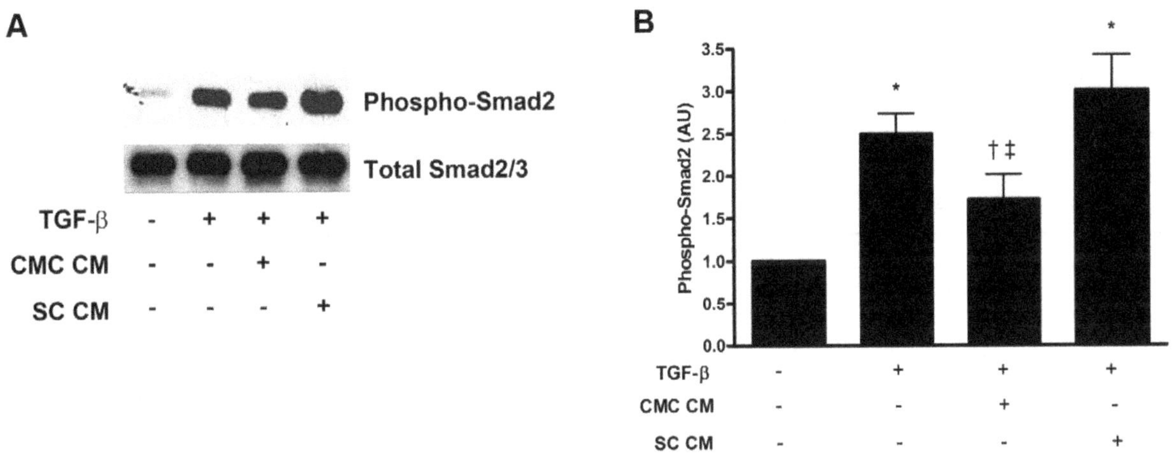

Figure 2. Intracellular TGF-β-induced Smad2 signalling. (a) Representative Western blot for phospho-Smad2 and total Smad2/3. (b) Quantitative analysis of Western blot for phospho-Smad2 (n = 5 independent experiments). * $p<0.05$ vs. control (no TGF-β, serum-free EBM-2 medium). † $p<0.05$ vs. TGF-β + serum-free EBM-2 medium. ‡ $p<0.05$ vs. SC-CM + TGF-β. Abbreviations: CMC CM: CMC conditioned medium. SC CM: SC conditioned medium. TGF-β: transforming growth factor-β. AU: arbitrary units.

mediated chronic kidney disease that also develops heart failure. In this model, the kidney and heart develop progressive fibrosis similar to many patients with CKD. Systolic blood pressure (SBP), urinary protein excretion and plasma creatinine were all elevated in SNX when compared with sham-operated animals at 8 weeks (Table 1). The kidneys receive approximately 20% of cardiac output such that infusing cells intra-arterially would be expected to deliver a greater number of cells to this site of injury than might be anticipated from intravenous administration. We therefore compared intra-arterial with intravenous routes of cell administration, with an *a priori* decision that if similar reductions in proteinuria were apparent, then the two groups would be considered as one, enabling greater statistical power for comparison with control animals. Administration of 10^6 CMCs attenuated the magnitude and progression of proteinuria in SNX rats to a near-identical extent whether infused by an intravenous or intra-arterial route. Indeed, for a range of functional and structural parameters in both the kidney and heart, outcomes were nearly identical for both routes of administration (Fig. S1). In addition to reducing proteinuria, cell therapy attenuated the increase in plasma creatinine in SNX rats, though it remained elevated in comparison to sham animals (Table 1). No mortality was seen in any treatment group after CMC or saline infusion.

CMC Infusion Ameliorates Fibrosis and Microvascular Rarefaction in the SNX Rat

To determine the structural correlates of the improved kidney function seen with CMC therapy, we examined the extent of glomerulosclerosis and tubulointerstitial fibrosis in SNX animals treated with syngeneic CMCs. Tubulointerstitial fibrosis, a major correlate of declining kidney function, was substantially increased in SNX rats, as was glomerulosclerosis. CMC-treated rats showed substantial reductions in the extent of fibrosis, both in the tubulointerstitium (Fig. 3) and in the glomerulus (Fig. 4).

Progressive fibrosis replaces normal renal parenchyma, including its constituent capillaries. Accordingly, we examined glomerular capillary density using immunolabelling for a glomerular endothelial cell antigen in SNX and CMC-treated SNX-rats. As expected, SNX rats experienced a significant reduction in glomerular capillary density, while CMC-treated SNX rats demonstrated preservation of glomerular capillaries (Fig. 5). With the consideration that the increased abundance of cells showing positive endothelial cell immunolabelling in CMC-treated SNX rats may reflect augmentation in antigenic expression rather than an increase in capillarity, a subset of SNX and CMC-treated SNX animals underwent fluorescence microangiography (FMA), demonstrating loss of both glomerular and peritubular capillaries (Fig. 5), along with their amelioration by CMC administration.

Chronic Diastolic Cardiac Dysfunction Is Improved by CMC Administration

Given the close association between kidney disease and heart failure, and the importance of chronic heart failure as a poor prognostic factor in CKD patients, we next examined pre-terminal (8 weeks post-surgery) cardiac function in SNX rats with and without CMC therapy, focussing particularly on diastolic function. SNX rats demonstrated chronic impairment of diastolic function as demonstrated by an elevated left ventricular end-diastolic pressure volume relationship (LV EDPVR), a marker of impaired left ventricular compliance (Fig. 6). When compared with untreated SNX animals, CMC-treated animals showed improvement in passive diastolic filling, as manifested by a reduction in LV EDPVR (Fig. 6).

CMC Infusion Ameliorates Cardiac Structural Damage in the Remnant Kidney Rat

One of the primary determinants of impaired left ventricular relaxation is the development of cardiac fibrosis. Accordingly, we examined the degree of cardiac matrix accumulation at 8 weeks post-surgery. As in the kidney, SNX lead to significant interstitial fibrosis in the heart. CMC treatment significantly attenuated the extent of cardiac fibrosis (Fig. 7). In addition, myocyte cross sectional area, indicative of cellular hypertrophy and thus worsened cardiac afterload, was increased in SNX rats and reduced by CMC administration (Fig. 8).

SCs Were without Effect on Cardio-Renal Function and Structure in the Remnant Kidney Rat

To ascertain whether the beneficial actions of CMCs in the SNX model tracked with their *in vitro* anti-fibrotic effects or whether it reflected a more generalizable attribute of bone marrow derived cells, we next examined the *in vivo* efficacy of marrow stromal cells in the SNX model. In contrast to CMCs, intravascular infusion of 10^6 SCs did not attenuate the structural or functional abnormalities in either the heart or kidney of SNX rats (Table S1 and Fig. S2).

In Vivo Tissue Localization of Infused CMCs

Given that both intravenous and intra-arterial CMC delivery had equivalent effects, and our *in vitro* results suggesting that CMCs release soluble antifibrotic factor(s) that inhibit TGF-β signalling in fibroblasts, we next sought to examine the abundance of the administered cells in the kidney and heart. Accordingly, CMCs were loaded with the vital cytoplasmic fluorophore CMTMR, and infused by tail vein injection into rats 4 weeks after 5/6 subtotal nephrectomy. While only rare CMTMR-labelled CMCs were

Table 1. Renal function at 8 weeks post-surgery.

	Sham	SNX	SNX–CMC iv	SNX–CMC ia	SNX - CMC
N	6	15	9	8	17
Urine protein (mg/day)	3.1×/÷1.1	64.0×/÷1.4*	9.3×/÷1.4†	8.8×/÷1.7†	9.0×/÷1.3†
Plasma creatinine (μmol/L)	32±2	81±11*	55±3†	62±5*	58±3*†
Systolic BP (mm Hg)	123±2	184±10*	172±6*	178±6*	175±4*

Abbreviations: SNX, SNX animal treated with phosphate-buffered saline; SNX–iv, SNX animal treated with intravenous CMC infusion; SNX–ia, SNX animal treated with intra-arterial CMC infusion; SNX–CMC, SNX animal treated with either intravenous or intra-arterial CMC infusion. Urine protein excretion is presented as geometric mean ×/÷ tolerance factors.
*$p<0.05$ versus sham-operated animals.
†$p<0.05$ versus SNX animals.

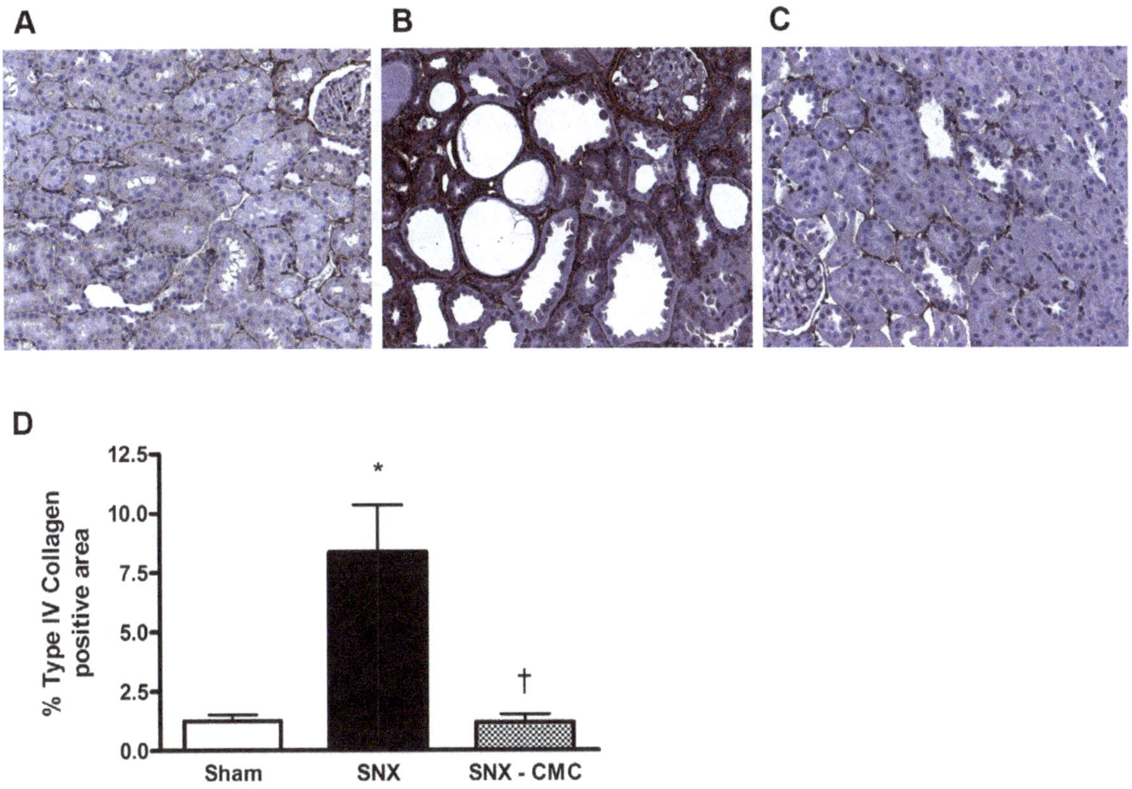

Figure 3. Tubulointerstitial renal cortical fibrosis. Kidney sections were immunolabelled for Type IV collagen 8 weeks post-surgery. (a–c) Representative cortical tubulointerstitial images. Original magnification × 160. (a) Sham animal. (b) SNX animal. (c) SNX–CMC animal. (d) Type IV collagen % positivity. * $p<0.05$ vs. sham operated animals. † $p<0.05$ vs. SNX animals.

detected in the kidneys and hearts of infused SNX animals at either early (1 day) or later (14 day) time points, CMTMR-labelled CMCs were abundant in the liver and spleen with a notable peak 4 days after administration but persistence throughout the time course of the study (Fig. 9).

Discussion

Despite current treatment, the incidence of end-stage renal disease continues to rise, with no major therapeutic advances to stall the progression of CKD since the introduction of renin-angiotensin system antagonists. In the present study, we show that declining GFR and worsening proteinuria, two of the cardinal laboratory indicators of progression towards end-stage kidney disease, were substantially attenuated by the administration of culture modified bone marrow derived cells in a widely used model of non-immune chronic kidney disease. Moreover, chronic heart failure, a common comorbidity in CKD that portends a poor prognosis, was also improved by cell therapy.

While CMCs have therapeutic effects in a range of diseases, the mechanisms by which they do so remain unclear. In the present study we explored their anti-fibrotic activity, focusing on the dominant prosclerotic factor TGF-ß, and the cells' *in vivo* efficacy in a model of chronic kidney disease that is characterized by clinically significant progressive scarring of both the kidney and the heart. CMCs, but not SCs, were shown to secrete factor(s) that inhibit TGF-ß receptor signalling and collagen production in cultured cells. Intriguingly, the beneficial effects seen *in vivo* with CMC infusion occurred despite minimal CMC localization to the kidney or heart, in either the acute or later settings, suggesting that diffusible factor(s), such as those identified in culture, may also be active in the *in vivo* setting. Indeed, rather than homing to the site of injury, exogenous CMCs were present in large numbers in the liver and spleen, suggesting that they may be preferentially sequestered by the reticulo-endothelial system.

In line with our limited understanding of how non-embryonic cell therapy might work, there has been considerable conjecture as to whether the administered cells differentiate [15], fuse with resident cells [16] or secrete paracrine factors [17]. Notwithstanding this debate, their efficacy has nevertheless been assumed to be dependent on cell homing to sites of injury [18]. As a consequence, techniques for increasing local cell delivery have been used increasingly in clinical trials in an attempt to maximize the therapeutic gain [19]. However, two studies in acute kidney injury models have suggested that circulating factors elaborated by bone marrow derived cells may account for the beneficial effects observed [20,21]. In the present study, we compared intravenous with intra-arterial CMC delivery, noting similar efficacy in a range of outcome measures with either mode of administration. Moreover, despite the observed benefits, CMCs were rarely present in the kidneys or hearts of treated SNX animals, whereas high numbers were found in the liver and spleen, suggesting that at least some of their effects may be mediated at a distance, possibly through the elaboration of diffusible factor(s) that inhibit(s) the actions of TGF-ß.

Glomerulonephritis, diabetes and hypertension account for the majority of chronic kidney disease in the developed world. However, despite this diverse range of etiologies, they are often characterized histopathologically by chronic cardiorenal fibrosis and microvascular rarefaction. Indeed, it is the extent of the

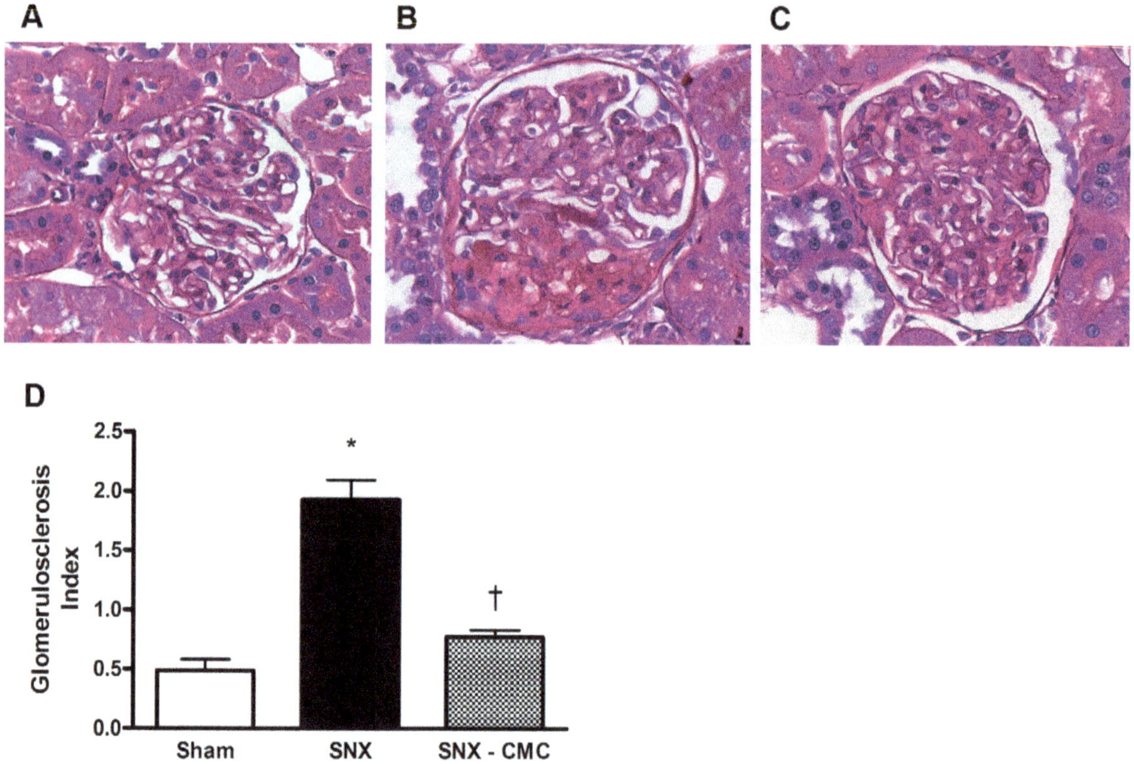

Figure 4. Glomerulosclerosis. PAS-stained kidney sections at 8 weeks post-surgery were used to assess the degree of glomerulosclerosis. (a–c) Representative glomerular images. Original magnification × 400. (a) Sham animal. (b) SNX animal. (c) SNX–CMC animal. (d) Glomerulosclerosis index (GSI). * $p<0.05$ vs. sham operated animals. † $p<0.05$ vs. SNX animals.

fibrosis, particularly in the renal interstitium, that correlates most closely with the decline in kidney function [22]. Similarly, in the heart, interstitial fibrosis, along with myocyte hypertrophy and capillary loss, are key components of adverse cardiac remodelling that affect cardiac geometry and function, particularly during diastole [23]. As in the kidney, fibrosis appears as a final common pathway in most forms of chronic cardiac disease, being present in diabetic [24] and uremic cardiomyopathies [25], ischaemic heart disease [23], and even in valvular heart disease where the extent of fibrosis correlates closely with left ventricular end-diastolic pressure and inversely with ejection fraction [26].

Consistent with its spectrum of activity in stimulating fibrosis, hypertrophy, podocyte injury, and capillary loss, elevated TGF-ß expression has been repeatedly demonstrated in studies of cardiac and renal disease in both humans and animal models [6], and in particular the 5/6 subtotally nephrectomised rat [27]. The central role of TGF-β in promoting fibrovascular pathology and subsequent organ dysfunction has been reinforced by multiple studies demonstrating the beneficial effects of blocking TGF-β for either chronic renal [28,29] or cardiac disease [30,31]. In the present study, we used ^{3}H-proline incorporation as a bioassay of fibroblast collagen production. In these studies, medium derived from CMCs, but not that from SCs, was found to suppress TGF-ß induced ^{3}H-proline incorporation, suggesting that soluble factor(s) released by CMCs, at least in part, mediate an anti-fibrotic effect.

To investigate how the culture modified medium was inhibiting TGF-ß induced ^{3}H-proline incorporation, we examined its well-described signalling pathway. Binding of TGF-ß to its type 2 receptor (TßR2), permits recruitment and activation of the type 1 receptor (TßR1), which in turn continues the signalling relay by phosphorylating and thereby activating the intermediate Smad2 [32]. In the present study, we show that conditioned medium from cultured CMCs reduced TGF-β-induced Smad2 phosphorylation, suggesting that factor(s) secreted into the medium by CMCs inhibited the activity of the TGF-ß receptor complex. In contrast to CMCs, conditioned medium from cultured SCs had comparatively minimal effects on TGF-ß induced ^{3}H-proline incorporation and Smad2 phosphorylation, suggesting that CMCs, and not SCs, are one of the principal BMDC populations that secrete these inhibitory factor(s).

A wide range of methods have been used to isolate and identify progenitor cells in bone marrow [33]. In the absence of specific and unique cell surface markers, we compared two major types of bone marrow derived cells based primarily on their *in vitro* adhesion and growth characteristics. Bone marrow cells were cultured on fibronectin-coated plates for 7 to 10 days, at which time they displayed many of the phenotypic and surface marker characteristics that are commonly associated with endothelial progenitor cells [33]. However, given the ambiguity surrounding the nomenclature of such cells, we used a more operational definition, referring to the cells that we used as early outgrowth, bone marrow derived, culture-modified cells (CMCs). The other broad category of bone marrow derived cells under investigation, mesenchymal or marrow stromal cells (SCs) were identified in this study by their plastic adherence and their ability to differentiate into osteoblasts, adipocytes, and chondroblasts, criteria used widely for their definition [34]. Since both the CMC and SC populations used in our studies were heterogeneous, the generalizability of our findings to other cell doses and other types of bone marrow derived cells, cultured under different conditions or administered in other disease settings, is uncertain.

Clinically, perhaps the most well known link between TGF-ß, fibrosis and renal dysfunction relates to angiotensin II, as agents

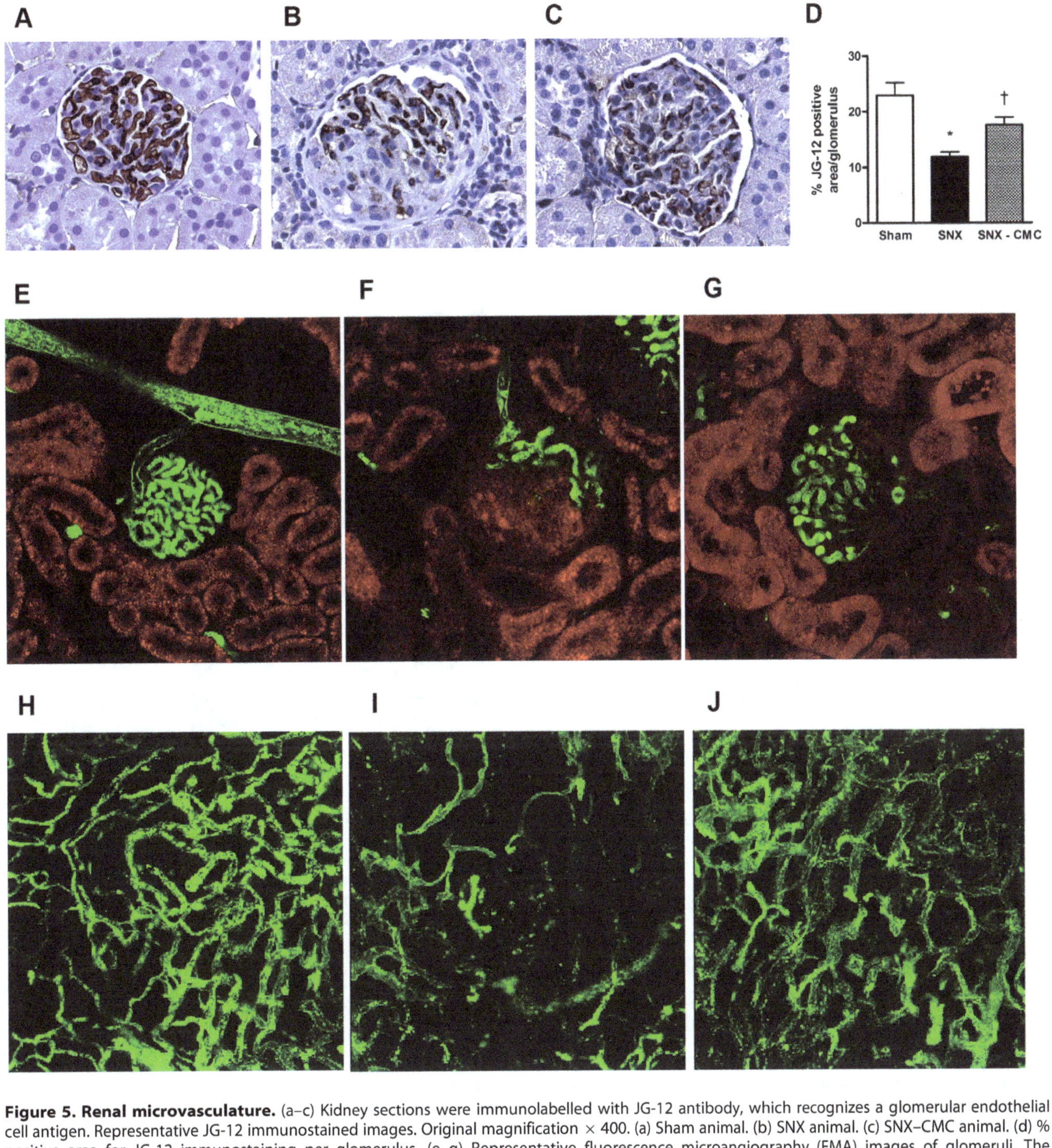

Figure 5. Renal microvasculature. (a–c) Kidney sections were immunolabelled with JG-12 antibody, which recognizes a glomerular endothelial cell antigen. Representative JG-12 immunostained images. Original magnification × 400. (a) Sham animal. (b) SNX animal. (c) SNX–CMC animal. (d) % positive area for JG-12 immunostaining per glomerulus. (e–g) Representative fluorescence microangiography (FMA) images of glomeruli. The autofluorescence of the surrounding renal cortex was captured and pseudocolourized red. The green fluorescence of the infused beads outlines microvascular structures. Original magnification × 40. (e) Sham animal. (f) SNX animal. (g) SNX–CMC animal. (h–j) Representative FMA images of peritubular capillaries. Each image is a flattened Z-stack of a 100 µm section taken with a confocal microscope. Original magnification × 75. (h) Sham animal. (i) SNX animal. (j) SNX–CMC animal. * $p<0.05$ vs. sham operated animals. † $p<0.05$ vs. SNX animals.

that block its formation and receptor binding are the cornerstones of current CKD management. While angiotensin converting enzyme (ACE) inhibitors and angiotensin receptor blockers (ARBs) were initially viewed as exerting their beneficial effects through primarily hemodynamic means, such as their ability to reduce intraglomerular pressure, more recent studies have emphasized the ability of these agents to reduce TGF-ß formation and attenuate fibrosis in the tubulointerstitium as well as the glomerulus, in both humans [35,36] and experimental animals [27,37]. Similarly, in the heart, beyond its haemodynamic effects, the ability of angiotensin II to induce TGF-ß expression [38] is thought to be a major contributor to the beneficial effects of renin-angiotensin system (RAS) blockade in heart failure [39,40].

To date, many of the studies showing beneficial effects of bone marrow derived cells have focussed on their pro-angiogenic actions. Consistent with these reports, the present study also showed that cell

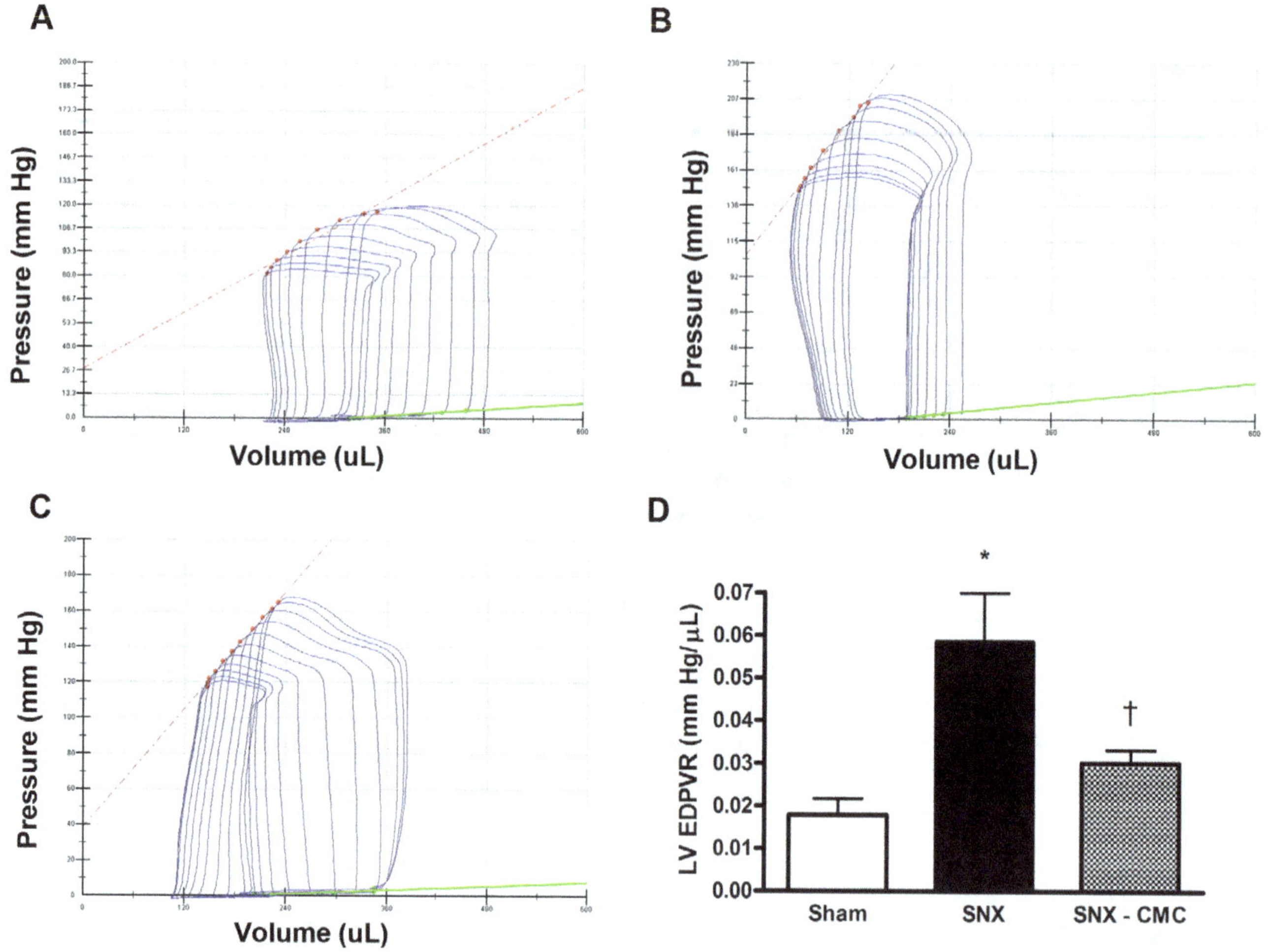

Figure 6. Invasive cardiac hemodynamic assessment at 8 weeks post-surgery. (a–c) Representative pressure-volume (PV) loops obtained 8 weeks post-surgery. Each loop is generated by the simultaneous measurement of left ventricular pressure and volume at all points in the cardiac cycle, enabling the measurement of cardiac functional parameters. Left ventricular end diastolic pressure volume relationship (LV EDPVR), a measure of passive LV relaxation, is represented by the slope of the tangent of the base of each PV loop (green lines). (a) Sham animal. (b) SNX animal. (c) SNX–CMC animal. (d) Quantitative analysis. * $p<0.05$ vs. sham operated animals. † $p<0.05$ vs. SNX animals.

therapy improved the microvasculature of the kidney as assessed by both immunohistochemical and angiographic techniques. While loss of the capillary microvasculature is a feature of the SNX model, as with CKD in humans, growth factors with primarily angiogenic effects, such as vascular endothelial growth factor (VEGF), do not attenuate proteinuria, hypertension or glomerulosclerosis despite preventing microvascular loss [41]. In contrast to VEGF, agents that target the pro-sclerotic factor TGF-β, either directly [29] or indirectly [28], have been shown to attenuate not only fibrosis and declining kidney function, but to also reduce proteinuria in models of CKD. Similarly, in the heart, agents that inhibit TGF-ß activity have also been shown to reduce fibrosis and cardiac dysfunction [30,31,42].

Functioning in tandem, the kidney and heart provide the physiological regulation of extracellular fluid volume, sodium homeostasis, blood pressure, cardiac output and glomerular filtration rate (GFR). In the setting of kidney disease, the resulting dysregulation affects cardiac function with increases in both pre- and afterload, along with the accumulation of waste products that characterizes the uraemic state. At a histopathological level, fibrosis and myocyte hypertrophy are features of cardiac tissue from both humans and animals with impaired kidney function that are thought to mediate the abnormal relaxation properties of the left ventricle in CKD [25,43,44]. In the present study, we found that CMC administration not only attenuated these pathological changes in cardiac structure but also led to improvements in diastolic filling. Importantly, these changes in cardiac function were assessed using load-insensitive techniques, an important consideration in the setting of the alterations in blood volume and arterial pressure seen in CKD.

As commonly seen with other therapeutic interventions in both the experimental and clinical settings, CMC administration led to a more dramatic reduction in proteinuria than in serum creatinine, reflecting the different pathogeneses of these two disease manifestations as well as the non-linear relationship between serum creatinine and GFR. Interestingly, while improvements in kidney filtration and proteinuria were observed with CMC treatment, systemic arterial pressure was unaffected, remaining significantly elevated above that of sham animals, as has been documented with other anti-TGF-β therapies in experimental renal disease [28]. These data suggest that the mechanisms underlying CMC-induced renal structural and functional changes in the 5/6 nephrectomy model are mostly independent of changes in systemic blood pressure. However, a

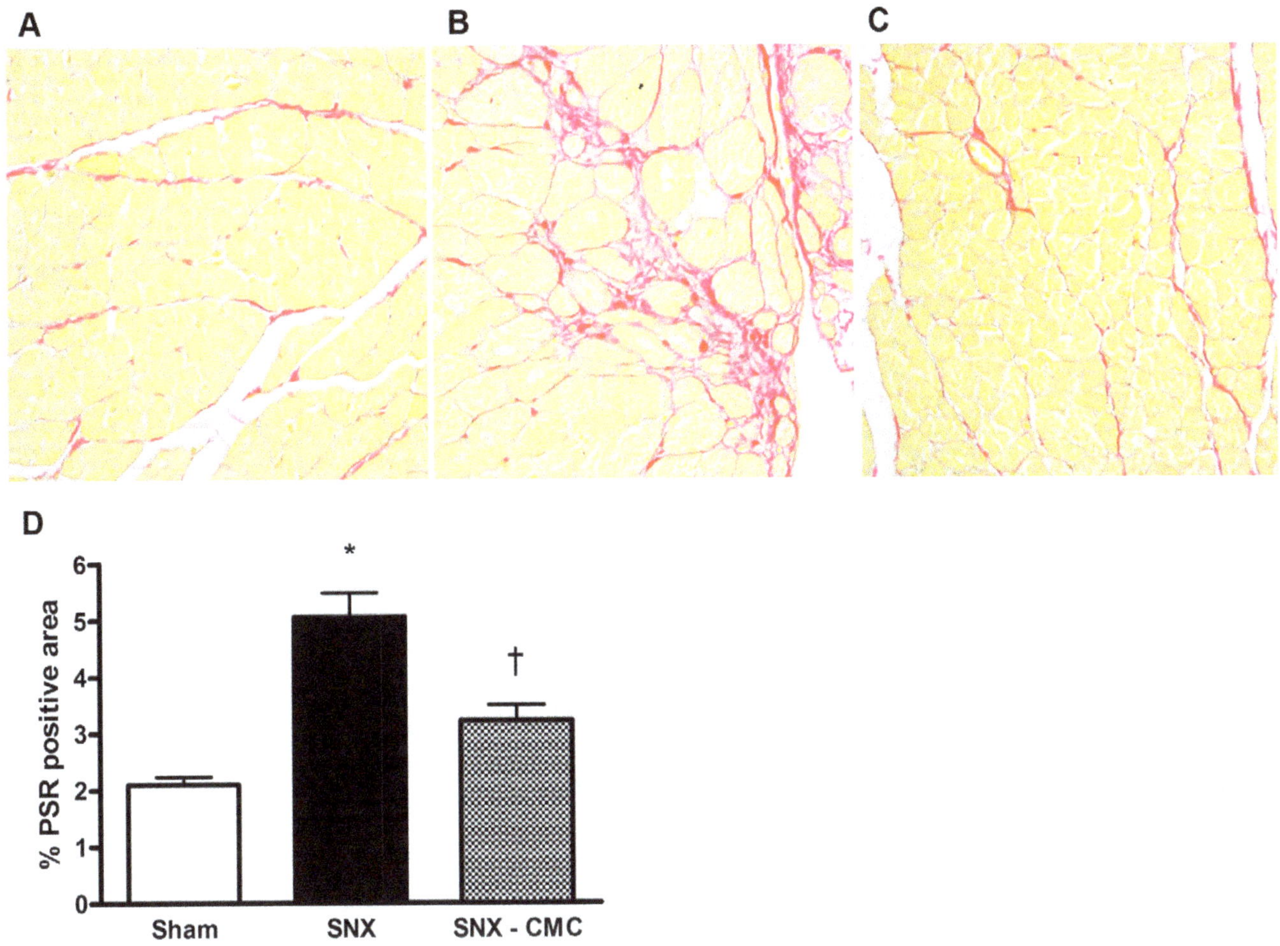

Figure 7. Cardiac fibrosis. (a–c) Representative picrosirius red stained heart sections at 8 weeks post-surgery. Original magnification × 160. (a) Sham animal. (b) SNX animal. (c) SNX–CMC animal. (d) Quantitative cardiac fibrosis analysis. * $p<0.05$ vs. sham operated animals. † $p<0.05$ vs. SNX animals. Abbreviations: PSR: picrosirius red.

modest trend towards blood pressure reduction was seen in CMC-treated animals at the end of the study, suggesting that this was a consequence of improved glomerular filtration rather than a cause. Importantly, given the well-recognized importance of systemic blood pressure control in the attenuation of renal disease progression [45], our data suggests that CMC infusion may provide additive benefit when used in combination with anti-hypertensive therapy.

In summary, to our knowledge, this study is the first to document the beneficial effects of exogenous CMCs in reducing the functional and structural manifestations of both renal and cardiac injury in a well-established model of chronic progressive cardio-renal disease. This study also suggests that CMCs may exert therapeutic effects not solely through localization to injured organs, but also from remote locations, and that specifically their anti-fibrotic activity may be mediated by the elaboration of soluble factor(s) that inhibit TGF-ß signalling.

Materials and Methods

Ethics Statement

All animal work was conducted according to the Canadian Council on Animal Care guidelines [46]. The specific experimental protocols were approved by the Animal Care Committee of St. Michael's Hospital.

CMCs and SCs Were Cultured from Bone Marrow Cells of Syngeneic Male F344 Rat Donors

CMCs were cultured as previously described [47]. Briefly, bone marrow cells were flushed from the femora and tibiae of 4 week old male Fischer 344 rats with sterile phosphate-buffered saline (PBS). The collected cells were centrifuged at 360 rcf for 10 min at 22°C. The supernatant was discarded, and the cell pellet was resuspended in differential endothelial cell culture medium (EGM-2, Clonetics Corp, Walkersville, MD). The cells were plated on human fibronectin-coated tissue culture flasks and incubated at 37°C with 5% CO_2 for 7 to 10 days to produce CMCs. Medium was changed every 2–3 days. Adherent CMCs adopted a typical cobblestone appearance in culture, and displayed positivity for a range of endothelial cell markers including binding of *Bandeiraea simplicifolia*-1 lectin, uptake of fluorescently labelled acetylated-LDL (DiI acLDL, Molecular Probes) and immunostaining for von Willebrand Factor (vWF) and vascular endothelial growth factor receptor type 2 (VEGFR-2), as previously described [47].

SCs were cultured as previously described [48]. Briefly, flushed bone marrow cells harvested as above were centrifuged at 360 rcf for 10 minutes at 22°C. The supernatant was discarded, and the cell pellet was resuspended in PBS supplemented with 0.5% bovine serum albumin and 2 mM EDTA (pH 7.2). The cells were then resuspended in Dulbecco's Modified Eagle Medium (DMEM,

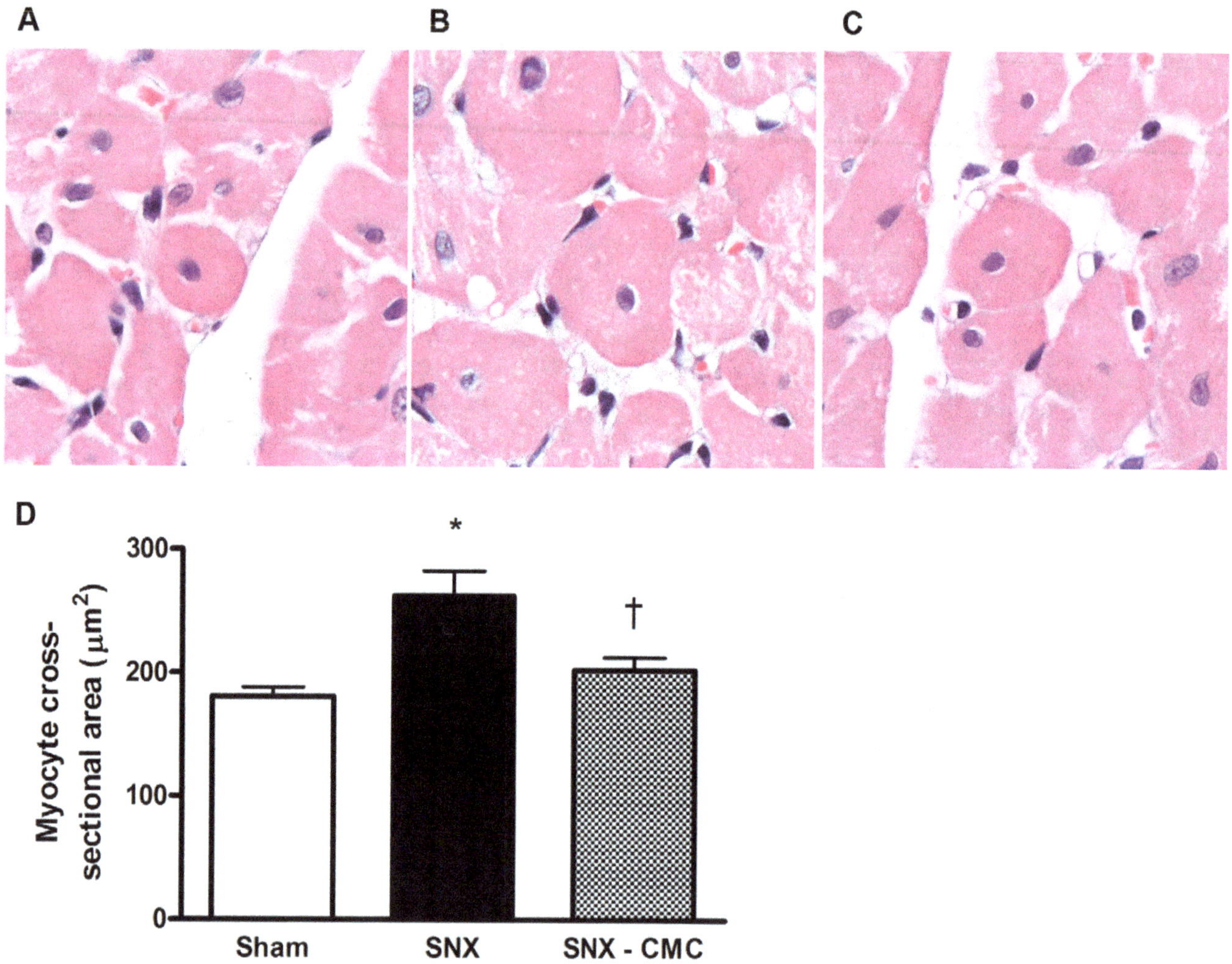

Figure 8. Cardiomyocyte cross-sectional area 8 weeks post-surgery. Original magnification × 400. (a) Sham animal. (b) SNX animal. (c) SNX–CMC animal. (d) Quantitative analysis of myocyte cross-sectional area. * $p<0.05$ vs. sham operated animals. † $p<0.05$ vs. SNX animals.

Gibco™; Invitrogen, Grand Island, NY), plated on plastic tissue culture flasks, and incubated at 37°C with 5% CO_2 to produce mesenchymal stromal cells (SCs). Medium was changed every 2–3 days. Cells used for experiments were between passages 2 and 6. The phenotype of the cells was confirmed through their plastic adherence and their ability to differentiate into chondroblasts, osteoblasts, and adipocytes [34].

Conditioned Medium Generation

CMC conditioned medium was generated by incubating subconfluent 10 day cultured CMCs with serum-free endothelial basal medium-2 (EBM-2) medium for 24 hr as previously described [17]. The medium was then collected and used for *in vitro* experiments. SC conditioned medium was generated similarly by incubating subconfluent passage 2–6 SCs with DMEM. Serum-free EBM-2 medium served as a control.

^{3}H-Proline Incorporation Assay

Neonatal cardiac fibroblasts were isolated from the hearts of 1-day-old Sprague-Dawley rat pups as previously described [42]. Cells were passaged twice and then seeded at a density of 50,000/well in DMEM. After 24 hr, fibroblasts were serum starved in DMEM supplemented with 0.5% bovine serum albumin (BSA), 150 uM L-ascorbic acid (Sigma-Aldrich), and 1% antibiotic/antimycotic mixture (Gibco™, Invitrogen), and then incubated with 0.5 mL of conditioned or unconditioned medium for 4 hr. For TGF-β stimulation experiments, TGF-β was added at a concentration of 20 ng/mL after the 4 hr pre-incubation with conditioned or unconditioned medium. The fibroblasts were then incubated with [^{3}H]-proline (1 μCi/well, L-[2,3,4,5-^{3}H]-proline; Amersham Biosciences) for 44 hours. Fibroblasts were then harvested, washed four times with PBS, solubilised in 0.75 ml of 1 M NaOH and then neutralized with 0.5 ml 1 M HCl. Incorporation of exogenous [^{3}H]-proline was measured using a liquid scintillation counter (LS 6000 Beckman Instruments, Inc) as previously described [49].

Western Blot Analysis

Neonatal cardiac fibroblasts were isolated and cultured as described above. After 24 hrs, fibroblasts were serum starved in DMEM supplemented with 0.5% bovine serum albumin (BSA), and 1% antibiotic/antimycotic mixture (Gibco™, Invitrogen), and then incubated with 0.5 mL of unconditioned medium, CMC CM, or SC CM for 4 hours. The fibroblasts were then stimulated with TGF-β 20 ng/mL for 2 hrs, and then lysed with Cell Lysis Buffer (Cell Signaling Technology). Cell lysates were probed for Smad2/3 (rabbit anti-rat, Catalog No. 3102) and phospho-Smad2 (rabbit anti-rat, Catalog No. 3104) using antibodies from Cells Signaling Technology after SDS-PAGE.

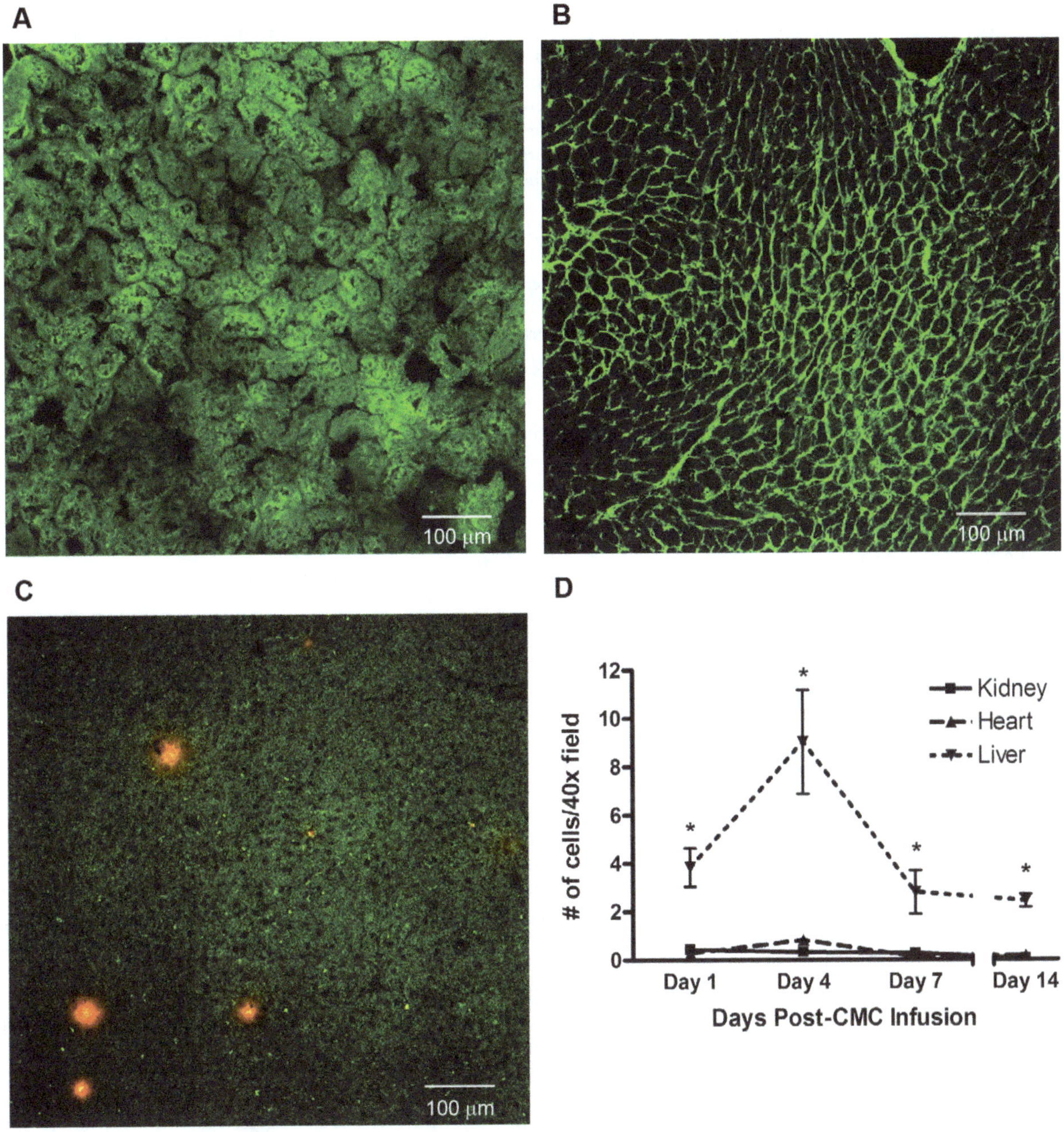

Figure 9. *In vivo* CMC tissue distribution 4 days post-infusion. (a–c): Representative confocal microscopy images of kidney, heart, and liver respectively at 4 days post-CMC infusion. Original magnification × 20. (a) Kidney cortex. (b) Heart. (c) Liver. (d) Time course of CMC retention in kidney, heart, and liver. n = 3 animals per time point. * $p<0.05$ vs. kidney.

Animals

Recipient (age 8–10 wks) and donor (age 3–4 wks) Fischer 344 rats were obtained (Charles River, Montreal, Quebec). Rats were maintained at the St. Michael's Hospital Animal Research Vivarium in a temperature-controlled (22°C) room with *ad libitum* access to commercial standard rat chow. All animal studies were approved by the St. Michael's Hospital Animal Ethics Committee in accordance with the Guide for the Care and Use of Laboratory Animals (NIH Publication No. 85-23, revised 1996).

Subtotal Nephrectomy Animal Model

Fischer 344 rats (Charles River, Montreal, Quebec) of 8 weeks of age were randomized to one-step subtotal 5/6 nephrectomy (n = 43) or sham surgery (n = 6), as previously described [27]. Briefly, animals were anesthetized with inhaled 2.5% isoflurane. The right kidney was removed via subcapsular nephrectomy. Infarction of approximately two thirds of the left kidney was achieved via selective ligation of 2 out of the 3 or 4 branches of the renal artery. Sham surgery consisted of laparotomy and manipulation of both kidneys before wound closure.

Cell Infusion

Four weeks after SNX, animals were randomized in a 1:1:2 fashion via a masked protocol to receive an infusion of: (1) 1×10^6 CMCs (intra-arterial injection), (2) 1×10^6 CMCs (intravenous injection), or (3) sterile phosphate-buffered saline (PBS, intravenous injection). For this procedure, animals were anesthetized with inhaled 2.5% isoflurane and either the left internal carotid artery (intra-arterial route) or right internal jugular vein (intravenous route) was cannulated with a PE50 catheter with the tip placed at the aortic arch or in the superior vena cava respectively. For PBS controls, PBS was infused via a single tail vein injection. On the day of infusion, CMCs were trypsinized and resuspended at a concentration of 10^6 cells/mL in sterile PBS. The total volume of infusion for each animal was 1 ml.

The *in vivo* study was predicated on the assumption that a clinically relevant effect of CMCs would be similar to that of angiotensin converting enzyme inhibitor therapy, with which an approximate 50% reduction in proteinuria is seen in the SNX model [27]. Having postulated that the intra-arterial and intravenous routes would result in similar reductions in proteinuria, we planned *a priori* should this be the case, the two intervention groups would be considered as one.

In a second cell infusion study, a further group of animals received 1×10^6 SCs by intravenous injection, as described above, using passage 2–6 SCs that had been trypsinized and resuspended in 1 mL of sterile PBS prior to administration.

Renal Functional Parameters

Body weight was determined weekly. Every two weeks, rats were individually housed in metabolic cages for 24 hr for subsequent determination of urine protein excretion using the benzethonium chloride method. Plasma creatinine was determined at sacrifice by the Jaffé method. Systolic blood pressure was measured in conscious rats using an occlusive tail-cuff plethysmograph attached to a pneumatic pulse transducer (Powerlab, ADInstruments, Colorado Springs, CO), as previously described [50].

Cardiac Catheterization

Cardiac catheterization and data analysis were performed as previously published [51]. In brief, a 2F miniaturized combined conductance catheter-micro-manometer (Model SPR-838 Millar instruments, Houston, TX) was inserted into the carotid artery to obtain aortic blood pressure, then advanced into the left ventricle until stable PV loops were obtained. Data were then acquired under steady state conditions and during preload reduction. The following functional parameters were then calculated (Millar analysis software PVAN 3.4): end diastolic volume, end diastolic pressure, end systolic pressure, ejection fraction, the slope of the end systolic pressure volume relationship, and the slope of the end diastolic pressure volume relationship (EDPVR).

Tissue Preparation and Histochemistry

At study end, rats were anesthetized with inhaled isoflurane 2.5%. The left renal artery was clamped and the remnant kidney removed, decapsulated, and sliced transversely before immersion fixation in 10% neutral buffered formalin, embedding in cryostat matrix (Tissue-Tek, Sakura, Kobe, Japan), or flash freezing in liquid nitrogen. The heart, liver, and spleen were also excised and stored in a similar manner. Formalin-fixed tissues were routinely processed, embedded in paraffin, and sectioned before staining with haematoxylin & eosin, Periodic acid-Schiff, and/or picrosirius red stains.

Immunohistochemistry

Glomerular endothelial cells were immunostained using the mouse anti-rat monoclonal antibody JG-12 (Bender Medsystems), which binds to endothelial cells of blood vessels but not to lymphatics in rat kidney [50]. Tubulointerstitial fibrosis was assessed by examining the accumulation of collagen type IV within the renal cortical tubulointerstitium. Type IV collagen deposition was detected by a goat anti-rat type IV collagen polyclonal antibody (Southern Biotech, Birmingham, AL), and quantified in six random non-overlapping 20x fields for each animal in a blinded fashion as previously described [52]. Immunohistochemistry was performed as previously described [53]. Omission of primary antisera served as the negative control.

Glomerulosclerosis Index

Glomerulosclerosis was assessed using a semi-quantitative technique in a blinded fashion as described previously [27]. In brief, the degree of sclerosis in each glomerulus was subjectively graded on a scale of 0–4: Grade 0, normal; Grade 1, sclerotic area up to 25% (minimal); Grade 2, sclerotic area 25–50% (moderate); Grade 3, sclerotic area 50–75% (moderate to severe) and Grade 4, sclerotic area 75–100% (severe). Glomerulosclerosis was defined as glomerular basement membrane thickening, mesangial hypertrophy and capillary occlusion. A glomerulosclerotic index (GSI) was then calculated using the formula:

$$GSI = \sum_{(i)=0}^{4} Fi\,(i)$$

Where Fi is the percentage of glomeruli in the rat with a given score (i).

Endothelial Cell Density

Glomerular capillary density was determined on JG-12 labelled kidney sections by computer-assisted image analysis (AIS; Analytical Imaging Station version 6.0, St. Catherines, ON, Canada). The percentage glomerular area positive for JG-12 immunostaining was determined in 30 randomly selected glomeruli from each rat in a blinded fashion as previously described [50].

Cardiac Matrix Deposition

The accumulation of matrix was quantified on picrosirius red stained heart sections using computer-assisted image analysis in a blinded fashion, as previously reported [54]. Briefly, 5 random non-overlapping fields from 6 animals per group were captured from the subendocardium and digitized using a BX50 microscope attached to a Fujix HC5000 digital camera. Digital images were then loaded onto a Pentium III IBM computer. An area of red on picrosirius red sections (for matrix) was selected for their color ranges. Calculation of the proportional area stained was then determined using image analysis, as described [54].

Myocyte Hypertrophy

The extent of cardiac myocyte hypertrophy, as measured by cross sectional area, was determined on haematoxylin-eosin stained sections in a blinded fashion, as previously published [55].

Fluorescence Microangiography

Renal (glomerular and tubulointerstitial) microvascular architecture was assessed 8 weeks post-surgery using a slightly modified fluorescence microangiography technique [56]. In brief, animals were anesthetized with inhaled isoflurane 2.5%. The right internal jugular vein was cannulated with a PE50 catheter and 100 U of unfractionated heparin was infused for systemic anticoagulation.

The abdominal aorta was cannulated with a 20G plastic catheter with the tip advanced to a point just distal to the renal artery origins. Whole body perfusion-exsanguination commenced at systolic blood pressure (SNX animals: 170–220 mm Hg, sham animals: 120 mm Hg) via the abdominal aorta with PBS (pH 7.4, 100 mL) to remove circulating blood, and the right internal jugular vein was simultaneously severed, allowing free flow of perfusate. The aorta proximal and distal to the renal artery origins was then clamped such that kidney perfusion was isolated. 5 ml of a pre-warmed (50°C) agarose (1%)–fluorescent microbead (10%) (0.02 µm diameter, Invitrogen) mixture was then infused via the 20G catheter into the aorta. After microbead infusion, the animal was cooled with ice for 10 mins, and then the kidney was harvested and immersed in neutral buffered formalin for 24 hrs at 4°C. 200 µm sections were then viewed using a confocal microscope at 20x optical zoom (Leica TCS SL, Leica, Richmond Hill, CA). Neurolucida software (MBF Bioscience, Willitson, VT) was used to digitally reconstruct glomerular and peritubular microvasculature.

CMTMR Labelling and CMC Tracking

CMCs cultured for 10 days as described were incubated with a 5 µM solution of 5-(and-6)-4-chloromethyl-benzoyl-amino-tetra-methylrhodamine (CMTMR, Invitrogen, Carlsbad, CA) for 30 min. 10^6 CMTMR- cells were infused via tail vein injection into SNX rats 4 weeks after surgery and animals were sacrificed at the time points described. The presence of CMTMR positive cells was determined on a Zeiss LSM510-META confocal microscope by counting CMTMR positive cells in 10 randomly selected 40× magnification fields in a 40 µm frozen section embedded in cryostat matrix (Tissue-Tek, Sakura, Kobe, Japan) [57].

Statistical Analysis

All data are shown as mean ± SEM unless otherwise stated. A minimum number of 3 independent experiments were performed for all *in vitro* experiments. Urine protein excretion is presented as geometric mean ×/÷ tolerance factors. Differences between groups were analyzed by ANOVA with post-hoc Fisher's Least Significant Difference. All statistics were performed using GraphPad Prism 4.00 for Windows (GraphPad Software, San Diego, CA) or SPSS 15.0 for Windows (SPSS, Chicago, IL). A change was considered statistically significant if $P<0.05$.

Supporting Information

Figure S1 Intravenous and intra-arterial CMC therapy resulted in similar renal and cardiac protection. (a) Proteinuria. (b) Systolic blood pressure. (c) Glomerulosclerosis. (d) Glomerular endothelial (JG-12) immunostaining. (e) Tubulointerstitial type IV collagen immunostaining. (f) Left ventricular end diastolic pressure-volume relationship. (g) Myocyte cross-sectional area. (h) Cardiac interstitial fibrosis. Abbreviations: SNX - iv: 5/6 nephrectomy (SNX) animal treated with intravenous CMC infusion. SNX - ia: SNX animal treated with intra-arterial CMC infusion. BP: blood pressure. LV EDPVR: left ventricular end diastolic pressure-volume relationship. PSR: picrosirius red.

Figure S2 Renal and cardiac parameters 8 weeks post-surgery in SNX and SNX - SC animals. (a) Tubulointerstitial type IV collagen immunostaining. (b) Glomerulosclerosis index. (c) Left ventricular end diastolic pressure-volume relationship. (d) Cardiac interstitial fibrosis. (e) Myocyte cross-sectional area. Abbreviations: LV EDPVR: left ventricular end diastolic pressure-volume relationship. PSR: picrosirius red. SNX: 5/6 subtotal nephrectomy animal treated with phosphate-buffered saline. SNX - SC: SNX animal treated with bone marrow-derived stromal cells.

Acknowledgments

The authors would like to thank Mr. C. Johnson, Ms. C. Botelho, and Ms. B. Stead for their technical support of the animal studies.

Author Contributions

Conceived and designed the experiments: DY KAC AA AK PAM DJS RG. Performed the experiments: DY KAC CL KT SLA YZ. Analyzed the data: DY KAC AA SLA YZ DJK. Contributed reagents/materials/analysis tools: AA CL MAK JT DJK HLP AK PAM DJS. Wrote the paper: DY KAC AA RG.

References

1. Wynn TA (2007) Common and unique mechanisms regulate fibrosis in various fibroproliferative diseases. J Clin Invest 117: 524–529.
2. Eddy AA (2005) Progression in chronic kidney disease. Adv Chronic Kidney Dis 12: 353–365.
3. Lopez B, Gonzalez A, Hermida N, Laviades C, Diez J (2008) Myocardial fibrosis in chronic kidney disease: potential benefits of torasemide. Kidney Int Suppl. pp S19–23.
4. Fried LF, Shlipak MG, Crump C, Bleyer AJ, Gottdiener JS, et al. (2003) Renal insufficiency as a predictor of cardiovascular outcomes and mortality in elderly individuals. J Am Coll Cardiol 41: 1364–1372.
5. Parfrey PS, Harnett JD, Barre PE (1991) The natural history of myocardial disease in dialysis patients. J Am Soc Nephrol 2: 2–12.
6. Border WA, Noble NA (1994) Transforming growth factor beta in tissue fibrosis. N Engl J Med 331: 1286–1292.
7. Lebrin F, Deckers M, Bertolino P, Ten Dijke P (2005) TGF-beta receptor function in the endothelium. Cardiovasc Res 65: 599–608.
8. Schultz Jel J, Witt SA, Glascock BJ, Nieman ML, Reiser PJ, et al. (2002) TGF-beta1 mediates the hypertrophic cardiomyocyte growth induced by angiotensin II. J Clin Invest 109: 787–796.
9. Lai KN, Leung JC, Chan LY, Saleem MA, Mathieson PW, et al. (2009) Podocyte injury induced by mesangial-derived cytokines in IgA nephropathy. Nephrol Dial Transplant 24: 62–72.
10. Yingling JM, Blanchard KL, Sawyer JS (2004) Development of TGF-beta signalling inhibitors for cancer therapy. Nat Rev Drug Discov 3: 1011–1022.
11. Burt RK, Loh Y, Pearce W, Beohar N, Barr WG, et al. (2008) Clinical applications of blood-derived and marrow-derived stem cells for nonmalignant diseases. JAMA 299: 925–936.
12. Kocher AA, Schuster MD, Szabolcs MJ, Takuma S, Burkhoff D, et al. (2001) Neovascularization of ischemic myocardium by human bone-marrow-derived angioblasts prevents cardiomyocyte apoptosis, reduces remodeling and improves cardiac function. Nat Med 7: 430–436.
13. Tateishi-Yuyama E, Matsubara H, Murohara T, Ikeda U, Shintani S, et al. (2002) Therapeutic angiogenesis for patients with limb ischaemia by autologous transplantation of bone-marrow cells: a pilot study and a randomised controlled trial. Lancet 360: 427–435.
14. Nakamura T, Torimura T, Sakamoto M, Hashimoto O, Taniguchi E, et al. (2007) Significance and therapeutic potential of endothelial progenitor cell transplantation in a cirrhotic liver rat model. Gastroenterology 133: 91–107 e101.
15. Orlic D, Kajstura J, Chimenti S, Bodine DM, Leri A, et al. (2001) Transplanted adult bone marrow cells repair myocardial infarcts in mice. Ann N Y Acad Sci 938: 221–229; discussion 229–230.
16. Nygren JM, Jovinge S, Breitbach M, Sawen P, Roll W, et al. (2004) Bone marrow-derived hematopoietic cells generate cardiomyocytes at a low frequency through cell fusion, but not transdifferentiation. Nat Med 10: 494–501.
17. Gnecchi M, Zhang Z, Ni A, Dzau VJ (2008) Paracrine mechanisms in adult stem cell signaling and therapy. Circ Res 103: 1204–1219.
18. Vandervelde S, van Luyn MJ, Tio RA, Harmsen MC (2005) Signaling factors in stem cell-mediated repair of infarcted myocardium. J Mol Cell Cardiol 39: 363–376.
19. Caplice NM, Gersh BJ, Alegria JR (2005) Cell therapy for cardiovascular disease: what cells, what diseases and for whom? Nat Clin Pract Cardiovasc Med 2: 37–43.

20. Bi B, Schmitt R, Israilova M, Nishio H, Cantley LG (2007) Stromal cells protect against acute tubular injury via an endocrine effect. J Am Soc Nephrol 18: 2486–2496.
21. Bruno S, Grange C, Deregibus MC, Calogero RA, Saviozzi S, et al. (2009) Mesenchymal stem cell-derived microvesicles protect against acute tubular injury. J Am Soc Nephrol 20: 1053–1067.
22. Nath KA (1992) Tubulointerstitial changes as a major determinant in the progression of renal damage. Am J Kidney Dis 20: 1–17.
23. Spinale FG (2007) Myocardial matrix remodeling and the matrix metalloproteinases: influence on cardiac form and function. Physiol Rev 87: 1285–1342.
24. Frustaci A, Kajstura J, Chimenti C, Jakoniuk I, Leri A, et al. (2000) Myocardial cell death in human diabetes. Circ Res 87: 1123–1132.
25. Amann K, Breitbach M, Ritz E, Mall G (1998) Myocyte/capillary mismatch in the heart of uremic patients. J Am Soc Nephrol 9: 1018–1022.
26. Hein S, Arnon E, Kostin S, Schonburg M, Elsasser A, et al. (2003) Progression from compensated hypertrophy to failure in the pressure-overloaded human heart: structural deterioration and compensatory mechanisms. Circulation 107: 984–991.
27. Wu LL, Cox A, Roe CJ, Dziadek M, Cooper ME, et al. (1997) Transforming growth factor beta 1 and renal injury following subtotal nephrectomy in the rat: role of the renin-angiotensin system. Kidney Int 51: 1553–1567.
28. Kelly DJ, Zhang Y, Gow R, Gilbert RE (2004) Tranilast attenuates structural and functional aspects of renal injury in the remnant kidney model. J Am Soc Nephrol 15: 2619–2629.
29. Ziyadeh FN, Hoffman BB, Han DC, Iglesias-De La Cruz MC, Hong SW, et al. (2000) Long-term prevention of renal insufficiency, excess matrix gene expression, and glomerular mesangial matrix expansion by treatment with monoclonal antitransforming growth factor-beta antibody in db/db diabetic mice. Proc Natl Acad Sci U S A 97: 8015–8020.
30. Kelly DJ, Zhang Y, Connelly K, Cox AJ, Martin J, et al. (2007) Tranilast attenuates diastolic dysfunction and structural injury in experimental diabetic cardiomyopathy. Am J Physiol Heart Circ Physiol 293: H2860–2869.
31. Kuwahara F, Kai H, Tokuda K, Kai M, Takeshita A, et al. (2002) Transforming growth factor-beta function blocking prevents myocardial fibrosis and diastolic dysfunction in pressure-overloaded rats. Circulation 106: 130–135.
32. Leask A, Abraham DJ (2004) TGF-beta signaling and the fibrotic response. Faseb J 18: 816–827.
33. Hirschi KK, Ingram DA, Yoder MC (2008) Assessing identity, phenotype, and fate of endothelial progenitor cells. Arterioscler Thromb Vasc Biol 28: 1584–1595.
34. Dominici M, Le Blanc K, Mueller I, Slaper-Cortenbach I, Marini F, et al. (2006) Minimal criteria for defining multipotent mesenchymal stromal cells. The International Society for Cellular Therapy position statement. Cytotherapy 8: 315–317.
35. Langham RG, Kelly DJ, Gow RM, Zhang Y, Cordonnier DJ, et al. (2006) Transforming growth factor-beta in human diabetic nephropathy: effects of ACE inhibition. Diabetes Care 29: 2670–2675.
36. Sakharova OV, Taal MW, Brenner BM (2001) Pathogenesis of diabetic nephropathy: focus on transforming growth factor-beta and connective tissue growth factor. Curr Opin Nephrol Hypertens 10: 727–738.
37. Border WA, Noble NA (1998) Interactions of transforming growth factor-beta and angiotensin II in renal fibrosis. Hypertension 31: 181–188.
38. Leask A (2007) TGFbeta, cardiac fibroblasts, and the fibrotic response. Cardiovasc Res 74: 207–212.
39. Kupfahl C, Pink D, Friedrich K, Zurbrugg HR, Neuss M, et al. (2000) Angiotensin II directly increases transforming growth factor beta1 and osteopontin and indirectly affects collagen mRNA expression in the human heart. Cardiovasc Res 46: 463–475.
40. Lapointe N, Blais C, Jr., Adam A, Parker T, Sirois MG, et al. (2002) Comparison of the effects of an angiotensin-converting enzyme inhibitor and a vasopeptidase inhibitor after myocardial infarction in the rat. J Am Coll Cardiol 39: 1692–1698.
41. Kang DH, Hughes J, Mazzali M, Schreiner GF, Johnson RJ (2001) Impaired angiogenesis in the remnant kidney model: II. Vascular endothelial growth factor administration reduces renal fibrosis and stabilizes renal function. J Am Soc Nephrol 12: 1448–1457.
42. Martin J, Kelly DJ, Mifsud SA, Zhang Y, Cox AJ, et al. (2005) Tranilast attenuates cardiac matrix deposition in experimental diabetes: role of transforming growth factor-beta. Cardiovasc Res 65: 694–701.
43. Amann K, Wiest G, Zimmer G, Gretz N, Ritz E, et al. (1992) Reduced capillary density in the myocardium of uremic rats–a stereological study. Kidney Int 42: 1079–1085.
44. Gross ML, Ritz E (2008) Hypertrophy and fibrosis in the cardiomyopathy of uremia–beyond coronary heart disease. Semin Dial 21: 308–318.
45. Klahr S, Levey AS, Beck GJ, Caggiula AW, Hunsicker L, et al. (1994) The effects of dietary protein restriction and blood-pressure control on the progression of chronic renal disease. Modification of Diet in Renal Disease Study Group. N Engl J Med 330: 877–884.
46. Olfert ED, Cross BM, McWilliam AA (1993) Guide to the Care and Use of Experimental Animals. Canadian Council on Animal Care.
47. Zhao YD, Courtman DW, Deng Y, Kugathasan L, Zhang Q, et al. (2005) Rescue of monocrotaline-induced pulmonary arterial hypertension using bone marrow-derived endothelial-like progenitor cells: efficacy of combined cell and eNOS gene therapy in established disease. Circ Res 96: 442–450.
48. Ortiz LA, Gambelli F, McBride C, Gaupp D, Baddoo M, et al. (2003) Mesenchymal stem cell engraftment in lung is enhanced in response to bleomycin exposure and ameliorates its fibrotic effects. Proc Natl Acad Sci U S A 100: 8407–8411.
49. Advani A, Gilbert RE, Thai K, Gow RM, Langham RG, et al. (2009) Expression, localization, and function of the thioredoxin system in diabetic nephropathy. J Am Soc Nephrol 20: 730–741.
50. Advani A, Kelly DJ, Advani SL, Cox AJ, Thai K, et al. (2007) Role of VEGF in maintaining renal structure and function under normotensive and hypertensive conditions. Proc Natl Acad Sci U S A 104: 14448–14453.
51. Connelly KA, Prior DL, Kelly DJ, Feneley MP, Krum H, et al. (2006) Load-sensitive measures may overestimate global systolic function in the presence of left ventricular hypertrophy: a comparison with load-insensitive measures. Am J Physiol Heart Circ Physiol 290: H1699–1705.
52. Kelly DJ, Chanty A, Gow RM, Zhang Y, Gilbert RE (2005) Protein kinase Cbeta inhibition attenuates osteopontin expression, macrophage recruitment, and tubulointerstitial injury in advanced experimental diabetic nephropathy. J Am Soc Nephrol 16: 1654–1660.
53. Advani A, Kelly DJ, Cox AJ, White KE, Advani SL, et al. (2009) The (Pro)renin receptor: site-specific and functional linkage to the vacuolar H+-ATPase in the kidney. Hypertension 54: 261–269.
54. Lehr HA, van der Loos CM, Teeling P, Gown AM (1999) Complete chromogen separation and analysis in double immunohistochemical stains using Photoshop-based image analysis. J Histochem Cytochem 47: 119–126.
55. Connelly KA, Kelly DJ, Zhang Y, Prior DL, Martin J, et al. (2007) Functional, structural and molecular aspects of diastolic heart failure in the diabetic (mRen-2)27 rat. Cardiovasc Res 76: 280–291.
56. Dutly AE, Kugathasan L, Trogadis JE, Keshavjee SH, Stewart DJ, et al. (2006) Fluorescent microangiography (FMA): an improved tool to visualize the pulmonary microvasculature. Lab Invest 86: 409–416.
57. Campbell AI, Kuliszewski MA, Stewart DJ (1999) Cell-based gene transfer to the pulmonary vasculature: Endothelial nitric oxide synthase overexpression inhibits monocrotaline-induced pulmonary hypertension. Am J Respir Cell Mol Biol 21: 567–575.

7

Increased Renal Versican Expression is Associated with Progression of Chronic Kidney Disease

Michael Rudnicki[1]*, Paul Perco[2], Hannes Neuwirt[1], Susie-Jane Noppert[1], Johannes Leierer[1], Judith Sunzenauer[1], Susanne Eder[1], Carlamaria Zoja[3], Kathrin Eller[1,4], Alexander R. Rosenkranz[1,4], Gerhard A. Müller[5], Bernd Mayer[2], Gert Mayer[1]

1 Medical University Innsbruck, Deptartment of Internal Medicine IV - Nephrology and Hypertension, Innsbruck, Austria, **2** Emergentec Biodevelopment GmbH, Vienna, Austria, **3** Mario Negri Institute for Pharmacological Research, Centro Anna Maria Astori, Science and Technology Park Kilometro Rosso, Bergamo, Italy, **4** Medical University of Graz, Deptartment of Internal Medicine, Clinical Division of Nephrology and Hemodialysis, Graz, Austria, **5** Georg-August-University Göttingen, Department of Medicine, Nephrology and Rheumatology, Göttingen, Germany

Abstract

Novel prognostic markers for progression of kidney disease are needed to distinguish patients who might benefit from a more aggressive nephroprotective therapy. Expression of the proteoglycan versican was evaluated in renal transcriptomics profiles and in an independent set of 74 renal biopsies. Versican levels were correlated to histologic damage scores and to renal outcome, and versican expression and regulation was evaluated *in vitro*. In transcriptomics profiles of renal tissue versican was positively correlated with (i) histological parameters in kidney biopsies, (ii) progressive decline of renal function in proteinuric kidney diseases, and (iii) impaired renal function and histology scores in diabetic nephropathy. In an independent cohort of 74 biopsies of glomerular diseases renal RNA levels of versican isoforms V0 and V1, but not V2 and V3 correlated significantly with creatinine after a mean follow up time of 53 months. Versican isoforms V0 and V1 together with serum creatinine at time of biopsy and the degree of glomerulosclerosis predicted 20% and 24% of the variability of creatinine at follow up, which was significantly more than serum creatinine and histological parameters alone (16%). However, when patients with acute kidney failure at time of biopsy (n = 5) were excluded, the additive predictive value of versican V1 was only marginally higher (35%) than creatinine and glomerulosclerosis alone (34%). Versican isoforms V0 and V1 were primarily expressed *in vitro* in proximal tubule cells and in fibroblasts. The results in humans were confirmed in three rodent models of kidney disease, in which renal versican expression was significantly upregulated as compared to corresponding controls. These data show for the first time an association of renal versican isoform V0 and V1 expression with progressive renal disease.

Editor: Jean-Claude Dussaule, Inserm, France

Funding: The research leading to these results has received funding from the European Community's Seventh Framework Programme (FP7/2007–2013) under the grant agreement 241544 (SysKid). The funders had no role in study design, data collection and analysis, decision to publish, or preparation of the manuscript.

Competing Interests: MR, PP, and GM filed a patent application on versican for prediction of progressive nephropathy in CKD patients (PCT/EP2010/057917: A method of diagnosing renal disorders). BM is co-owner, and PP is employee of emergentec biodevelopment GmbH. This does not alter the authors' adherence to all the PLoS ONE policies on sharing data and materials. All other authors have nothing to disclose.

* E-mail: michael.rudnicki@i-med.ac.at

Introduction

Progression of chronic kidney disease (CKD) is associated with increased morbidity and mortality, reduced quality of life, and major challenges for healthcare systems [1]. Clinical features predicting a poor prognosis include impaired renal function, hypertension and nephrotic range proteinuria at presentation [2] as well as during follow-up [3,4]. Histopathological changes such as the degree of tubular atrophy and interstitial fibrosis have been shown to better predict long-term renal survival than the extent of glomerular damage even in primary glomerular diseases [5]. To further enhance the prediction of progression of CKD various genes and proteins have been identified as molecular biomarker candidates of kidney damage, and their clinical significance has recently been reviewed in detail [6].

High-throughput transcriptomics experiments together with integrative bioinformatics led to the identification of additional novel biomarker candidates. Henger et al. identified a marker set of nine genes (Chemokine (C-C motif) ligand 21, interleukin 8, matrix metalloproteinase 3, 7 and 9, urokinase R, chemokine (C-X-C motif) receptor 5, integrin beta 4, and pleiotrophin), which predicted a progressive course of CKD [7]. Perco et al. showed that histology of zero-hour preimplant biopsies explained only 14% of the variability of one year creatinine whereas a combination of three biomarkers (NLR family, pyrin domain containing 2, immunoglobulin J polypeptide, and the regulator of G-protein signaling 5) without clinical covariables explained 28% [8]. Recently, our group identified activation of intracellular *vascular endothelial growth factor signaling* and *hypoxia response* pathways in microdissected proximal tubule cells from patients with progressive CKD using microarrays and pathway analysis tools. The expression levels of hypoxia-inducible factor-1 alpha and vascular endothelial growth factor-A were significantly superior in predicting clinical outcome as compared to proteinuria, renal function, and degree of histological damage [9].

In the latter two datasets the hyaluronan binding proteoglycan versican (VCAN) – also termed chondroitin sulphate proteoglycan 2 (CSPG2) - showed a significant correlation with progressive decline of post-bioptical renal function in patients with CKD on the one hand and with increased histological damage on the other hand. The aim of the present study was to characterize versican as a novel renal biomarker predicting progressive decline of kidney function in patients with proteinuric nephropathies.

Results

Versican is a Marker of Renal Injury and Impaired Renal Function

Data are summarized in table 1. In the histogenomics data set by Perco et al. the expression levels of versican showed significant associations to the degree of acute tubular injury (2.55 fold upregulation), tubular atrophy (2.10 fold upregulation), as well as interstitial fibrosis (1.94 fold upregulation) in zero-hour preimplant renal biopsies [8] (figure S1). Rudnicki et al. analyzed global gene expression in microdissected human proximal tubular epithelial cells isolated from 21 patients with various proteinuric nephropathies. In the array raw data set versican showed a significant mean upregulation by 69% in 3 of 4 versican spots on the arrays when stable (n = 14) and progressive subjects (n = 7) were compared (figure S2) [9]. In kidney biopsies from patients with diabetic nephropathy (DN) versican expression was increased 1.4 fold as compared to patients with minimal change disease (MCD) ($p<0.05$) (figure S3) [10]. In the 13 diabetic DN biopsies renal versican expression was furthermore significantly correlated with serum creatinine at time of biopsy (spot 1: $R = 0.70$, $p = 0.008$, spot 2: $R = 0.58$, $p = 0.04$) and with chronic histological damage (spot 1: $R = 0.68$, $p = 0.01$, spot 2: $R = 0.62$, $p = 0.03$) (figures S4 and S5).

However, neither of these studies confirmed the results by real-time PCR or analyzed the expression of the specific versican isoforms V0, V1, V2 and V3 in the respective context covered by each study.

Renal Versican Expression Correlates with Progressive Decline of Kidney Function

To further characterize renal expression of versican isoforms and the association with clinical parameters we analyzed the expression of versican isoforms V0, V1, V2 and V3 in an independent cohort of 74 patients with various proteinuric kidney diseases (table 2). We did not detect any expression of V2 in these samples, and V3 did not show any correlation with laboratory, clinical or histological parameters (data not shown). No significant correlation of V0 and V1 to age, creatinine, eGFR or proteinuria at time of biopsy was detected, although the correlation of V1 to creatinine at biopsy was of borderline significance ($R = 0.220$, $p = 0.06$, table 3). However, both isoforms V0 and V1 did significantly correlate with serum creatinine at time of follow-up (V0 $R = 0.337$, $p = 0.003$; V1 $R = 0.387$, $p = 0.001$), but not with eGFR or proteinuria. Regarding histological characteristics no significant correlation of V0 or V1 levels with the histological diagnosis, and the degree of tubular atrophy/interstitial fibrosis (TAIF), interstitial inflammation (II), or glomerulosclerosis (GS) was observed. However, V1 levels showed a borderline significant correlation with the degree of TAIF ($R = 0.208$, $p = 0.075$) and II ($R = 0.199$, $p = 0.092$) (table 3). We classified the set of 74 patients as stable or progressive according to doubling of serum creatinine or reaching of end-stage renal disease (ESRD) during follow-up. As shown in figure 1A the expression of V0 and V1 was higher in progressive disease (V0:1.56 fold, $p = 0.034$; V1:1.67 fold,

Table 1. Microarray data sets used to evaluate the expression of versican in renal pathologies.

Reference	Disease	N	Age (years)	Creatinine (mg/dl)	Tissue	Comparison	Versican upregulation	Significance level [c]
[8]	Zero-hour transplant biopsies	82	47±16	n.a.	Whole kidney	Acute tubular injury [b] Tubular atrophy [b] Interstitial fibrosis [b]	+2.55 fold +2.10 fold +1.94 fold	P<0.05
[9]	Proteinuric nephropathies [a]	31	38±15	1.7±1.2	Microdissected PTECs from renal biopsies	Progressive vs stable kidney disease	+1.69 fold	P<0.05 in 3 of 4 versican spots
[10]	LD, CD, MCD, DN	24	47±16	1.4±1.2	Tubulointerstitium from renal biopsies	DN vs MCD DN: Pearson correlation with serum creatinine DN: Pearson correlation with histology score	+1.4 fold R = 0.70 R = 0.68	P<0.05 P<0.05 P<0.05

DN diabetic nephropathy, MCD minimal change disease, LD living donors, CD cadaveric donors, PTECs proximal tubular epithelial cells. [a] Proteinuric glomerular diseases included focal segmental glomerulosclerosis (FSGS), MCD, IgA nephropathy (IGAN), lupus nephritis (LN), rapid-progressive glomerulonephritis (RPGN), membranoproliferative glomerulonephritis (MPGN), ANCA associated vasculitis (AAV) and hypertensive nephropathy (HTN). Mean values and standard deviations are shown. [b] Refer to the text for definition of the histological classes. [c] In (8) samples with low and high histological damage were compared and in (9) stable and progressive samples were compared. A two-tailed t-test was performed. In (10) samples from MCD and DN were compared (two tailed t-test), and also a Pearson correlation of creatinine at biopsy and histology score in DN with versican levels was calculated.

$p = 0.011$). Versican V0 and V1 levels did not correlate to eGFR slope (calculated as delta ml/min/1.73 m^2 per year), neither in the whole group nor when analysis was restricted to subjects with eGFR values <60 ml/min/1.73 m^2 (data not shown). In the stable cohort 5 patients were identified who had acute renal failure (ARF) at time of biopsy. Since data on renal function of these patients was not available before biopsy, ARF was defined as a decrease of creatinine during follow-up of more than 50%. These 5 patients had a creatinine at time of biopsy of 5.37±1.25 mg/dl and 1.40±0.32 mg/dl after a follow-up time of 55±19 months. When these 5 patients were excluded from the stable cohort, renal function at time of biopsy was significantly different between the stable and the progressive cohort (table 2). V0 and V1 significantly correlated with creatinine at time of biopsy and at time of follow-up, while no significant correlations were found with age and proteinuria. Regarding histological parameters no significant correlations of V0 and V1 with the diagnosis were identified. However, V0 correlated significantly with the degree of GS, while V1 correlated significantly with the degree of TAIF and showed a borderline significant correlation with the degree of II (table 4). As shown in figure 1B the expression of V0 and V1 was still higher in progressive disease (V0:1.52 fold, $p = 0.051$; V1:1.64 fold, $p = 0.018$) although the level of significance was borderline in the case of V0.

Versican Predicts Future Renal Function

Creatinine at time of biopsy ($p = 0.002$) and the degree of GS ($p = 0.006$), but neither the degree of proteinuria, nor the extent of TAIF or II were significantly associated with adverse renal outcome. The isoforms V0 and V1 correlated with creatinine at follow-up resulting in R^2 values of 0.1026 ($p = 0.0033$) and 0.1421 ($p = 0.0006$), respectively. The combination of the two parameters GS and creatinine at time of biopsy (model 1) resulted in an adjusted R^2 of 0.1619 ($p = 0.0009$). Addition of V0 to this model resulted in an adjusted R^2 of 0.2012 ($p = 0.0004$) (model 2). The model with the highest adjusted R^2 of 0.2438 ($p = 0.0001$) included the variables GS, creatinine at time of biopsy, and V1 (model 3). The model with both isoforms together with GS and creatinine at time of biopsy (model 4) did not further increase the predictive value (table 5). We also analyzed the prediction of future renal function using the same variables after exclusion of the 5 patients with AKI. In this analysis creatinine at time of biopsy became a strong predictor of creatinine at follow-up with an adjusted R^2 of 0.34. Although glomerulosclerosis and both versican isoforms also showed significant associations with creatinine at follow-up, the addition of glomerulosclerosis and either V0 or V1 or both isoforms to creatinine did not increase the predictive value of creatinine to a significant extent (table 6).

Immunohistochemical Staining Shows Pronounced Versican Expression in the Tubulointerstitial Compartment

Next we evaluated the potential origin of versican expression by immunohistochemistry in a healthy control and in representative biopsies from patients with proteinuric nephropathies. We found ubiquitous versican protein expression in the glomerular and in the tubulointerstitial compartment as well as in blood vessels (figure 2). Glomerular expression was rather weak, and the tubular expression was more pronounced at the basolateral membrane. In areas of marked interstitial fibrosis versican expression was also increased showing a fibrillar pattern. In renal blood vessels no expression of versican was detected in the intima, but there was a strong signal in the media and in the adventitia. In healthy renal tissue versican expression was generally lower than in the diseased cases. A weak signal was seen mainly in the tubulointerstitium.

Versican is Expressed in Renal Epithelial Cells and in Fibroblasts in vitro

We further analyzed cell and organ specificity of versican expression. Human proximal tubule cell line HK2 and human skin fibroblast (SF) cell line showed highest expression of V0 and V1 (figure 3). Apart from this relatively similar expression pattern in these three cell lines, we also detected cell type specific differences in expression between the isoforms V0 and V1. Human kidney fibroblasts TK-173, leukocytes, and the epithelial cell line A431 showed a V0 expression which was approximately 5 to 25 times less than in HK2 cells. The expression of V0 was extremely low in prostate epithelial cells, colon epithelial cells, smooth muscle cells and also in control ("healthy") kidney tissue (0.06% to 0.3% as compared to HK2). The results were similar for V1 (0.01% to 7% as compared to HK2), with the exception that V1 expression was also very low in kidney fibroblasts and leukocytes (0.01% to 0.08% as compared to HK2). We did not detect any versican expression in endothelial cells.

TGF-ß1 Upregulates Versican in Fibroblasts

Based on the high basal expression of versican in tubule cells and in fibroblasts we next examined the effect of angiotensin (Ang) II, platelet-derived growth factor (PDGF)-AB and transforming growth factor (TGF) beta-1 on the expression of all versican isoforms in HK-2 and TK-173 cells. We selected these ligands because of their known regulatory effect on versican expression in smooth-muscle cells, and their well-established profibrotic and proinflammatory characteristics. When HK-2 and TK-173 cells were treated with Ang II or PDGF-AB, we did not detect any regulation of any of the versican isoforms. However, treatment with TGF beta-1 resulted in a significant upregulation of V0 and V1 by approx. 3.5 fold in the fibroblast cell line TK-173. We did not detect any significant effect of TGF-ß1 on versican isoform expression in the proximal tubule cell line HK-2 (figure 4).

Versican is Upregulated in Rodent Models of Kidney Diseases

We determined the relevance of our findings by analyzing renal versican mRNA expression in mouse and rat models resembling human glomerular pathologies. The expression values in corresponding controls were arbitrarily set to 1. Versican was upregulated 3.5 fold ($p = 0.02$) in mice with accelerated nephrotoxic serum nephritis, a model of proliferative glomerulonephritis, after 14 days (figure 5). In rats with adriamycin-induced nephropathy, that mimics aspects of human MCD and focal-segmental glomerulosclerosis (FSGS), a 1.5 fold ($p = 0.03$) increase in versican mRNA as compared to controls was found at 21 days. Finally, a highly significant upregulation of renal versican, i.e. 8.0 fold ($p<0.001$) increase over control, was observed in rats with Passive Heymann Nephritis (PHN) - a severe model of proteinuric nephropathy which partly resembles human membranous nephropathy (MN) - studied at 6 months. In ADR and in PHN nephropathy versican expression was also increased on the protein level (figure 6).

Discussion

In this work we describe the two versican isoforms V0 and V1 as novel biomarker candidates with the potential to predict progression of CKD already at an early stage.

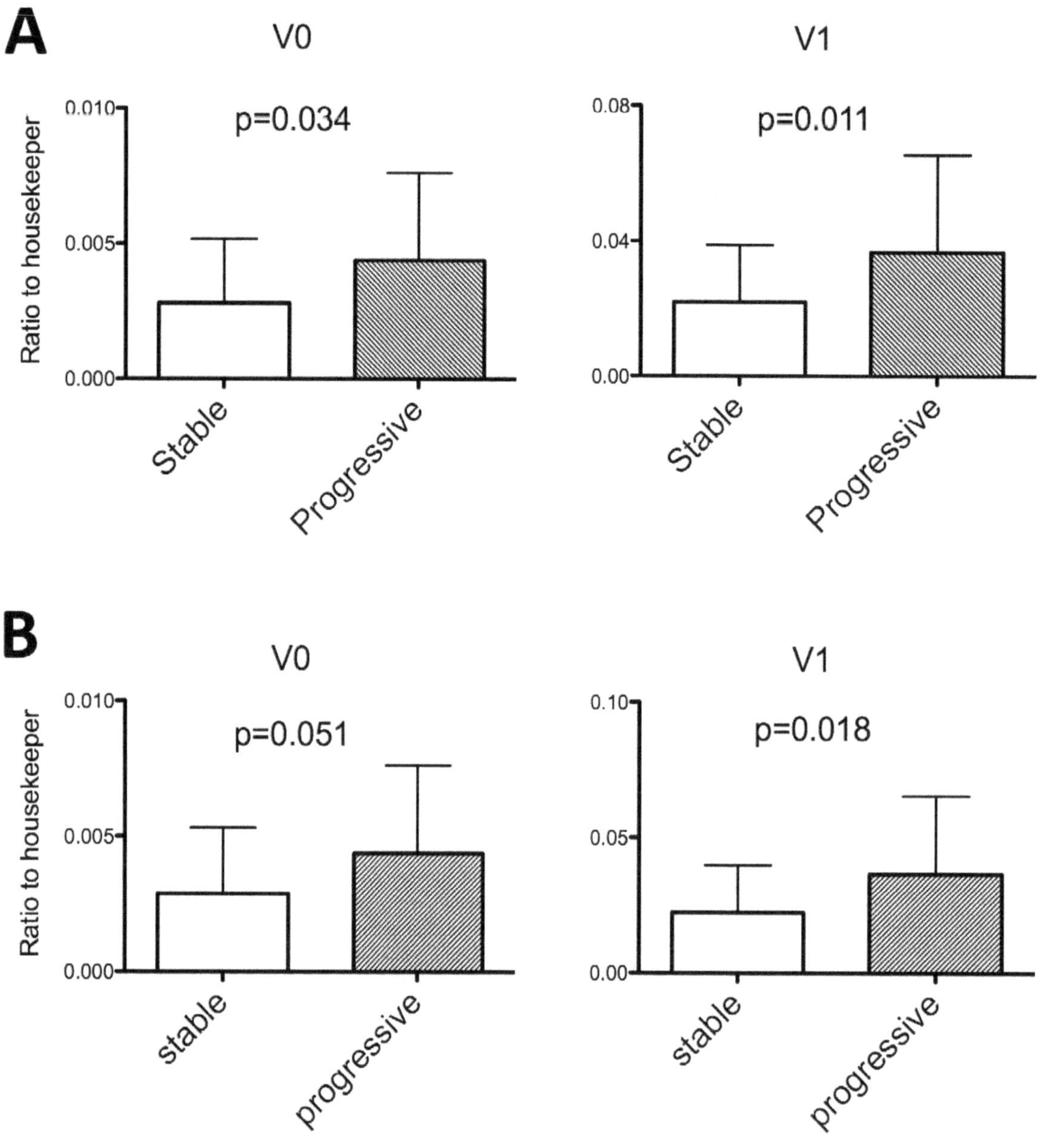

Figure 1. Versican isoform V0 and V1 expression correlates with progression of chronic kidney disease. (A) Whole patient cohort, (B) Patients without ARF. Mean values and standard deviation are shown. p-values of a two-tailed t-test are indicated.

Versican is an extracellular matrix (ECM) protein belonging to the family of hyaluronan-binding proteoglycans showing expression in a variety of connective tissues. Four splice variants of human versican have been identified (V0, V1, V2 and V3), which result from alternative splicing of the two central exons 7 and 8 encoding the central glycosaminoglycan carrying regions, glycosaminoglycan alpha (GAG-α) and beta (GAG-β) [11]. It is V0 and V1, which are the predominant versican isoforms in stroma tissues of most cancers [12,13,14], while V2 expression seems to be restricted to the central nervous tissue [15]. V3 does not contain any GAG attachment sites and has been proposed to act as a regulatory protein [16]. Versican is involved in cell proliferation, cell adhesion, migration, and extracellular matrix assembly [17]. The expression of versican in smooth muscle cells is induced by various mitogens such as transforming growth factor beta-1, platelet derived growth factor, epidermal growth factor, basal fibroblast growth factor, and interleukin 1 beta via phosphatidylinositol 3-kinase–protein kinase B signaling, and is regulated by downstream transcription factors such as cAMP-responsive element binding protein, nuclear factor-kB (NF-kB), and p53 [18].

We identified versican as a marker of histological damage in zero-hour biopsies, of progressive decline of renal function in CKD and in DN in publicly available transcriptomics data sets. Furthermore, versican V0 and V1 levels significantly increased the predictive value of conventional clinical and histological risk factors for renal disease progression in an independent cohort of patients with proteinuric renal diseases. In the field of cancer research several authors have previously identified high levels of tissue versican expression as an indicator for poor outcome in malignant diseases such as prostate cancer [19] and breast cancer [12]. Data on the association of versican expression with clinical outcome in kidney disease are scarce. In a genomics analysis in

Table 2. Patients included in the analysis of versican expression.

Clinical characteristics	All patients [n = 74]	All stable [n = 58]	Stable w/o ARF [n = 53]	Progressive [n = 16]	*p* *	*p* **
Sex (m/f)	49/25	36/22	33/20	13/3	NA	NA
Age (years)	48±16	48±17	48±17	47±14	n.s.	n.s.
Biopsy creatinine (mg/dl)	1.89±1.47	1.76±1.45	1.42±0.88	2.37±1.48	n.s.	0.003
Biopsy proteinuria (g/g)	3.46±3.35	3.42±3.63	3.62±3.72	3.61±2.00	n.s.	n.s.
Follow up time (months)	53±22	55±20	55±20	45±27	n.s.	n.s.
Endpoint: ESRD	12	0	0	12	NA	NA
Endpoint: Doubling creatinine	4	0	0	4	NA	NA
Follow up creatinine (mg/dl)	2.51±2.62	1.34±0.72	1.34±0.74	6.76±2.64	<0.001	<0.001
Follow up proteinuria (g/g)	1.27±1.78	0.65±0.79	0.67±0.80	3.43±2.43	<0.001	<0.001
Diagnosis						
DN	3	1	1	2	NA	NA
HTN	7	4	3	3	NA	NA
IGAN	19	13	12	6	NA	NA
MCD	10	10	10	0	NA	NA
FSGS	7	5	5	2	NA	NA
Vasculitis	6	6	5	0	NA	NA
MN	8	5	5	3	NA	NA
IN	4	4	3	0	NA	NA
LN	2	2	2	0	NA	NA
MPGN	2	2	2	0	NA	NA
Goodpasture	2	2	1	0	NA	NA
other	3	3	3	0	NA	NA
RPGN	1	1	1	0	NA	NA

ESRD end-stage renal disease, 2 x creatinine doubling of serum creatinine. Proteinuria was measured as protein/creatinine ratio in g/g. Mean values and standard deviations are shown. Differences between the means were analyzed by a two-tailed t-test. n.s. not significant (p>0.05), NA not applicable. For abbreviation of the histological diagnosis see the *Experimental Procedures* section. ARF Acute Renal Failure. * *all stable vs progressive.* ** *stable w/o ARF vs progressive.*

Table 3. Clinical and histological correlations of versican isoforms V0 and V1 in the whole CKD cohort.

	V0		V1	
	Pearson R	**p**	**Pearson R**	**p**
Biopsy				
Creatinine	0.191	0.103	0.220	0.060
Proteinuria	0.140	0.239	0.044	0.711
Age	−0.008	0.944	−0.040	0.733
Follow up				
Creatinine	0.337	0.003	0.387	0.001
Proteinuria	0.079	0.557	0.028	0.833
Histology				
Diagnosis	ANOVA	0.163	ANOVA	0.174
Degree of TAIF	0.104	0.378	0.208	0.075
Degree of II	0.131	0.268	0.199	0,092
Degree of GS	0.146	0.222	−0.062	0,605

TAIF tubular atrophy/interstitial fibrosis, II Interstitial inflammation, GS glomerular sclerosis.

Table 4. Clinical and histological correlations of versican isoforms V0 and V1 in the CKD cohort excluding patients with ARF.

	V0		V1	
	Pearson R	**p**	**Pearson R**	**p**
Biopsy				
Creatinine	0.352	0.003	0.380	0.001
Proteinuria	0.123	0.317	0.026	0.832
Age	-0.023	0.848	−0.054	0.657
Follow up				
Creatinine	0.331	0.006	0.381	0.001
Proteinuria	0.067	0.625	0.020	0.903
Histology				
Diagnosis	ANOVA	0.080	ANOVA	0.132
Degree of TAIF	0.166	0.180	0.253	0.039
Degree of II	0.169	0.168	0.231	0.058
Degree of GS	0.256	0.036	0.028	0.824

TAIF tubular atrophy/interstitial fibrosis, II Interstitial inflammation, GS glomerular sclerosis.

Table 5. Versican isoforms predict the clinical course on top of traditional risk factors – analysis of the whole cohort.

Whole cohort (n = 74)			
	Creatinine at follow-up		
Univariate model	**parameter estimate**	**p-value**	**adj R^2**
Creatinine at biopsy	0.6372	0.0019	0.1155
Proteinuria at biopsy	0.0249	0.7930	<0
TAIF	0.4871	0.1520	0.0150
II	0.3773	0.2440	0.0053
GS	0.8050	0.0045	0.0983
Versican V0	339.3458	0.0033	0.1026
Versican V1	49.9941	0.0006	0.1421
	Creatinine at follow-up		
Model 1	**parameter estimate**	**p-value**	**adj R^2**
Creatinine at biopsy	0.5004	0.0149	
GS	0.5768	0.0429	
total		0.0009	0.1619
	Creatinine at follow-up		
Model 2	**parameter estimate**	**p-value**	**adj R^2**
GS	0.5284	0.0579	
Creatinine at biopsy	0.4294	0.0342	
Versican V0	232.2049	0.0411	
total		0.0004	0.2012
	Creatinine at follow-up		
Model 3	**parameter estimate**	**p-value**	**adj R^2**
GS	0.6947	0.0119	
Creatinine at biopsy	0.3414	0.0894	
Versican V1	41.2212	0.0052	
total		0.0001	0.2438
	Creatinine at follow-up		
Model 4	**parameter estimate**	**p-value**	**adj R^2**
Creatinine at biopsy	0.3364	0.0978	
GS	0.7207	0.0141	
Versican V0	−51.2110	0.7789	
Versican V1	46.5995	0.0552	
total		0.0002	0.2333

For abbreviations see table 3 or 4.

Table 6. Versican isoforms predict the clinical course on top of traditional risk factors – analysis of the dataset without ARF patients.

Dataset without ARF patients (n = 69)			
	Creatinine at follow-up		
Univariate model	**parameter estimate**	**p-value**	**adj R^2**
Creatinine at biopsy	1.4115	<0.001	0.3382
Proteinuria at biopsy	0.0155	0.8752	<0
TAIF	0.6018	0.0962	0.0265
II	0.4850	0.1595	0.0151
GS	0.8082	0.0056	0.0984
Versican V0	332.0354	0.0055	0.0960
Versican V1	48.4368	0.0013	0.1322
	Creatinine at follow-up		
Model 1	**parameter estimate**	**p-value**	**adj R^2**
Creatinine at biopsy	1.3211	<0.001	
GS	0.1545	0.5750	
total		<0.001	0.3417
	Creatinine at follow-up		
Model 2	**parameter estimate**	**p-value**	**adj R^2**
GS	0.1612	0.5870	
Creatinine at biopsy	1.2331	<0.001	
Versican V0	102.0562	0.9310	
total		<0.001	0.3403
	Creatinine at follow-up		
Model 3	**parameter estimate**	**p-value**	**adj R^2**
GS	0.2684	0.3527	
Creatinine at biopsy	1.1344	<0.001	
Versican V1	19.2900	0.1999	
total		<0.001	0.3486
	Creatinine at follow-up		
Model 4	**parameter estimate**	**p-value**	**adj R^2**
Creatinine at biopsy	1.1313	<0.001	
GS	0.2790	0.3638	
Versican V0	−19.0025	0.9135	
Versican V1	21.3068	0.3745	
Total		<0.001	0.3382

For abbreviations see table 3 or 4.

ageing kidneys, Melk et al. found renal versican RNA levels to be increased 2.90 fold in kidney tissue from older patients as compared to samples from adults. The highest differential versican expression (3.64 fold) was observed between samples with higher and lower degree of histological damage, thus also indicating a correlation with histological damage [20]. In kidney transplantation Einecke et al. evaluated global gene expression in 105 renal biopsies [21]. Versican was one of the most significant genes, which predicted renal graft loss with a 3.42 times higher expression in failed grafts as compared to censored grafts. Interestingly, in our independent cohort of 74 patients with various renal histologies versican expression levels did not correlate with the degree of TAIF, II or GS, although the correlation of V0 with glomerulosclerosis and of V1 with TAIF and II reached significant levels after exclusion of patients with ARF (see below). This association of versican with histological

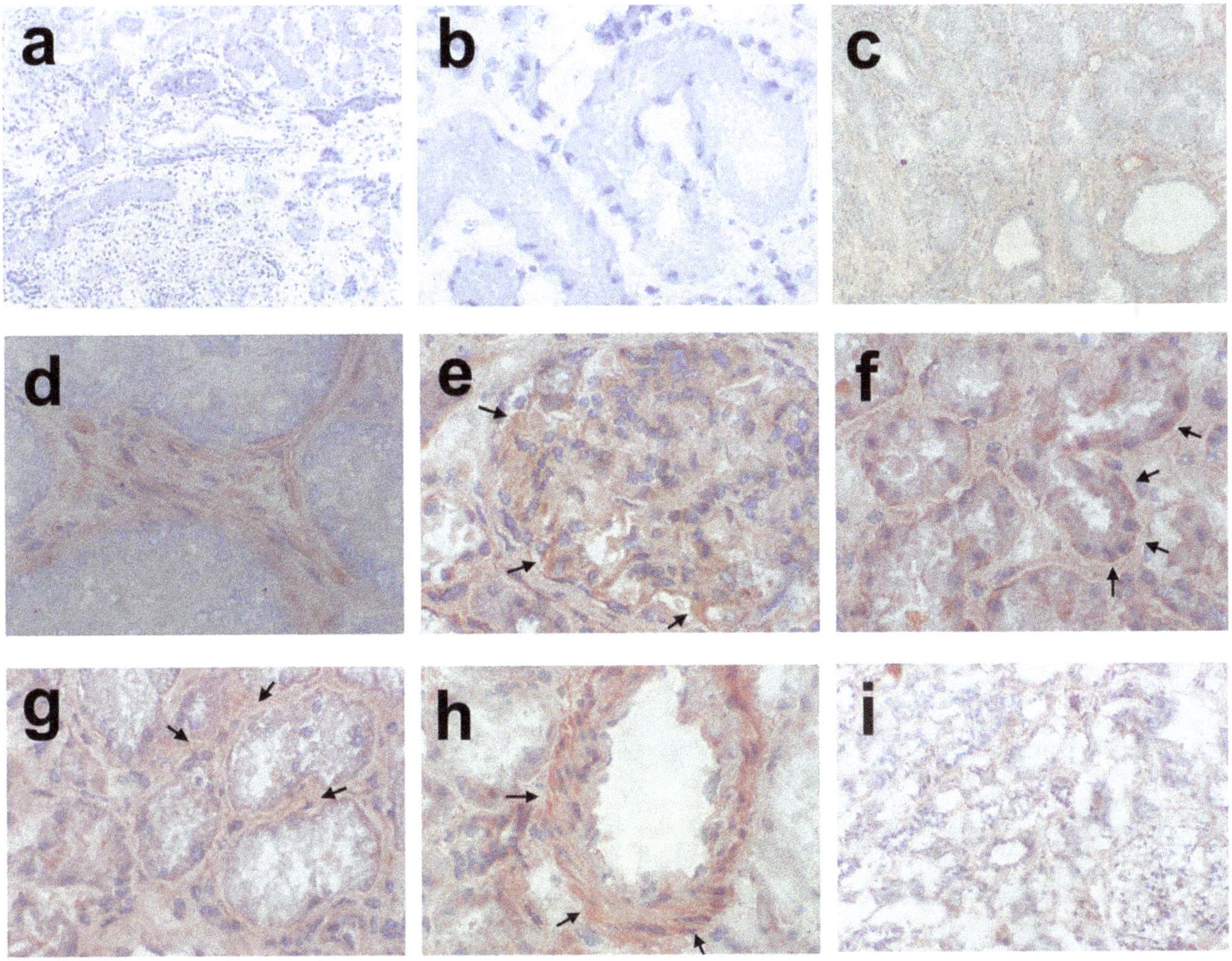

Figure 2. Immunohistochemical staining of versican in positive controls, in human biopsy samples of IgA-Nephropathy (IgAN) and WHO Class IV Lupus Nephritis (LN4) and in healthy kidney tissue. Representative images are shown. a) negative control 100x, b) isotype control 400x, c) and d) positive control in prostate cancer samples (100x and 400x), e) glomerular (LN4, stable), f) tubular (LN4, stable), g) interstitial (IgAN, stable), h) vascular (IgAN, stable) expression (all 400x) of versican in human biopsy samples of renal disease, and i) healthy kidney tissue from a tumor nephrectomy (100x).

injury is in line with findings from several authors where (not isoform specific) versican expression was increased in renal tissue with high degree of histological injury [8,10,20]. This association is further supported by the borderline significant correlation of versican levels with serum creatinine at time of biopsy (which became significant after exclusion of ARF patients) in our cohort and in the findings from Schmid et al. [10]. Therefore, we cannot rule out the possibility that the predictive characteristics of versican V0 and V1 expression values on progression of renal failure are not – at least in part – due to increased damage of kidney tissue and poor kidney function already at time of biopsy.

Versican levels did neither correlate with proteinuria nor did proteinuria predict adverse renal outcome. This lack of association of chronic histological changes and of proteinuria with prognosis might point to a selection bias in which patients with an acute form of glomerulonephritis and not a chronic presentation undergo kidney biopsy, thus limiting the generalizability of these results. To address this issue we identified 5 patients with ARF at time of biopsy in the stable cohort. Although these patients showed lower renal versican V0 and V1 expression than other stable patients as well as the progressive cohort, the differences did not reach statistical significance (data not shown). After exclusion of these 5 patients V0 and V1 levels were still higher in progressive subjects (V0 $p = 0.051$, V1 $p = 0.018$). Furthermore, V0 and V1 showed positive correlations to creatinine at time of biopsy and to the degree of histological damage. However, then the predictive value of creatinine at time of biopsy increased substantially ($R^2 = 0.34$), and was not improved by the degree of glomerulosclerosis or V0 or V1 levels to a significant extent. These results in patients without ARF are in line with published data, which show that basal renal function is a robust marker for prediction of progression of CKD. However, in the clinical setting of deteriorated renal function at time of biopsy it is often difficult to predict future renal function. In this setting renal versican expression might serve as a potential candidate to predict worse renal outcome.

Results in humans were reproduced in three animal models of nephropathies in which renal versican expression was significantly increased in diseased animals as compared to controls. Analysis of versican RNA expression *in vitro* showed significantly higher expression levels of V0 and V1 in renal tubule cells and in fibroblasts than in other cell lines. These findings were corrobo-

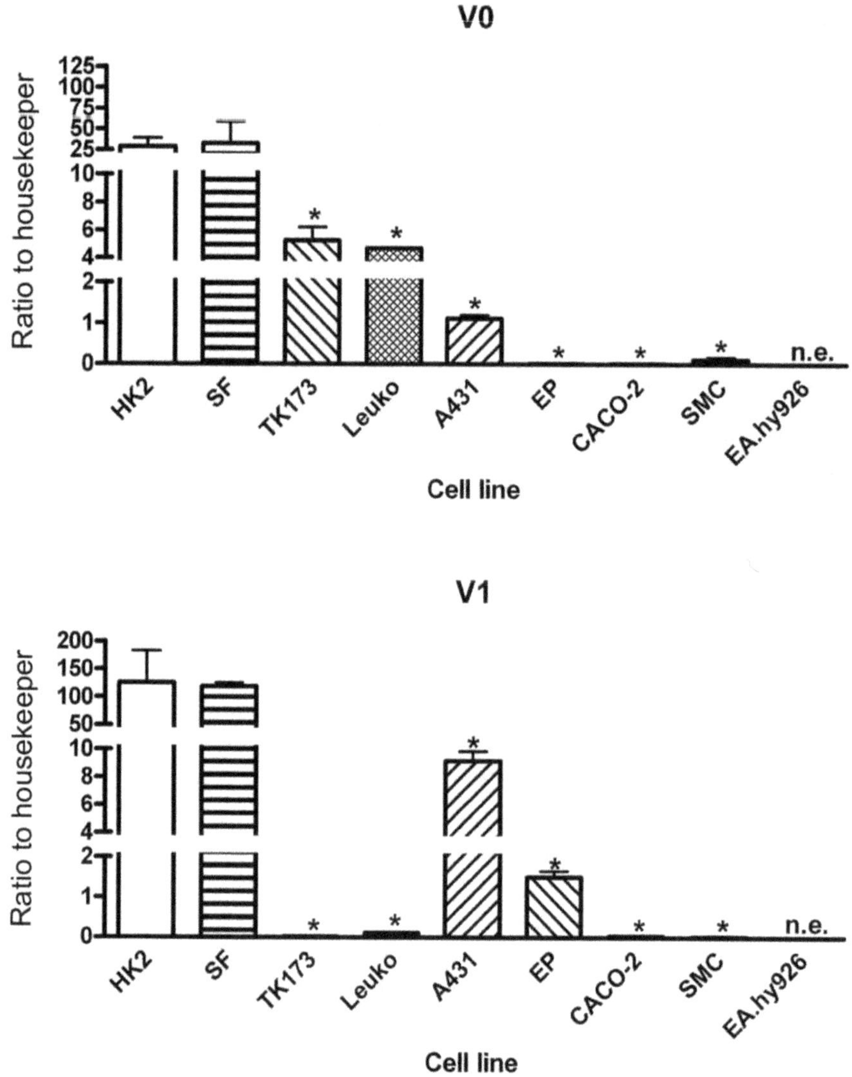

Figure 3. Expression of versican mRNA in vitro. Versican is expressed in various renal and non-renal cell lines. HK2 renal proximal tubule cells, SF primary skin fibroblasts, TK173 kidney fibroblasts, A431 epidermoid carcinoma cell line, EP prostate epithelial cells, CACO2 colon carcinoma cells, CMS primary smooth muscle cells, EA.hy926 endothelial cells. The expression values are shown as ratio to PPIA. The mean and the standard deviation from n = 3 experiments is shown. * $p<0.05$ as compared to HK2 cells measured by a two-tailed t-test. n.e. not expressed.

rated in biopsies from patients with IgA nephropathy (IgAN) and Lupus nephritis showing versican protein expression mainly in tubule cells, the ECM and interstitial fibroblasts. Bode-Lesniewska et al. showed that the V0 and V1 isoforms of versican are expressed in various tissues and epithelial cells, but not in renal tubules and glomeruli [22]. However, versican was detected in the surrounding interstitial tissue and in sclerosed glomeruli. These contradicting results could be explained by the fact that renal tubular expression of versican might only be activated in the diseased state. This hypothesis is supported by our findings of very low versican expression in control kidney tissue. Similar to our results a higher expression of versican in the fibromuscular stroma was reported in prostate cancer tissue [19] and in the stroma of nodules in benign prostatic hyperplasia [23] but not in prostate epithelial cells when compared with healthy prostate samples. These studies suggest that versican is mainly expressed in fibroblasts, and also deposited as part of the ECM, respectively.

We detected an induction of versican expression in fibroblasts by TGF beta-1. It has been proposed that versican might be involved in epithelial-mesenchymal-transition (EMT) and mesenchymal-epithelial-transition (MET). In NIH3T3 fibroblasts V1 but not V2 induced MET with a switch in cadherin expression from N- to E-cadherin, reduced expression of vimentin, and increased expression of occludin resulting in a polarized and epithelial phenotype [24]. Furthermore, V1 enhanced cell proliferation, modulated cell cycle progression, and inhibited apoptosis via the activation of epithelial growth factor receptor expression, modulation of its downstream pathways and by inducing degradation of the cyclin-dependent kinase inhibitor p27 [25]. In the context of progressive renal disease these observations would suggest "protective" characteristics of at least versican isoform V1, in which overexpression in fibroblasts induces an epithelial phenotype and enhances gap junction communications.

On the other hand it was shown that versican binds to adhesion molecules on the surface of leukocytes such as P- and L-selectins, and also CD44 [26]. Furthermore, the chondroitin sulphate chains of versican mediate the binding of several chemokines involved in the recruitment of mononuclear leukocytes [27]. Together with

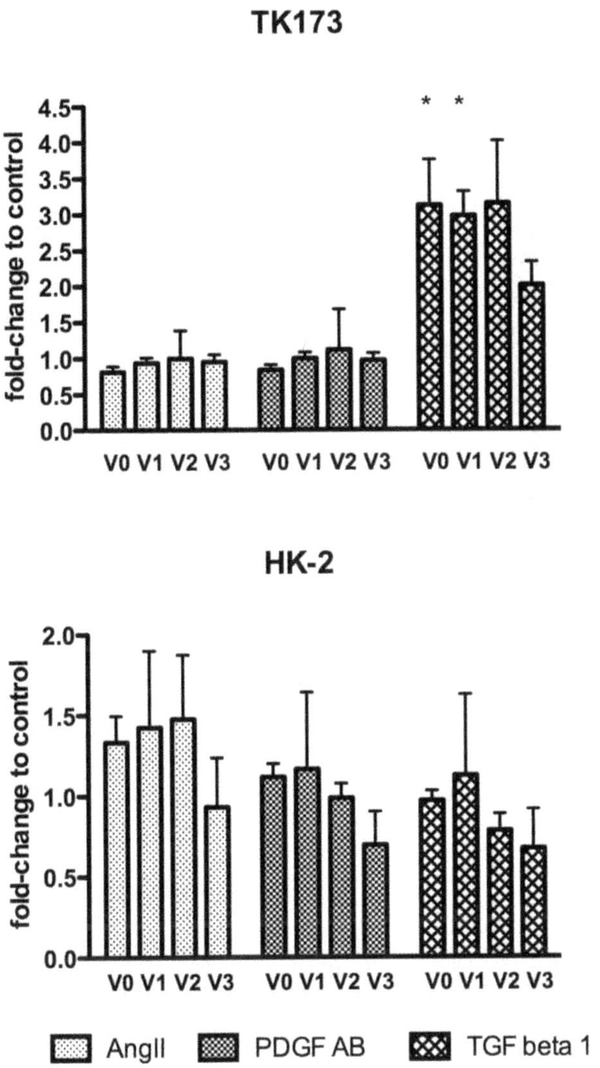

Figure 4. Versican regulation in fibroblasts and tubule cells. TK-173 and HK-2 cells were treated with Ang II, PDGF-AB and TGF-ß1 for 24 hours. After RNA isolation all 4 versican isoforms were analyzed by real-time PCR (n = 3 assays per ligand). Results shown are mean ratios to the housekeeper gene PPIA ± standard deviation. *$p<0.05$ as compared to controls.

versicans ability to bind to ECM components [28] increased versican levels might hence sustain an inflammatory microenvironment, thus promoting fibrogenesis and progression of CKD.

In conclusion, we identified renal expression of versican isoforms V0 and V1 as markers for unfavourable renal prognosis. Due to the highly interactive characteristics of versican this molecule represents a promising candidate for further studies of renal pathologies. However, before versican levels can be used as a prognostic marker candidate these findings have to be replicated in an independent cohort of well characterized patients with sufficient statistical power.

Materials and Methods

Ethics Statement

Before performing a routine kidney biopsy due to a clinical indication a written informed consent is obtained from every patient. Usually two biopsy cores are retrieved, one for routine histological analysis, which is fixed immediately with formalin and embedded in paraffin, and one for immunofluorescence analysis, which is embedded in Tissue-Tek®OCT™ (Sakura, Alphen aan den Rijn, the Netherlands) compound and processed as cryocut sections. After the diagnostic workup is finished the surplus cryocut sections are stored at −80°C. The Institutional Review Board of the Medical University of Innsbruck has accredited the use of surplus material from routine kidney biopsies for research purposes.

Microarray Data Sets on Versican Expression in Kidney Tissue

We extracted versican RNA expression values from three transcriptomics studies in the context of kidney transplantation [8], chronic kidney disease [9] and diabetic nephropathy [10]. Versican levels were investigated in the context of the clinical questions of the respective papers (table 1). Raw data from the array experiments and supplemental figures are accessible via www.microarray.at.

Patients and Kidney Biopsies of the Validation Cohort

We used kidney biopsies obtained from 74 patients with proteinuric renal diseases during their routine diagnostic workup. Diagnoses included focal segmental glomerulosclerosis (FSGS), minimal change disease (MCD), IgA nephropathy (IGAN), lupus nephritis (LN), rapid-progressive glomerulonephritis (RPGN), membranoproliferative glomerulonephritis (MPGN), ANCA associated vasculitis (AAV), hypertensive nephropathy (HTN), membranous nephropathy (MN), Goodpasture syndrome, interstitial nephritis (IN) and other. Clinical follow-up data is summarized in table 2. Progressive disease was defined as doubling of serum creatinine during follow-up or end-stage renal disease. All other patients were defined as stable. An independent pathologist scored the degree of tubular atrophy/interstitial fibrosis (TAIF), glomerular sclerosis (GS) and interstitial inflammation (II) following a semiquantitative grading system on haematoxylin/eosin and periodic-acid-Schiff- or Pearse-stained sections.

Correlation of Versican Isoform mRNA Levels with Clinical Parameters and Outcome

Correlations of versican isoforms V0 and V1 were calculated to (i) clinical parameters at time of biopsy (age, creatinine, eGFR-MDRD, proteinuria), (ii) clinical parameters at follow-up (creatinine, eGFR-MDRD, proteinuria), and (iii) histological parameters (diagnosis, degree of TAIF, GS and II). The Pearson correlation coefficient was used for all analyses except for the correlation of versican levels with histological diagnosis for which an ANOVA test was used. We determined the strength of versican isoforms V0 and V1 along with traditional risk factors for progression such as creatinine at time of biopsy, proteinuria, degree of TAIF, GS and II to predict patient outcome. Creatinine at follow-up was used as outcome variable in the linear regression models.

RNA Isolation and Real-time PCR

RNA was isolated using the RNeasy® Micro Kit (Qiagen, Hilden, Germany). RNA was reverse transcribed into cDNA with the High Capacity cDNA reverse Transcription kit (Applied Biosystems, Carlsbad, CA). Preamplification was performed using TaqMan® Gene Expression Assays (*vide infra*) and the TaqMan® PreAmp Master Mix. The preamplified cDNA was analyzed in duplicates on the 7500 Fast Real-Time PCR System (Applied Biosystems, Carlsbad, CA) using the following inventoried

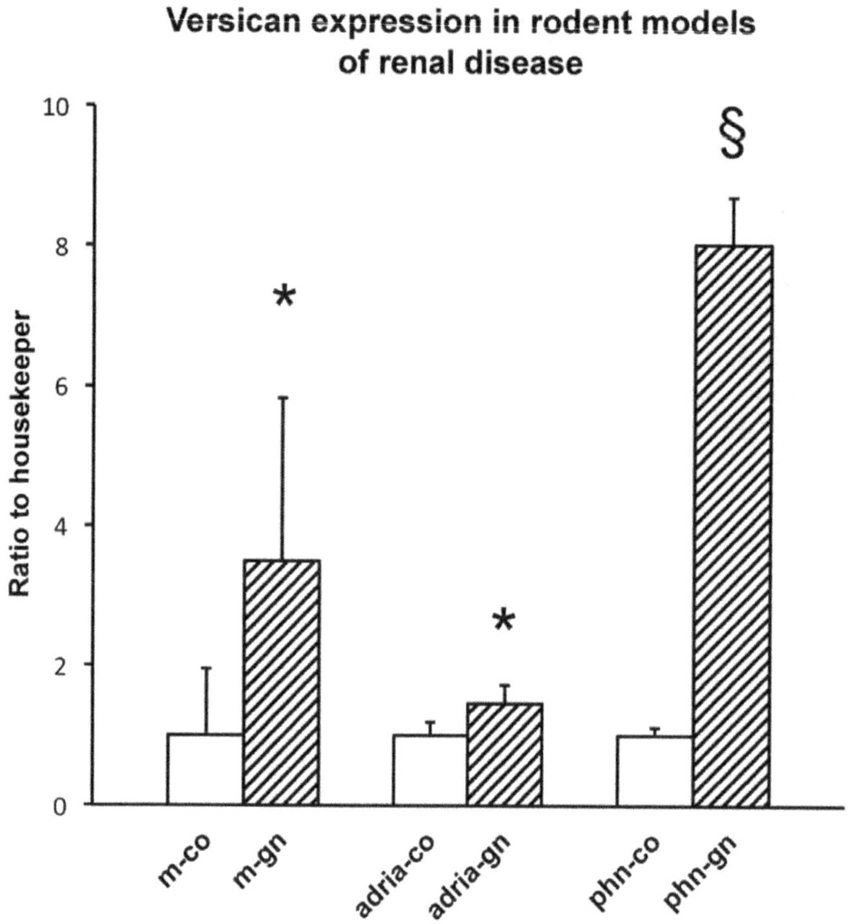

Figure 5. Versican expression in rodent models of renal disease. Versican is significantly upregulated in various mouse and rat models of glomerulonephritis. Mean values and standard deviations are shown. Two-tailed t-test was performed. * $p<0.05$, § $p<0.001$, co controls, gn glomerulonephritis, m mouse, phn Passive Heyman Nephritis, adria Adriamycin rats.

TaqMan® Gene Expression Assays: PPIA (cyclophilin A; Hs99999904_m1), VCAN0 (Hs01007944_m1), VCAN1 (Hs01007937_m1), VCAN2 (Hs01007943_m1) and VCAN3 (Hs01007941_m1). The relative amounts of transcripts for each gene were normalized to the reference gene cyclophilin A (PPIA).

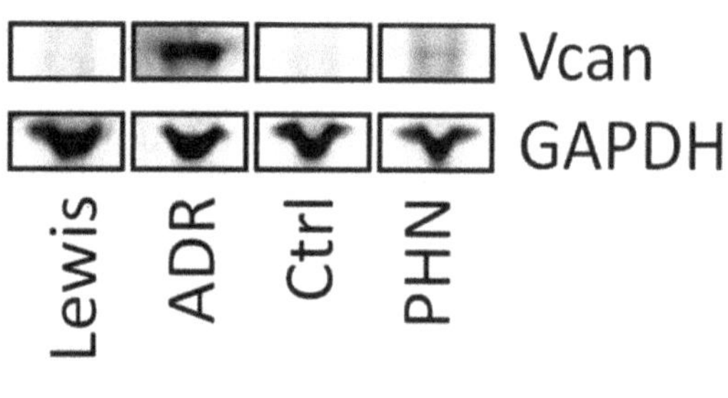

Figure 6. Expression of versican protein in vivo. Versican protein expression is induced in two rat models of glomerulonephritis (Adriamycin-induced glomerulonephritis (ADR) and Passive Heymann Nephritis (PHN)) compared to respective controls, Lewis and Ctrl. Versican expression was analyzed in 6 samples of each group. Figure 6 shows one representative sample each.

Cell Culture

Human renal proximal tubule cells (HK2), colon carcinoma cells (CACO2), epidermoid carcinoma cells (A431), and human endothelial cells (EA.hy926) were purchased from the American Type Culture Collection. The human kidney fibroblast cell line TK-173 was provided by Gerhard A. Müller, Göttingen, Germany [29]. Immortalized prostate epithelial cells (EP156T, EP153T) [30], primary smooth muscle cells (SMC) [31] and primary skin fibroblasts (SF) [32] were obtained from Helmut Klocker at the Department of Experimental Urology from the Medical University Innsbruck. Leukocyte cDNA was obtained from the Human MTC™ Panel I and Panel II (Clontech, Mountain View, CA). Kidney tissue was obtained from the unaffected part of a kidney, which was nephrectomized due to renal cell carcinoma. HK-2 cells were cultured in keratinocyte-serum-free medium (KSFM) containing 10% FCS, 5 ng/ml recombinant epidermal growth factor (rEGF), and 0.05 mg/ml bovine pituitary extract (BPE) and 1% PenStrep. TK173 fibroblasts were cultured in DMEM containing 10% FCS, 1% Glutamax (Life Technologies Corporation, Carlsbad, CA) and 1% PenStrep. After 24 h in serum-free medium HK-2 and TK173 cells were cultured for 24 h in the presence of angiotensin (Ang) II (10^{-7} mM), platelet-derived growth factor (PDGF)-AB (10 ng/ml) or transforming growth factor (TGF) beta-1 (10 ng/ml). RNA isolation and quantitative real-time PCR of the versican isoforms was performed as described above, but RNA was not pre-amplified.

Versican Immunohistochemistry

Frozen sections from six patients (3 IgAN, 3 class IV lupus nephritis) were stained for human versican protein. Two patients (both IgAN) showed severe renal function impairment and a progressive course of disease, while the other 4 showed conserved renal function and a stable course of disease. As healthy control tissue we used an unaffected part of a tumor nephrectomy specimen. The sections were fixed in cold acetone. The sections were then incubated at 4°C overnight with a 1:400 dilution of the primary antibody (rabbit anti-human Versican, sc-25831, Santa Cruz, CA). Versican was detected by the Vectastain Elite ABC Kit (Vector Laboratories, Burlingame, CA). This system uses a biotin-conjugated secondary antibody (1:1000), avidin and biotinylated horseradish peroxidase, and 3-amino-9-ethylcarbazole (AEC) as the chromogen for visualization. All sections were counterstained with hematoxylin.

Animal Models of Renal Disease

We investigated versican expression in 3 rodent models of renal disease: (A) Accelerated anti-glomerular basement membrane nephritis was induced in n = 8 mice as described previously [33], and n = 8 untreated animals served as controls. In brief, 8- to 12-wk-old male C57Bl/6J mice were obtained from Charles River (Sulzfeld, Germany). The animals were preimmunized subcutaneously with 2 mg/ml rabbit IgG (Jackson Immuno Research Laboratories, West Grove, PA) dissolved in incomplete Freund's adjuvant (Sigma, St. Louis, MI) and nonviable desiccated *Mycobacterium tuberculosis* H37a (Difco Laboratories, Detroit, MI). After 5 days, heat-inactivated rabbit anti-mouse GBM antiserum was injected *via* the tail vein. The animals were sacrificed after 14 days. Austrian veterinary authorities approved these animal experiments (GZ 66.011/0.111–11/10b/2008; Bundesministerium für Wissenschaft und Forschung). (B) Passive Heymann Nephritis (PHN) was induced in n = 5 2-month old male Sprague-Dawley rats (Charles River Italia s.p.a., Calco, Italy) by a single intravenous injection of 0.4 ml/100 g body weight of rabbit anti-Fx1A antibody, followed 7 days later by unilateral nephrectomy to accelerate the onset of renal damage [34]. Animals were sacrificed after 6 months. Age-matched Sprague–Dawley rats (n = 5) were used as control. (C) Adriamycin nephropathy was induced in n = 5 male Lewis rats (Charles River Italia s.p.a., Calco, Italy) by a single intravenous injection of ADR (Adriblastina, Pfizer Italia s.r.l, Latina, Italy) at the dose of 5 mg/kg [35]. Five Lewis rats intravenously injected with saline served as controls. Animals were sacrificed after 21 days. Animal care and treatment were in accordance with current law [36]. Animal studies were submitted to and approved by the Institutional Animal Care and Use Committee of "Mario Negri" Institute, Milan, Italy. Renal expression of versican was analyzed by real-time PCR following the above outlined protocol using the inventoried TaqMan Gene Expression Assays for mouse versican (Mm01283063_m1), mouse 18s ribosomal RNA (Mm03928990_g1), rat versican (Rn01493755_m1) and rat cyclophilin A (Rn00690933_m1). The TaqMan Gene Expression Assays for mouse-versican and rat-versican used in this study are not isoform-specific but rather allow the detection of the expression of any of the known versican isoforms.

Western Blot

The protocol has been previously published [37]. In brief, 1×1×2 mm blocks of rat kidney tissue were lysed in 250 µl of SDS sample buffer (NuSep Inc., Bogart, GA). 15 µl per lane were resolved using 4 to 12% Bis-Tris gels (Invitrogen, Leek, The Netherlands) and transferred onto a nitrocellulose membrane (Invitrogen). Primary antibody (rabbit anti-human versican, sc-25832, Santa Cruz Biotechnology Inc., Santa Cruz, CA) was incubated at 4°C over night. After washing, membranes were incubated with fluorescence-labeled secondary antibodies (Molecular Probes, Eugene, OR) and subsequently scanned using the Odyssey infrared imaging system (LiCor Biosciences, Lincoln, NE).

Supporting Information

Figure S1 Versican expression in zero-hour preimplant renal biopsies. Data were extracted from the publication by Perco et al. Increased versican expression is found in biopsies with a higher level of histological damage, such as glomerulosclerosis (gs), arteriolosclerosis (as), interstitial fibrosis (if), interstitial inflammation (ii), tubular atrophy (ta) and acute tubular injury (ati). The degree of histological damage was assessed using a semiquantitative grading system: 0 - no; 1 - minor; 2 - moderate; 3– severe. Samples with grade 0 were defined as "low" in gs, as, if, ii and ta, while samples with grades 1–3 were defined as "high". In the case of ati samples with grade 0–1 were defined "low" and samples with grades above 2 were defined as "high". * depicts significant differences.

Figure S2 Versican expression in microdissected tubule cells from human subjects with stable and progressive course of CKD. Data extracted from microarray raw data from our group [9]. The accession numbers represent four different versican spots on the arrays. Three of those four showed significant differences in expression. * $p<0.05$.

Figure S3 Versican expression in living donors, minimal change disease, cadaveric donors and in diabetic nephropathy. Data extracted from the raw data provided by Schmid et al [10]. NM_004385 and BF218922 represent two different spots on the respective microarrays. * $p<0.05$

Figure S4 Versican expression and serum creatinine at time of biopsy in diabetic nephropathy. Data extracted from the raw data provided by Schmid et al [10].

Figure S5 Versican expression and histology score in diabetic nephropathy. Data extracted from the raw data provided by Schmid et al [10].

Acknowledgments

We kindly thank Prof. Dieter Zimmermann (Zürich, Switzerland) for sharing his expertise on versican research with our group. We are also grateful to Helmut Klocker (Innsbruck, Austria) for providing cell cultures for the in vitro experiments.

Author Contributions

Conceived and designed the experiments: MR PP BM GM. Performed the experiments: MR HN SJN JS SE KE JL. Analyzed the data: MR PP. Contributed reagents/materials/analysis tools: HN KE ARR GAM CZ. Wrote the paper: MR PP GM.

References

1. Meguid El Nahas A, Bello AK (2005) Chronic kidney disease: the global challenge. Lancet 365: 331–340.
2. D'Amico G (1992) Influence of clinical and histological features on actuarial renal survival in adult patients with idiopathic IgA nephropathy, membranous nephropathy, and membranoproliferative glomerulonephritis: survey of the recent literature. Am J Kidney Dis 20: 315–323.
3. Hladunewich MA, Troyanov S, Calafati J, Cattran DC (2009) The natural history of the non-nephrotic membranous nephropathy patient. Clin J Am Soc Nephrol 4: 1417–1422.
4. Reich HN, Troyanov S, Scholey JW, Cattran DC (2007) Remission of proteinuria improves prognosis in IgA nephropathy. J Am Soc Nephrol 18: 3177–3183.
5. Meyer TW (2003) Tubular injury in glomerular disease. Kidney Int 63: 774–787.
6. Kronenberg F (2009) Emerging risk factors and markers of chronic kidney disease progression. Nat Rev Nephrol 5: 677–689.
7. Henger A, Kretzler M, Doran P, Bonrouhi M, Schmid H, et al. (2004) Gene expression fingerprints in human tubulointerstitial inflammation and fibrosis as prognostic markers of disease progression. Kidney Int 65: 904–917.
8. Perco P, Kainz A, Wilflingseder J, Soleiman A, Mayer B, et al. (2009) Histogenomics: association of gene expression patterns with histological parameters in kidney biopsies. Transplantation 87: 290–295.
9. Rudnicki M, Perco P, Enrich J, Eder S, Heininger D, et al. (2009) Hypoxia response and VEGF-A expression in human proximal tubular epithelial cells in stable and progressive renal disease. Lab Invest 89: 337–346.
10. Schmid H, Boucherot A, Yasuda Y, Henger A, Brunner B, et al. (2006) Modular activation of nuclear factor-kappaB transcriptional programs in human diabetic nephropathy. Diabetes 55: 2993–3003.
11. Dours-Zimmermann MT, Zimmermann DR (1994) A novel glycosaminoglycan attachment domain identified in two alternative splice variants of human versican. J Biol Chem 269: 32992–32998.
12. Ricciardelli C, Brooks JH, Suwiwat S, Sakko AJ, Mayne K, et al. (2002) Regulation of stromal versican expression by breast cancer cells and importance to relapse-free survival in patients with node-negative primary breast cancer. Clin Cancer Res 8: 1054–1060.
13. Sakko AJ, Ricciardelli C, Mayne K, Tilley WD, Lebaron RG, et al. (2001) Versican accumulation in human prostatic fibroblast cultures is enhanced by prostate cancer cell-derived transforming growth factor beta1. Cancer Res 61: 926–930.
14. Nikitovic D, Zafiropoulos A, Katonis P, Tsatsakis A, Theocharis AD, et al. (2006) Transforming growth factor-beta as a key molecule triggering the expression of versican isoforms v0 and v1, hyaluronan synthase-2 and synthesis of hyaluronan in malignant osteosarcoma cells. IUBMB Life 58: 47–53.
15. Dours-Zimmermann MT, Maurer K, Rauch U, Stoffel W, Fassler R, et al. (2009) Versican V2 assembles the extracellular matrix surrounding the nodes of ranvier in the CNS. J Neurosci 29: 7731–7742.
16. Miquel-Serra L, Serra M, Hernandez D, Domenzain C, Docampo MJ, et al. (2006) V3 versican isoform expression has a dual role in human melanoma tumor growth and metastasis. Lab Invest 86: 889–901.
17. Theocharis AD (2008) Versican in health and disease. Connect Tissue Res 49: 230–234.
18. Wight TN, Merrilees MJ (2004) Proteoglycans in atherosclerosis and restenosis: key roles for versican. Circ Res 94: 1158–1167.
19. Ricciardelli C, Mayne K, Sykes PJ, Raymond WA, McCaul K, et al. (1998) Elevated levels of versican but not decorin predict disease progression in early-stage prostate cancer. Clin Cancer Res 4: 963–971.
20. Melk A, Mansfield ES, Hsieh SC, Hernandez-Boussard T, Grimm P, et al. (2005) Transcriptional analysis of the molecular basis of human kidney aging using cDNA microarray profiling. Kidney Int 68: 2667–2679.
21. Einecke G, Reeve J, Sis B, Mengel M, Hidalgo L, et al. (2010) A molecular classifier for predicting future graft loss in late kidney transplant biopsies. J Clin Invest 120: 1862–1872.
22. Bode-Lesniewska B, Dours-Zimmermann MT, Odermatt BF, Briner J, Heitz PU, et al. (1996) Distribution of the large aggregating proteoglycan versican in adult human tissues. J Histochem Cytochem 44: 303–312.
23. True LD, Hawley S, Norwood TH, Braun KR, Evanko SP, et al. (2009) The accumulation of versican in the nodules of benign prostatic hyperplasia. Prostate 69: 149–158.
24. Sheng W, Wang G, La Pierre DP, Wen J, Deng Z, et al. (2006) Versican mediates mesenchymal-epithelial transition. Mol Biol Cell 17: 2009–2020.
25. Sheng W, Wang G, Wang Y, Liang J, Wen J, et al. (2005) The roles of versican V1 and V2 isoforms in cell proliferation and apoptosis. Mol Biol Cell 16: 1330–1340.
26. Kawashima H, Hirose M, Hirose J, Nagakubo D, Plaas AH, et al. (2000) Binding of a large chondroitin sulfate/dermatan sulfate proteoglycan, versican, to L-selectin, P-selectin, and CD44. J Biol Chem 275: 35448–35456.
27. Hirose J, Kawashima H, Yoshie O, Tashiro K, Miyasaka M (2001) Versican interacts with chemokines and modulates cellular responses. J Biol Chem 276: 5228–5234.
28. Wu YJ, La Pierre DP, Wu J, Yee AJ, Yang BB (2005) The interaction of versican with its binding partners. Cell Res 15: 483–494.
29. Schuttert JB, Liu MH, Gliem N, Fiedler GM, Zopf S, et al. (2003) Human renal fibroblasts derived from normal and fibrotic kidneys show differences in increase of extracellular matrix synthesis and cell proliferation upon angiotensin II exposure. Pflugers Arch 446: 387–393.
30. Kogan I, Goldfinger N, Milyavsky M, Cohen M, Shats I, et al. (2006) hTERT-immortalized prostate epithelial and stromal-derived cells: an authentic in vitro model for differentiation and carcinogenesis. Cancer research 66: 3531–3540.
31. Massoner P, Haag P, Seifarth C, Jurgeit A, Rogatsch H, et al. (2008) Insulin-like growth factor binding protein-3 (IGFBP-3) in the prostate and in prostate cancer: local production, distribution and secretion pattern indicate a role in stromal-epithelial interaction. The Prostate 68: 1165–1178.
32. Klocker H, Kaspar F, Eberle J, Uberreiter S, Radmayr C, et al. (1992) Point mutation in the DNA binding domain of the androgen receptor in two families with Reifenstein syndrome. American journal of human genetics 50: 1318–1327.
33. Rosenkranz AR, Mendrick DL, Cotran RS, Mayadas TN (1999) P-selectin deficiency exacerbates experimental glomerulonephritis: a protective role for endothelial P-selectin in inflammation. J Clin Invest 103: 649–659.
34. Zoja C, Corna D, Camozzi D, Cattaneo D, Rottoli D, et al. (2002) How to fully protect the kidney in a severe model of progressive nephropathy: a multidrug approach. Journal of the American Society of Nephrology : JASN 13: 2898–2908.
35. Remuzzi G, Zoja C, Remuzzi A, Rossini M, Battaglia C, et al. (1985) Low-protein diet prevents glomerular damage in adriamycin-treated rats. Kidney international 28: 21–27.
36. Zoja C, Corna D, Gagliardini E, Conti S, Arnaboldi L, et al. (2010) Adding a statin to a combination of ACE inhibitor and ARB normalizes proteinuria in experimental diabetes, which translates into full renoprotection. American journal of physiology Renal physiology 299: F1203–1211.
37. Bellezza I, Neuwirt H, Nemes C, Cavarretta IT, Puhr M, et al. (2006) Suppressor of cytokine signaling-3 antagonizes cAMP effects on proliferation and apoptosis and is expressed in human prostate cancer. The American journal of pathology 169: 2199–2208.

8

Aortic Calcification and Femoral Bone Density are Independently Associated with Left Ventricular Mass in Patients with Chronic Kidney Disease

Colin D. Chue[1,2], Nadezhda A. Wall[3], Nicola J. Crabtree[4], Daniel Zehnder[5], William E. Moody[1,2], Nicola C. Edwards[1,2], Richard P. Steeds[2], Jonathan N. Townend[2], Charles J. Ferro[6]*

1 School of Clinical and Experimental Medicine, College of Medical and Dental Sciences, University of Birmingham, Birmingham, United Kingdom, **2** Department of Cardiology, Queen Elizabeth Hospital Birmingham, Birmingham, United Kingdom, **3** School of Immunity and Infection, College of Medical and Dental Sciences, University of Birmingham, Birmingham, United Kingdom, **4** Department of Endocrinology, Birmingham Children's Hospital, Birmingham, United Kingdom, **5** Clinical Sciences Research Institute, University of Warwick, Coventry, United Kingdom, **6** Department of Nephrology, Queen Elizabeth Hospital Birmingham, Birmingham, United Kingdom

Abstract

Background: Vascular calcification and reduced bone density are prevalent in chronic kidney disease and linked to increased cardiovascular risk. The mechanism is unknown. We assessed the relationship between vascular calcification, femoral bone density and left ventricular mass in patients with stage 3 non-diabetic chronic kidney disease in a cross-sectional observational study.

Methodology and Principal Findings: A total of 120 patients were recruited (54% male, mean age 55±14 years, mean glomerular filtration rate 50±13 ml/min/1.73 m^2). Abdominal aortic calcification was assessed using lateral lumbar spine radiography and was present in 48%. Mean femoral Z-score measured using dual energy x-ray absorptiometry was 0.60±1.06. Cardiovascular magnetic resonance imaging was used to determine left ventricular mass. One patient had left ventricular hypertrophy. Subjects with aortic calcification had higher left ventricular mass compared to those without (56±16 vs. 48±12 g/m^2, P = 0.002), as did patients with femoral Z-scores below zero (56±15 vs. 49±13 g/m^2, P = 0.01). In univariate analysis presence of aortic calcification correlated with left ventricular mass (r = 0.32, P = 0.001); mean femoral Z-score inversely correlated with left ventricular mass (r = −0.28, P = 0.004). In a multivariate regression model that included presence of aortic calcification, mean femoral Z-score, gender and 24-hour systolic blood pressure, 46% of the variability in left ventricular mass was explained (P<0.001).

Conclusions: In patients with stage 3 non-diabetic chronic kidney disease, lower mean femoral Z-score and presence of aortic calcification are independently associated with increased left ventricular mass. Further research exploring the pathophysiology that underlies these relationships is warranted.

Editor: Xing-Ming Shi, Georgia Health Sciences University, United States of America

Funding: This work was funded by an unrestricted educational grant from Genzyme Corporation. Genzyme Corporation had no role in study design, data collection and analysis, decision to publish, or in preparation of the manuscript.

Competing Interests: The authors have read the journal's policy and have the following conflicts: CJF, JNT, RPS and CDC are recipients of an unrestricted educational grant from Genzyme Corporation. CJF and CDC have received lecture fees and advisory board fees from Genzyme Corporation. This does not alter the authors' adherence to all the PLoS ONE policies on sharing data and materials.

* E-mail: charles.ferro@uhb.nhs.uk

Introduction

Cardiovascular morbidity and mortality are increased in patients with chronic kidney disease (CKD) and have an independent inverse relationship with glomerular filtration rate (GFR) [1]. There is accumulating evidence that much of this increased risk is due to underlying structural heart disease, such as left ventricular hypertrophy (LVH), leading to arrhythmia and heart failure [2,3]. Left ventricular mass (LVM) assessed as a continuous variable is increasingly recognised as an important prognostic marker [4], and reductions in LVM are associated with improved outcome in patients with increased cardiovascular risk [5].

Patients with CKD have deranged bone-mineral metabolism, with increased levels of the phosphaturic hormone fibroblast growth factor 23 (FGF-23) and parathyroid hormone (PTH) arising from impaired renal excretion of phosphate and impaired vitamin D activation [6]. Bone mineral density (BMD) measured using dual-energy x-ray absorptiometry (DEXA) scanning is commonly reduced in patients with CKD [7] and is an independent predictor of cardiovascular mortality in dialysis patients [8]. Vascular calcification is also highly prevalent in CKD [9] and end stage kidney disease (ESKD) [10] and is associated with increased mortality [11,12]. The mechanism by which reduced BMD and vascular calcification might influence cardiovascular outcome in CKD is unknown. We therefore explored the relationship between femoral BMD, vascular calcification and LVM, measured using the gold-standard technique of cardiovascular magnetic resonance imaging, in a cohort of patients with stage 3 non-diabetic CKD.

Methods

Objectives

To determine the relationship between femoral bone density, presence of vascular calcification and LVM in patients with stage 3 non-diabetic CKD.

Participants

Subjects were recruited from the renal clinics at the Queen Elizabeth Hospital Birmingham, UK, from 2009 to 2011. Patients were included if aged 18–80 years with stage 3 CKD (GFR 30–59 mL/min/1.73 m^2) [13] and no change in medication in the preceding three months. Patients with heart failure, atrial fibrillation, moderate or severe valvular disease, uncontrolled hypertension (office blood pressure >140/90 mmHg), total serum cholesterol >5.5 mmol/L whether on or off treatment and diabetes mellitus were excluded. Patients receiving treatment with a phosphate binder or vitamin D analogue were also excluded.

Data collection

Demographic data including body mass index and heart rate were recorded. Routine haematological and biochemical parameters were measured. Serum calcium levels were corrected for serum albumin. GFR was estimated (eGFR) using the four-variable Modification of Diet in Renal Disease formula with serum creatinine recalibrated to be traceable to an isotope derived mass spectroscopy method [14]. High sensitive C-reactive protein (hsCRP) was measured using a validated immunoassay (IBL International GMBH, Hamburg, Germany). Albuminuria was measured using a spot albumin: creatinine ratio. Calcium-phosphate homeostasis was assessed through measurement of the phosphatonin FGF-23, its soluble co-receptor klotho, and vitamin D. Fibroblast growth factor 23 was measured using a two-site enzyme-linked immunosorbent assay (Kainos Laboratories Inc., Tokyo, Japan). Soluble serum α-klotho was determined using a solid phase sandwich immunoassay (Immuno-Biological Laboratories Co., Japan). 1,25-dihydroxyvitamin D was measured using immunoextraction followed by quantitation by immunoassay (Immunodiagnostic Systems Ltd, Tyne and Wear, UK). 25-hydroxyvitamin D was measured by liquid chromatography-tandem mass spectrometry. Urinary fractional excretion of phosphate was calculated from 24-hour urine collections using the equation [(urine phosphate x serum creatinine)/(urine creatinine x serum phosphate)] x100, which allows correction for incomplete urine collections over 24-hours and standardises urinary phosphate excretion according to degree of renal impairment [15]. Office brachial blood pressure (BP) was recorded in the non-dominant arm in triplicate following 15 minutes of supine rest using a validated oscillometric sphygmomanometer (Dinamap ProCare 200, GE Healthcare, United Kingdom) [16] according to British Hypertension Society guidelines [17]. All subjects underwent twenty-four hour ambulatory BP measurement (Meditech ABPM-04, PMS Instruments, Maidenhead, United Kingdom). Arterial stiffness was assessed using the gold-standard measurement of carotid-femoral pulse wave velocity (PWV, SphygmoCor, AtCor Medical, Sydney) as previously described using a high fidelity micromanometer (SPC-301, Millar Instruments, Texas) to sequentially record electrocardiographically-gated carotid and femoral waveforms following 15 minutes of supine rest [18].

Assessment of bone density

Dual energy x-ray absorptiometry scanning (Hologic QDR Series 4500 with Discovery Software version 11.02:03, Hologic Europe, Zaventem, Belgium) was used to assess BMD of both proximal femurs (femoral neck, Ward's region, trochanteric region). All scans were reported by an experienced bone densitometry clinical scientist blinded to clinical data. T-scores that refer to the young adult reference mean calculated from the manufacturer's database (based on the National Health and Nutrition Examination Survey (NHANES) population) [19] were determined. Osteopenia and osteoporosis were defined according to the World Health Organisation definitions (normal bone T-score >-1, osteopenia T-score -1 to -2.5 and osteoporosis T-score <-2.5). The BMD of each subject was standardised by calculating the difference between the observed and predicted values (sourced from the manufacturer's reference database based on the NHANES population) [19] divided by the square root of the estimated variance. This derived standard score, or Z-score, is a measure of the deviation from the expected population mean, adjusted for the covariance on a scale with zero mean and unit standard deviation, so that 95% of the normal population will have a Z-score between -2 and 2 [20]. Coefficients of variation in our clinic are 1.1%.

Assessment of aortic calcification

The presence and extent of abdominal aortic calcification were assessed using a lateral lumbar spine radiograph and validated semi-quantitative scoring method as previously described [21]. This semi-quantitative technique shows good correlation with electron beam computed tomography assessment [22]. The abdominal aorta adjacent to the L1-L4 vertebra was divided into four sections using the midpoint of each intervertebral space as a boundary. The anterior and posterior aortic walls of each section were scored out of 3 according to the extent of calcification present with a maximum score of 24 for the entire abdominal aorta. All radiographs were analysed and scored by two independent observers. Any discordance in the presence or absence of calcification between the two observers resulted in re-assessment of that radiograph and evaluation by a radiologist to reach a final consensus.

Cardiovascular magnetic resonance imaging

Cardiovascular magnetic resonance imaging was performed on a 1.5 Tesla scanner (Symphony, Siemens, Erlangen, Germany). Serial contiguous short axis cines were piloted from the vertical long axis and horizontal long axis of the left ventricle (electrocardiographically-gated, steady-state free precession imaging [True-FISP]; temporal resolution 40–50 ms, repetition time 3.2 ms, echo time 1.6 ms, flip angle 60°, slice thickness 7 mm) in accordance with previously validated methodologies [23]. Analysis was performed offline (Argus Software, Siemens, Erlangen, Germany) by a single observer for measurement of left ventricular function, volumes and LVM [23], which was indexed to body surface area (LVMI; Mosteller formula, BSA (m^2) = $\sqrt{}$((weight (kg) × height (cm))/3600). Left ventricular hypertrophy was defined as an LVMI greater than age and gender corrected limits [23].

Ethics

West Midlands Research Ethics Committee approved the study and written informed consent was obtained from each participant. The study was conducted in accordance with the *Declaration of Helsinki* and the principles of *Good Clinical Practice.*

Table 1. Demographic data for all subjects and according to presence or absence of abdominal aortic calcification.

	All Patients (n = 120)	Calcification (n = 57)	No Calcification (n = 63)	P
Age	55±14	63±11	47±12	<0.001
Males (%)	65 (54)	38 (67)	27 (43)	0.01
History of cardiovascular disease (%)	13 (11)	12 (21)	1 (2)	0.002
Smokers (%)	64 (53)	38 (68)	26 (41)	0.007
Body mass index (kg/m^2)	29.0±5.5	29.2±3.5	28.9±6.9	0.71
Office systolic blood pressure (mmHg)	128±17	133±17	123±15	0.001
Office diastolic blood pressure (mmHg)	71±11	71±12	72±10	0.61
Pulse pressure (mmHg)	57±17	62±19	52±13	<0.001
24-hour systolic blood pressure (mmHg)	124±12	127±12	121±12	0.007
24-hour diastolic blood pressure (mmHg)	71±9	70±8	72±9	0.19
24-hour pulse pressure (mmHg)	53±11	57±12	49±8	<0.001
Heart rate (bpm)	63±10	62±12	63±9	0.82

Data are mean±standard deviation or frequency (%). Analysed using unpaired t-tests or χ^2.

Statistical methods

All data were analysed using SPSS version 19 (SPSS Inc, Chicago, Il, USA). Data are shown as mean±standard deviation, frequency (percentage) or median (interquartile range). Data distribution was tested using the Kolmogorov-Smirnov test and normality plots. Normally distributed variables were analysed using unpaired t-tests and χ^2. Variables not normally distributed were log transformed prior to analysis (serum triglycerides, hsCRP, PTH, FGF-23, albumin-creatinine ratio, urinary fractional excretion of phosphate and PWV). Analysis of variance with *post hoc* Tukey was conducted to assess the impact of mean hip Z-score and presence of vascular calcification on LVMI. Pearson correlation and linear regression were used to assess the relationship between two continuous variables. Colinearity between variables was assessed by examining the variance inflation factor; a value >5 indicated colinearity. A Type I error rate below 5% (P<0.05) was considered statistically significant.

Table 2. Renal diagnoses.

Renal Diagnosis	Frequency (%)
Hypertensive nephropathy	16 (13)
IgA nephropathy	13 (11)
Reflux nephropathy	12 (10)
Adult polycystic kidney disease	12 (10)
Systemic vasculitis	13 (11)
Focal segmental glomerulosclerosis	8 (7)
Nephrectomy for neoplasm	5 (4)
Other glomerulonephritis	7 (6)
Other	30 (25)
Unknown	4 (3)

Data are frequency (percentage).

Reproducibility

Intraobserver variability for LVMI was determined by random selection of twelve scans (10% of the cohort) for repeat analysis by the same observer. Interobserver variability for aortic calcification score was determined by comparing calcification scores between two observers for all 120 subjects. Variability of LVMI and aortic calcification score was determined using an intraclass correlation coefficient and two-way random effects model.

Results

Participants

Of the 1297 patients with non-diabetic CKD screened in the outpatient renal clinics, 602 met the study entry criteria. In total 494 patients were approached to take part in the CRIB-PHOS

Table 3. Medication use.

Medication	Frequency (%)
ACEI	64 (53)
ARB	32 (27)
ACEI and/or ARB	92 (77)
Aspirin	23 (19)
Statin	53 (44)
Other lipid lowering therapy	6 (6)
β-blocker	20 (17)
Calcium-channel blocker	33 (28)
Diuretic	32 (27)
α-blocker	17 (14)
Calcium supplement	8 (7)
Bisphosphonate	9 (8)
Prednisolone	18 (15)
Immunosuppressant	23 (19)

Data are frequency (percentage). ACEI, angiotensin converting enzyme inhibitor; ARB, angiotensin receptor blocker.

Table 4. Biochemical data for all subjects and according to presence or absence of abdominal aortic calcification.

	All Patients (n = 120)	Calcification (n = 57)	No Calcification (n = 63)	P
eGFR (mL/min/1.73m^2)	50±13	48±13	52±13	0.09
Total cholesterol (mmol/L)	4.9±1.2	4.8±1.1	5.0±1.3	0.32
Triglycerides (mmol/L)	1.16 (0.84–2.00)	1.39 (0.98–2.15)	0.98 (0.73–1.40)	0.01
hsCRP (μg/mL)	2.21 (1.15–6.37)	3.02 (1.13–8.52)	1.96 (1.15–5.96)	0.54
Phosphate (mmol/L)	1.03±0.16	1.03±0.17	1.03±0.17	0.98
Phosphate >1.4mmol/L (%)	4 (3)	2 (4)	2 (3)	1.00
Calcium (mmol/L)	2.21±0.09	2.23±0.09	2.19±0.10	0.04
Parathyroid hormone (ng/L)[a]	52 (38–71)	55 (42–72)	47 (35–71)	0.14
Parathyroid hormone >65ng/L (%)[a]	36 (32)	18 (36)	18 (29)	0.54
Alkaline phosphatase (mmol/L)	182±56	188±58	177±55	0.25
Fibroblast growth factor 23 (pg/mL)	67.6 (50.3–85.2)	67.0 (52.8–86.2)	67.6 (45.7–83.3)	0.34
Klotho (pg/mL)	943 ± 396	951 ± 471	936 ± 317	0.84
1,25-dihydroxyvitamin D (pmol/L)	76.0 ± 31.0	74.3 ± 26.9	77.6 ± 34.5	0.57
25-hydroxyvitamin D (nmol/L)	55.6 ± 30.5	53.9 ± 29.5	57.2 ± 31.5	0.56
Albumin: creatinine ratio (mg/mmol)	6 (1–48)	8 (1–43)	3 (1–53)	0.86
Urinary fractional excretion of phosphate	21 (13–32)	19 (14–29)	21 (12–34)	0.74

[a]Data available for 112 subjects. Data are mean±standard deviation, frequency (%) or median (interquartile range). Analysed using unpaired t-tests or χ^2. eGFR, estimated glomerular filtration rate; hsCRP, high sensitive C-reactive protein.

study; 374 declined to participate and therefore 120 were recruited. Demographic data for these 120 subjects are shown in Table 1. The mean age of all participants was 55±14 years with 54% male. Renal diagnoses and medication use are detailed in Tables 2 and 3. Patients were on a mean of 1.7±1.2 antihypertensive agents with 77% receiving either an angiotensin converting enzyme inhibitor and/or an angiotensin receptor blocker. Biochemical data are shown in Table 4. Three per cent of patients had a serum phosphate above 1.4 mmol/L, the upper limit of normal for our assay. Thirty-six patients (32%) had a PTH value above the upper limit of normal for our assay (65 ng/L) and two had a PTH above twice the upper limit of normal. No patients had a serum calcium concentration greater than 2.60 mmol/L. Pulse wave velocity, left ventricular mass and bone density data are shown in Table 5. Ten patients (8%) had osteopenia, of which six were over the age of 50 years; no patients were overtly osteoporotic. Ten patients (8%) had a Z-score of less than −1; mean Z-score was 0.60±1.06. Almost half (48%) of all participants had detectable calcification of the aorta, with a median calcification score of 4 (range 1–18). Only one patient (1%) had LVH.

Aortic calcification

A comparison of demographics between patients with calcification and those without is shown in Table 1. Those with calcification were significantly older, more likely to be male and more likely to have a history of cardiovascular disease and smoking compared to those without. The only biochemical differences were higher serum triglycerides and higher serum calcium concentrations in patients with aortic calcification; there was no difference in serum phosphate, total cholesterol, hsCRP or eGFR (Table 4).

Table 5. Arterial stiffness, left ventricular mass and bone mineral density data for all subjects and according to presence or absence of abdominal aortic calcification.

	All Patients (n = 120)	Calcification (n = 57)	No Calcification (n = 63)	P
Pulse wave velocity (m/s)	8.9 (7.4–11.2)	10.0 (8.3–12.9)	8.0 (6.7–9.4)	<0.001
Pulse wave velocity$_{adj}$ (m/s)	9.1 (7.9–10.8)	10.4 (8.6–12.9)	8.2 (6.8–9.5)	<0.001
Left ventricular ejection fraction (%)	74±7	75±8	74±6	0.20
Left ventricular mass (g)	101±30	111±30	93±28	0.001
Left ventricular mass index (g/m^2)	52±13	57±14	48±11	0.001
Mean femoral bone mineral density (g/cm^2)	1.00±0.14	1.02±0.14	0.98±0.13	0.20
Mean femoral T-score	0.03±0.96	0.04±0.95	0.02±0.98	0.89
Mean femoral Z-score	0.60±1.06	0.77±1.04	0.45±1.06	0.10

Data are mean±standard deviation or median (interquartile range). Analysed using unpaired t-tests.

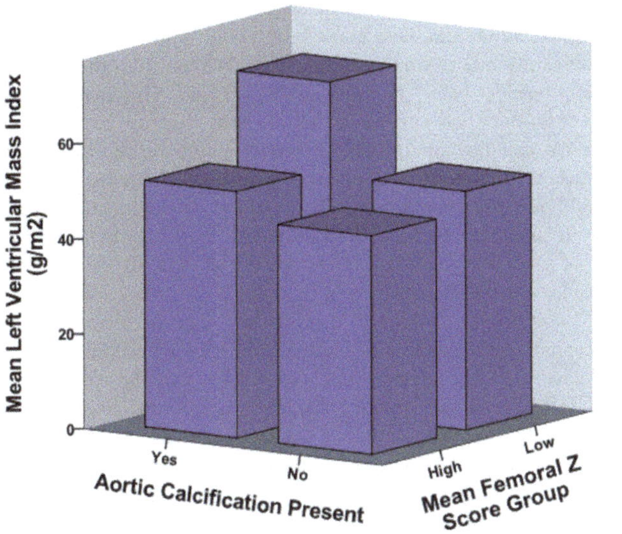

Figure 1. The relationship between aortic calcification, mean femoral Z-scores and left ventricular mass index. Both low mean femoral Z-score (below zero) and presence of aortic calcification were significantly associated with increased left ventricular mass index ($P<0.001$, two-way analysis of variance).

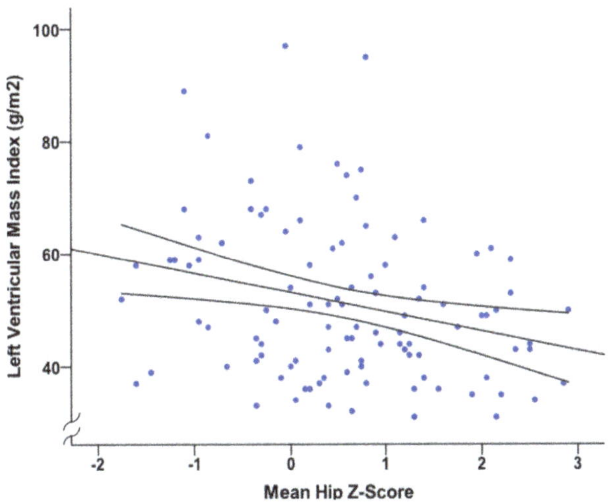

Figure 2. The relationship between mean femoral Z-score and left ventricular mass index. Data analysed using Pearson correlation ($r^2=0.072$, $P=0.006$).

There were also no significant differences in FGF-23, klotho or vitamin D. Individuals with calcification had stiffer arteries with significantly higher PWV (10.0 (8.3–12.9) vs. 8.0 (6.7–9.4) m/s, $P<0.001$) compared to those without (Table 5). Mean LVMI was also higher in patients with calcification (57 ± 14 vs. 48 ± 11 g/m^2, $P=0.001$). There was no significant difference in parameters of femoral bone density between the groups.

Effects of bone density and vascular calcification on left ventricular mass

Subjects were divided into two groups of high or low mean femoral Z-score according to whether their mean femoral Z-score was above or below zero (the standardised mean for the population). Patients in the high mean femoral Z-score group were older (58 ± 12 vs. 45 ± 13 years, $P<0.001$), heavier (mean weight 87 ± 15 vs. 74 ± 14 kg, $P<0.001$) and had significantly lower LVMI than those in the low Z-score group (50 ± 12 vs. 57 ± 15 g/m^2, $P=0.02$). There were no other demographic or biochemical differences between the groups; in particular there were no significant differences in markers of bone metabolism or inflammation. A two-way analysis of variance was used to explore the effect of high or low Z-scores and the presence or absence of aortic calcification on LVMI. Both Z-score grouping and presence of aortic calcification had significant effects on LVMI ($P<0.001$; Figure 1).

Correlates of left ventricular mass

In univariate analyses mean femoral Z-score and presence of aortic calcification correlated with LVMI ($r=-0.28$, $P=0.004$ and $r=0.32$, $P=0.001$ respectively; Figure 2 and Table 6). All variables that significantly correlated with LVMI in univariate analyses were entered into a multiple regression model (Table 6), with 24-hour systolic BP used as the most strongly correlated variable for BP. The model explained 46% of the variability in LVMI ($P<0.001$). Gender, 24-hour systolic BP, presence of aortic calcification and mean femoral Z-score emerged as independent predictors of LVMI, with systolic BP, presence of calcification and mean femoral Z-score each contributing to 4% of the variation in LVMI. Substitution of 24-hour systolic BP with office systolic BP made no appreciable difference to the model.

Reproducibility

Intraobserver variability for LVMI was excellent with an intraclass correlation coefficient of 0.992 (0.981–0.997, $P<0.001$). Interobserver variability for aortic calcification was also low with an intraclass correlation coefficient of 0.917 (0.883–0.941, $P<0.001$).

Discussion

In this cross-sectional observational study of patients with stage 3 non-diabetic CKD a significant independent inverse relationship between femoral bone density Z-scores and LVMI was demonstrated. Furthermore, the presence of aortic calcification was associated with increased aortic stiffness and significantly greater LVMI independent of bone density. Our findings highlight important links between bone disease, vascular calcification and LVM, a prognostically important cardiovascular variable.

Several population studies have linked reduced bone density and osteoporotic fractures with cardiovascular disease, especially heart failure, although the mechanisms are unknown [24,25,26,27]. Our findings suggest that underlying structural heart disease may be an important link. The presence of LVH as a marker of increased cardiovascular risk is well accepted, but the value of LVM as a continuous variable that has a graded relationship with cardiovascular risk is being increasingly recognised [4,28]. Only one other study to date has demonstrated an association between BMD and LVM. This cross-sectional study of 460 healthy individuals showed BMD to be an independent predictor of echocardiographically-derived LVMI in post-menopausal women but not in men [29].

Coronary artery calcification independently correlated with LVMI in a study of 118 haemodialysis patients [30]. Most of the patients in this study (75%) had established LVH on echocardiography. Our data extends these findings to include patients with early stage CKD, almost all of which had normal LVM. Vascular calcification has been shown to be a predictor of adverse cardiovascular outcome in several populations [11,12]. This has

Table 6. Univariate and multivariate analyses with left ventricular mass index as the outcome variable.

	Univariate		Multivariate	
	r	P	B	95% CI
Gender	−0.50	<0.001	−0.34	−13.45–−4.48
Office systolic blood pressure (mmHg)[a]	0.31	0.001		
24-hour systolic blood pressure (mmHg)	0.40	<0.001	0.23	0.07–0.43
24-hour pulse pressure (mmHg)[a]	0.30	0.002		
Parathyroid hormone (ng/L)	0.23	0.019	0.09	−4.66–17.37
Albumin: creatinine ratio (mg/mmol)	0.25	0.01	0.12	−0.54–3.43
Presence of aortic calcification	0.32	0.001	0.21	0.89–10.12
Mean femoral Z-score	−0.28	0.004	−0.23	−4.75–−0.85

[a]24-hour systolic blood pressure was used as the strongest correlating variable representing blood pressure in the model. Data analysed using Pearson correlation (univariate) and enter linear regression (multivariate). All variables that correlated significantly with left ventricular mass index in univariate analysis were entered into the multivariate regression model. R^2 for model = 0.46, P<0.001. For gender 0 = male, 1 = female. β, standardised coefficient; 95% CI, 95% confidence interval.

often been attributed to a high atherosclerotic burden. Our data also supports a contributory role for increased LVM.

Arterial stiffness is a powerful predictor of poor cardiovascular outcome [12] and a number of studies, including our own, have shown a relationship between vascular calcification and increased arterial stiffness in CKD [31] and ESKD patients [32,33,34]. Increased arterial stiffness is characterised by augmented systolic BP and pulse pressure, which can increase afterload on the left ventricle, thus promoting ventricular stiffening, hypertrophy and fibrosis [3]. Despite higher PWV in patients with calcification, we did not demonstrate an association between arterial stiffness and LVM. A relationship between arterial stiffness and LVMI has previously been demonstrated in ESKD patients [35], but this is not a consistent finding [36]. The near-normal PWV and LVM of our cohort may have masked any potential underlying relationship between these two variables.

Several reports from the general population have demonstrated an inverse association between severity of vascular calcification and bone density [37,38,39], with a similar relationship also being reported in dialysis patients using coronary artery calcification scoring [40,41]. Evidence of such a relationship in the early stage CKD population is limited. In a cross-sectional analysis of 48 patients with CKD (mean GFR 35±10 mL/min/1.73 m^2), Toussaint *et al* demonstrated an inverse correlation between femoral arterial calcification (but not aortic calcification) assessed using computed tomography (CT) and femoral BMD measured using DEXA scanning [31]. Filgueira *et al* divided 72 patients with stage 2–4 CKD into tertiles of vertebral bone density measured using CT and found those in the lowest bone density tertile to have significantly higher coronary artery calcification than those in the other tertiles [42]. In our study we did not demonstrate a relationship between bone density and presence or extent of vascular calcification. These differences may be explained by our exclusion of diabetic patients, the relative absence of established renal bone disease and relatively preserved kidney function in our cohort (mean GFR 50±13 mL/min/1.73 m^2) together with our use of a less sensitive semi-quantitative technique for detection of vascular calcification.

Abnormalities of mineral metabolism, such as elevated serum phosphate and calcium-phosphate product, have been identified as risk factors for the presence or progression of vascular calcification in CKD patients in a number of studies [41], but this finding is not consistent [9,31]. Similarly FGF-23 has been linked to calcification of peripheral arteries but not of the aorta [43]. Serum calcium and triglycerides were higher amongst patients with calcification in our cohort but there were no significant differences in serum phosphate, PTH, FGF-23, klotho, vitamin D, cholesterol or alkaline phosphatase between groups. Our study does not support a role for FGF-23, klotho or vitamin D as a mediator of increased LVM in the setting of vascular calcification and reduced bone density, but this requires confirmation with larger numbers of patients. Serum levels of calcium and phosphate are poor markers of total body calcium and phosphate content, and the prevalence of hyperphosphataemia amongst our cohort was low, most likely reflecting relatively preserved kidney function.

Limitations

Our study was observational and cross-sectional in design and thus subject to potential confounding from missing variables. We can only report associations and not infer causality. The use of lateral lumbar spine radiography and a semi-quantitative scoring method to assess severity of aortic calcification is not as sensitive as other modalities such as CT scanning and is therefore likely to have underestimated the prevalence of vascular calcification in our cohort. Nevertheless we were still able to demonstrate an independent relationship between severity of vascular calcification and LVM using this method.

Conclusion

In patients with stage 3 non-diabetic CKD lower femoral bone density Z-scores and presence of vascular calcification are independently associated with increased LVM. Further studies into the mechanisms and potential effect of treatments that maintain bone density and attenuate progression of vascular calcification on LVM are warranted.

Author Contributions

Conceived and designed the experiments: CJF JNT RPS CDC. Performed the experiments: CDC NAW WEM NCE RPS. Analyzed the data: CDC NAW NJC DZ RPS. Contributed reagents/materials/analysis tools: NJC DZ RPS. Wrote the paper: CDC CJF NAW WEM NCE JNT RPS.

References

1. Van Biesen W, De Bacquer D, Verbeke F, Delanghe J, Lameire N, et al. (2007) The glomerular filtration rate in an apparently healthy population and its relation with cardiovascular mortality during 10 years. Eur Heart J 28: 478−483.
2. Foley RN, Parfrey PS, Harnett JD, Kent GM, Martin CJ, et al. (1995) Clinical and echocardiographic disease in patients starting end-stage renal disease therapy. Kidney Int 47: 186−192.
3. Chue CD, Townend JN, Steeds RP, Ferro CJ (2010) Arterial stiffness in chronic kidney disease: causes and consequences. Heart 96: 817−823.
4. Schillaci G, Verdecchia P, Porcellati C, Cuccurullo O, Cosco C, et al. (2000) Continuous relation between left ventricular mass and cardiovascular risk in essential hypertension. Hypertension 35: 580−586.

5. Devereux RB, Wachtell K, Gerdts E, Boman K, Nieminen MS, et al. (2004) Prognostic significance of left ventricular mass change during treatment of hypertension. JAMA 292: 2350−2356.
6. Elder G (2002) Pathophysiology and recent advances in the management of renal osteodystrophy. J Bone Miner Res 17: 2094−2105.
7. Rix M, Andreassen H, Eskildsen P, Langdahl B, Olgaard K (1999) Bone mineral density and biochemical markers of bone turnover in patients with predialysis chronic renal failure. Kidney Int 56: 1084−1093.
8. Taal MW, Roe S, Masud T, Green D, Porter C, et al. (2003) Total hip bone mass predicts survival in chronic hemodialysis patients. Kidney Int 63: 1116−1120.
9. Russo D, Palmiero G, De Blasio AP, Balletta MM, Andreucci VE (2004) Coronary artery calcification in patients with CRF not undergoing dialysis. Am J Kidney Dis 44: 1024−1030.
10. Goodman WG, Goldin J, Kuizon BD, Yoon C, Gales B, et al. (2000) Coronary-artery calcification in young adults with end-stage renal disease who are undergoing dialysis. N Engl J Med 342: 1478−1483.
11. Adragao T, Pires A, Lucas C, Birne R, Magalhaes L, et al. (2004) A simple vascular calcification score predicts cardiovascular risk in haemodialysis patients. Nephrol Dial Transplant 19: 1480−1488.
12. Blacher J, Guerin AP, Pannier B, Marchais SJ, London GM (2001) Arterial calcifications, arterial stiffness, and cardiovascular risk in end-stage renal disease. Hypertension 38: 938−942.
13. (2002) K/DOQI clinical practice guidelines for chronic kidney disease: evaluation, classification, and stratification. Am J Kidney Dis 39: S1−266.
14. Levey AS BJ, Lewis JB, Greene T, Rogers N, Roth D (1999) A more accurate way to estimate glomerular filtration rate from serum creatinine: a new prediction equation. Modification of Diet in Renal Disease Study Group. Annals of Internal Medicine 130: 461−470.
15. Isakova T, Wahl P, Vargas GS, Gutierrez OM, Scialla J, et al. (2011) Fibroblast growth factor 23 is elevated before parathyroid hormone and phosphate in chronic kidney disease. Kidney Int 79: 1370−1378.
16. Reinders A, Reggiori F, Shennan AH (2006) Validation of the DINAMAP ProCare blood pressure device according to the international protocol in an adult population. Blood Press Monit 11: 293−296.
17. Williams B, Poulter NR, Brown MJ, Davis M, McInnes GT, et al. (2004) Guidelines for management of hypertension: report of the fourth working party of the British Hypertension Society, 2004-BHS IV. J Hum Hypertens 18: 139−185.
18. Edwards NC, Steeds RP, Stewart PM, Ferro CJ, Townend JN (2009) Effect of spironolactone on left ventricular mass and aortic stiffness in early-stage chronic kidney disease: a randomized controlled trial. J Am Coll Cardiol 54: 505−512.
19. Looker AC, Wahner HW, Dunn WL, Calvo MS, Harris TB, et al. (1998) Updated data on proximal femur bone mineral levels of US adults. Osteoporos Int 8: 468−489.
20. Seeman E, Hopper JL, Bach LA, Cooper ME, Parkinson E, et al. (1989) Reduced bone mass in daughters of women with osteoporosis. N Engl J Med 320: 554−558.
21. Kauppila LI, Polak JF, Cupples LA, Hannan MT, Kiel DP, et al. (1997) New indices to classify location, severity and progression of calcific lesions in the abdominal aorta: a 25-year follow-up study. Atherosclerosis 132: 245−250.
22. Bellasi A, Ferramosca E, Muntner P, Ratti C, Wildman RP, et al. (2006) Correlation of simple imaging tests and coronary artery calcium measured by computed tomography in hemodialysis patients. Kidney Int 70: 1623−1628.
23. Maceira AM, Prasad SK, Khan M, Pennell DJ (2006) Normalized left ventricular systolic and diastolic function by steady state free precession cardiovascular magnetic resonance. J Cardiovasc Magn Reson 8: 417−426.
24. Sennerby U, Melhus H, Gedeborg R, Byberg L, Garmo H, et al. (2009) Cardiovascular diseases and risk of hip fracture. JAMA 302: 1666−1673.
25. Gerber Y, Melton LJ 3rd, Weston SA, Roger VL (2011) Association between myocardial infarction and fractures: an emerging phenomenon. Circulation 124: 297−303.
26. Jankowska EA, Jakubaszko J, Cwynar A, Majda J, Ponikowska B, et al. (2009) Bone mineral status and bone loss over time in men with chronic systolic heart failure and their clinical and hormonal determinants. Eur J Heart Fail 11: 28−38.
27. Tanko LB, Christiansen C, Cox DA, Geiger MJ, McNabb MA, et al. (2005) Relationship between osteoporosis and cardiovascular disease in postmenopausal women. J Bone Miner Res 20: 1912−1920.
28. Turakhia MP, Schiller NB, Whooley MA (2008) Prognostic significance of increased left ventricular mass index to mortality and sudden death in patients with stable coronary heart disease (from the Heart and Soul Study). Am J Cardiol 102: 1131−1135.
29. Lim YH, Shin J, Lee JU, Lim HK, Hong S, et al. (2010) Bone Mineral Density is an Independent Determinant of Left Ventricular Mass Index in the General Female Population. Korean Circ J 40: 573−580.
30. Yildiz A, Memisoglu E, Oflaz H, Yazici H, Pusuroglu H, et al. (2005) Atherosclerosis and vascular calcification are independent predictors of left ventricular hypertrophy in chronic haemodialysis patients. Nephrol Dial Transplant 20: 760−767.
31. Toussaint ND, Lau KK, Strauss BJ, Polkinghorne KR, Kerr PG (2008) Associations between vascular calcification, arterial stiffness and bone mineral density in chronic kidney disease. Nephrol Dial Transplant 23: 586−593.
32. Sigrist M, Bungay P, Taal MW, McIntyre CW (2006) Vascular calcification and cardiovascular function in chronic kidney disease. Nephrol Dial Transplant 21: 707−714.
33. Haydar AA, Covic A, Colhoun H, Rubens M, Goldsmith DJ (2004) Coronary artery calcification and aortic pulse wave velocity in chronic kidney disease patients. Kidney Int 65: 1790−1794.
34. Guerin AP, London GM, Marchais SJ, Metivier F (2000) Arterial stiffening and vascular calcifications in end-stage renal disease. Nephrol Dial Transplant 15: 1014−1021.
35. Nitta K, Akiba T, Uchida K, Otsubo S, Otsubo Y, et al. (2004) Left ventricular hypertrophy is associated with arterial stiffness and vascular calcification in hemodialysis patients. Hypertens Res 27: 47−52.
36. Roman MJ, Ganau A, Saba PS, Pini R, Pickering TG, et al. (2000) Impact of arterial stiffening on left ventricular structure. Hypertension 36: 489−494.
37. Schulz E, Arfai K, Liu X, Sayre J, Gilsanz V (2004) Aortic calcification and the risk of osteoporosis and fractures. J Clin Endocrinol Metab 89: 4246−4253.
38. Kiel DP, Kauppila LI, Cupples LA, Hannan MT, O'Donnell CJ, et al. (2001) Bone loss and the progression of abdominal aortic calcification over a 25 year period: the Framingham Heart Study. Calcif Tissue Int 68: 271−276.
39. Banks LM, Lees B, MacSweeney JE, Stevenson JC (1994) Effect of degenerative spinal and aortic calcification on bone density measurements in post-menopausal women: links between osteoporosis and cardiovascular disease? Eur J Clin Invest 24: 813−817.
40. Braun J, Oldendorf M, Moshage W, Heidler R, Zeitler E, et al. (1996) Electron beam computed tomography in the evaluation of cardiac calcification in chronic dialysis patients. Am J Kidney Dis 27: 394−401.
41. Moe SM (2006) Vascular calcification and renal osteodystrophy relationship in chronic kidney disease. Eur J Clin Invest 36 Suppl 2: 51−62.
42. Filgueira A, Carvalho AB, Tomiyama C, Higa A, Rochitte CE, et al. (2011) Is coronary artery calcification associated with vertebral bone density in nondialyzed chronic kidney disease patients? Clin J Am Soc Nephrol 6: 1456−1462.
43. Inaba M, Okuno S, Imanishi Y, Yamada S, Shioi A, et al. (2006) Role of fibroblast growth factor-23 in peripheral vascular calcification in non-diabetic and diabetic hemodialysis patients. Osteoporos Int 17: 1506−1513.

9

Association of Chronic Kidney Disease and Peripheral Artery Disease with Inappropriate Left Ventricular Mass

Ho-Ming Su[1,3,4], Tsung-Hsien Lin[1,4], Po-Chao Hsu[1], Chee-Siong Lee[1,4], Wen-Hsien Lee[1], Szu-Chia Chen[2,3,4]*, Wen-Chol Voon[1,4], Wen-Ter Lai[1,4], Sheng-Hsiung Sheu[1,4]

1 Division of Cardiology, Department of Internal Medicine, Kaohsiung Medical University Hospital, Kaohsiung Medical University, Kaohsiung, Taiwan, 2 Division of Nephrology, Department of Internal Medicine, Kaohsiung Medical University Hospital, Kaohsiung Medical University, Kaohsiung, Taiwan, 3 Department of Internal Medicine, Kaohsiung Municipal Hsiao-Kang Hospital, Kaohsiung Medical University, Kaohsiung, Taiwan, 4 Faculty of Medicine, College of Medicine, Kaohsiung Medical University, Kaohsiung, Taiwan

Abstract

Inappropriate left ventricular mass index (LVM) may develop as a response to particular hemodynamic and metabolic alterations. Inappropriate LVM and peripheral artery disease (PAD) characterized by abnormally low or high ankle-brachial index (ABI) are common in chronic kidney disease (CKD) patients, in whom there may be a close and cause-effect relationship. The aim of this study is to assess whether CKD and abnormal ABI has an independent and additive association with inappropriate LVM. A total of 1110 patients were included in the study. Inappropriate LVM was defined as observed LVM more than 28% of the predicted value. The ABI was measured using an ABI-form device. PAD was defined as ABI <0.9 or ≥ 1.3 in either leg. Multivariate analysis showed that patients with estimated glomerular filtration rate (eGFR) <45 ml/min/1.73 m^2 (odds ratio [OR], 1.644; $P = 0.011$) and PAD (OR, 2.082; $P = 0.002$) were independently associated with inappropriate LVM. The interaction between eGFR <45 ml/min/1.73 m^2 and PAD on inappropriate LVM was statistically significant ($P = 0.044$). Besides, eGFR<45 ml/min/1.73 m^2 (change in observed/predicted LVM, 19.949; $P<0.001$) and PAD (change in observed/predicted LVM, 11.818; $P = 0.003$) were also significantly associated with observed/predicted LVM. Our findings show that eGFR <45 ml/min/1.73 m^2 and PAD are independently and additively associated with inappropriate LVM and observed/predicted LVM. Assessments of eGFR and ABI may be useful in identifying patients with inappropriate LVM.

Editor: Angelo Scuteri, INRCA, Italy

Funding: The authors have no support or funding to report.

Competing Interests: The authors have declared that no competing interests exist.

* E-mail: scarchenone@yahoo.com.tw

Introduction

A condition of growth of myocardium exceeding the hemodynamic needs has been reported and called inappropriate left ventricular mass (LVM). Predicted LVM for sex, height$^{2.7}$, and hemodynamic load can be used as an inappropriate reference for the observed LVM [1,2]. Recently, the presence of inappropriate LVM has been found in a significant proportion of patients with arterial hypertension, aortic stenosis, or chronic kidney disease (CKD) and has been reported to have a negative impact on cardiovascular prognosis [1,3–7]. Therefore, identifying patients with inappropriate LVM for aggressive treatment interventions is important.

Left ventricular hypertrophy (LVH) is not only highly prevalent in CKD patients but also often inappropriate [1,6,7]. Besides, high prevalence of peripheral artery disease (PAD) characterized by abnormal ankle-brachial index (ABI) is frequently noted in patients with CKD [8,9]. Abnormally low and high ABIs are affected by or linked to various risk factors for LVH, such as arterial stiffness, hypertension, and coexisting atherosclerosis [10,11]. There may be a close and cause-effect relationship between CKD, PAD and inappropriate LVM. However, there are limited studies to evaluate the association of CKD and PAD with inappropriate LVM. Accordingly, the aim of this study is to assess whether CKD and abnormal ABI has an independent and additive association with inappropriate LVM.

Subjects and Methods

Study Patients and Design

Study subjects were randomly included from a group of patients who arranged for echocardiographic examinations at Kaohsiung Municipal Hsiao-Kang Hospital. Patients with significant aortic or mitral valve disease, atrial fibrillation, or inadequate image visualization were excluded. We did not include all patients consecutively because ABI and blood pressures must be measured within 5 min after the completion of an echocardiographic examination. A total of 1110 patients (mean age 61.3±13.8 years, 646 males/464 females) were included.

Ethics Statement

The study protocol was approved by the institutional review board of the Kaohsiung Medical University Hospital (KMUH-IRB-20120131). Informed consents have been obtained in written form from patients and all clinical investigation was conducted according to the principles expressed in the Declaration of

Helsinki. The patients gave consent for the publication of the clinical details.

Evaluation of Cardiac Structure and Function

The echocardiographic examination was performed by one experienced cardiologist with a VIVID 7 (General Electric Medical Systems, Horten, Norway), with the participant respiring quietly in the left decubitus position. The cardiologist was blind to the other data. Two-dimensional and two-dimensionally guided M-mode images were recorded from the standardized views. The echocardiographic measurements included left ventricular internal diameter in diastole (LVIDd), left ventricular posterior wall thickness in diastole (LVPWTd), interventricular septal wall thickness in diastole (IVSTd), E-wave deceleration time, transmitral E wave velocity and transmitral A wave velocity. Left ventricular ejection fraction (LVEF) was measured by the modified Simpson's method. Left ventricular relative wall thickness (LVRWT) was calculated as the ratio of 2×LVPWTd/LVIDd. Observed LVM was calculated using Devereux-modified method, i.e. LVM = 1.04× [(IVSTd + LVIDd + LVPWTd)^3– LVIDd^3] –13.6 g [12]. Predicted LVM was estimated using the following equation [2]: predicted LVM = 55.37+6.64×height (m$^{2.7}$) +0.64×stroke work - 18.07×sex (in which sex was coded as male = 1 and female = 2). Stroke work was estimated as systolic blood pressure times stroke volume product and converted in gram meters by multiplying by 0.0144. Inappropriate LVM was also assessed as the ratio between observed and predicted LVM (observed/predicted LVM). LVM was defined 'inappropriate' when observed LVM was more than 28% of the predicted value (i.e. observed/predicted LVM >128%) [1,2].

Assessment of ABI

The values of ABI were measured by using an ABI-form device (VP1000; Colin Co. Ltd., Komaki, Japan), which automatically and simultaneously measured blood pressures in both arms and ankles using an oscillometric method [13–15]. The ABI was calculated by the ratio of the ankle systolic blood pressure divided by the arm systolic blood pressure. The ABI measurement was done once in each patient. PAD was defined as ABI <0.9 or ≥1.3 in either leg.

Collection of Demographic, Medical and Laboratory Data

Demographic and medical data, including age, gender and comorbid conditions were garnered from medical records or interviews with patients. Body mass index (BMI) was calculated as the ratio of weight in kilograms divided by square of height in meters. Blood samples were obtained within 1 month of enrollment. Laboratory data were measured from fasting blood samples using an autoanalyzer (Roche Diagnostics GmbH, D-68298 Mannheim COBAS Integra 400). Serum creatinine was measured by the compensated Jaffé (kinetic alkaline picrate) method in a Roche/Integra 400 Analyzer (Roche Diagnostics, Mannheim, Germany) using a calibrator traceable to isotope-dilution mass spectrometry [16]. The value of estimated glomerular filtration rate (eGFR) was calculated using the 4-variable equation in the Modification of Diet in Renal Disease (MDRD) study [17]. In addition, information regarding antihypertensive medications including angiotensin converting enzyme inhibitors (ACEI), angiotensin II receptor blockers (ARB), β-blockers, calcium channel blockers and diuretics during the study period was obtained from medical records.

Statistical Analysis

Statistical analysis was performed using SPSS 15.0 for windows (SPSS Inc. Chicago, USA). Data are expressed as percentages, mean ± standard deviation or median (25th–75th percentile) for triglyceride. Multiple comparisons among the study groups were performed by one-way analysis of variance (ANOVA) followed by post hoc test adjusted with a Boneferroni correction. The differences between patients with appropriate and inappropriate LVM were checked by Chi-square test for categorical variables or by independent t-test for continuous variables. Age, sex and non-echocardiographic variables which were significantly different between patients with appropriate and inappropriate LVM were selected for multivariate analysis. Hence, the adjusted covariates included age, sex, diabetes mellitus (DM), hypertension, coronary artery disease, PAD, mean arterial pressure, pulse pressure, BMI, log triglyceride, eGFR <45 ml/min/1.73 m^2, 4 study groups and medication including ACEI and/or ARB, β-blocker and diuretic use. Multiple logistic and linear regression analyses were used to identify the factors associated with inappropriate LVM and observed/predicted LVM. A difference was considered significant if the P value was less than 0.05.

Results

As can be seen in Table 1, the comparison of baseline and echocardiographic characteristics between patients with appropriate and inappropriate LVM, we studied 1110 patients (646 men and 464 women, mean age 61.3±13.8 years). The prevalence of inappropriate LVM was 68.3% and the value of observed/predicted LVM of all patients was 153.2±48.3%. Compared with patients with appropriate LVM, patients with inappropriate LVM were significantly associated with more male, higher prevalence of DM, higher prevalence of hypertension, higher prevalence of coronary artery disease, higher prevalence of PAD, lower mean arterial pressure, lower pulse pressure, higher BMI, higher triglyceride, lower eGFR, higher prevalence of eGFR <45 mL/min/1.73 m^2, more ACEI and/or ARB use, more β-blocker use, more diuretic use, lower LVEF and higher LVRWT. The prevalence of eGFR <45 mL/min/1.73 m^2 was higher in patients with inappropriate LVM (19.3% and 25.7%, P=0.019), but the prevalence of eGFR <60 mL/min/1.73 m^2 was comparable between the two groups (47.4% and 52.6%, P=0.107).

The study population was further classified into four groups according to eGFR ≥45 or <45 ml/min/1.73 m^2 and with/without PAD. Groups 1, 2, 3 and 4 were made up of patients with eGFR ≥45 ml/min/1.73 m^2 without PAD, eGFR <45 ml/min/1.73 m^2 without PAD, eGFR ≥45 ml/min/1.73 m^2 with PAD and eGFR <45 ml/min/1.73 m^2 with PAD, respectively. The comparison of clinical characteristics among the study groups was shown in Table 2. There were 737, 199, 110 and 644 patients in groups 1, 2, 3 and 4, respectively. The observed/predicted LVM in groups 1, 2, 3 and 4 were 147.3±43.6, 162.1±58.3, 159.2±46.5 and 182.7±52.8%, respectively. Additionally, the prevalence of inappropriate LVM in groups 1, 2, 3 and 4 were 64.7%, 70.4%, 78.2% and 87.5%, respectively.

Relation of eGFR <45 ml/min/1.73 m^2 and PAD to Inappropriate LVM and Observed/predicted LVM

Table 3 shows the odds ratio (OR) estimates for inappropriate LVM and the unstandardized coefficient β estimates for observed/predicted LVM with adjustment for age, sex, DM, hypertension, coronary artery disease, PAD, mean arterial pressure, pulse pressure, BMI, log triglyceride, eGFR <45 mL/min/1.73 m^2 and medication including ACEI and/or ARB, β-blocker and diuretic

Table 1. Comparison of baseline and echocardiographic characteristics between patients with appropriate and inappropriate left ventricular mass.

Characteristics	All patients (n = 1110)	Appropriate LVM (n = 352)	Inappropriate LVM (n = 758)
Age (year)	61.3±13.8	60.9±14.3	61.4±13.5
Male gender (%)	58.2	52.3	60.9*
Diabetes mellitus (%)	29.1	23.9	31.5*
Hypertension (%)	71.1	66.5	73.7*
Coronary artery disease (%)	19.8	15.3	21.9*
PAD (%)	15.7	9.4	18.6**
Mean arterial pressure (mmHg)	97.2±14.0	99.7±13.0	96.0±14.3**
Pulse pressure (mmHg)	58.6±14.6	61.2±14.3	57.4±14.5**
Body mass index (kg/m^2)	26.1±4.0	24.8±3.5	26.7±4.1**
Laboratory parameters			
Albumin (g/dL)	4.07±0.45	4.12±0.43	4.05±0.46
Fasting glucose (mg/dL)	114.2±41.5	112.7±41.2	115.0±41.6
Triglyceride (mg/dL)	124 (86–186)	118 (83–171)	128 (87–190.75)*
Total cholesterol (mg/dL)	191.2±43.8	193.1±42.8	190.3±44.2
Hematocrit (%)	40.2±5.6	40.2±5.0	40.1±5.9
Baseline eGFR (mL/min/1.73 m^2)	57.0±20.7	59.2±19.7	56.0±21.1*
eGFR <45 mL/min/1.73 m^2 (%)	23.7	19.3	25.7*
eGFR <60 mL/min/1.73 m^2 (%)	51.0	47.4	52.6
Medications			
ACEI and/or ARB use (%)	56.8	46.1	61.5**
β-blocker use (%)	43.5	38.0	46.0*
Calcium channel blocker use (%)	36.8	33.0	38.6
Diuretic use (%)	28.8	16.5	34.5**
Echocardiographic data			
Observed/predicted LVM (%)	153.2±48.3	108.7±16.6	173.8±44.0**
LVEF (%)	60.9±14.5	65.6±10.2	58.7±15.6**
LVRWT	0.38±0.09	0.35±0.07	0.40±0.09**
E-wave deceleration time (ms)	204.8±67.1	201.4±60.0	206.4±70.2
E/A	1.01±0.52	1.01±0.47	1.00±0.55

Abbreviations. LVM, left ventricular mass; PAD, peripheral artery disease; eGFR, estimated glomerular filtration rate; ACEI, angiotensin converting enzyme inhibitor; ARB, angiotensin II receptor blocker; LVEF, left ventricular ejection fraction; LVRWT, left ventricular relative wall thickness; E, transmitral E wave velocity; A, transmitral A wave velocity.
*P<0.05, **P<0.001 compared to patients with appropriate LVM.

use. In the multivariate logistic analysis, eGFR <45 mL/min/1.73 m^2 (OR, 1.644; 95% confidence interval [CI], 1.120 to 2.414; P=0.011) and PAD (OR, 2.082; 95% CI, 1.311 to 3.307; P=0.002) were significantly associated with inappropriate LVM. The interaction between eGFR <45 ml/min/1.73 m^2 and PAD on inappropriate LVM was statistically significant (OR, 2.982; 95% CI, 1.456 to 6.104; P=0.003). As for the relation of eGFR <45 mL/min/1.73 m^2 and PAD to observed/predicted LVM, the multivariate linear analysis shows eGFR <45 mL/min/1.73 m^2 (change in observed/predicted LVM, 19.949; 95% CI 13.098 to 26.800; P<0.001) and PAD (change in observed/predicted LVM, 11.818; 95% CI, 4.144 to 19.493; P=0.003) were independently associated with observed/predicted LVM.

Relation of Study Groups to Inappropriate LVM and Observed/predicted LVM

Table 4 displays the OR estimates for inappropriate LVM and the unstandardized coefficient β estimates for observed/predicted LVM with adjustment for age, sex, DM, hypertension, coronary artery disease, 4 study groups, mean arterial pressure, pulse pressure, BMI, log triglyceride, and medication including ACEI and/or ARB, β-blocker and diuretic use. In the multivariate logistic analysis, group 2 (OR, 1.626; 95% CI, 1.078 to 2.453; P=0.020; *vs.* group 1), group 3 (OR, 2.042; 95% CI, 1.201 to 3.471; P=0.008; *vs.* group 1) and group 4 (OR, 3.592; 95% CI, 1.481 to 8.712; P=0.005; *vs.* group 1) were significantly associated with inappropriate LVM. As for the relation of study groups to observed/predicted LVM, the multivariate linear analysis shows group 2 (change in observed/predicted LVM, 20.293; 95% CI 12.725 to 27.862; P<0.001; *vs.* group 1), group 3 (change in observed/predicted LVM, 12.356; 95% CI, 3.186 to 21.526; P=0.008; *vs.* group 1) and group 4 (change in observed/predicted LVM, 30.865; 95% CI, 17.796 to 43.934; P<0.001; *vs.* group 1) were independently associated with observed/predicted LVM.

Table 2. Comparison of baseline and echocardiographic characteristics among 4 study groups.

Characteristics	*Group 1* (n = 737)	*Group 2* (n = 199)	*Group 3* (n = 110)	*Group 4* (n = 64)
Age (year)	59.0±13.2	65.4±13.1*	63.4±15.1*	70.3±12.5*#
Male gender (%)	57.3	55.3	72.7*†	53.1
Diabetes mellitus (%)	22.8	40.2*	27.3	70.3*†#
Hypertension (%)	66.5	78.9	76.1	92.2*
Coronary artery disease (%)	17.6	19.2	38.2*†	15.6#
Mean arterial pressure (mmHg)	96.5±13.2	100.4±16.3*	95.1±13.9†	98.2±14.2
Pulse pressure (mmHg)	56.1±13.2	64.1±16.3*	59.4±15.1†	68.8±14.3*#
Body mass index (kg/m^2)	26.2±3.9	25.4±3.8	26.3±4.1	26.5±5.3
Laboratory parameters				
Albumin (g/dL)	4.18±0.37	3.90±0.50*	4.07±0.53	3.79±0.49*#
Fasting glucose (mg/dL)	111.7±37.7	119.0±50.4	116.0±46.1	128.8±43.3*
Triglyceride (mg/dL)	122.5 (84.75–183)	125.5 (90–189.75)	138 (84.5–210.5)	116.5 (87.25–169)
Total cholesterol (mg/dL)	194.9±44.1	180.4±42.5*	188.0±43.0	186.9±39.6
Hematocrit (%)	42.0±4.3	35.8±6.1*	40.5±5.7*†	34.1±5.5*#
Baseline eGFR (mL/min/1.73 m^2)	66.3±13.3	29.0±12.7*	63.4±12.5†	25.9±12.3*#
Medications				
ACEI and/or ARB use (%)	54.1	61.8	57.3	71.9*
β-blocker use (%)	42.4	48.7	45.5	35.9
Calcium channel blocker use (%)	31.0	48.2*	40.9	60.9*#
Diuretic use (%)	24.7	36.4*	26.4	56.3*†#
Echocardiographic data				
Observed/predicted LVM (%)	147.3±43.6	162.1±58.3*	159.2±46.5	182.7±52.8*†#
Inappropriate LVM (%)	64.7	70.4	78.2*	87.5*
LVEF (%)	62.3±13.6	58.8±16.2*	59.2±15.1	60.0±15.6
Relative wall thickness	0.38±0.09	0.38±0.09	0.37±0.10	0.41±0.10#
E-wave deceleration time (ms)	198.0±59.9	215.9±79.9*	224.1±76.8*	216.1±74.6
E/A	1.02±0.53	0.94±0.51	0.97±0.45	1.06±0.56

Groups 1, 2, 3 and 4 were made up of patients with eGFR ≥45 ml/min/1.73 m^2 without PAD, eGFR <45 ml/min/1.73 m^2 without PAD, eGFR ≥45 ml/min/1.73 m^2 with PAD and eGFR <45 ml/min/1.73 m^2 with PAD, respectively. Abbreviations are the same as in Table 1.
*$P<0.05$ compared with group 1;
†$P<0.05$ compared with group 2;
#$P<0.05$ compared with group 3.

Discussion

In the present study, we evaluated the association of CKD and PAD with inappropriate LVM and observed/predicted LVM and found eGFR <45 ml/min/1.73 m^2 and PAD were independently and additively associated with inappropriate LVM and observed/predicted LVM. In addition, patients with coexistence of eGFR <45 ml/min/1.73 m^2 and PAD had the highest value of observed/predicted LVM among 4 study groups.

The ABI is reported to be a good marker for atherosclerosis and an ABI <0.9 is useful in the diagnosis of peripheral artery occlusive disease (PAOD) [18–20]. In addition, an ABI ≥1.3 is considered to indicate medial artery calcification (MAC) [21]. High prevalence of PAOD and increased MAC are frequently

Table 3. Multivariate analyses of eGFR <45 mL/min/1.73 m^2 and PAD to inappropriate LVM and observed/predicted LVM.

Parameters	inappropriate LVM		observed/predicted LVM	
	Odds ratio (95% CI)	*P*	Unstandardized coefficient β (95% CI)	*P*
eGFR <45 mL/min/1.73 m^2	1.644 (1.120–2.414)	0.011	19.949 (13.098–26.800)	<0.001
PAD	2.082 (1.311–3.307)	0.002	11.818 (4.144–19.493)	0.003

Multivariate model: adjusted for age, sex, diabetes mellitus, hypertension, coronary artery disease, PAD, mean arterial pressure, pulse pressure, body mass index, log triglyceride, eGFR <45 mL/min/1.73 m^2 and medication including ACEI and/or ARB, β-blocker and diuretic use. Abbreviations are the same as in Table 1.

Table 4. Multivariate analyses of study groups to inappropriate LVM and observed/predicted LVM.

Parameters	inappropriate LVM		observed/predicted LVM	
	Odds ratio (95% CI)	*P*	Unstandardized coefficient β (95% CI)	*P*
Group 1	1		1	
Group 2	1.626 (1.078–2.453)	0.020	20.293 (12.725–27.862)	<0.001
Group 3	2.042 (1.201–3.471)	0.008	12.356 (3.186–21.526)	0.008
Group 4	3.592 (1.481–8.712)	0.005	30.865 (17.796–43.934)	<0.001

Multivariate model: adjusted for age, sex, diabetes mellitus, hypertension, coronary artery disease, 4 study groups, mean arterial pressure, pulse pressure, body mass index, log triglyceride and medication including ACEI and/or ARB, β-blocker and diuretic use. Groups 1, 2, 3 and 4 were made up of patients with eGFR ≥45 ml/min/1.73 m^2 without PAD, eGFR <45 ml/min/1.73 m^2 without PAD, eGFR ≥45 ml/min/1.73 m^2 with PAD and eGFR <45 ml/min/1.73 m^2 with PAD, respectively. Abbreviations are the same as in Table 1.

noted in patients with CKD [8,9], which may through multiple pathogenic mechanisms involved, including deranged calcium/phosphate balance, secondary hyperparathyroidism, homocysteine, lipoprotein(a) metabolism, alterations in inflammatory and coagulation pathways, fluid overload, alterations in the angiotensin and endothelin systems, malnutrition, uremic toxins, oxidative stress and insulin resistance [22–26]. Moreover, either abnormally low or high ABI can predict overall and cardiovascular mortality in patients with chronic renal failure [27,28]. In our study, eGFR <45 ml/min/1.73 m^2 and PAD were independently and additively associated with inappropriate LVM and observed/predicted LVM even after adjustment for many confounding factors. Hence, it suggested that CKD and PAD might have a synergic effect on inappropriate LVM.

Another finding of our study was that when compared between the two groups without PAD, only the group with eGFR <45 ml/min/1.73 m^2 was associated with inappropriate LVM. Recently, we also consistently demonstrated a significant trend for a stepwise increase in the observed/predicted LVM and in the prevalence of inappropriate LVM corresponding to advancement in CKD stages in CKD patients. Moreover, increased observed/predicted LVM was significantly associated with increased cardiovascular events in this population [7]. The possible mechanisms is that the hemodynamic and metabolic disturbances in patients with CKD may synergistically activate a variety of pathophysiological alterations including hemodynamic abnormalities (i.e. increased preload and afterload) and non-hemodynamic abnormalities (i.e. neuro-hormonal stressors, factors promoting myocardial fibrosis and atherosclerosis) and thus result in the excessive growth of LVM [29–33].

Similarly, when compared between the two groups without CKD, only the group with PAD was associated with inappropriate LVM. Previous studies demonstrated that the ABI value in the LVH group was significantly lower than that in the non-LVH group [34,35]. In addition, Ix JH et al. [36] evaluated the association between abnormally low or high ABI and LVMI in 4972 MESA (multi-Ethic Study of atherosclerosis) participants without clinical cardiovascular disease. They found either abnormally low or high ABI was significantly associated with greater left ventricular mass index. Our recent study in CKD patients also showed patients with abnormal ABIs had a greater LVMI [37]. These results suggested that low and high ABI might be related to LVH. Atherosclerosis directly caused a decrease in blood perfusion in the lower extremities and an increase in arterial wall stiffness, contributing to arterial distensibility, and then final progressed to LVH [9,38,39].

The definition and classification for CKD was proposed by the National Kidney Disease National Kidney Foundation Kidney Disease Outcomes Quality Initiative (NKF-KDOQI) in 2002 [40]. CKD was defined based on the presence of kidney damage or eGFR <60 ml/min/1.73 m^2 for more than 3 months, irrespective of cause. The high prevalence of early CKD stages may represent over-diagnosis of kidney disease and lead to the potential for overuse of substantially resources. Some have proposed a lower eGFR threshold (30 or 45 *vs.* 60 ml/min/1.73 m^2) to define the presence of CKD or to subdivide stage 3 into stage 3a (45–59 ml/min/1.73 m^2) and 3b (30–44 ml/min/1.73 m^2) [41,42]. In our study, eGFR <45 ml/min/1.73 m^2 was significantly associated with inappropriate LVM ($P=0.019$), but eGFR <60 ml/min/1.73 m^2 did not achieve significance ($P=0.107$). This finding supported the suggestion to lower the eGFR threshold for defining CKD. However, our study was only a cross-sectional one and lacked prognosis data. Thus, longer follow-up is required to clarify whether eGFR <45 ml/min/1.73 m^2 is a better prognostic parameter than eGFR <60 ml/min/1.73 m^2.

De Simone et al. [6] had evaluated the relations between inappropriate LVM and renal function in patients with CKD without known cardiac disease and found the prevalence of inappropriate LVM was higher in CKD patients than in healthy controls (43% *vs.* 10%, $P<0.001$). Besides, prevalence of inappropriate LVM paralleled the severity of renal dysfunction ranging from 10% in stage 1 CKD patients to 100% in stage 5 CKD patients. Nardi et al. [1] also investigated the comparison of the prevalence of inappropriate LVM between hypertensive patients with or without CKD. They found that the prevalence of inappropriate LVM was 52.5% in patients with CKD vs. 30.5% in hypertensive patients with normal renal function ($P<0.001$). In our study, the prevalence of inappropriate LVM was up to 68.3%. Because our study subjects were included from patients who arranged for echocardiographic examinations, they frequently had multiple comorbidities, such as DM, hypertension, coronary artery disease, PAD and CKD, which might partially explain the high prevalence of inappropriate LVM in our study.

There were several limitations to our study. Predicted LVM is calculated by age, gender, height and stroke work. Thus, a single blood pressure measurement may have a great impact on the calculation of predicted LVM. Average ambulatory blood pressure over 24 h may be more closely related to LVM than single clinic blood pressure measurement. In addition, treatment with antihypertensive drugs can potentially influence left ventricular geometry and functional parameters. In particular, the use of diuretics may reduce left ventricular diameter and thus cause a greater prevalence of inappropriate LVM. For ethical reason, we didn't hold any drugs at the time of echocardiographic evaluation. However, in order to elucidate the influence of drugs, we had added different classes of antihypertensive drugs in the analysis and still found CKD and PAD had a significant association with inappropriate LVM and observed/predicted LVM.

In conclusion, our study demonstrated that eGFR <45 ml/min/1.73 m^2 and PAD were independently and additively associated with inappropriate LVM and observed/predicted LVM. The combination of CKD and PAD might have a synergic effect on inappropriate LVM. Assessments of eGFR and ABI may be useful in identifying patients with inappropriate LVM.

Author Contributions

Conceived and designed the experiments: H-MS S-CC. Performed the experiments: H-MS T-HL P-CH C-SL W-HL S-CC. Analyzed the data: H-MS S-CC. Contributed reagents/materials/analysis tools: H-MS T-HL P-CH C-SL W-HL S-CC W-CV W-TL S-HS. Wrote the paper: H-MS S-CC.

References

1. Nardi E, Palermo A, Mule G, Cusimano P, Cottone S, et al. (2009) Left ventricular hypertrophy and geometry in hypertensive patients with chronic kidney disease. J Hypertens 27: 633–641.
2. de Simone G, Devereux RB, Kimball TR, Mureddu GF, Roman MJ, et al. (1998) Interaction between body size and cardiac workload: Influence on left ventricular mass during body growth and adulthood. Hypertension 31: 1077–1082.
3. Chinali M, De Marco M, D'Addeo G, Benincasa M, Romano C, et al. (2007) Excessive increase in left ventricular mass identifies hypertensive subjects with clustered geometric and functional abnormalities. J Hypertens 25: 1073–1078.
4. de Simone G, Palmieri V, Koren MJ, Mensah GA, Roman MJ, et al. (2001) Prognostic implications of the compensatory nature of left ventricular mass in arterial hypertension. J Hypertens 19: 119–125.
5. de Simone G, Verdecchia P, Pede S, Gorini M, Maggioni AP (2002) Prognosis of inappropriate left ventricular mass in hypertension: The mavi study. Hypertension 40: 470–476.
6. Cioffi G, Tarantini L, Frizzi R, Stefenelli C, Russo TE, et al. (2011) Chronic kidney disease elicits excessive increase in left ventricular mass growth in patients at increased risk for cardiovascular events. J Hypertens 29: 565–573.
7. Chen SC, Chang JM, Liu WC, Chen YY, Chen LI, et al. (2012) The ratio of observed to predicted left ventricular mass is independently associated with increased cardiovascular events in patients with chronic kidney disease. Hypertens Res 35: 832–838.
8. de Vinuesa SG, Ortega M, Martinez P, Goicoechea M, Campdera FG, et al. (2005) Subclinical peripheral arterial disease in patients with chronic kidney disease: Prevalence and related risk factors. Kidney Int Suppl 93: S44–47.
9. Leskinen Y, Salenius JP, Lehtimaki T, Huhtala H, Saha H (2002) The prevalence of peripheral arterial disease and medial arterial calcification in patients with chronic renal failure: Requirements for diagnostics. Am J Kidney Dis 40: 472–479.
10. Aboyans V, Ho E, Denenberg JO, Ho LA, Natarajan L, et al. (2008) The association between elevated ankle systolic pressures and peripheral occlusive arterial disease in diabetic and nondiabetic subjects. J Vasc Surg 48: 1197–1203.
11. Niederhoffer N, Lartaud-Idjouadiene I, Giummelly P, Duvivier C, Peslin R, et al. (1997) Calcification of medial elastic fibers and aortic elasticity. Hypertension 29: 999–1006.
12. Devereux RB, Alonso DR, Lutas EM, Gottlieb GJ, Campo E, et al. (1986) Echocardiographic assessment of left ventricular hypertrophy: Comparison to necropsy findings. Am J Cardiol 57: 450–458.
13. Tomiyama H, Yamashina A, Arai T, Hirose K, Koji Y, et al. (2003) Influences of age and gender on results of noninvasive brachial-ankle pulse wave velocity measurement–a survey of 12517 subjects. Atherosclerosis166: 303–309.
14. Yamashina A, Tomiyama H, Takeda K, Tsuda H, Arai T, et al. (2002) Validity, reproducibility, and clinical significance of noninvasive brachial-ankle pulse wave velocity measurement. Hypertens Res 25: 359–364.
15. Yokoyama H, Shoji T, Kimoto E, Shinohara K, Tanaka S, et al. (2003) Pulse wave velocity in lower-limb arteries among diabetic patients with peripheral arterial disease. J Atheroscler Thromb 10: 253–258.
16. Vickery S, Stevens PE, Dalton RN, van Lente F, Lamb EJ (2006) Does the id-ms traceable mdrd equation work and is it suitable for use with compensated jaffe and enzymatic creatinine assays? Nephrol Dial Transplant 21: 2439–2445.
17. Levey AS, Bosch JP, Lewis JB, Greene T, Rogers N, et al. (1999) A more accurate method to estimate glomerular filtration rate from serum creatinine: A new prediction equation. Modification of diet in renal disease study group. Ann Intern Med 130: 461–470.
18. Fishbane S, Youn S, Flaster E, Adam G, Maesaka JK (1996) Ankle-arm blood pressure index as a predictor of mortality in hemodialysis patients. Am J Kidney Dis 27: 668–672.
19. Fowkes FG, Housley E, Cawood EH, Macintyre CC, Ruckley CV, et al. (1991) Edinburgh artery study: Prevalence of asymptomatic and symptomatic peripheral arterial disease in the general population. Int J Epidemiol 20: 384–392.
20. Newman AB, Tyrrell KS, Kuller LH (1997) Mortality over four years in shep participants with a low ankle-arm index. J Am Geriatr Soc 45: 1472–1478.
21. Orchard TJ, Strandness DE, Jr (1993) Assessment of peripheral vascular disease in diabetes. Report and recommendations of an international workshop sponsored by the american heart association and the american diabetes association 18–20 september 1992, new orleans, louisiana. Diabetes Care 16: 1199–1209.
22. Levin A, Djurdjev O, Barrett B, Burgess E, Carlisle E, et al. (2001) Cardiovascular disease in patients with chronic kidney disease: Getting to the heart of the matter. Am J Kidney Dis 38: 1398–1407.
23. Shinohara K, Shoji T, Tsujimoto Y, Kimoto E, Tahara H, et al. (2004) Arterial stiffness in predialysis patients with uremia. Kidney Int 65: 936–943.
24. O'Hare A, Johansen K (2001) Lower-extremity peripheral arterial disease among patients with end-stage renal disease. J Am Soc Nephrol 12: 2838–2847.
25. O'Hare AM, Hsu CY, Bacchetti P, Johansen KL (2002) Peripheral vascular disease risk factors among patients undergoing hemodialysis. J Am Soc Nephrol 13: 497–503.
26. Webb AT, Franks PJ, Reaveley DA, Greenhalgh RM, Brown EA (1993) Prevalence of intermittent claudication and risk factors for its development in patients on renal replacement therapy. Eur J Vasc Surg 7: 523–527.
27. Guerrero A, Montes R, Munoz-Terol J, Gil-Peralta A, Toro J, et al. (2006) Peripheral arterial disease in patients with stages iv and v chronic renal failure. Nephrol Dial Transplant 21: 3525–3531.
28. Ono K, Tsuchida A, Kawai H, Matsuo H, Wakamatsu R, et al. (2003) Ankle-brachial blood pressure index predicts all-cause and cardiovascular mortality in hemodialysis patients. J Am Soc Nephrol 14: 1591–1598.
29. Ritz E (2006) Heart and kidney: Fatal twins? Am J Med 119: S31–39.
30. Levin A, Singer J, Thompson CR, Ross H, Lewis M (1996) Prevalent left ventricular hypertrophy in the predialysis population: Identifying opportunities for intervention. Am J Kidney Dis 27: 347–354.
31. Levin A, Thompson CR, Ethier J, Carlisle EJ, Tobe S, et al. (1999) Left ventricular mass index increase in early renal disease: Impact of decline in hemoglobin. Am J Kidney Dis 34: 125–134.
32. Scandinavian Simvastatin Survival Group (1994) Randomised trial of cholesterol lowering in 4444 patients with coronary heart disease: The scandinavian simvastatin survival study (4s). Lancet 344: 1383–1389.
33. Hunter JJ, Chien KR (1999) Signaling pathways for cardiac hypertrophy and failure. N Engl J Med 341: 1276–1283.
34. Devereux RB, Reichek N (1977) Echocardiographic determination of left ventricular mass in man. Anatomic validation of the method. Circulation 55: 613–618.
35. Fu W, Ye C, Mei C, Rong S, Wang W (2006) Reverse correlation between ankle-brachial index and left ventricular hypertrophy in patients on maintenance haemodialysis. Nephrology (Carlton) 11: 9–14.
36. Ix JH, Katz R, Peralta CA, de Boer IH, Allison MA, et al. (2010) A high ankle brachial index is associated with greater left ventricular mass mesa (multi-ethnic study of atherosclerosis). J Am Coll Cardiol 55: 342–349.
37. Su HM, Lin TH, Hsu PC, Chu CY, Lee WH, et al. (2012) Abnormally low and high ankle-brachial indices are independently associated with increased left ventricular mass index in chronic kidney disease. PLoS One (In press).
38. Roman MJ, Ganau A, Saba PS, Pini R, Pickering TG, et al. (2000) Impact of arterial stiffening on left ventricular structure. Hypertension 36: 489–494.
39. Roman MJ, Pickering TG, Schwartz JE, Pini R, Devereux RB (1995) Association of carotid atherosclerosis and left ventricular hypertrophy. J Am Coll Cardiol 25: 83–90.
40. Levey AS, Coresh J, Bolton K, Culleton B, Harvey KS, et al. (2002) Initiative KDOQ. K/DOQI clinical practice guidelines for chronic kidney disease: Evaluation, classification, and stratification. Am J Kidney Dis 39: S1–266.
41. Eckardt KU, Berns JS, Rocco MV, Kasiske BL (2009) Definition and classification of ckd: The debate should be about patient prognosis–a position statement from kdoqi and kdigo. Am J Kidney Dis 53: 915–920.
42. Levey AS, de Jong PE, Coresh J, El Nahas M, Astor BC, et al. (2011) The definition, classification, and prognosis of chronic kidney disease: A kdigo controversies conference report. Kidney Int 80: 17–28.

10

Swimming Exercise Prevents Fibrogenesis in Chronic Kidney Disease by Inhibiting the Myofibroblast Transdifferentiation

Chiung-Chi Peng[1,2,3]*, Kuan-Chou Chen[4,5], Chiu-Lan Hsieh[6], Robert Y. Peng[7]

1 Graduate Institute of Clinical Medicine, College of Medicine, Taipei Medical University, Taipei, Taiwan, **2** Department of Physical Therapy, Graduate Institute of Rehabilitation Science, China Medical University, Taichung, Taiwan, **3** Graduate Institute of Rehabilitation Science, China Medical University, Taichung, Taiwan, **4** Department of Urology, School of Medicine, College of Medicine, Taipei Medical University, Taipei, Taiwan, **5** Department of Urology, Shuang Ho Hospital, Taipei Medical University, Zhonghe, Taipei, Taiwan, **6** Graduate Institute of Biotechnology, National Changhua University of Education, 1, Changhua City, Taiwan, **7** Research Institute of Biotechnology, Hungkuang University, Shalu County, Taichung, Taiwan

Abstract

Background: The renal function of chronic kidney disease (CKD) patients may be improved by a number of rehabilitative mechanisms. Swimming exercise training was supposed to be beneficial to its recovery.

Methodology/Principal Findings: Doxorubicin-induced CKD (DRCKD) rat model was performed. Swimming training was programmed three days per week, 30 or 60 min per day for a total period of 11 weeks. Serum biochemical and pathological parameters were examined. In DRCKD, hyperlipidemia was observed. Active mesangial cell activation was evidenced by overexpression of PDGFR, P-PDGFR, MMP-2, MMP-9, α-SMA, and CD34 with a huge amount collagen deposition. Apparent myofibroblast transdifferentiation implicating fibrogenesis in the glomerular mesangium, glomerulonephritis and glomeruloscelorosis was observed with highly elevated proteinuria and urinary BUN excretion. The 60-min swimming exercise but not the 30 min equivalent rescued most of the symptoms. To quantify the effectiveness of exercise training, a physical parameter, i.e. "the strenuosity coefficient" or "the myokine releasing coefficient", was estimated to be 7.154×10^{-3} pg/mL-J.

Conclusions: The 60-min swimming exercise may ameliorate DRCKD by inhibiting the transdifferentiation of myofibroblasts in the glomerular mesangium. Moreover, rehabilitative exercise training to rescue CKD is a personalized remedy. Benefits depend on the duration and strength of exercise, and more importantly, on the individual physiological condition.

Editor: Krisztian Stadler, Pennington Biomedical Research Center, United States of America

Funding: The authors want to show their gratitude to the financial supports issued by the National Science Council (NSC 99-2320-B-038-011-MY3 and 99-2320-B-039-034) and those offered by Chinese Medical University (CMU99-N1-09 & CMU100-TS-07). The funders had no role in study design, data collection and analysis, decision to publish, or preparation of the manuscript.

Competing Interests: The authors have declared that no competing interests exist.

* E-mail: misspeng@ms2.hinet.net

Introduction

Chronic kidney disease (CKD) usually is associated with impaired cardiac and vascular functions, reduced muscle mass, attenuated muscle strength and power, and an apparent decreased tolerance to exercise [1]. Increasing awareness has prescribed exercise designed to restore certain extent of physical performance and quality of life under those conditions. Numerous interventions involving the aerobic and the resistance exercise training, either the treadmill running or swimming, have been reported beneficial to CKD [2,3,4]. Appreciating and understanding the function of exercise is vital to understanding how to prevent CKD which leads to end stage renal disease (ESRD). Pedersen & Fischer indicated strenuous exercise stimulates the myokine (interleukin-6, IL-6) release. The myokine IL-6 in priority is consumed intramuscularly under the influence of AMPK [5]. Different strength and duration of exercise can differentially release different kinds of cytokines [5,6,7]. Highly trained athletes usually exhibit a chronic mild hypercortisolism and activation of proinflammatory cytokine IL-6 [8]. IL-6 and TNF-α are produced as a consequence of inflammation [9]. Under many pathological conditions, IL-6 and TNF-α usually are counteracting [10,11,12].

PDGF is one of important cytokines involved in mesangial proliferation and renal fibrogenesis in glomerulonephritis and anti-Thy1 nephritis [13,14]. Almost all experimental and human renal diseases are characterized by altered expression of components of the PDGF system. Infusion or systemic overexpression of PDGF-B or PDGF-D induces prominent proliferative changes of mesangial and renal fibrosis [4]. While the action of PDGF is determined by the relative expression of PDGF alpha-receptors (PDGFR-α) and beta-receptors (PDGFR-β) on the surface of myofibroblasts. These receptors are induced during fibrogenesis, thereby amplifying biological responses to PDGF [7].

PDGFR and alpha-smooth muscle actin (α-SMA) are two markers of mesangial cell activation. Both signs are significantly correlated with the interstitial damage (interstitial infiltrate and fibrosis) [15].

In normal kidneys and in patients with mild histological lesions, the interstitial area showed scattered peritubular cells positive for PDGFR-β and α-SMA, with distribution resembling the capillary network. α-SMA is strikingly increased in patients with moderate to severe lesions, particularly in areas of tubulointerstitial fibrosis [15].

CD34, a sialomucin-type glycophosphoprotein acting as an adhesion molecule, is a marker of haematopoietic stem cells (HSCs) and leukemic cells [16,17,18,19]. CD34 is concentrated mostly in mesangial area and endothelial surfaces in glomeruli [18]. Overexpression of CD34 reflects the pathogenesis of glomerular alterations (e.g. glomerulonephritis) related to age, diabetes, and the severity of the disease [18,20,21]. Matrix metalloproteinase-2 (MMP-2) and -9 (MMP-9) may regulate collagen accumulation in CKD inflammatory sites, thus allowing cyst enlargement and limiting the severity of interstitial fibrosis [22].

It has raised evidences showing that chronic training from middle age to old age increases blood oxidative damage [23]. Exercise tends to increase oxidative stress as evidenced by stimulated production of MDA and concomitant downregulation of superoxide dismutase (SOD) [24], similar effect was reported by Coelho et al. (2010) [25]. Long-term exercise could increase damage markers like protein carbonyl content and lipid peroxidation in plasma and erythrocytes [23]. However, the efficiency may depend on the optimal type, frequency, intensity, and duration of the physical activity [26]. Controversial literature revealed chronic exercise appears to be an effective strategy to attenuate the age-related decline in the elderly [23]. Jia et al. (2012) demonstrated that long-term aerobic exercise could remarkably improve hemorheological property and the oxidative stress with hypercholesterolemia [27]. Overall, sport in general applied at moderate loads has predominantly positive effect on the health of humans especially concerning cardiovascular and metabolic diseases [28]. Swimming exercise at 30°C (considered as a cold exposure) evidently revealed beneficial cold specific changes, like increased dehydrogenase [29] and enhanced Ca^{2+}-activated myofibril ATPase activities [30]. In addition, exercise increases blood flow and oxygen supply [31]. Exercise training alters the vascular reactivity, enhances endothelium-dependent and -independent renal vasodilation [32]. Literature also indicated that nitric oxide can play an alternative role affecting the blood flow [31].

Considering swimming exercise may improve the flow of blood, oxygen and nutrients to kidneys, we hypothesize swimming exercise may help maintain renal health by excreting toxic metabolites, suppressing renal inflammation, reducing oxidative stress, and inhibiting fibrogenesis to improve CKD. We performed this study using the doxorubicin-Sprague-Dawley rat CKD model.

Materials and Methods

Chemicals and Kits

The biochemical tests conducted with the specific enzymatic colorimetric assay kits were all provided by Roche, either located at Switzerland or USA. The reagents IFCC and P-5-P were used for assay of GOT and GPT. Octacalcium phosphate (OCP) and UV were used for the determination of serum calcium and phosphate ions. For other determinations we used BCG for serum albumin, CHOD for cholesterol, lipase-glycerol oxidase for triglycerides; KINETIC for serum BUN, picric acid for creatinine (Jaffe reaction), colorimetric oxidase for uric acid, and Sirius Red for collagen staining. Doxorubicin (DR) was a product of Pfizer (Milano, Italia). Pro-PREP lysis buffer was purchased from the iNtRON Biotechnology (Seongnam, Korea). The kits for other determinations included SOD and TBARS from Cayman (Michigan, USA), the rat IL-6 EIA Kit from PeproTech (NJ, USA), and the rat TNF-α Kit from the R&D Systems Inc. (MN, USA). The sources of the antibodies used in this experiment were: PDGF Receptor β (1:1000), phosphor-PDGF Receptor β (1:1000) and β-actin from Cell Signaling (MA, USA); phosphor-PI3K (1:500) from Santa Cruz (CA, USA); α-Smooth Muscle Actin (1:1000) from Sigma-Aldrich Co. (MO, USA); CD34 (1:400) from Leica (Germany). Chemiluminescent HRP Substrate was the product of Millipore (MA, USA). Sodium dodecyl sulfate (SDS) and polyacrylamide gel (PAGE) were products of Sigma Aldrich (MO, USA).

Animal CKD Model

This experimental protocol was approved by the Institutional Animal Care and Use Committee (IAUCC), China Medical University (Taichung, Taiwan). The Principles of Laboratory Animal Care (NIH publication) were followed. Thirty six 4-week old Sprague-Dawley adult male rats (BioLASCO Taiwan Co., Ltd. Resources) having body weight 220–250 g were used in the study. In the first week, these rats were fed ordinary laboratory chow and acclimated in the animal room conditioned at 23°C±1°C and RH 50–60% with a 12-h/12-h light/dark cycle. The animals had free access to water and pellet chow containing 1.8–2.2% of calcium, 1.1% of phosphorus and 2650 kcal/kg energy. These rats were randomly assigned to six groups: the Normal sedentary (Normal), the doxorubicin induced CKD (DRCKD) sedentary, the 30 min swimming (Swim 30), the DRCKD+30 min swimming (DRCKD+Swim 30), the 60 min swimming (Swim 60); and the DRCKD+60 min swimming (DRCKD+Swim 60). These six groups were separately housed in twelve colony cages, 3 rats in each.

Swimming Exercise Training Protocol

In the second week, the pre-swimming exercise for acclimation was started in an experimental swimming pool (30°C, water depth: 44 cm; radius 120 cm). A gradual progression protocol was applied beginning with swimming for 5 min to 10 min, and then gradually extended to 20, 30, 40, 50 min per day. CKD was induced by a single s.c. 7.5 mg/kg of doxorubicin after the pre-swimming acclimation [33]. The actual swimming experiment was started on the next day after the doxorubicin injection according to Osato et al. with slight modification [4]. From the third week on, the rats were subjected to 30 min- and 60 min-swimming training exercises respectively, 3 days/week for a total period of 11 weeks. During the whole course, the sedentary rats were remained in the cage under the same environmental condition and inspected daily. At two-week intervals, after having been collected the blood samples, rats were transferred to metabolic cage, one in each, and the urine samples were collected. The samples obtained were subjected to biochemical and immuno- analyses for a duration of 11 weeks. The body weights were assessed by regularly recording every week. After euthanized, the ratio of kidney weight to body weight (KW/BW) was taken. On finishing the experiment, rats were euthanized and the kidneys were excised and subjected to pathological examinations.

Serum and Urinary Biochemical Parameters

The serum levels of GPT, GOT, cholesterol, triglycerides, BUN, uric acid, creatinine, and albumin were assayed with each specific kit provided by Roche (Switzerland). The serum calcium and phosphate levels were assayed with the specific kits (Roche, USA) by following the manufacturer's instruction. The superoxide dismutase (SOD) and the thiobarbituric acid reactive substance (TBARs) were assayed with the commercial ELISA kits provided by Cayman Chemical Co. (Michigan, USA). The optical density was taken by the SYSMEX K-1000 Automated Hematology Analyzer (GMI, MN, USA). The blood cell counting for erythrocytes, leukocytes, and platelets was conducted using the SYSMEX K-1000 Automated Hematology Analyzer (GMI, MN, USA).

Gelatinolytic Zymography

The expression of matrix metalloproteinases MMP-2 and MMP-9 were assayed according to Leber and Balkwill [34]. Briefly, the plasma was centrifuged for 10 minutes at 3000×g. The supernatant serum (10 μL) was loaded onto a 7.5% SDS-PAGE copolymerized with 0.1% gelatin and subjected to electrophoresis under 100 V for 1.5 h. In order to remove SDS, the gel was washed twice, each time with 2.5% TritonX-100 solution for 30 min, and then rinsed with the incubation buffer (0.05 M Tris-HCl buffer, pH 8.0, 5 mM $CaCl_2$ plus 5 mM $ZnCl_2$). The mixture was incubated at 37°C overnight. The gel was stained with Coomasie Blue at room temperature for 2 h as directed by Leber and Balkwill [34]. Gelatinases in the serum can be detected as unstained gelatin degraded zones on the gel. The amount expressed was quantified with a densitometer (ImagePro Plus 5.0 Media Cybernetics, Bethesda, MD).

Cytokine Expression

After the swimming training was completed, the rats were subjected to intraperitoneal ketamine and xylasine anesthesia and the blood samples were immediately withdrawn from the abdominal aorta. The levels of IL-6 and TNF-α were measured by the Rat IL-6 EIA KIT provided by PeproTech Inc. (NJ, USA) and the Rat TNF-α KIT by R&D Systems Inc. (MN, USA) according to the manufacturer's instruction. The minimal detectable limits instructed by the manufacturers for IL-6 and TNF-α are 62 and 5 $pg{\cdot}mL^{-1}$, respectively.

Western Blotting

Frozen samples of renal cortex tissues (approximately 100 mg at −80°C) were homogenized with 1 mL of Pro-PREP lysis buffer (pH 7.2) in a homogenizer (T10 basic, The IKA Company, Germany). The homogenate was centrifuged at 12000×g for 20 min at 4°C and the supernatant was collected as tissue sample lysate. The lysate was heated at 100°C for 10 min before loading and separated on precasted 7.5% SDS-PAGE. The proteins were electrotransferred onto the PVDF membrane in transfer buffer for 1 hour. The nonspecific binding to the membrane was blocked with 5% nonfat milk in TBS buffer for 1 hour at room temperature. The membranes were then incubated for 16 hours at 4°C with various primary antibodies. After extensive washing in TBS buffer, the membranes were incubated for 1 hour at room temperature with the secondary antibody in blocking buffer containing 5% nonfat milk. The PVDF membranes were then washed with TBS buffer and the signals were visualized using the Luminescent Image Analyzer LAS-4000 (Fujifilm, Tokyo, Japan). Levels of PDGFR, P-PDGFR, and α-SMA were analyzed by each specific immunoassay according to the manufacturer's instruction. β-actin was used as reference protein.

Glomerular Volume

The glomerular volume was calculated according to Weibel (Eq. 1) [35].

$$\mathbf{GV} = \boldsymbol{\beta}/k \times (\mathbf{GA})^{3/2}$$

Where GV = glomerular volume (mm^3); GA = cross-sectional tuft area (mm^2); β is the shape coefficient for a sphere (in this paper = 1.38); ***k*** is the size distribution coefficient (in this paper = 1.1).

Histochemical Examination

Kidneys were fixed by immersion with 10% formalin in PBS (pH 7.4) at 4°C for 24 hours and processed for paraffin embedding. Paraffin sections were dewaxed in xylene and rehydrated in a series of ethanol washes. The nuclei of these specimens were stained with Weigert's Haematoxylin (Sigma-Aldrich, MO, USA), and the collagen content was stained with Sirius Red (Sigma-Aldrich, MO, USA).

CD34 and α-SMA Immunohistochemical Examination

Paraffin-embedded sections, 3 μm thickness, were deparaffinized in xylene, rehydrated in graded ethanol, and washed in 0.1 mol/L phosphate-buffered saline (PBS, pH = 7.5). The sections were then incubated with 3% H_2O_2 for 10 min at room temperature and washed for three times with distilled water. Antigen retrival was performed by heating the sections twice in 200 mL for 1×Antigen Retrival Citrate Buffer in microwave over at 98°C for 8 min. After cooling, the sections were blocked with 1% normal goat serum in PBS for 20 min.

Then the slides were incubated with primary antibodies against α-SMA and CD34 at 4°C for 16 h, and the sections were washed in PBS, incubated with the Post Primary Rabbit anti mouse IgG (Bond^{TM} Polymer Refine Detection kit, Leica Ltd, UK) for 20 min at room temperature. After incubation, the sections were rinsed in PBS and developed by 0.04% 3,3-diaminobenzidine tetrahydrochloride (Bond^{TM} Polymer Refine Detection kit, Leica Ltd, UK). Finally, all sections were then counterstained with hematoxylin and visualized using an Olympus light microscope. Quantitative analysis was performed using an Image-ProPLUS (Meyer Instruments, USA) analysis system at ×400 magnification. Thirty glomeruli in the cortex and the cortex-medulla junctions were randomly scanned. The integrated optical density (IOD) was measured. The sum of the IOD was obtained and the mean value calculated [36].

Statistics

Data obtained in the same group were analyzed by Duncan's multiple range tests with computer statistical software SAS 9.0 (SAS Institute Inc., Cary, NC, USA). Significance of difference was judged by a confidence level of $p<0.05$.

Results

Body Weight Gain Affected by Swimming Exercise

The body weight increase of the three normal controls was very comparable. The body weight increased from 290–300 g at the initial to around 440 g at week 11. All DR-induced rats showed no gain in body weight through the entire course. Conversely, from week 8 on, they showed a slight decline in body weight until to 260 g despite of the exercise or the non-exercise (Fig. 1A).

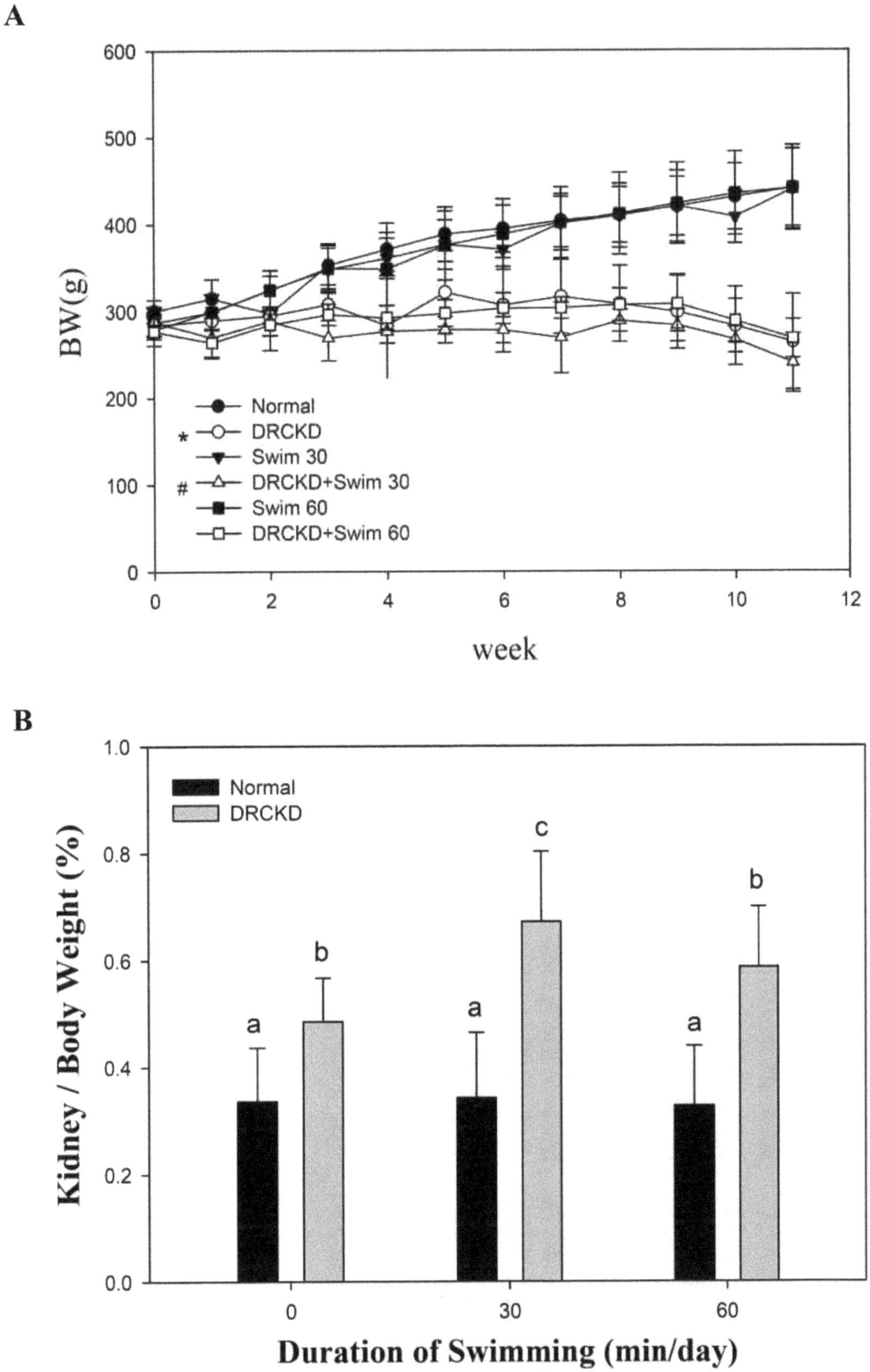

Figure 1. The time course change of body weight (A), the ratio of kidney weight/body weight (B) affected by swimming exercise in different rat groups.

The Kidney Weight Affected by Swimming Exercise

All DR-induced rats showed serious swelling of kidneys due to renal edema. The ratio of kidney to body weight (Kw/Bw) for the sedentary group was 0.33. The value was raised to 0.49, 0.67 and 0.59 in groups DRCKD, DRCKD+30 min and DRCKD+60 min swimming exercise, respectively. Apparently, although the 60 min swimming showed better effect, swimming exercise could only partially ameliorate the renal edema status (Fig. 1B).

Effect of Swimming Exercise on the Appearance of Rat Kidneys

The outer appearance of normal rat kidneys revealed regular reddish color, contrasting with those pale and whitish kidneys of DRCKD rats (Fig. 2). Serious cortex swelling with large liquid-containing cysts were found in the kidneys of 30 min swimming rats, indicating that 30 min swimming exercise failed to alleviate the DRCKD status (Fig. 2). As contrast, the DRCKD+60 min swimming exercise had improved to some extent, although still remaining swollen with edema in the final stage of experiment, much of the physiological and biochemical parameters shown in the following sections revealed that the 60 min swimming exercise in fact displayed better outcome.

Swimming Exercise only Partially Restored the Swollen Glomeruli

DR induced renal edema. The glomeruli were swollen to almost destroyed and the surrounding mesangial tissues also became thickened due to swelling. Only the 60 min swimming exercise was shown able to restore most of the status (Fig. 3A). Quantitatively, the glomerular volume of all three normal groups remained unchanged at 1.20 mm^3, DR significantly increased the glomerular volume to 1.89 mm^3 with apparent edema and inflammation [5]. On receiving swimming training, the values for the 30 min and 60 min swimming groups reduced to 1.54 and 1.33 mm^3, respectively, implicating that 60 min swimming exercise was feasibly beneficial to restore the renal edema status (Fig. 3B).

Effect of Collagen Deposition in Renal Interstitial Tissue by Swimming Exercise

DR induced huge amount of collagen deposition in the interstitial tissue of kidney (Fig. 4A, b) accompanied with very large extent of glomerular swelling, only the 60 min swimming exercise was able to ameliorate the deposition (Fig. 4A, B, C, D, E, F) when compared with Fig. 4A, B, C, D. The spectral density of Sirius staining was quantified as Figure 4B.

MMP-9 Expression Affected by Swimming Exercise

The matrix metalloproteinases MMP-2 and MMP-9 were all shown upregulated by DR, MMP-9 was completely, while MMP-2 was only slightly suppressed by the 60 min swimming exercise (Fig. 5).

Serum Interleukin-6 and TNF-α Levels Affected by Swimming Exercise

DRCKD significantly upregulated production of IL-6 to 9.8 ng/mL. Either the 30 min- or the 60 min swimming exercise was shown able to downregulate the level to 7.4–7.5 ng/mL. When compared with the three normal groups, swimming exercise was found unable to restore the level of IL-6 (Fig. 6A). As a contrast, the level of the normal sedentary renal tissue TNF-α was 918 pg/mL and that of DRCKD sedentary was 260 pg/mL. The 60 min swimming exercise was seen able to upregulate its level to 405 pg/mL only, which was still far below the value of the 60 min swimming group, 850 pg/mL. In summary, the 60 min swimming exercise was able to partially improve but could not have completely rescued the DRCKD damages in view of the expression of IL-6 and TNF-α (Fig. 6B).

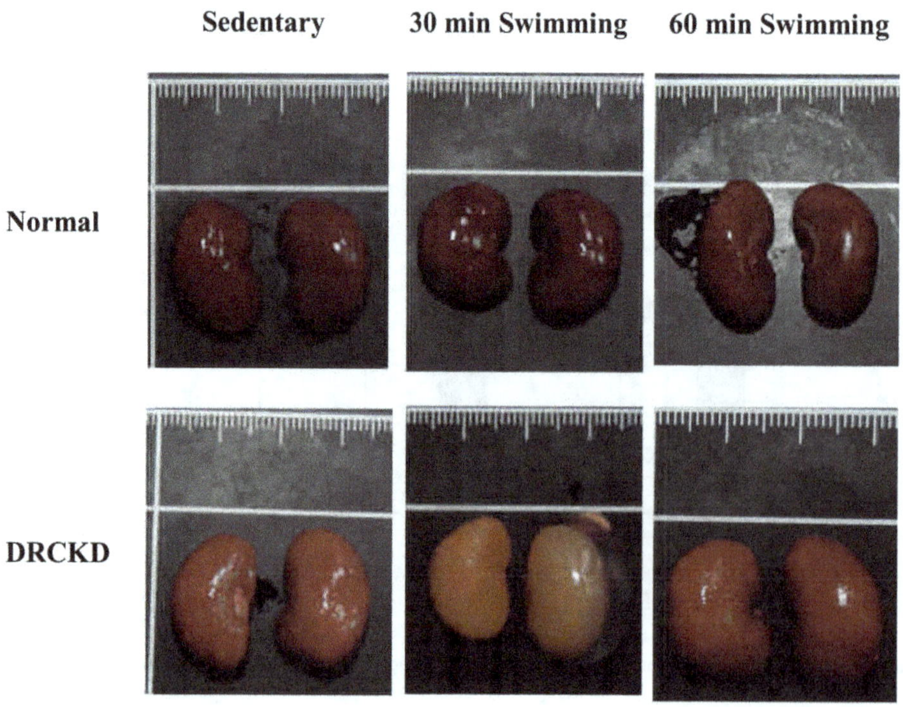

Figure 2. Damages of kidneys induced by doxorubicin secured by swimming exercise.

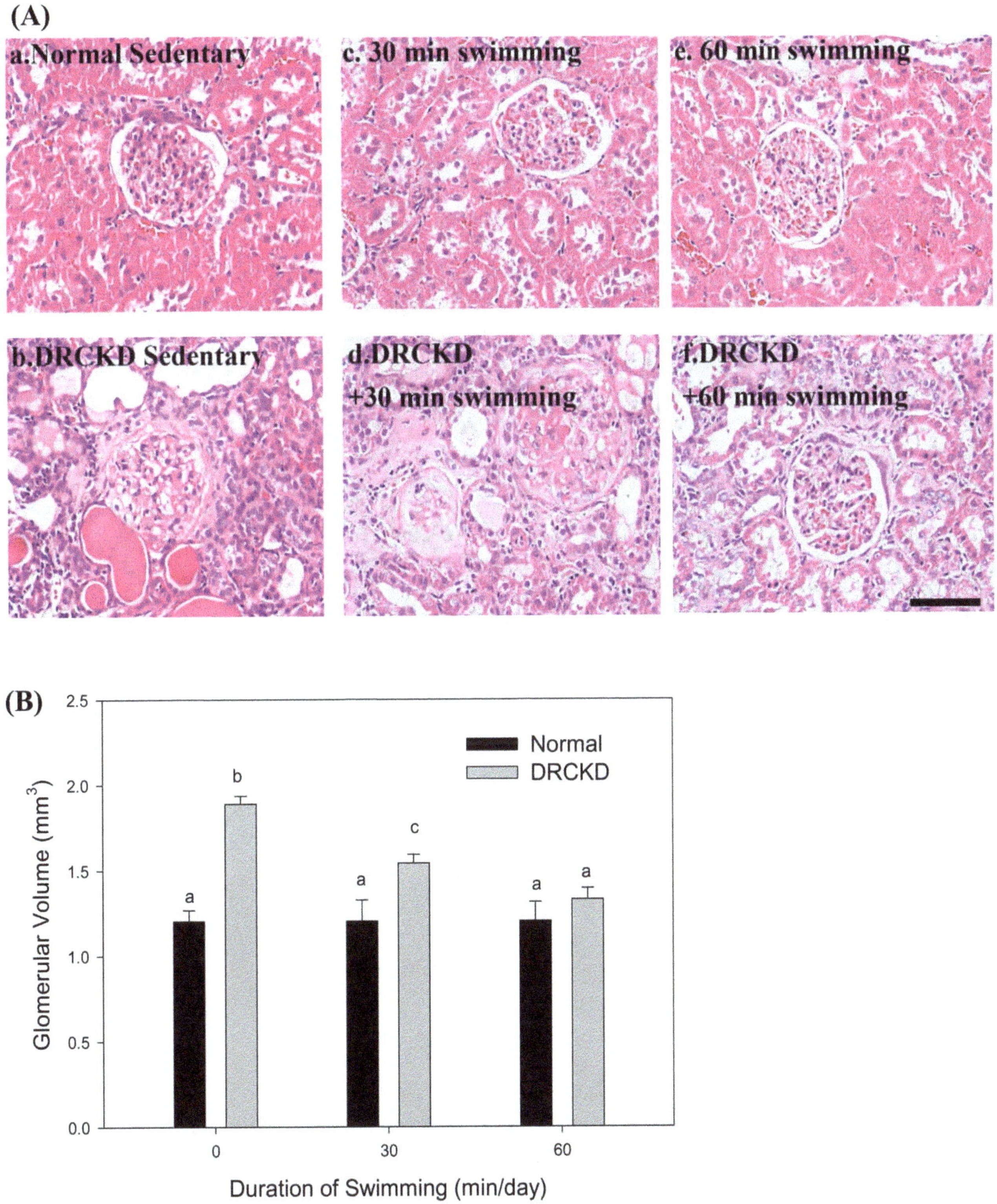

Figure 3. Histochemical examination on the renal cells by Hematoxylin-Eosin staining (A) and the glomerular swelling status (glomerular volume) (B) secured by swimming exercise (magnification ×400). (3A)The six illustrations are: (a) the Normal sedentary; (b) DRCKD sedentary; (c) 30 min swimming; (d) DRCKD+30 min swimming; (e) 60 min swimming; (f) DRCKD+60 min swimming. The pathological findings are: focal, minimal to severe/high, chronic progressive nephrosis (CPN) accompanied with renal cell necrosis, regeneration, hyaline casts, polycysts, and membranous glomerulonephritis with interstitial fibrosis. The glomerular tubules were destroyed by the inflammatory edema and swelling (b and d). The partial recovery by 30 min swimming exercise (d), but more completely secured by the 60 min swimming exercise training (f), in which the DRCKD (b) has been greatly improved to a status with only slight to severe minimal membranous glomerulonephritis and interstitial fibrosis (magnification ×400) (bar = 100 μm).

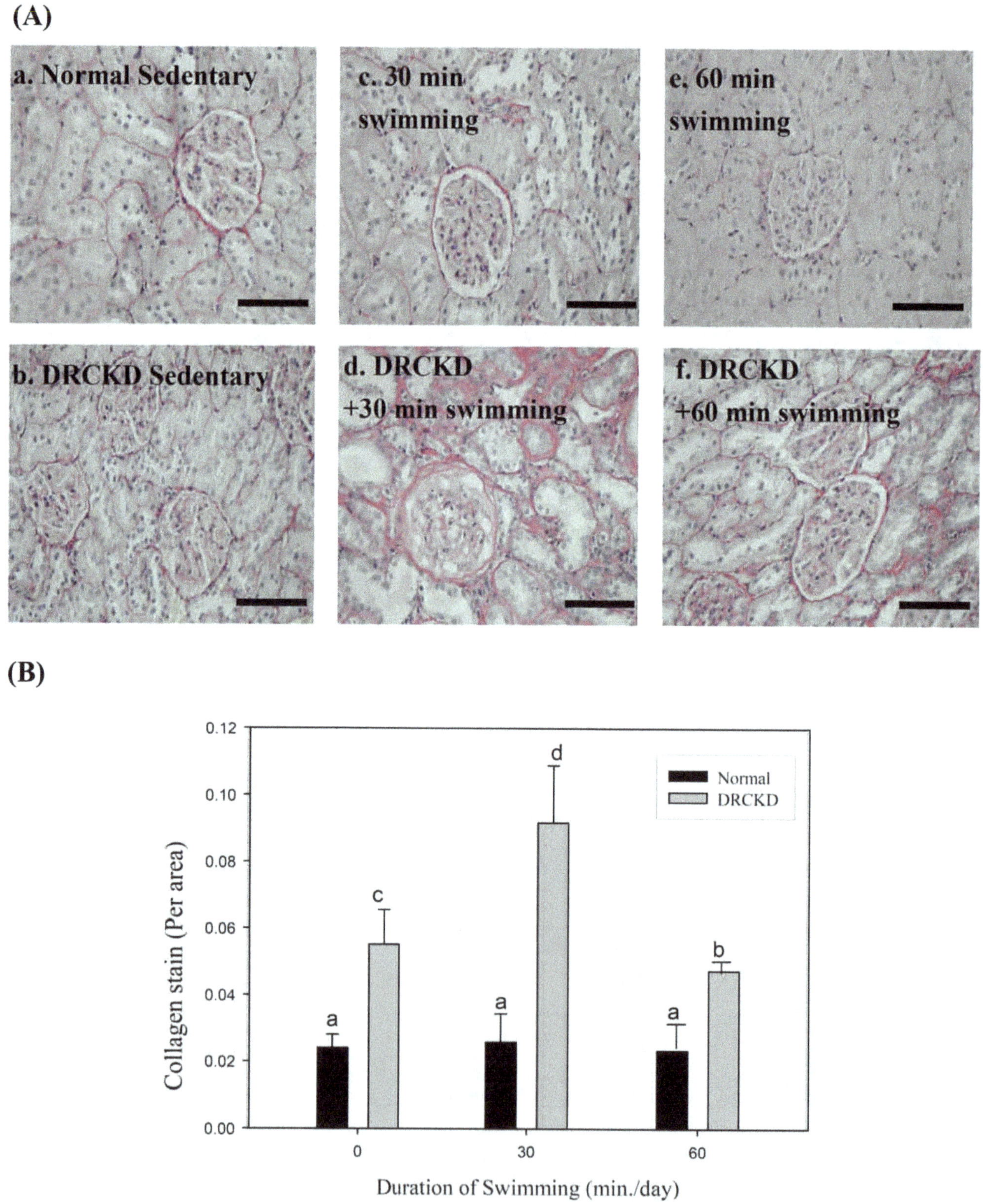

Figure 4. Histochemical examination on the collagen deposition in renal interstitial tissues by Sirius Red stain. (A) Collagen deposition in the renal interstitial tissues (shown in red coloration) was secured by swimming exercise (Magnification ×400). The six illustrations are: (a) the Normal sedentary; (b) DRCKD sedentary; (c) 30 min swimming; (d) DRCKD+30 min swimming; (e) 60 min swimming; (f) DRCKD+60 min swimming. In the early stage of CKD (b), the area of collagen deposition was broader than the normal sedentary group (a). The 30-min swimming exercise enhanced (d), but the 60 min swimming exercise ameliorated such pathological event (f) (magnification ×400) (bar = 100 μm). **(B)** The spectral density of Sirius staining was quantified by Image ProPLUS.

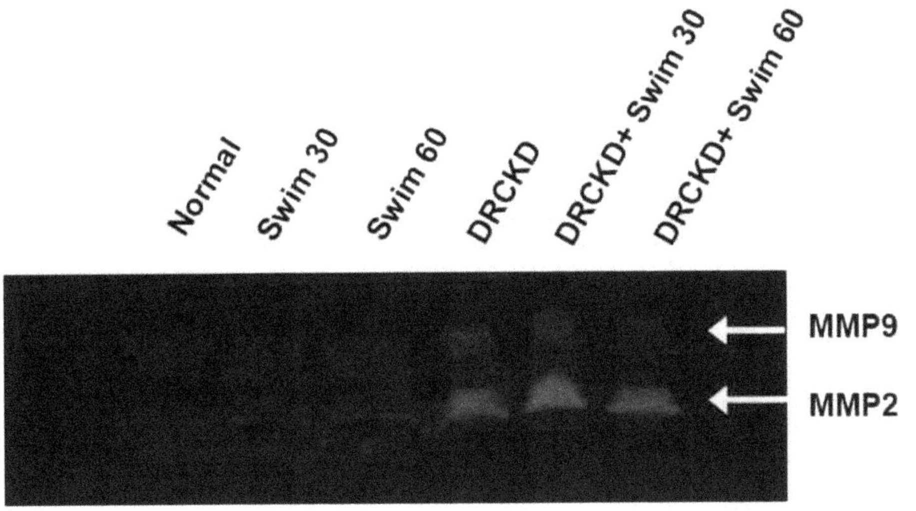

Figure 5. The gelanolytic zymography of the matrix metalloproteinases, MMP-2 and MMP-9. The level of MMP-9 induced by doxorubicin was secured by swimming exercise.

Serum GPT and GOT Levels Affected by Swimming Exercise

Although at week 11, DRCKD groups showed slightly higher levels of serum GPT and GOT, reaching respectively 104 U/mL and 176 U/mL, however, by referring to the normal ranges 28–132 U/mL and 59–247 U/mL for GPT and GOT respectively, swimming exercise did not show any effect on the level of these two parameters (Table 1).

Serum Calcium and Phosphate Levels Affected by Swimming Exercise

Similar result was found for serum calcium. Swimming did not alter the level of serum calcium when compared with the normal range 5.3–13.0 mg/dL (Table 2). In contrast, the serum phosphate level of was slightly elevated in groups DRCKD and DRCKD+30 min swimming, reaching 13.6 and 14.4 mg/dL, respectively. DRCKD+60 min swimming exercise significantly reduced the serum phosphate level to 8.6 mg/mL, almost approaching the normal value 5.3–8.3 mg/dL (Table 2).

Serum Cholesterol and Triglyceride Levels Affected by Swimming Exercise

The serum cholesterol and triglyceride were all raised by DR induction, reaching 238, 350, and 348 mg/dL, respectively in groups of DRCKD, DCKD+30 min swimming, and DRCKD+60 min swimming. Comparing with the normal sedentary (44 mg/dL), the 30 min swimming (41 mg/dL), and the 60 min swimming group (50 mg/dL), neither swimming exercise was able to ameliorate the hyperlipidemic status induced by DRCKD in comparison with the normal level for cholesterol, 40–130 mg/dL; and 26–145 mg/dL for triglyceride) (Table 2).

Serum BUN Affected by Swimming Exercise

The DRCKD raised serum BUN level up to 94 mg/dL at week 11. Moderate swimming exercise (30 min swimming) failed to suppress the elevation of BUN. While the aerobic 60 min swimming exercise only partially suppressed the serum level of BUN to 48 mg/mL, 2 folds over the normal range 15–21 mg/dL (Table 3).

Serum Uric Acid Level Affected by Swimming Exercise

The serum uric acid levels in all groups were not affected by swimming exercise, all remaining within the normal range 1–6 mg/dL (Hospital clinical data) (Table 3).

Swimming Exercise Failed to Restore the Serum Creatinine Level

DR induced slight elevation of serum creatinine, the levels raised to 1.0–1.1 mg/dL at week 11. Swimming exercise did not show any effect on its restoration when referring to the normal serum creatinine range for SD rats 0.2–0.8 mg/dL (Table 3).

Swimming Exercise was Unable to Restore Serum Albumin Decrease

DR induced hypoalbuminemia. At week 11, the serum albumin levels were all decreased in the DRCKD rats, ranging from 2.4–2.6 g/dL (Table 3). Swimming exercise failed to restore this trend comparing with the normal range 3.4–4.8 g/dL. The levels remained at 2.4, 2.2, and 2.6 g/dL, respectively in groups DRCKD, DRCKD+30 min swimming, and DRCKD+60 min swimming, comparing with 3.5 g/dL exhibited by the normal sedentary group (Table 3).

Urinary Parameters Were All Improved

Urinary protein, creatinine, and BUN levels were all partially improved but not completely by swimming exercise training at Week 11. The urinary protein was reduced from 828 to 507, and 258 mg/dL in groups DRCKD, DRCKD+30 min swimming, and DRCKD+60 min swimming, comparing to 20–23 mg/dL of the three normal groups (Table 4). The creatinine levels of all groups except the normal sedentary were very comparable, exhibiting values between 51–72 mg/dL. Interestingly, the normal sedentary group still remained at 128 mg/dL comparing to 125–143 mg/dL of the initial values for all groups (Table 4). As for the level of urinary BUN, after swimming exercise, the value of DRCKD group was reduced from 257 mg/dL for DRCKD to 198 and 140 mg/dL in groups DRCKD+30 min- and DRCKD+60 min swimming exercise, respectively (Table 4).

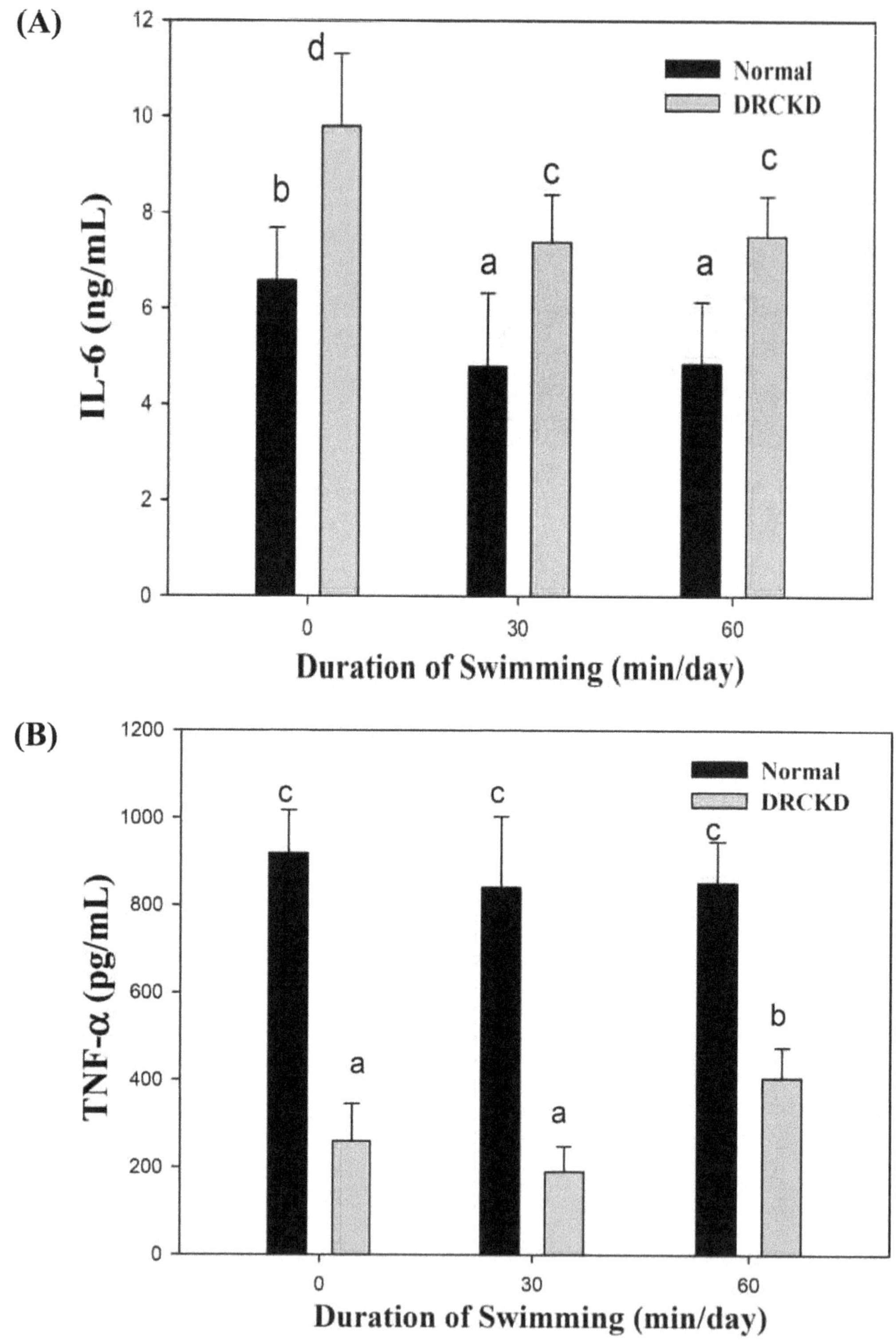

Figure 6. Levels of serum IL-6 (A) and tissue TNF-α (B) affected by swimming exercise.

Swimming Exercise Sustained Antioxidative Strength and Reduced Oxidative Stress

DRCKD inhibited the activity of SOD to 38 U/mL at week 4, and 45 U/mL at week 11. Although the 30 min swimming group did not show any effect, the 60 min swimming exercise significantly activated the SOD levels to 82 U/mL in the 60 min controls, comparing to 56–62 U/mL of the normal sedentary group (Table 5). Nonetheless in the DRCKD groups, swimming exercise failed to show any beneficial effect, implicating that although swimming exercise is able to strengthen the *in vivo* antioxidative bioactivity in the healthy control groups, it may fail to restore the antioxidative strength like SOD in the DRCKD rats.

Table 1. Serum GPT and GOT Affected by Swimming Exercise.*,†

Parameter	Week 4	Week 11
Serum GPT (U/mL)		
Normal	$44\pm5^{b,A}$	$58\pm4^{d,C}$
DRCKD	$49\pm5^{c,A}$	$104\pm7^{e,D}$
30 min swimming	$44\pm4^{b,B}$	$41\pm4^{a,A}$
DRCKD+30 min swimming	$44\pm3^{b,A}$	$54\pm5^{c,B}$
60 min swimming	$38\pm4^{a,A}$	$40\pm5^{a,B}$
DRCKD+60 min swimming	$50\pm6^{c,B}$	$46\pm4^{b,A}$
Serum GOT (U/mL)		
Normal	$93\pm4^{e,A}$	$96\pm5^{d,B}$
DRCKD	$57\pm5^{a,A}$	$176\pm9^{e,D}$
30 min swimming	$74\pm4^{c,A}$	$79\pm6^{c,B}$
DRCKD+30 min swimming	$62\pm5^{b,C}$	$39\pm4^{a,B}$
60 min swimming	$85\pm6^{d,B}$	$77\pm7^{c,A}$
DRCKD+60 min swimming	$83\pm6^{d,C}$	$41\pm5^{b,A}$

*Different superscripts in upper case in the same row indicate significant difference between time intervals. Different superscripts in lower case in the same column indicate the significant difference between different groups (n = 6). Significant level $p<0.05$. Data for week 0 were unavailable.
†Normal ranges for GOT and GPT are 59–247 U/mL and 28–132 U/mL, respectively. (data source from the National Laboratory Animal Center, Taipei, Taiwan).

Table 2. Serum biochemical parameters affected by swimming exercise.*,†

Parameter	Week 0	Week 11
Serum calcium ion (mg/dL)		
Normal	$11.4\pm1.2^{a,C}$	$11.3\pm1.2^{c,C}$
DRCKD	$11.3\pm1.3^{a,C}$	$9.8\pm0.6^{a,A}$
30 min swimming	$11.4\pm1.2^{a,C}$	$10.7\pm1.0^{b,B}$
DRCKD+30 min swimming	$11.2\pm1.2^{a,C}$	$10.7\pm1.1^{b,B}$
60 min swimming	$11.2\pm1.4^{a,C}$	$10.6\pm1.0^{b,B}$
DRCKD+60 min swimming	$11.4\pm1.5^{a,D}$	$12.0\pm1.0^{d,C}$
Serum phosphate (mg/dL)		
Normal	$9.9\pm0.6^{b,D}$	$9.2\pm0.8^{b,C}$
DRCKD	$10.3\pm1.4^{c,D}$	$13.6\pm1.7^{d,E}$
30 min swimming	$9.2\pm1.2^{a,C}$	$9.4\pm0.7^{c,C}$
DRCKD+30 min swimming	$9.3\pm1.3^{a,B}$	$14.4\pm1.8^{e,D}$
60 min swimming	$10.1\pm1.5^{c,D}$	$9.1\pm0.6^{b,C}$
DRCKD+60 min swimming	$9.5\pm1.4^{a,C}$	$8.6\pm0.5^{a,B}$
Serum cholesterol (mg/dL)		
Normal	$79\pm2^{b,D}$	$44\pm2^{b,B}$
DRCKD	$75\pm2^{a,A}$	$238\pm14^{d,B}$
30 min swimming	$80\pm2^{b,E}$	$41\pm2^{a,B}$
DRCKD+30 min swimming	$82\pm2^{c,A}$	350 ± 14^{e}
60 min swimming	$96\pm3^{e,E}$	$50\pm2^{c,B}$
DRCKD+60 min swimming	$87\pm3^{d,A}$	$348\pm13^{f,D}$
Serum triglyceride (mg/dL)		
Normal	$38\pm2^{c,C}$	$42\pm2^{b,D}$
DRCKD	$34\pm2^{b,A}$	$170\pm3^{d,B}$
30 min swimming	$33\pm1^{a,A}$	$44\pm2^{c,C}$
DRCKD+30 min swimming	$32\pm2^{a,A}$	$192\pm7^{e,B}$
60 min swimming	$39\pm3^{d,B}$	$41\pm2^{a,C}$
DRCKD+60 min swimming	$45\pm3^{e,A}$	$255\pm11^{f,C}$

Swimming exercise did not show any effect in the 30 min- and 60 min swimming groups. DRCKD significantly raised the level of TBARs to 53 μM comparing to 20–24 μM of the normal sedentary group. Amazingly, the moderate 30 min swimming exercise further enhanced the level to 80 μM at week 4 and to 100 μM at week 11. Conversely, the 60 min swimming exercise suppressed the formation of TBARs significantly to 58–59 μM, an implication in the beneficial effect of aerobic exercise, the 60 min swimming, on the oxidative damages occurring on the lipoproteins like low density lipoprotein (Table 5).

Swimming Exercise more Prominently Affected Platelet Counts

By referring to the normal red blood cell (RBC) count $(7.0\text{–}10.0)\times10^6/\mu L$ for the Sprague Dawley rats, doxorubicin moderately suppressed the erythrocyte formation, the lowest count was seen with the DRCKD+30 min swimming group $(5.8\pm0.5)\times10^6/\mu L$ (Table 6). Unlike the RBC, the leukocyte (the white blood cell, WBC) count in all DRCKD rats revealed to be with normal count except the 30 min swimming exercise, which was raised to high peak count $25\pm5\times10^3/\mu L$. As a contrast, the WBC level was restored to normal $(17\pm5)\times10^3/\mu L$ by the 60 min swimming exercise (Table 6). The reason why the RBC concentration was not apparently affected, while the WBC count in the DRCKD+30 min swimming exercise was so highly raised is worth investigation. Similarly, the platelet count was significantly raised to $(1445\pm589)\times10^3/\mu L$ and $(1513\pm137)\times10^3/\mu L$ in groups DRCKD and DRCKD+30 min swimming training, respectively. Only the 60 min swimming program was able to restore the platelet count to $(1016\pm475)\times10^3/\mu L$ [The normal range is $(500\text{–}1300)\times10^3/\mu L$] (Table 6).

Swimming Training Downregulated PDGFR and P-PDGFR in DRCKD Rats

In the three control groups, the levels of PDGF and PDGFR were very comparable. DR apparently upregulated, while swimming exercise downregulated, the levels of PDGFR and P-PDGFR in DR treated groups (Fig. 7).

Swimming Training Downregulated CD34 and α-SMA in DRCKD Rats

Immunohistochemical examination revealed that a tremendous number of myofibroblasts undergoing transdifferential fibrogenesis were apparently emerging mostly in the mesangium of glomerulli, less amount on the epithelia of convoluted tubules, as evidenced by the expression of CD34 (Fig. 8A) and α-SMA (Fig. 7 & 8B). Partial recovery was found in the DRCKD+30 min swimming exercise group, contrasting to the complete amelioration in the DRCKD+60 min swimming exercise subjects (Fig. 8).

Table 3. Serum biochemical parameters affected by swimming exercise*,† (continued).

Parameter	Week 0	Week 11
Serum BUN (mg/dL)		
Normal	$15\pm3^{d,B,}$	$14\pm2^{a,A}$
DRCKD	$13\pm1^{c,A}$	$94\pm4^{e,E}$
30 min swimming	$12\pm1^{b,A}$	$17\pm2^{b,C}$
DRCKD+30 min swimming	$13\pm1^{c,A}$	$100\pm5^{f,E}$
60 min swimming	$13\pm1^{c,A}$	$18\pm2^{c,C}$
DRCKD+60 min swimming	$10\pm1^{a,A}$	$48\pm3^{d,E}$
Serum uric acid (mg/dL)		
Normal	$3.4\pm0.2^{b,B}$	$2.0\pm0.1^{c,B}$
DRCKD	$2.7\pm0.1^{a,D}$	$2.1\pm0.1^{c,B}$
30 min swimming	$3.3\pm0.2^{b,D}$	$1.4\pm0.1^{a,C}$
DRCKD+30 min swimming	$4.8\pm0.2^{e,D}$	$3.0\pm0.1^{d,C}$
60 min swimming	$3.8\pm0.2^{c,C}$	$1.7\pm0.1^{b,B}$
DRCKD+60 min swimming	$4.6\pm0.3^{d,D}$	$2.0\pm0.1^{c,A}$
Serum creatinine (mg/dL)		
Normal	$0.5\pm0.1^{a,A}$	$0.5\pm0.1^{a,A}$
DRCKD	$0.7\pm0.1^{b,A}$	$1.0\pm0.1^{c,D}$
30 min swimming	$0.5\pm0.1^{a,A}$	$0.5\pm0.1^{a,A}$
DRCKD+30 min swimming	$0.5\pm0.1^{a,A}$	$1.1\pm0.1^{d,D}$
60 min swimming	$0.5\pm0.1^{a,A}$	$0.8\pm0.1^{b,D}$
DRCKD+60 min swimming	$0.5\pm0.1^{a,A}$	$1.1\pm0.1^{d,C}$
Serum albumin (g/dL)		
Normal	$4.4\pm0.7^{c,C}$	$3.5\pm0.7^{e,A}$
DRCKD	$4.4\pm0.5^{c,C}$	$2.4\pm0.6^{a,A}$
30 min swimming	$4.4\pm0.6^{c,D}$	$3.4\pm0.6^{d,A}$
DRCKD+30 min swimming	$4.1\pm0.7^{b,D}$	$2.2\pm0.4^{a,A}$
60 min swimming	$4.4\pm0.7^{c,D}$	$3.4\pm0.7^{d,A}$
DRCKD+60 min swimming	$4.0\pm0.4^{a,E}$	$2.6\pm0.5^{c,A}$

*Different superscripts in upper case in the same row indicate significant difference between time intervals. Different superscripts in lower case in the same column indicate the significant difference between different groups (n = 6). Significant level $p<0.05$.

†The normal serum levels are: calcium ion, 5.3–13.0 mg/dL; phosphate, 5.3–8.3 mg/dL; cholesterol, 40–130 mg/dL; triglyceride, 26–145 mg/dL; BUN, 15–21 mg/dL; uric acid, 1–6 mg/dL (human standard); creatinine, 0.2–0.8 mg/dL; albumin, 3.8–4.8 g/dL (data source from the National Laboratory Animal Center, Taipei, Taiwan).

Discussion

DR Reduced Weight Gain Due to "Protein-energy Malnutrition"

Potential mechanisms of muscle wasting in renal failure can occur through the insulin and IGF-1 receptor-mediated signaling via the insulin receptor substrate (IRS)/phosphoinositide-3 kinase (PI3K)/Akt pathway, which drives anabolic, anticatabolic, and antiapoptotic processes, potentially leading to a catabolic state with body weight loss [2]. Moreover, a reduction in circulating amino acid levels, as is often seen in renal failure patients, would reduce the anabolic stimulus functioning via this pathway as well [2,9].

Low grade exercise or too short the period of exercise could stimulate proinflammatory cytokines known to inhibit directly anabolic activity of GH→IGF-1 axis, resulting in the body weight loss [37]. As seen, 60 min swimming exercise retained higher body

Table 4. Urinary biochemical parameters.*

Parameter	Week 0	Week 11
Protein, mg/dL		
Normal	$20\pm12^{a,A}$	$24\pm12^{a,A}$
DRCKD	$22\pm13^{a,A}$	$828\pm26^{f,B}$
30 min swimming	$21\pm11^{a,A}$	$100\pm24^{b,B}$
DRCKD+30 min swimming	$22\pm12^{a,A}$	$507\pm32^{e,B}$
60 min swimming	$23\pm10^{a,A}$	$113\pm25^{c,B}$
DRCKD+60 min swimming	$22\pm14^{a,A}$	$258\pm32^{d,B}$
Creatinine, mg/dL		
Normal	$125\pm24^{b,A}$	$128\pm33^{e,A}$
DRCKD	$138\pm21^{c,B}$	$58\pm28^{b,A}$
30 min swimming	$128\pm22^{b,B}$	$51\pm34^{a,A}$
DRCKD+30 min swimming	$143\pm34^{d,B}$	$67\pm27^{c,A}$
60 min swimming	$121\pm18^{a,B}$	$67\pm34^{c,A}$
DRCKD+60 min swimming	$125\pm27^{b,B}$	$72\pm23^{d,A}$
BUN, mg/dL		
Normal	$55\pm15^{a,A}$	$60\pm18^{a,A}$
DRCKD	$60\pm16^{a,A}$	$257\pm14^{d,B}$
30 min swimming	$60\pm13^{a,A}$	$62\pm17^{a,A}$
DRCKD+30 min swimming	$57\pm15^{a,A}$	$198\pm14^{c,B}$
60 min swimming	$56\pm16^{a,A}$	$58\pm16^{a,A}$
DRCKD+60 min swimming	$55\pm17^{a,A}$	$140\pm14^{b,B}$

*Data expressed in mean±SD from triplicates (n = 6). The superscripts in lower case indicate significance of difference in the same column, and those in upper case indicate significance in the same row.

Table 5. The oxidative stress in DRCKD and antioxidative power of swimming exercise.

Parameter	Week 4	Week 11
SOD (U/mL)		
Normal	$56\pm3^{d,A}$	$62\pm5^{d,B}$
DRCKD	$38\pm3^{b,A}$	$45\pm5^{c,B}$
30 min swimming	$56\pm7^{d,A}$	$60\pm2^{d,B}$
DRCKD+30 min swimming	$30\pm6^{a,B}$	$27\pm2^{a,A}$
60 min swimming	$82\pm2^{e,A}$	$82\pm2^{e,A}$
DRCKD+60 min swimming	$45\pm5^{c,B}$	$42\pm1^{b,A}$
TBARS (μM)		
Normal	$24\pm1^{b,B}$	$20\pm5^{a,A}$
DRCKD	$53\pm3^{c,A}$	$53\pm3^{d,A}$
30 min swimming	$23\pm6^{a,A}$	$23\pm3^{b,A}$
DRCKD+30 min swimming	$80\pm6^{e,A}$	$100\pm7^{f,B}$
60 min swimming	$24\pm5^{b,A}$	$24\pm2^{c,A}$
DRCKD+60 min swimming	$59\pm4^{d,A}$	$58\pm4^{e,A}$

*Different superscripts in upper case in the same row indicate significant difference between time intervals. Different superscripts in lower case in the same column indicate the significant difference between different groups (n = 6). Significant level $p<0.05$. Data for week 0 were unavailable.

Table 6. Blood cell count affected by swimming exercise.#

Parameter	Blood cell counts at week 11		
Cell	RBC ($\times10^6/\mu L$)	WBC ($\times10^3/\mu L$)	Platelet ($\times10^3/\mu L$)
	(Normal range: 7.0–10.0)#	(Normal range: 6.0–17.0) #	(Normal range: 500–1300) #
Normal	7.4 ± 0.1^b	10 ± 4^c	875 ± 136^a
DRCKD	6.4 ± 1.7^a	8 ± 0^c	$1445\pm589^{a,b}$
30 min swimming	7.6 ± 0.6^b	$13\pm2^{b,c}$	796 ± 112^a
DRCKD+30 min swimming	5.8 ± 0.5^a	25 ± 5^a	1513 ± 137^a
60 min swimming	6.8 ± 1.4^b	9 ± 3^c	643 ± 67^a
DRCKD+60 min swimming	6.4 ± 0.5^b	17 ± 5^b	$1016\pm475^{a,b}$

#Values in each column with different superscripts of lower case (a to c) indicate significantly different with each other at significant level $p<0.05$.

weight than the 30 min equivalent (Fig. 1), indicating higher quality of 60 min swimming training in this regard (Fig. 1). As evidenced, severe body weight loss was seen in the DRCKD victims, a status similar to the "protein-energy malnutrition" described by Fock et al. [38].

Kidneys Enlarged in DRCKD but Glomerular Volume Restored by Swimming Exercise Training

The kidneys of DRCKD rats exhibited severe renal swelling and edema, and more surprisingly, the rats having received swimming exercise revealed much more enlarged kidneys (Fig. 1), implicating the glomerular blood flow had not been recovered by swimming exercise. Speculatively, the blood flow in the kidneys of CKD rats and the GFR improved by swimming exercise elicited a transient swelling in the early stage of recovery [39,40]. This secondary renal swelling could in turn release or compensate in part the burden caused by DRCKD in the renal interstitial tissue. As evidenced, the ratio Kw/Bw finally was reduced to 0.59 by the strenuous DRCKD+60 min swimming exercise at week 11 (Fig. 2B). Similar trend was seen in the glomerular volume (GV) change (Fig. 3B), underlying the 60 min swimming exercise training exhibiting better effect in improving the DRCKD status.

Serum and Urinary BUN not Effectively Reduced by Aerobic Exercise Training

As evidenced by serum and urinary BUN, the trend in improving renal function by exercise was apparently observed in DRCKD rats, yet still incomplete (Table 3; Table 4). Exercise positively increases blood flow, oxygen and nutrient transport to kidneys to help maintain renal health [2,3], an implication in the *in vivo* actively proceeding catabolic nature of DRCKD [2,9].

Swimming Exercise Ineffective in Restoring Serum Albumin and Proteinuria

More often, the glomerular filtration rate (GFR) will be greatly reduced in CKD patients, and concomitantly, proteinuria and glomerular hypertension may be evoked [41]. Proteinuria is a risk factor for progression of chronic renal failure (CRF), which is very common in CKD patients [42]. The reasons that swimming exercise failed to ameliorate the serum albumin level may be due to i) the enhanced renal excretion, resulting increased factional

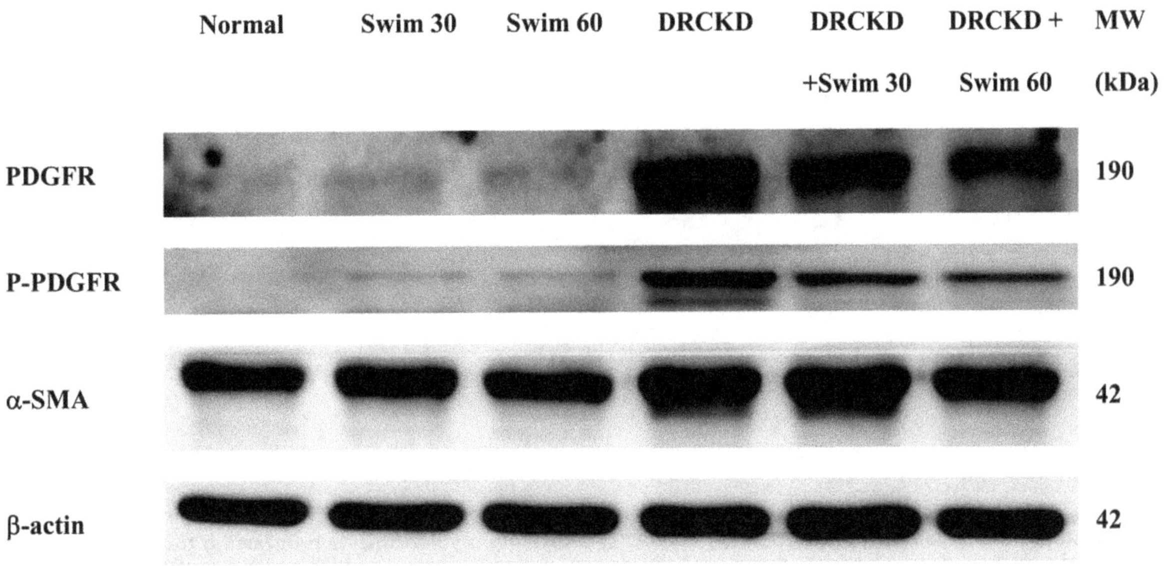

Figure 7. Western blotting for PDGFR, P-PDGFR, and α-SMA in DRCKD rat kidneys which were restored by swimming exercise.

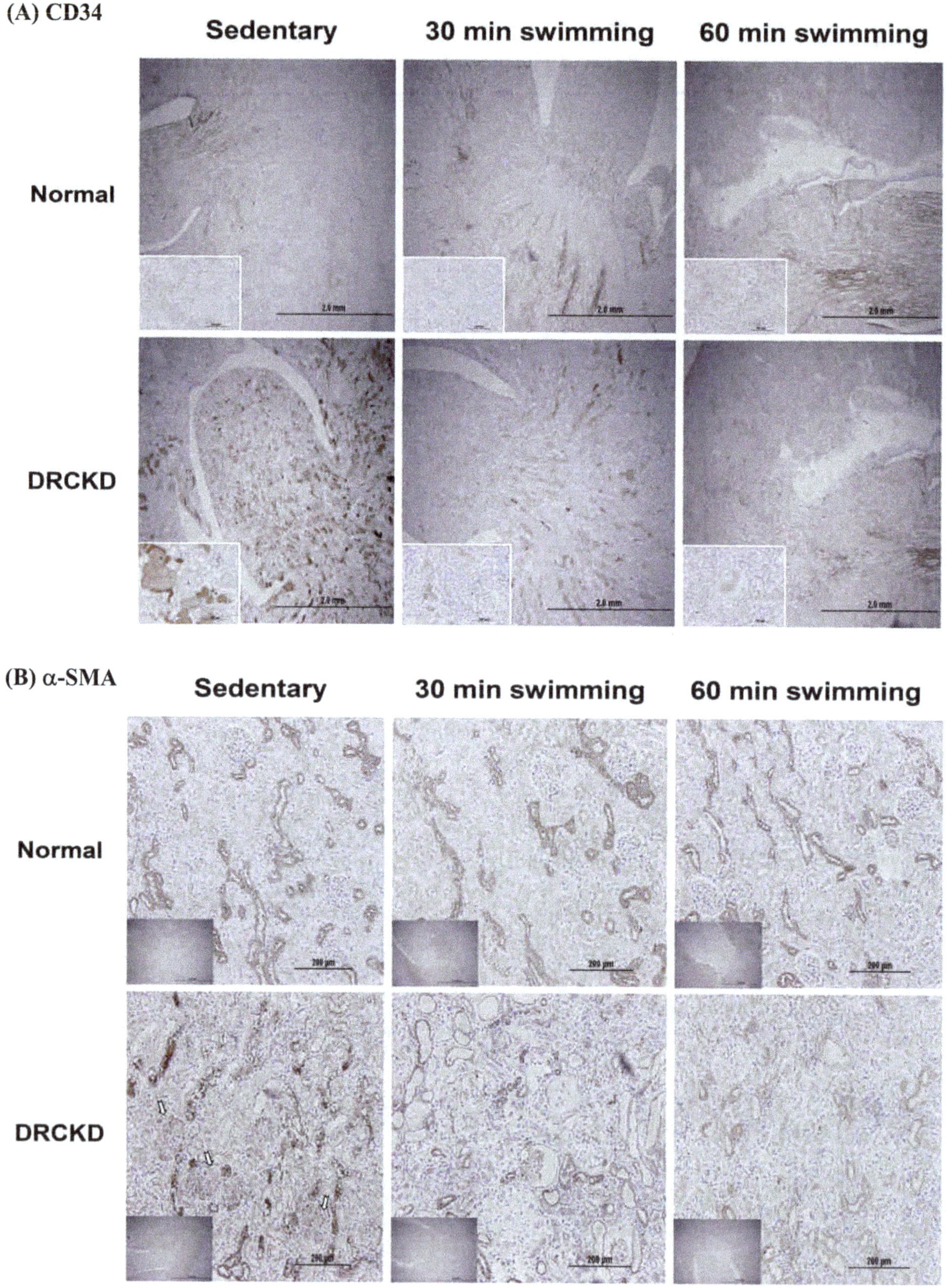

Figure 8. Immunohistochemical examination of CD34 (A) α-SMA (B) indicating myofibroblasts progressing transdifferentiation fibrogenesis. The myofibroblasts are emerging in the mesangium of glomeruli and on the epithelia of the tubule convolutes. (magnification: CD34×40; α-SMA ×200).

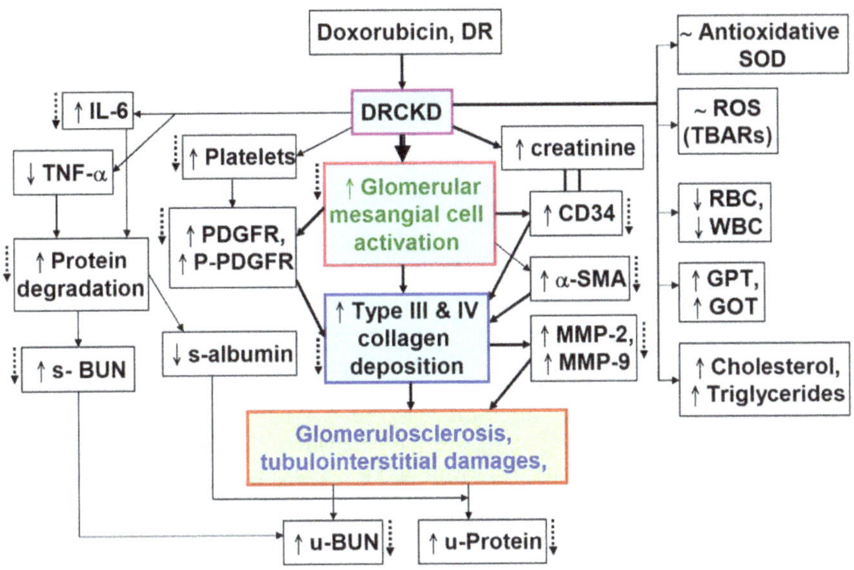

Figure 9. A summary of the signaling in DRCKD and the ameliorating effect of 60-min swimming exercise. DR induced chronic kidney disease (CKD) and activated glomerular mesangial cells, increasing platelets counts, upregulating PDGF and PDGFR, overexpressed CD34, α-SMA and MMP-2 and MMP-9, causing type III and type IV collagen deposition in the interstitium of glomeruli, resulting glomerulosclerosis and tubulointerstitial damages (solid arrows inside the box). 60-min swimming exercise may ameliorate the status of CKD (dotted arrows outside the box).

clearance of albumin [43], and ii) the increased catabolic effect [2,9] (Table 3).

Upregulation of MMP-2 and MMP-9 in DRCKD Reduced by Swimming Exercise

Tubular cell epithelial-mesenchymal transition (EMT) is a fundamental contributor to renal fibrosis. In moderate and severe tubulo-interstitial damage, increased expression of MMP-2 had been noted [44]. MMP-2 may regulate collagen accumulation at those sites (Fig. 4, 5) [45]. During severe tubulo-interstitial damage, highly upregulated MMP-2 may contribute the pathological basement membrane splitting and disruption of type–IV collagen [44]. Similar yet lesser expression was also seen with MMP-9. Thus, swimming exercise was able to partially ameliorate the CKD status.

Oppositely Regulated Status of IL-6 and TNF-α during Exercise Performing

In some occasion of catabolic status, the chronic inflammation associated with renal failure often can lead to elevated levels of TNF-α and IL-6. But this was not the case with our experiment (Fig. 6). IL-6 is a well known fibroblast growth factor [46], often reported to be associated with fibrosis [47]. Both cytokines are known to induce muscle atrophy. One possible mechanism for this effect is negative modulation of IRS/PI3K/Akt signaling that effectively reduces cellular sensitivity to IGF-1 and insulin [2,9,48]. Speculatively, the 60 min swimming exercise could not trigger the production of IL-6 (myokine), hence the total IL-6 level was downregulated by swimming (Fig. 6). Reducing adipose tissue mass, through weight loss in association with exercise, can lower TNF-α and IL-6 levels and increase adiponectin concentrations [49]. Similarly, IL-6 upregulates the number of TNF-alpha receptors, resulting in suppressed hepatic TNF-α levels [50]. Conversely, the mechanism behind the downregulation of adiponectin during exercise had been ascribed to the high quality exercise-induced upregulation of (myokine) IL-6 expression [51,52,53]. Swimming significantly downregulated IL-6 or upregulated TNF-α (Fig. 6), an implication in the beneficial effect of swimming exercise. To summarize, different extent of exercise exerts differently in strength [5].

Swimming Exercise was a Good Hypolipidemic Agent, However Ineffective Toward the Hyperlipidemic Status Induced by DRCKD

In the DRCKD groups, we observed that the cholesterol and triglyceride levels were unsuppressed by swimming exercise, a result contrary to Osato et al. [4]. There is recent evidence of a link between IL-6 and AMP-activated protein kinase (AMPK). AMPK activation stimulates fatty acid oxidation and increases glucose uptake [54]. We speculate that DR may have highly activated the enzymes malonyl transferase and mevalonate kinase, and exercise might have used up some adipose tissue and cholesterol without inhibiting these enzymes (Table 2).

Doxorubicin Upregulated PDGFR and P-PDGFR, Swimming Exercise Ameliorated Progressive Renal Disease

Growth factors have been demonstrated to be important mediators of extracellular matrix (ECM) accumulation in glomerulonephritis (GN). TGF-β, PDGF and basic fibroblast growth factor have been shown to promote ECM accumulation, tubulointerstitial hyperplasia and fibrosis [55]. Mesangial cells produce PDGF, and various growth factors induce mesangial proliferation via induction of PDGF-B chain synthesis. Glomerular mesangial matrix accumulation characterizes many progressive renal diseases [56,57]. DR overexpressed PDGFR and P-PDGFR, causing a pre-fibrotic status in kidney (Fig. 3A), while swimming training downregulated PDGFR and P-PDGFR in an intensity-responsive fashion (Fig. 7). Studies have demonstrated that overactivity of PDGF-BB in scarless fetal wounds induces fetal wound fibrosis [22,58–60].

In chronic inflammatory conditions, the stimulatory effect of PDGF on connective tissue cells may lead to tissue fibrosis, consistent with our data (Fig. 3A and 4) [57], to extend, the use of anti-PDGF-B can be a good therapeutic approach to progressive renal disease [56].

The Antioxidative Nature of Swimming Exercise

Silveira et al. hypothesized that after acute bouts of moderate exercise, activation of the sympathetic nervous system would lead to activation of nuclear factor-κB (NF-κB) biochemical pathways via the Ras/ERK cascade with concomitant rise in NADPH oxidase activity and generation of reactive oxygen species [9], in some circumstances, elevation of cortisol and cathecholamines in plasma could be involved [61].

Superoxide dismutase (SOD) is an *in vivo* cellular antioxidant enzyme which acts as a catalyst in the process of dismutation of superoxide into oxygen and hydrogen peroxide. SOD works as an antioxidant because it outcompetes the damaging reactions of superoxide on genetic material. SOD has been proven to be very effective in the treatment of colonic inflammation. Also, the antioxidant properties of SOD may make it an important treatment for inflammatory bowel disease [62].

DRCKD inhibited the activity of SOD, while DRCKD+60 min swimming group was shown able to partially recover its level. Such a result was totally not seen in the DRCKD+30 min swimming, implicating the aerobic exercise was more effective to evoke the cellular antioxidative capability.

Similarly, DRCKD significantly boosted the level of TBARs to 53 μM comparing to 20–24 μM of the normal sedentary group. The moderate 30 min swimming exercise further enhanced the level to 80 μM at week 4 and to 100 μM at week 11. Conversely, 60 min swimming exercise significantly suppressed the formation of TBARs to 58–59 μM, again implicating the beneficial effect of aerobic exercise (Table 5). Data consistent with Aslan et al. (1998), the MDA level after the 5 week training program was lower than the MDA level after acute exercise period but was still higher than sedentary period [63].

DRCKD Upregulated CD34 and α-SMA

CD34 is a marker of haematopoietic progenitor cells, stromal precursors, vascular endothelial cells, and a variety of stromal tumour cells. At the level of extraglomerular or intraglomerular mesangium, CD34 may signal either the presence of HSCs, or conversely, may be a marker of transdifferentiation [19]. Immunohistochemical co-staining of CD34 and α-SMA has been used to study various glomerulonephritis (GN) as a transformed mesangial cell marker [64]. In normal glomeruli, all cell types were negative for CD34, but in glomeruli in mesangial proliferative glomerulonephritis, CD34 is expressed exclusively in mesangial cells in parallel to α-SMA expression (Fig. 8A and 8B) [64]. Alternatively, Gluhovschi et al. indicated CD34 does not significantly correlate with mesangial α-SMA [19]. Swimming exercise at 60 min program restored its level to normal (Fig. 8A). Recent studies of Galeano et al. (2007) found that a genetic defect affecting sialic acid biosynthesis causes hematuria, proteinuria, and structural glomerular defects leading to animal death within days after birth [65]. α-SMA is a specific marker of mesangial cell activation [66], while it seems to have a better correlation with serum creatinine [19]. α-SMA plays key roles in glomerular remodeling [67], 60 min swimming training restored it to normal level (Fig. 7, 8B). The experimental results are summarized in Fig. 9.

To quantify the efficiency of different exercises on (myokine) IL-6 release, we elucidated a mathematical model (See 'Support Information S1"). Mathematical evaluation pointed out that 60 min swimming exercise does not release myokine. Instead, it directly consumes plasma IL-6 in proportional to the work expenditure. The consumption coefficient for swimming exercise $\mathbf{K'}_{swim}$ was −0.1098 pg/mL-J. While from the 60 min treadmill exercise we showed the "strenuosity coefficient" or "the myokine releasing coefficient" to have a magnitude 7.154×10^{-3} pg/mL-J (See 'Support Information S1"), which apparently was not achievable by the swimming exercise, implicating the differential benefits being dependent on duration- and strength of exercise.

In summary, exercise represents a physical stress that challenges homeostasis. The challenges including the clinical, the patient's, systemic and the environment factors involve most of the relevant physiological, biochemical, and immunological parameters. Exercise rehabilitation for CKD patients is a personalized rehabilitation in nature. Bergamaschi et al. (1997) pointed out the participation of other associated factors in the experimental model must be carefully inspected [41,6]. Thus, an optimum benefit only can be achieved provided a perfect rehabilitation design is available.

Conclusion

The 60 min swimming exercise training is more effective than the 30 min alternative in improving the DRCKD status. The 60 min swimming exercise prevents fibrosis of glomerular mesangium by inhibiting mesangial cell activation and CD34 expression, and simultaneously, by downregulating IL-6, PDGF, PDGFR, P-PDGFR, α-SMA, and dysregulating MMPs to suppress myofibroblast transdifferentiation. To quantify the critical effective condition for myokine IL-6 release, we have elucidated a mathematical index "The strenuosity coefficient" or "The myokine releasing coefficient" with a magnitude 7.154×10^{-3} pg/mL-J, and only above this value, the myokine IL-6 can be released during exercise.

Author Contributions

Conceived and designed the experiments: C-CP. Performed the experiments: C-CP. Analyzed the data: K-CC. Contributed reagents/materials/analysis tools: C-LH. Wrote the paper: RYP.

References

1. Painter P (2008) Exercise in Chronic Disease: Physiological Research Needed. Exercise and Sport Sciences Review. 83–90. www.acsm-essr.org
2. Adams GR, Vaziri ND (2006) Skeletal muscle dysfunction in chronic renal failure: effects of exercise. Am J Physiol Renal Physiol 290: F753–F761.
3. Johansen KL (2007) Exercise in the End-Stage Renal Disease Population. J Am Soc Nephrol 18: 1845–1854.
4. Osato S, Onoyama K, Okuda S, Sanai T, Hori K, et al. (1990) Effect of swimming exercise on the progress of renal dysfunction in rat with focal glomerulosclerosis. Nephron 55: 306–311.
5. Pedersen BK, Fischer CP (2007) Beneficial health effects of exercise – the role of IL-6 as a myokine. Trends Pharmacol Sci 28: 152–155.
6. Steensberg A, Keller C, Starkie RL, Osada T, Febbraio MA, et al. (2002) IL-6 and TNF-α expression in, and release from, contracting human skeletal muscle. Am J Physiol Endocrinol Metab 283: E1272–E1278.

7. Duzova H, Karakoc Y, Emre MH, Dogan ZY, Kilinc E (2009). Effects of acute moderate and strenuous exercise bouts on IL-17 production and inflammatory response in trained rats. J Sports Sci Med 8: 219–224.
8. Carrero JJ, Yilmaz MI, Lindholm B, Stenvinkel P (2008) Cytokine dysregulation in chronic kidney disease: How can we treat it? Blood Purif 26: 291–299.
9. Silveira EMS, Rodrigues MF, Krause MS, Vianna DR, Almeida BS, et al.(2007) Acute exercise stimulates macrophage function: possible role of NF-kB pathways. Cell Biochem Funct 25: 63–73.
10. Berk BC, Abe JI, Min W, Surapisitchat J, Yan C (2011) Endothelial atheroprotective and anti-inflammatory mechanisms. Ann NY Acad Sci 947: 93–111.
11. Boo YC, Sorescu G, Boyd N, Shiojima I, Walsh K, et al. (2002). Shear stress stimulates phosphorylation of endothelial nitric-oxide synthase at Ser^{1179} by Akt-independent mechanisms: role of protein kinase Am J Biol Chem 277: 3388–3396.
12. Bowman T, Garcia R, Turkson J, Jove R (2000) STATs in oncogenesis. Oncogene 19: 2474–2488.
13. Bruunsgaard H (2005) Physical activity and modulation of systemic low-level inflammation. J Leukoc Biol 78: 819–835.
14. Bloomfield SA, Coyle EF (1993) Bed rest, detraining and retention of training-induced adaptations. In: Resource Manual for Guidelines for Exercise Testing and Prescription (2nd ed), J. L. Durstine, P. L. Painter, J. L. Roitman, L. D. Zwiren (eds.). Philadelphia: Lea and Febiger, 115–128.
15. Ranieri E, Gesualdo L, Grandaliano G, Maiorano E, Schena FP (2001) The role of alpha-smooth muscle actin and platelet-derived growth factor-beta receptor in the progression of renal damage in human IgA nephropathy. J Nephrol 14: 253–262.
16. Fackler MJ, Krause DS, Smith OM, Civin CI, May WS (1995) Full length but not truncated CD34 inhibits hematopoietic cell differentiation of M1 cells. Blood 85: 3040–3047.
17. Bauheter S, Singer MS, Henzel W, Hemmerich S, Renz M, et al. (2003). Binding of L-selectin to the vascular sialomucin CD34. Science 262: 436–438.
18. Acevedo LM, Londono I, Oubaha M, Ghitescu L, Bendayan M (2008) Glomerular CD34 expresssion in short- and long-term diabetes. J Hitochem Cychem 56: 605–614.
19. Gluhovschi C, Gluhovschi G, Potencz E, Herman D, Trandafirescu V, et al. (2008) What is the significance of CD34 immuostaining in the extraglomerular and intraglomerula mesangium? Virchows Arch 453: 321–328.
20. Chebotareva NV, Proppe D, Rudolf P, Kozlovskaia IV (2002) Clinical significance of expression of the smooth muscle actin-alpha and CD34 antigen in mesangial cells in glomerulonephritis. Ter Arkh 74: 27–31.
21. Pusztaszeri MP, Seelentag W, Bossman FT (2006) Immunohitochemical expression of endothelial markers CD31, CD34, von Willebrand Factor, and Fli-1 in normal human tissues. J Histochem Cytochem 54: 385–395.
22. Peltonen J, Hsiao LL, Jaakkola S, Sollberg S, Aumailley M, et al. (1991) Activation of collagen gene expression in keloids: co-localization of type I and VI collagen and transforming growth factor-beta 1 mRNA. J Invest Dermatol 97: 240–248.
23. de Gonzalo-Calvo D, Fernández-García B, de Luxán-Delgado B, Rodríguez-González S, García-Macia M, et al. (2012) Chronic training increases blood oxidative damage but promotes health in elderly men. Age (Dordr). 2012 Jan 4. [Epub ahead of print].
24. Peng CC, Chen KC, Lu HY, Peng RY (2012) Treadmill exercise improved adriamycin-induced nephropathy. J Biol Regul Homeost Agents (in press).
25. Coelho BL, Rocha LG, Scarabelot KS, Scheffer DL, Ronsani MM, et al. (2010) Physical exercise prevents the exacerbation of oxidative stress parameters in chronic kidney disease. J Ren Nutr 20: 169–175.
26. Stump CS (2011) Physical Activity in the Prevention of Chronic Kidney Disease. Cardiorenal Med 1: 164–173. Epub 2011 Jul 25.
27. Jia B, Wang X, Kang A, Wang X, Wen Z, et al. (2012) The effects of long term aerobic exercise on the hemorheology in rats fed with high-fat diet. Clin Hemorheol Microcirc. 2012 Jan 3. [Epub ahead of print].
28. Vierck HB, Darvin ME, Lademann J, Reißhauer A, Baack A, et al. (2012) The influence of endurance exercise on the antioxidative status of human skin. Eur J Appl Physiol. 2012 Jan 22. [Epub ahead of print].
29. Harri M, Kuusela P (1986) Is swimming exercise or cold exposure for rats? Acta Physiol Scand 126: 189–197.
30. Belcastro AN, Maybank P, Rossiter M, Secord D (1985) Effect of endurance swimming on rat cardiac myofibrillar ATPase with experimental diabetes. Can J Physiol Pharamcol 63: 1202–1205.
31. Tschakovsky ME, Joyner MJ (2008) Nitric oxide and muscle blood flow in exercise. Appl Physiol Nutr Metab 33: 151–161.
32. De Moraes, R., Gioseffi G., Nóbrega AC, Tibiriçá E (2004) Effect of exercise training on the vascular reactivity of the whole kidney circulation in rabbits. J Appl Physiol 97: 683–688.
33. Bertani T, Poggi A, Pozzoni R, Delaini F, Sacchi G, et al. (1982) Adriamycin-induced nephrotic syndrome in rats: sequence of pathologic events. Lab Invest 46: 16–23.
34. Leber TM, Balkwill FR (1997) Zymography: a single-step staining method for quantitation of proteolytic activity on substrate gels. Anal Biochem 249: 24–28.
35. Weibel ER (1979) Stereological methods. In: Practical Methods for Biological Morphometry. London: Academic. pp 51–57.
36. Liang Y, Li YJ (2009) Expression of JAKs/STATs pathway molecules in rat model of rapid focal segmental glomerulosclerosis. Pediatr Nephrol 24: 1667–1671.
37. Nemet D, Oh Y, Kim HS (2002) Effect of intensive exercise on inflammatory cytokines and growth mediators in adolescent boys. Pediatrics 110: 681–689.
38. Fock RA, Vinolo MA, de Moura Sá Rocha V, de Sá Rocha LC, Borelli P (2007) Protein-energy malnutrition decreases the expression of TLR-4/MD-2 and CD14 receptors in peritoneal macrophages and reduces the synthesis of TNF-alpha in response to lipopolysaccharide (LPS) in mice. Cytokine 40: 105–114.
39. Poortmans JR (1995) Renal response to exercise in healthy and diseased patients. Nephrologie 16: 317–324.
40. Heifets M, Davis TA, Tegtmeyer E, Klahr S (1987) Exercise training ameliorates progressive renal disease in rats with subtotal nephrectomy. Kidney Int 32: 815–820.
41. Bergamaschi CT, Boim MA, Moura LA, Piçarro IC, Schor N (1997) Effects of long-term training on the progression of chronic renal failure in rats. Med Sci Sports Exerc 29: 169–174.
42. Bonegio RG, Fuhro R, Wang Z, Valeri CR, Andry C, et al. (2005) Rapamycin ameliorates proteinuria-associated tubulointerstitial inflammation and fibrosis in experimental membranous nephropathy. J Am Soc Nephrol 16: 2063–2072.
43. Jeansson M, Bjorck K, Tenstad O, Haraldsson B (2009) Adriamycicn alters glomerular endothelium to induce proteinuria. J Am Soc Nephrol 20: 114–122.
44. Aresu L, Benali S, Garbisa S, Gallo E, Castagnaro M (2011) Matrix mettaloproteinases and their role in the renal epithelial mesanchymal transition. Histol Histopathol 26: 307–313.
45. Rankin CA, Itoh Y, Tian C, Ziemer DM, Calvet JP, et al. (1999) Matrix metalloproteinase-2 in a murine model of infantile-type polycystic kidney disease. J Am Soc Nephrol 10: 210–217.
46. Hasegawa M, Fujimoto M, Takehara K, Sato S (2005) Pathogenesis of systemic sclerosis: altered B cell function is the key linking systemic autoimmunity and tissue fibrosis. J Dermatol Sci 39: 1–7.
47. Zeisberg EM, Potenta SE, Sugimoto H, Zeisberg M, Kalluri R (2008) Fibrosis in kidney fibrosis emerge via endothelial-to-mesenchymal transition. J Am Soc Nephrol 19: 2282–2287.
48. Stitt TN, Drujan D, Clarke BA, Panaro F, Timofeyva Y, et al. (2004) The IGF-1/PI3K/Akt pathway prevents expression of muscle atrophy-induced ubiquitin ligases by inhibiting FOXO transcription factors. Mol Cell 14: 395–403.
49. Olszanecka-Gliniaowicz M, Zahorska-Markiewicz B, Janowska J (2006) The effect of weight loss on serum concentrations of nitric oxide, TNF-alpha and soluble TNF-alpha receptors. Endokrynol Pol 57: 87–493.
50. Platel D, Bernard A, Mack G, Guiguet M (1996) Interleukin 6 upregulates TNF-alpha-dependent C3-stimulating activity through enhancement of TNF-alpha specific binding on rat liver epithelial cells. Cytokine 8: 895–899.
51. Bruun JM, Lihn AS, Verdic C, Pedersen SB, Toubro S, et al. (2003) Regulation of adiponectin by adipose tissue-derived cytokines: *in vivo* and *in vitro* investigations in humans. Am J Physiol Endocrinol Metab 285: E527–E533.
52. Fasshauer M, Kralisch S, Klier M, Lossner U, Bluher M, et al. (2003a) Adiponectin gene expression and secretion is inhibited by interleukin-6 in 3T3-L1 adipocytes. Biochem Biophys Res Commun 301: 1045–1050.
53. Fasshauer M, Paschke R (2003b) Regulation of adipocytokines and insulin resistance. Diabetologia 46: 1594–1603.
54. Kahn BB, Alquier T, Carling D, Hardie DG (2005) AMP-activated protein kinase: ancient energy gauge provides clues to modern understanding of metabolism. Cell Metab 1: 15–25.
55. Tang WW, Ulich TR, Lacey DL, Hill DC, Qi M, et al. (1996) Platelet-derived growth factor-BB induces renal tubulointerstitial myofibroblast formation and tubulointestitial fibrosis. Am J Pathol 148: 1169–1180.
56. Ostendorf T, Kunter U, Gröne HJ, Bahlmann F, Kawachi H, et al. (2001) Specific anatagonism of PDGF prevents renal scarring in experimental glomerulonephritis. J Am Soc Nephrol 12: 909–918.
57. Martinet Y, Rom WN, Grotendorst GR, Martin GR, Crystal RG (1987) Exaggerated spontaneous release of platelet-derived growth factor by alveolar macrophages from patients with idiopathicpulmonary fibrosis. N Engl J Med 317: 202–209.
58. Rubin K, Tingdtrom A, Hansson GK, Larsson E, Ronnstrand L, et al. (1988) Induction of B-type receptors for platelet-derived growth factor in vascular inflammation: Possible implications for development of vascular proliferative lesions. Lancet 1: 1353–1356.
59. Kulozik M, Hogg A, Lankat-Buttgereit B, Krieg T (1990) Co-localization of transforming growth factor beta 2 with alpha 1(I) procollagen mRNA in tissue sections of patients with systemic sclerosis. J Clin Invest 86: 917–922.
60. Ghahary A, Shen YJ, Scott PG, Gong Y, Tredget EE (1993) Enhanced expression of mRNA for transforming growth factor-beta, type I and type III procollagen in human post-burn hypertrophic scar tissues. J Lab Clin Med 22: 465–473.
61. Mastorakos G, Pavlatou M, Diamanti-Kandarakis E, Chrousos GP (2005) Exercise and the stress system. Hormones 4: 73–89.
62. Vouldoukis I, Lacan D, Kamate C, Coste P, Calenda A, et al. (2004) Antioxidant and anti-inflammatory properties of a Cucumis melo LC. extract rich in superoxide dismutase activity. J Ethnopharmacol 94: 67–75.
63. Aslan R, Sekeroglu MR, Tarkçioglu M, Bayiroglu F, Ismail Meral I (1998) Effect of acute and regular exercise on antioxidative enzymes, tissue damage markers and membrane lipid peroxidation of erythrocytes in sedentary students. Tr J Med Sci 28: 411–414.

64. Naruse K, Fulieda M, Miyazaki E, Hayashi Y, Kuroda N, et al. (1999) CD34 expressions as a novel marker of transformed mesangial cells in biopsied glomerular diseases. J Pathol 189: 105–111.
65. Galeano B, Klootwijk R, Manoli I, Sun M, Ciccone C, et al. (2007) Mutation in the key enzyme of sialic acid biosynthesis causes severe glomerula proteinuria and is rescued by N-acetylmannosamine. J Clin Invest 117: 1585–1594.
66. Johnson RJ, Iida H, Alpers CE, Majesky MW, Schwartz SM, et al. (1991) Expression of smooth muscle cell phenotype by rat mesangial cells in immune complex nephritis. Alpha smooth muscle actin is a marker of mesangial cell proliferation. J Clin Invest 87: 847–858.
67. Ichimura K, Kurihara H, Sakai T (2006) Involvement of mesangial cells expressing α-smooth muscle actin during restorative glomerular remodeling in Thy-1.1 nephritis. J Histochem Cytochem 54: 1291–1301.
68. Li KW (2009) Relationship between the Measured Friction Coefficient and Tread Groove Depth on Footwear Pad under Different Floor and Surface Conditions. J Occup Safety Health 17: 18–28.

11

Modification of Diet in Renal Disease (MDRD) Study and CKD Epidemiology Collaboration (CKD-EPI) Equations for Taiwanese Adults

Ling-I Chen[1☯], **Jinn-Yuh Guh**[1,4☯], **Kwan-Dun Wu**[3], **Yung-Ming Chen**[3], **Mei-Chuan Kuo**[1,4], **Shang-Jyh Hwang**[1,4], **Tzu-Hui Chen**[2], **Hung-Chun Chen**[1,4*]

1 Division of Nephrology, Department of Internal Medicine, Kaohsiung Medical University Hospital, Kaohsiung, Taiwan, **2** Department of Nursing, Kaohsiung Medical University Hospital, Kaohsiung, Taiwan, **3** Department of Internal Medicine, National Taiwan University Hospital, Taipei, Taiwan, **4** Faculty of Renal Care, College of Medicine, Kaohsiung Medical University, Kaohsiung, Taiwan

Abstract

Background: Estimated glomerular filtration rate (eGFR) using the Modification of Diet in Renal Disease (MDRD) study or the Chronic Kidney Disease Epidemiology Collaboration (CKD-EPI) equations may not be accurate for Asians; thus, we developed modified eGFR equations for Taiwanese adults.

Methods: This cross-sectional study compared the Taiwanese eGFR equations, the MDRD study, and the CKD-EPI equations with inulin clearance (C_{in}). A total of 695 adults including 259 healthy volunteers and 436 CKD patients were recruited. Participants from the Kaohsiung Medical University Hospital were used as the development set (N = 556) to develop the Taiwanese eGFR equations, whereas participants from the National Taiwan University Hospital were used as the validation set (N = 139) for external validation.

Results: The Taiwanese eGFR equations were developed by using the extended Bland-Altman plot in the development set. The Taiwanese MDRD equation was $1.309 \times MDRD^{0.912}$, Taiwanese CKD-EPI was $1.262 \times CKD\text{-}EPI^{0.914}$ and Taiwanese four-level CKD-EPI was $1.205 \times$four-level $CKD\text{-}EPI^{0.914}$. In the validation set, the Taiwanese equations had the lowest bias, the Taiwanese equations and the Japanese CKD-EPI equation had the lowest RMSE, whereas the Taiwanese and the Japanese equations had the best precision and the highest P_{30} among all equations. However, the Taiwanese MDRD equation had higher concordance correlation than did the Taiwanese CKD-EPI, the Taiwanese four-level CKD-EPI and the Japanese equations. Moreover, only the Taiwanese equations had no proportional bias among all of the equations. Finally, the Taiwanese MDRD equation had the best diagnostic performance in terms of ordinal logistic regression among all of the equations.

Conclusion: The Taiwanese MDRD equation is better than the MDRD, CKD-EPI, Japanese, Asian, Thai, Taiwanese CKD-EPI, and Taiwanese four-level CKD-EPI equations for Taiwanese adults.

Editor: Jean-Claude Dussaule, INSERM, France

Funding: This study was supported by the Bureau of Health Promotion (DOH99-HP-1107), Department of Health, R.O.C. (Taiwan). The funders had no role in study design, data collection and analysis, decision to publish, or preparation of the manuscript.

Competing Interests: The authors have declared that no competing interests exist.

* E-mail: chenhc@kmu.edu.tw

☯ These authors contributed equally to this work.

Introduction

The abbreviated Modification of Diet in Renal Disease (MDRD) study equation [1] was derived from Caucasians and African Americans with chronic kidney diseases (CKD) [2] and is not accurate for Asians [3–6] or when the estimating equations for glomerular filtration rate (eGFR) are above 60 mL/min/1.73 m^2 [7]. Thus, some Asian countries have developed their own eGFR equations [5,8–11]. However, many equations were derived solely from CKD patients, thereby having limitations in application to the general population [12,13]. For example, the MDRD equation underestimated the gold standard GFR measured by inulin clearance (C_{in}) for those with C_{in} of greater than 60 mL/min/1.73 m^2 in a recent Japanese study [4].

The Chronic Kidney Disease-Epidemiology Collaboration (CKD-EPI) equation may be more accurate than the MDRD Study equation, particularly at higher levels of GFR and in populations without CKD [14,15]. Thus, the Kidney Disease Improving Global Outcomes (KDIGO) 2012 guidelines recommend using the CKD-EPI equation in adults unless an alternative equation has been shown to be more accurate in the local population [16]. Additionally, the four-level CKD-EPI equation (Black, Asian, Native American and Hispanic, White and other) may improve accuracy for Asians [17].

Taiwan has a high prevalence (11.93%) and a low awareness (3.54%) of CKD [18]. In order to diagnose CKD by an eGFR equation with better accuracy based on the native data, we used C_{in} as the gold standard to develop modified Taiwanese eGFR equations from a cohort of CKD and healthy people and compared the performance between the original and the modified MDRD Study and the CKD-EPI equations.

Materials and Methods

We recruited adults aged over 18 years to sign informed consents from the Kaohsiung Medical University Hospital and the National Taiwan University Hospital. Subjects with acute renal failure, allergy to inulin, pregnancy, problems in voiding, amputation, congestive heart failure, cirrhosis with ascites, use of cimetidine or trimethoprim, oliguria, and those who had ever received any renal replacement therapy were excluded. Healthy volunteers were enrolled according to the percentage of age distribution in Taiwanese reported by the Ministry of the Interior of Taiwan. CKD was diagnosed and classified according to the K/DOQI clinical guidelines [1]. The ratio of the number of the CKD patients to healthy volunteers was approximately 2:1 in this study.

Ethics Statement

The study protocol was approved by the Institutional Review Board of the Kaohsiung Medical University Hospital (KMUH-IRB-960304) and National Taiwan University Hospital (NTUH-IRB-201002031M). Informed consents were obtained in written form from patients and all clinical investigations were conducted according to the principles expressed in the Declaration of Helsinki. The patients gave consent for the publication of the clinical details.

Inulin clearance

All subjects underwent procedures to measure C_{in} at the Kaohsiung Medical University Hospital or the National Taiwan University Hospital with the same protocol after the approval by the Ethics Committee in each respective hospital. C_{in} was calculated from serum inulin, urine inulin concentration, and urine volume collected in each time period. The protocol has been described before [9,19]. Briefly, after overnight fasting, the subject drank 500 mL of water 30 minutes before intravenous injection of inulin (40 mL 10% inulin in 360 mL 0.54% NaCl with a final concentration of 1%, Fuji Yakuhin Co. Ltd., Saitama, Japan). Just before the infusion, complete urine collection and blood sampling were performed in an ordinary way. To maintain hydration, 60 mL of water was drunk at 30 and 60 minutes after the start of inulin infusion. The rate of inulin infusion was 300 mL/hour for the first 30 min and 100 mL/hour for the following 60 min.

Blood samples for serum inulin concentration were collected at 45 min and 75 min after the start of inulin infusion. Urine samples for urinary inulin concentration were collected between 30 and 60 min and between 60 and 90 min after the patient completely voided the bladder at 30 min. The first and second urinary excretions of inulin were added, assuming the total amount as a single urine collection between 30 and 90 min [9]. This value was then used with the mean of the first (45 minutes) and second (75 minutes) serum inulin concentrations to calculate C_{in} as the measured GFR (mL/min/1.73 m^2) [9]. Note that this abbreviated method for the calculation of C_{in} has been shown to be equivalent to the full 2-hour C_{in} protocol [9].

Serum inulin was measured by an enzymatic method by using a commercial kit (Diacolor Inulin; Toyobo Co, Osaka, Japan) with Hitachi 7180 auto-analyzer at the Kaohsiung Medical University Hospital. The steady-state of serum inulin concentrations was reached at 45 min (22.2 [21.5, 22.9] mg/dL) and 75 min (21.6 [21.1, 22.1] mg/dL) because the coefficient of variation was only 2.9%. This result was similar to a previous study [9].

Measurement of creatinine and estimated GFR

Serum creatinine (SCr) was measured by the IDMS-traceable enzymatic method in a Roche Cobas Integra 400 at the Kaohsiung Medical University Hospital. The eGFR values were calculated by the IDMS-traceable MDRD equation: $175 \times SCr^{-1.154} \times Age^{-0.203} \times 0.742$ (if female), the CKD-EPI equation: $141 \times \min(SCr/\kappa, 1)^{\alpha} \times \max(SCr/\kappa, 1)^{-1.209} \times 0.993^{Age} \times 1.018$ [if female] where κ is 0.7 for females and 0.9 for males, α is −0.329 for females and −0.411 for males, min indicates the minimum of SCr/κ or 1, and max indicates the maximum of SCr/κ or 1, and the four-level CKD-EPI equation [17]: $141 \times \min(SCr/\kappa, 1)^{\alpha} \times \max(SCr/\kappa, 1)^{-1.210} \times 0.993^{Age} \times 0.993$ [if female] $\times 1.05$ [if Asian] where κ is 0.7 for females and 0.9 for males, α is −0.328 for females and −0.412 for males, min indicates the minimum of SCr/κ or 1, and max indicates the maximum of SCr/κ or 1.

Additionally, the Japanese modifications of MDRD (=0.808×MDRD) and CKD-EPI (=0.813×CKD-EPI) [10], Asian (Chinese, Malays and Indians in Singapore) modifications of MDRD (=1.086×MDRD) and CKD-EPI (=1.049×CKD-EPI) [11] and Thai modification of MDRD (=1.129×MDRD) [20] were calculated.

Statistical analysis

Continuous data were expressed as the mean ± standard error of the mean or mean (95% confidence interval) unless stated otherwise. Linear regression was expressed as the prediction equation ± standard deviation of prediction. The 95% prediction interval was calculated as the estimate ±2 standard deviations of prediction. Note that the 95% prediction interval is always wider than the 95% confidence interval because the former estimates the scatter of the data whereas the latter estimates only the mean [21]. Continuous variables were compared by unpaired *t*-tests whereas categorical variables were compared by χ^2 tests unless stated otherwise. All eGFR equations were compared to the Taiwanese MDRD equation.

The Taiwanese equations were generated from the whole development set by using linear regression of the difference on the average (i.e. the extended Bland-Altman plot in the MethComp package in R, which was designed specifically for method comparison studies) [22] of the log-transformed C_{in} and the MDRD, CKD-EPI and four-level CKD-EPI equations.

Internal validation of the Taiwanese equations was performed by 2,000 bootstraps in which the subjects were drawn at random with replacement [23]. Hence, subjects may be represented zero or many times in a bootstrap sample. The Taiwanese equations were trained in the sampled subjects and tested in the original development set in each bootstrap step. Afterwards, the difference of RMSE between the bootstrap and the test samples was subtracted from the RMSE of the original development set [23].

For the validation set, eGFR equations were assessed for accuracy and agreement. Accuracy was measured as the percentage within 30% of C_{in} (P_{30}), bias, precision, and the root mean squared error (RMSE) [24]. The bias was defined as the median difference between C_{in} and eGFR (C_{in} - eGFR) with negative values indicating overestimation of C_{in}. Precision was expressed as the interquartile range of the bias. RMSE was defined as the square root of the average squared difference of C_{in} and eGFR. RMSE was compared by using 2,000 bootstrap samples to derive the standard errors of the differences of RMSE [11].

Because P_{30} and bias were compared between the paired data, P_{30} was compared by the exact McNemar test, whereas bias was compared by the Wilcoxon signed rank test.

Agreement between two continuous variables (C_{in} and eGFR) was measured by the concordance correlation coefficient (r) [25] and the Bland-Altman plot [22,26]. Concordance correlation was compared by Zou's method [27]. Note that the comparison of two r's (r of C_{in} and eGFR1 and r of C_{in} and eGFR2) requires a third r (r of eGFR1 and eGFR2). Diagnostic performance of the eGFR equations for the classification of CKD stages (according to C_{in} or eGFR alone, disregarding proteinuria) was assessed by ordinal logistic (generalized ordered logit) regression and chance-corrected agreement (kappa coefficient, a measure of the agreement between two categorical variables) [28]. Ordinal logistic regressions (C_{in}-defined CKD category and eGFR was the dependent and independent variable, respectively) (Methods S1) were compared by the Akaike information criterion (AIC) where a model with the lowest AIC is the best model [29]. Note that the AIC is an information-theoretic approach in which there are no null hypothesis significance tests to choose the lowest AIC [29]. Instead, the Akaike weight (*wi*) is used to weigh the evidence of each model [29,30].

$$wi = \frac{\exp(-(AICi - \min(AIC))/2)}{\sum_{k=1}^{K} \exp(-(AICi - \min(AIC))/2)}$$

Here, exp denotes the exponential, *AICi* denotes the *AIC* for the *i*th model whereas min (*AIC*) denotes the minimal *AIC* for the *K* models.

Analyses were computed by using the R (version 3.0.0; Free Software Foundation, Boston, MA) and the Stata software (version 13.0, StataCorp LP, College Station, TX).

Results

Characteristics of the Participants in the Development and Validation Sets

From April, 2008 to October, 2009, a total of 300 persons were recruited from the Kaohsiung Medical University Hospital where 11 subjects were excluded due to incomplete data. From Oct. 2009 to June 2011, a total of 406 persons were recruited from either the Kaohsiung Medical University Hospital or the National Taiwan University Hospital. Thus, a total of 695 participants which included 259 healthy volunteers and 436 CKD patients were recruited.

Participants from the Kaohsiung Medical University Hospital (located in the southern Taiwan) were used as the development set (N = 556) to develop the Taiwanese eGFR equations whereas participants from the National Taiwan University Hospital were used as the validation set (N = 139) for the external validation of the Taiwanese eGFR equations. Note that this was a geographical external validation set [31], in that the National Taiwan University Hospital is a different hospital located in Northern Taiwan. As shown in Table 1, there were no healthy volunteers, and the participants were older in the validation set.

Determination and bootstrap cross-validation of the Taiwanese eGFR equations in the development set

Taiwanese eGFR equations were determined by using linear regression of the difference on the average (i.e. the extended Bland-Altman plot) in the development set [22]. Taiwanese eGFR equations were $1.309 \times MDRD^{0.912}$ for the Taiwanese MDRD (Fig. 1A), $1.262 \times CKD\text{-}EPI^{0.914}$ for the Taiwanese CKD-EPI (Fig. 1B) and $1.205 \times$four-level $CKD\text{-}EPI^{0.914}$ for the Taiwanese four-level CKD-EPI (Fig. 1C) in the (anti-logged) original units, respectively. In 2,000 bootstraps of the development set, RMSE of the Taiwanese MDRD (11.7) was lower than that of the Taiwanese CKD-EPI (13.7) and Taiwanese four-level CKD-EPI (18.3). Note that RMSE of internal validation was lower than that of the external validation. However, the results of internal validation are usually too optimistic and external validation is necessary for the generalizability of prediction rules [32].

Accuracy of eGFR for the validation set

Accuracy was assessed by P_{30}, bias, precision and the RMSE. We found P_{30} for all of the equations except that of the Japanese equations, Taiwanese CKD-EPI or Taiwanese four-level CKD-EPI equations was lower than that of the Taiwanese MDRD equation for the whole set (Table 2) and those with $C_{in} \geq 60$ mL/min/1.73 m^2 (Table3). In contrast, only P_{30} of the four-level CKD-EPI, Asian CKD-EPI and Thai MDRD equations were lower than that of the Taiwanese MDRD equation for those with $C_{in} < 60$ mL/min/1.73 m^2 (Table 4)

The Taiwanese equations had the lowest bias among all of the equations for the whole set (Table 2), those with $C_{in} \geq 60$ mL/min/1.73 m^2 (Table 3) and those with $C_{in} < 60$ mL/min/1.73 m^2 (Table 4). The Taiwanese and the Japanese equations had the best precision (19–20 mL/min/1.73 m^2) among all of the equations for the whole set (Table 2). The Taiwanese equations, the Japanese CKD-EPI equation, and the MDRD equation had the lowest RMSE among all equations for the whole set (Table 2). In contrast, the Taiwanese MDRD equation and the Japanese equations had the lowest RMSE for those with $C_{in} < 60$ mL/min/1.73 m^2 (Table 4). However, the Taiwan MDRD equation had lower RMSE than did all equations except the Taiwanese CKD-EPI, Taiwanese four-level CKD-EPI, MDRD and CKD-EPI equations for those with $C_{in} \geq 60$ mL/min/1.73 m^2 (Table 3).

Agreement between C_{in} and eGFR for the validation set

The agreement between C_{in} and the eGFR equations was assessed by concordance correlation and the Bland-Altman plot for the validation set. We found that concordance correlation of the Taiwanese MDRD equation (0.823) was higher ($P < 0.05$) than those of the Japanese MDRD (0.803), Taiwanese CKD-EPI (0.78), Taiwanese four-level CKD-EPI (0.78), Thai MDRD (0.772) and Japanese CKD-EPI (0.771) equations, but was not different from that of the MDRD (0.826), CKD-EPI (0.798), Asian MDRD (0.794), Asian CKD-EPI (0.782),or four-level CKD-EPI (0.781), for the whole set.

The concordance correlation of the Taiwanese MDRD equation (0.757) was higher ($P < 0.05$) than those of the Taiwanese CKD-EPI (0.729), Taiwanese four-level CKD-EPI (0.728), MDRD (0.685), CKD-EPI (0.628), Asian MDRD (0.627), Asian CKD-EPI (0.593), four-level CKD-EPI (0.59) and Thai MDRD (0.598) equations, but was not different from that of the Japanese MDRD (0.771) or Japanese CKD-EPI (0.746) equation, for those with $C_{in} < 60$ mL/min/1.73 m^2.

The concordance correlation of the Taiwanese MDRD (0.537) was higher ($P < 0.05$) than those of the Taiwanese four-level CKD-EPI (0.39) and Taiwanese CKD-EPI (0.388) and Japanese CKD-EPI (0.378) equations, but was not different from that of the MDRD (0.571), Asian MDRD (0.522), Japanese MDRD (0.502), Thai MDRD (0.489), CKD-EPI (0.464), four-level CKD-EPI (0.447) or Asian CKD-EPI (0.446), for those with $C_{in} \geq 60$ mL/min/1.73 m^2.

Table 1. Clinical characteristics of the participants.

Clinical characteristics	Development set (n = 556)	Validation set (n = 139)	P
Age (years)	47±0.7	51±1	0.006
Men (%)	47.1	51	0.40
Height (cm)	163±0.4	163±0.8	0.96
Weight (kg)	64±0.5	62±1	0.14
Body surface area (m^2)	1.69±0.01	1.67±0.01	0.28
CKD clinic patient (%)	53.4	100.0	<0.001
Diabetes mellitus (%)	12.0	12.2	0.95
Serum creatinine (mg/dL)	1.52±0.05	1.43±0.1	0.45
C_{in} (mL/min/1.73 m^2)	67±1.6	68.8±3.0	0.56
C_{in}<60 mL/min/1.73 m^2 (%)	43.5	42.5	0.82

Abbreviations: CKD, chronic kidney disease; C_{in}, inulin clearance.

In the Bland-Altman plot of the original data (data not shown), there were increasing scatters of differences with increasing eGFR (i.e. V-shaped limits of agreement) for all of the equations. Moreover, there were negative correlations between the difference and the mean for the MDRD, CKD-EPI and four-level CKD-EPI equations respectively. These findings violated the assumptions of the homogeneity of the scatter of differences and a constant bias for the Bland-Altman plot [22,26,33]. Thus, the Bland-Altman plot of the difference of the log-transformed data on the ordinate [33] was shown in Fig. 2. Note that the anti-log of the difference between two log-transformed data is the ratio of the two data in the original units. The geometric mean ratio (95% limit of agreement) in the original units of the Taiwanese MDRD (A), Taiwanese CKD-EPI (B), Taiwanese four-level CKD-EPI (C), MDRD (D), CKD-EPI (E) and four-level CKD-EPI (F) equations was 1.023 (0.58, 1.79), 1.025 (0.57, 1.8), 1.025 (0.57, 1.8), 0.93 (0.5, 1.7), 0.91 (0.49, 1.7), 0.86 (0.46, 1.6), respectively.

Regression lines and the 95% prediction intervals of the extended Bland-Altman plot of the log-transformed C_{in} and the log-transformed Taiwanese MDRD (Fig. 3A), Taiwanese CKD-EPI (Fig. 3B), Taiwanese four-level CKD-EPI (Fig. 3C), MDRD (Fig. 3D), CKD-EPI (Fig. 3E) and four-level CKD-EPI (Fig. 3F) in the (anti-logged) original units are shown in Fig. 3.

The slope (95% confidence interval) of the Taiwanese MDRD, Taiwanese CKD-EPI, Taiwanese four-level CKD-EPI, MDRD, CKD-EPI, four-level CKD-EPI, Japanese MDRD, Japanese CKD-EPI, Asian MDRD, Asian CKD-EPI and Thai MDRD was 0.99 (0.92, 1.06), 1.008 (0.93, 1.08), 1.007 (0.93, 1.08), 0.9 (0.83, 0.96), 0.92 (0.85, 0.99), 0.92 (0.85, 0.99), 0.9 (0.83, 0.96), 0.92 (0.85, 0.99), 0.9 (0.83, 0.96), 0.92 (0.85, 0.99) and 0.9 (0.83, 0.96), respectively. Note that only the Taiwanese equations had no proportional bias (i.e. they had slopes that were not different from 1).

Diagnostic performances of the eGFR equations for the classification of CKD stages for the validation set

Diagnostic performance of the eGFR equations for the classification of CKD stages was assessed by the ordinal logistic regression and the kappa coefficients [28]. We found that all the eGFR equations had similar kappa values compared with that of the Taiwanese MDRD equation for the whole set (Table 2), those with $C_{in} \geq 60$ mL/min/1.73 m^2 (Table 3) and those with $C_{in} <$ 60 mL/min/1.73 m^2 (Table 4).

In ordinal logistic regression, the Taiwanese MDRD equation had the lowest AIC (230.7) compared to those of the MDRD (231.4), CKD-EPI (232), four-level CKD-EPI (232.2), Taiwanese CKD-EPI (231.4), Taiwanese four-level CKD-EPI (231.5), Japanese MDRD (231.4), Japanese CKD-EPI (232), Asian MDRD (231.4), Asian CKD-EPI (232) and Thai MDRD (231.4) equations. Moreover, the Taiwanese MDRD equation had the highest Akaike weight (0.14) compared to those of the MDRD (0.097), CKD-EPI (0.07), four-level CKD-EPI (0.07), Taiwanese CKD-EPI (0.098), Taiwanese four-level CKD-EPI (0.09), Japanese MDRD (0.097), Japanese CKD-EPI (0.07), Asian MDRD (0.097), Asian CKD-EPI (0.07) and Thai MDRD (0.097) equations. Thus, the Taiwanese MDRD equation had the best diagnostic performance.

Discussion

In this study, the Taiwanese equations had the lowest bias, the Taiwanese equations and the Japanese CKD-EPI equation had the lowest RMSE, whereas the Taiwanese and the Japanese equations had the best precision and the highest P_{30}. The Taiwanese MDRD equation had higher concordance correlation than the Taiwanese CKD-EPI, Taiwanese four-level CKD-EPI and the Japanese equations. Moreover, only the Taiwanese equations had no proportional bias among all of the equations. Finally, the Taiwanese MDRD equation had the best diagnostic performance in terms of ordinal logistic regression among all of the equations.

We found that the MDRD, CKD-EPI, four-level CKD-EPI, Asian equations, and Thai MDRD equations overestimated GFR, whereas the Japanese equations underestimated GFR. In contrast, the Taiwanese equations had very low bias in that the Taiwanese equations had the lowest bias among all equations.

The Taiwanese and the Japanese equations had similar performances in terms of P_{30} and precision in that they had the highest P_{30} and the best precision among all equations. Moreover, the Taiwanese equations and the Japanese CKD-EPI equation had the lowest RMSE among all equations. However, the Taiwanese equations had lower biases than those of the Japanese equations and the Taiwanese MDRD equation had lower RMSE than those of the Japanese equations for those with $C_{in} \geq 60$ mL/min/1.73 m^2. Note that P_{30} is an arbitrary measure of accuracy whereas dichotomization (i.e., P_{30}) of continuous variables introduces biases [34]. In contrast, bias and RMSE are standard

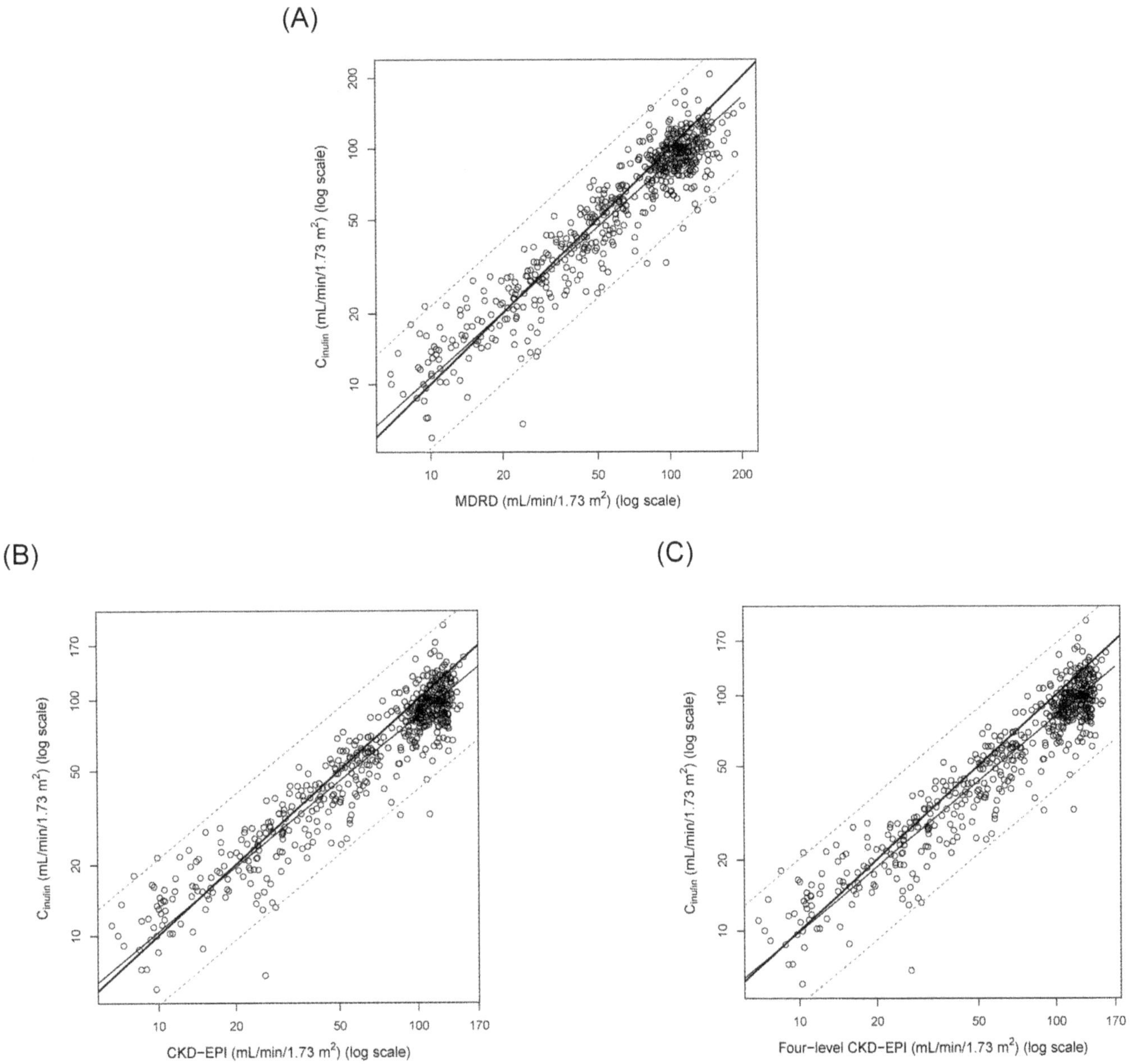

Figure 1. Determination of the Taiwanese eGFR equations in the development set. Taiwanese eGFR equations were derived by using linear regression of the differences on the average (i.e. the extended Bland-Altman plot). C_{in} and the eGFR equations were log-transformed and plotted on the log-scale. The regression line (thin solid line) and its 95% prediction interval (dotted lines) were plotted along with the identity (thick solid diagonal) line. (A) The regression equation of the Taiwanese MDRD equation was $1.309\times MDRD^{0.912}$ in the (anti-logged) original unit. (B) The regression equation of the Taiwanese CKD-EPI equation was $1.262\times CKD\text{-}EPI^{0.914}$ in the original unit. (C) The regression equation of the Taiwanese four-level CKD-EPI equation was $1.205\times$four-level $CKD\text{-}EPI^{0.914}$ in the original unit.

measures of model accuracy [35]. Moreover, the Taiwanese MDRD equation had higher concordance correlation than the Japanese equations. Finally, the Japanese, but not the Taiwanese equations, had proportional bias. Thus, the Taiwanese MDRD equation is better than the Japanese equations.

In the Bland-Altman plot, the 95% limits of agreement were too wide to draw conclusions. Nonetheless, only the Taiwanese equations had no proportional bias among all equations in the extended Bland-Altman plot [22].

Surprisingly, the Taiwanese MDRD equation had similar kappa value with the other equations. This finding can be explained by the fact that eGFR is a continuous variable and that the eGFR-defined CKD stage is an arbitrary categorical variable whereas dichotomization of continuous predictor variables introduces biases [34]. In contrast, the Taiwanese MDRD equation-derived eGFR (a continuous variable) had the best diagnostic performance in terms of the lowest AIC and the highest Akaike weight in the ordinal logistic regression.

Many (but not all) studies found that the CKD-EPI equation was more accurate than the MDRD equation [6,24,36-38]. For example, the Japanese CKD-EPI equation was better than the Japanese MDRD equation [10]. The CKD-EPI equation was also better than the MDRD and four-level CKD-EPI equations in a Chinese study [39]. However, the CKD-EPI equation was not

Table 2. Performance of the eGFR equations for the validation set.

	P_{30} (%)	Bias (mL/min/1.73 m^2)	Precision (mL/min/1.73 m^2)	RMSE (mL/min/1.73 m^2)	Kappa
MDRD	63.3*	−5.4**	23	23.3	0.437
CKD-EPI	60.4**	−8.0**	25	24.2#	0.38
Four-level CKD-EPI	52.5**	−12.0**	29	26.1*	0.38
Japanese MDRD	71.2	5.8**	19	23.7#	0.48
Japanese CKD-EPI	70.5	4.0**	20	23.4	0.494
Asian MDRD	56.8**	−11.0**	28	27.0**	0.435
Asian CKD-EPI	54.0**	−11.0**	28	26.0**	0.38
Thai MDRD	52.5**	−14.0**	32	29.0**	0.435
Taiwanese MDRD	73.4	0.17	19	21.4	0.495
Taiwanese CKD-EPI	73.4	0.42	20	23.0	0.549
Taiwanese four-level CKD-EPI	74.1	0.24	20	23.0	0.549

Abbreviations and definitions: MDRD, Modification of Diet in Renal Disease; CKD-EPI, Chronic Kidney Disease Epidemiology Collaboration; P_{30}, the percentage within 30% of inulin clearance; bias, median difference of inulin clearance and estimated GFR (C_{in} − eGFR); precision, interquartile range of the bias; RMSE, root mean square error; Kappa, kappa coefficients of the eGFR equations for the classification of CKD stages.
#P<0.05 versus Taiwanese MDRD;
*p<0.01 versus Taiwanese MDRD;
**P<0.001 versus Taiwanese MDRD.

better than the MDRD study equation for diabetic patients [37,38]. In this study, the Taiwanese CKD-EPI and Taiwanese four-level CKD-EPI equations were worse than the Taiwanese MDRD equation especially for those with C_{in}<60 mL/min/1.73 m^2

The differences in ethnicity, study population and the use of different reference GFR methods may account for this discrepancy. For example, our study and the Japanese study [10] used the gold standard C_{in} as the reference GFR, whereas the MDRD and CKD-EPI equation used urinary clearance of iothalamate, which overestimates C_{in} [40-42]. In contrast, the Singapore and the Thai studies [11,20] used plasma technetium-^{99m}-labeled diethylenetriamine penta-acetate (^{99m}Tc-DTPA) clearance, which also overestimates C_{in} [43,44].

The strengths of this study were the use of the gold standard (C_{in}) as the reference GFR, the inclusion of healthy volunteers, and the validation of the Taiwanese eGFR equations using an external validation set. One of the limitations of this study was that there were no healthy volunteers in the validation set. However, the mean C_{in} was similar and the proportion of subjects with C_{in}< 60 mL/min/1.73 m^2 was also similar between the development and the validation set. The other limitation was that the participants were older in the external validation set. However, differences in case mix is not a great concern for external

Table 3. Performance of the eGFR equations for the participants with C_{in}≥60 mL/min/1.73 m^2 in the validation set.

	P_{30} (%)	Bias (mL/min/1.73 m^2)	Precision (mL/min/1.73 m^2)	RMSE (mL/min/1.73 m^2)	Kappa
MDRD	65.0*	−9.2**	30	27.0	0.257
CKD-EPI	65.0*	−12.0**	26	26.7	0.205
Four-level CKD-EPI	57.5**	−16.6**	26	28.4#	0.205
Japanese MDRD	78.8	8.6**	26	27.9#	0.28
Japanese CKD-EPI	81.3	5.2**	26	28.7#	0.29
Asian MDRD	60.0*	−17.0**	30	31.1#	0.26
Asian CKD-EPI	57.5**	−16.0**	26	28.3#	0.26
Thai MDRD	55.0**	−22.0**	31	33.9#	0.26
Taiwanese MDRD	81.3	2.1	28	25.8	0.271
Taiwanese CKD-EPI	81.3	1.2	26	27.5	0.33
Taiwanese four-level CKD-EPI	81.3	1.4	26	27.5	0.33

Abbreviations and definitions: MDRD, Modification of Diet in Renal Disease; CKD-EPI, Chronic Kidney Disease Epidemiology Collaboration; P_{30}, the percentage within 30% of inulin clearance; bias, median difference of inulin clearance and estimated GFR (C_{in} − eGFR); precision, interquartile range of the bias; RMSE, root mean square error; Kappa, kappa coefficients of the eGFR equations for the classification of CKD stages.
#P<0.05 versus Taiwanese MDRD;
*p<0.01 versus Taiwanese MDRD;
**P<0.001 versus Taiwanese MDRD.

Table 4. Performance of the eGFR equations for the participants with C_{in}<60 mL/min/1.73 m^2 in the validation set.

	P_{30} (%)	Bias (mL/min/1.73 m^2)	Precision (mL/min/1.73 m^2)	RMSE (mL/min/1.73 m^2)	Kappa
MDRD	61.0	−1.7**	17	17.0**	0.356
CKD-EPI	54.0	−3.1**	21	20.3**	0.31
Four-level CKD-EPI	45.8*	−5.0**	24	22.6**	0.31
Japanese MDRD	61.0	3.9**	13	12.3	0.424
Japanese CKD-EPI	56.0	2.4**	15	13.9	0.407
Asian MDRD	52.5	−4.8**	21	20.2**	0.365
Asian CKD-EPI	49.0#	−5.1**	24	22.4**	0.291
Thai MDRD	49.0*	−5.6**	23	21.9**	0.365
Taiwanese MDRD	62.7	−0.58	15	13.2	0.429
Taiwanese CKD-EPI	62.7	−0.61	15	14.7*	0.411
Taiwanese four-level CKD-EPI	64.4	−0.62	15	14.8*	0.411

Abbreviations and definitions: MDRD, Modification of Diet in Renal Disease; CKD-EPI, Chronic Kidney Disease Epidemiology Collaboration; P_{30}, the percentage within 30% of inulin clearance; bias, median difference of inulin clearance and estimated GFR (C_{in} − eGFR); precision, interquartile range of the bias; RMSE, root mean square error; Kappa, kappa coefficients of the eGFR equations for the classification of CKD stages.
#P<0.05 versus Taiwanese MDRD;
*p<0.01 versus Taiwanese MDRD;
**P<0.001 versus Taiwanese MDRD.

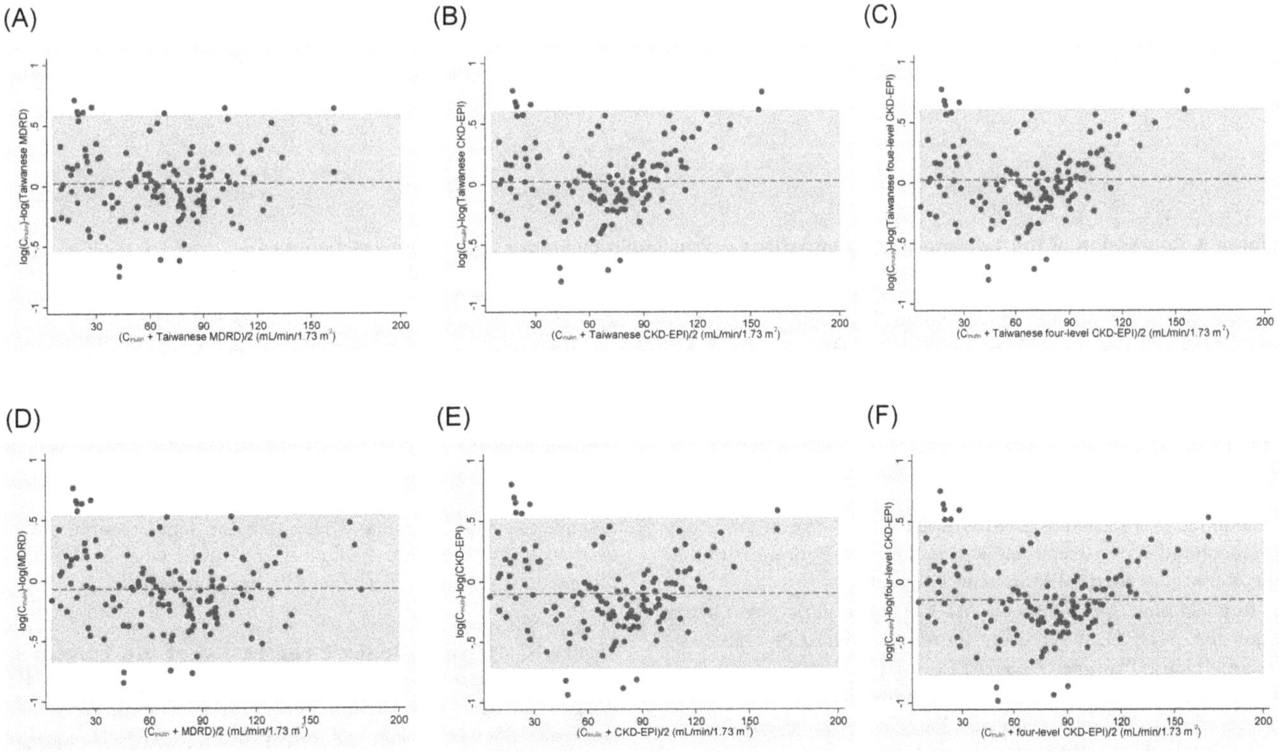

Figure 2. Bland-Altman plot of eGFR equations versus inulin clearance (C_{in}) for the validation set. The difference of log-transformed C_{in} and eGFR equation (ordinate) was plotted against the mean of C_{in} and each respective eGFR equation (abscissa). The mean difference was shown as a dotted horizontal line whereas the 95% limit of agreement was shown as the shaded area. Note that the anti-log of the difference between two log-transformed data is the ratio of the two data in the original units. Bland-Altman plot of (A) The geometric mean ratio (95% limit of agreement) was 1.023 (0.58, 1.79) for the Taiwanese MDRD in the original unit, (B) The geometric mean ratio (95% limit of agreement) was 1.025 (0.57, 1.8) for the Taiwanese CKD-EPI in the original unit, (C) The geometric mean ratio (95% limit of agreement) was 1.025 (0.57, 1.8) for the Taiwanese four-level CKD-EPI, (D) The geometric mean ratio (95% limit of agreement) was 0.93 (0.5, 1.7) for the MDRD in the original unit, (E) The geometric mean ratio (95% limit of agreement) was 0.91 (0.49, 1.7) for the CKD-EPI in the original unit and (F) The geometric mean ratio (95% limit of agreement) was 0.86 (0.46, 1.6) for the four-level CKD-EPI in the original unit.

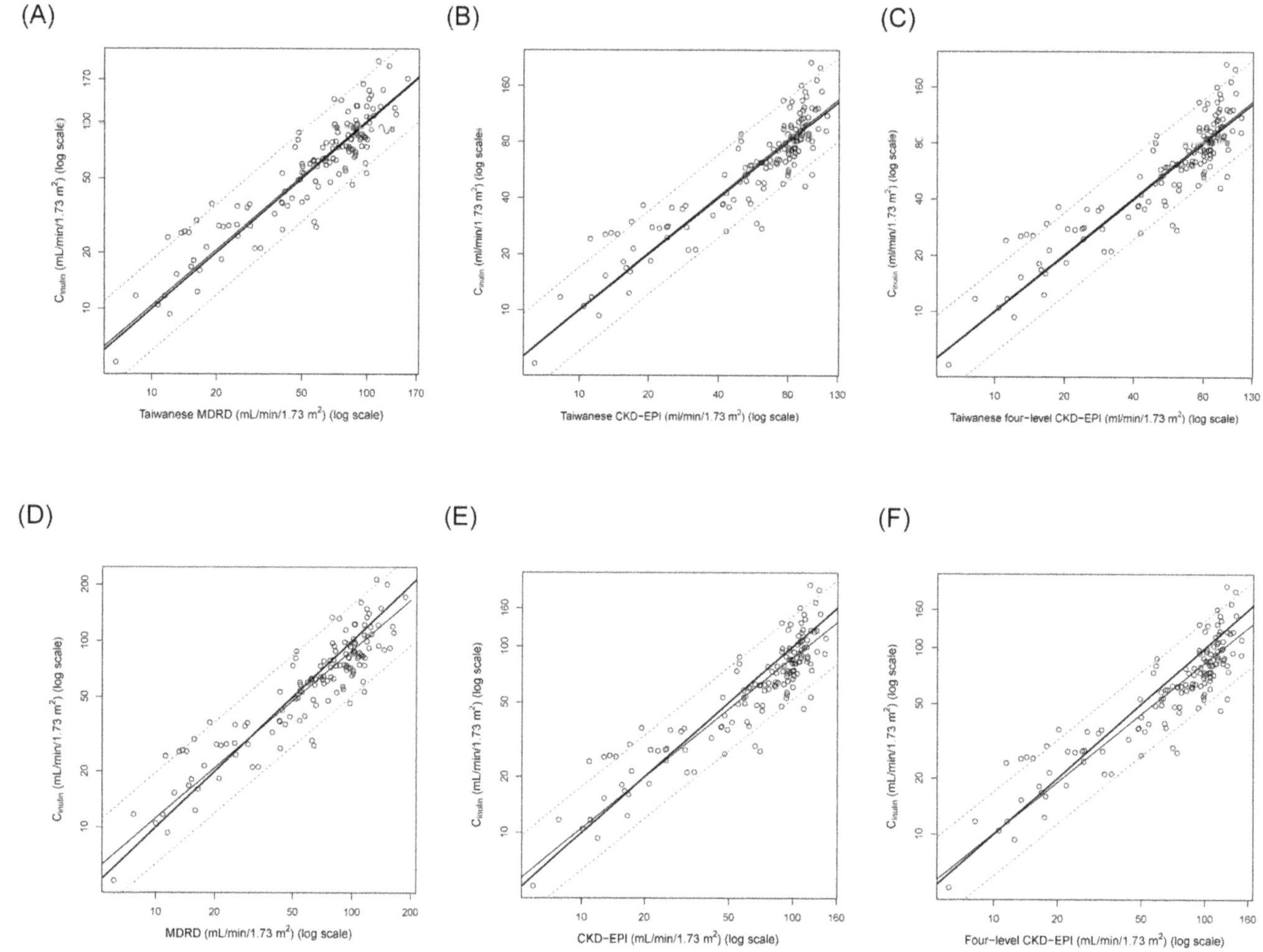

Figure 3. Regression of the Taiwanese eGFR equations versus inulin clearance (C_{in}) in the validation set. C_{in} and the eGFR equations were log-transformed and plotted on the log-scale in the regression derived from the extended Bland-Altman plot. The regression line (thin solid line) and its 95% prediction interval (dotted lines) were plotted along with the identity (thick solid diagonal) line. (A) The slope (95% confidence interval) was 0.99 (0.92, 1.06) and the regression equation of the Taiwanese MDRD was 1.06×Taiwanese $MDRD^{0.99}$ in the anti-logged (original) unit. (B) The slope was 1.008 (0.93, 1.08) and the regression equation of the Taiwanese CKD-EPI was 0.99×Taiwanese $CKD\text{-}EPI^{1.01}$ in the original unit. (C) The slope was 1.007 (0.93, 1.08) and the regression equation of the Taiwanese four-level CKD-EPI was 0.99×Taiwanese four-level $CKD\text{-}EPI^{1.01}$ in the original unit. (D) The slope was 0.9 (0.83, 0.96) and the regression equation of the MDRD equation was 1.41×$MDRD^{0.9}$ in the original unit. (E) The slope was 0.92 (0.85, 0.99) and the regression equation of the CKD-EPI equation was 1.28×$CKD\text{-}EPI^{0.92}$ in the original unit. (F) The slope was 0.92 (0.85, 0.99) and the regression equation of the four-level CKD-EPI was 1.22×four-level $CKD\text{-}EPI^{0.92}$ in the original unit.

validation [31]. Finally, both hospitals used the same study protocol and serum creatinine and inulin were both measured at the Kaohsiung Medical University Hospital.

In conclusion, the Taiwanese MDRD equation performs better than the MDRD, CKD-EPI, four-level CKD-EPI, Japanese, Asian, Thai, Taiwanese CKD-EPI, and Taiwanese four-level CKD-EPI equations for Taiwanese adults. Thus, further studies are required to determine its clinical applications (e.g. correlations with complications and prognosis) in Taiwan.

Supporting Information

Figure S1 Logistic regression for C_{in}-defined CKD stage 1 in the validation set. Linear regression (the oblique line) and logistic regression (the S-shaped sigmoid curve) of the Taiwanese MDRD equation for the prediction of the probability ($\pi(x)$) of inulin clearance (C_{in})-defined CKD stage 1 (the dots on the vertical axis, yes = 1, no = 0). Note that the probability of CKD stage 1 increases as eGFR increases and that the logistic curve always predicts $\pi(x)$ to be within the limit of zero and 1 whereas the linear regression line can predict $\pi(x)$ to be less than zero.

Figure S2 Ordinal logistic regression of the Taiwanese MDRD equation for the prediction of C_{in}-defined CKD stages in the validation set. Ordinal logistic regression (generalized ordered logit) of the Taiwanese MDRD equation was performed by the cumulative logit model. (A) Cumulative probability of C_{in}-defined CKD stages and the logistic curves. Note that the cumulative probability of CKD stage 1, stage 1–2, stage 1–3 and stage 1–4 increases as eGFR increases. (B) Taiwanese MDRD equation was used to predict the log(odds) (logit) of the probability of CKD stage 1, stage 1–2, stage 1–3 and stage 1–4. Note that the non-linear relationship between cumulative probability and eGFR in (A) had been transformed to be a linear ($\alpha+\beta x$) relationship. The odds ratio (95% confidence interval) of one unit increase in x was calculated as exp(β), which was 1.09 (1.05, 1.13), 1.11 (1.07, 1.15), 1.14 (1.08, 1.21) and 2.01 (1.06, 3.82) for stage 1, stage 1–2, stage 1–3 and stage 1–4, respectively.

Methods S1 Supplemental methods-ordinal logistic regression.

Acknowledgments

We would like to thank Drs. Seiichi Matsuo, Enyu Imai, Masaru Horio, and Yoshinari Yasuda for their assistance with inulin clearance testing and measurement.

Author Contributions

Conceived and designed the experiments: L-IC J-YG H-CC. Performed the experiments: L-IC J-YG H-CC T-HC Y-MC K-DW. Analyzed the data: J-YG. Contributed reagents/materials/analysis tools: M-CK S-JH T-HC Y-MC K-DW. Wrote the paper: L-IC J-YG.

References

1. National-Kidney-Foundation (2002) K/DOQI clinical practice guidelines for chronic kidney disease: evaluation, classification, and stratification. Am J Kidney Dis 39: S1–S266.
2. Levey AS, Bosch JP, Lewis JB, Greene T, Rogers N, et al. (1999) A more accurate method to estimate glomerular filtration rate from serum creatinine: a new prediction equation. Modification of Diet in Renal Disease Study Group. Ann Intern Med 130: 461–470.
3. Zuo L, Ma Y-C, Zhou Y-H, Wang M, Xu G-B, et al. (2005) Application of GFR-estimating equations in Chinese patients with chronic kidney disease. Am J Kidney Dis 45: 463–472.
4. Imai E, Horio M, Nitta K, Yamagata K, Iseki K, et al. (2007) Estimation of glomerular filtration rate by the MDRD study equation modified for Japanese patients with chronic kidney disease. Clin Exp Nephrol 11: 41–50.
5. Ma YC, Zuo L, Chen JH, Luo Q, Yu XQ, et al. (2006) Modified glomerular filtration rate estimating equation for Chinese patients with chronic kidney disease. J Am Soc Nephrol 17: 2937–2944.
6. Earley A, Miskulin D, Lamb EJ, Levey AS, Uhlig K (2012) Estimating equations for glomerular filtration rate in the era of creatinine standardization: a systematic review. Ann Intern Med 156: 785–795.
7. Stevens L, Coresh J, Feldman H, Greene T, Lash J, et al. (2007) Evaluation of the modification of diet in renal disease study equation in a large diverse population. JASN 18: 2749–2757.
8. Imai E, Horio M, Nitta K, Yamagata K, Iseki K, et al. (2007) Modification of the Modification of Diet in Renal Disease (MDRD) Study equation for Japan. Am J Kidney Dis 50: 927–937.
9. Horio M, Imai E, Yasuda Y, Hishida A, Matsuo S, et al. (2009) Simple sampling strategy for measuring inulin renal clearance. Clin Exp Nephrol 13: 50–54.
10. Horio M, Imai E, Yasuda Y, Watanabe T, Matsuo S (2010) Modification of the CKD epidemiology collaboration (CKD-EPI) equation for Japanese: accuracy and use for population estimates. Am J Kidney Dis 56: 32–38.
11. Teo BW, Xu H, Wang D, Li J, Sinha AK, et al. (2011) GFR estimating equations in a multiethnic Asian population. Am J Kidney Dis 58: 56–63.
12. Rule A, Larson T, Bergstralh E, Slezak J, Jacobsen S, et al. (2004) Using serum creatinine to estimate glomerular filtration rate: accuracy in good health and in chronic kidney disease. Ann Intern Med 141: 929–937.
13. Poggio E, Wang X, Greene T, Van Lente F, Hall P (2005) Performance of the modification of diet in renal disease and Cockcroft-Gault equations in the estimation of GFR in health and in chronic kidney disease. JASN 16: 459–466.
14. Levey A, Stevens L, Schmid C, Zhang YL, Castro A, et al. (2009) A new equation to estimate glomerular filtration rate. Ann Intern Med 150: 604–612.
15. Stevens L, Schmid C, Greene T, Zhang YL, Beck G, et al. (2010) Comparative performance of the CKD Epidemiology Collaboration (CKD-EPI) and the Modification of Diet in Renal Disease (MDRD) Study equations for estimating GFR levels above 60 mL/min/1.73 m2. Am J Kidney Dis 56: 486–495.
16. KDIGO (2013) Definition, identification, and prediction of CKD progression. Kidney Int 61: 63–72.
17. Stevens L, Claybon M, Schmid C, Chen J, Horio M, et al. (2011) Evaluation of the Chronic Kidney Disease Epidemiology Collaboration equation for estimating the glomerular filtration rate in multiple ethnicities. Kidney Int 79: 555–562.
18. Hsu C-C, Hwang S-J, Wen C-P, Chang H-Y, Chen T, et al. (2006) High prevalence and low awareness of CKD in Taiwan: a study on the relationship between serum creatinine and awareness from a nationally representative survey. Am J Kidney Dis 48: 727–738.
19. Orita Y, Gejyo F, Sakatsume M, Shiigai T, Maeda Y, et al. (2005) [Estimation of glomerular filtration rate by inulin clearance: comparison with creatinine clearance]. Nihon Jinzo Gakkai Shi 47: 804–812.
20. Praditpornsilpa K, Townamchai N, Chaiwatanarat T, Tiranathanagul K, Katawatin P, et al. (2011) The need for robust validation for MDRD-based glomerular filtration rate estimation in various CKD populations. Nephrology, dialysis, transplantation 26: 2780–2785.
21. Altman DG, Gardner MJ (1988) Calculating confidence intervals for regression and correlation. Br Med J (Clin Res Ed) 296: 1238–1242.
22. Carstensen B (2010) Comparing methods of measurement: Extending the LoA by regression. Stat Med 29: 401–410.
23. Seel RT, Steyerberg EW, Malec JF, Sherer M, Macciocchi SN (2012) Developing and evaluating prediction models in rehabilitation populations. Arch Phys Med Rehabil 93: S138–153.
24. Delanaye P, Pottel H, Botev R, Inker LA, Levey AS (2013) Con: Should we abandon the use of the MDRD equation in favour of the CKD-EPI equation? Nephrol Dial Transplant 28: 1396–1403; discussion 1403.
25. Barchard KA (2012) Examining the reliability of interval level data using root mean square differences and concordance correlation coefficients. Psychol Methods 17: 294–308.
26. Atkinson G, Nevill AM (1998) Statistical methods for assessing measurement error (reliability) in variables relevant to sports medicine. Sports Med 26: 217–238.
27. Zou GY (2007) Toward using confidence intervals to compare correlations. Psychol Methods 12: 399–413.
28. Gilchrist J (2009) Weighted 2×2 kappa coefficients: recommended indices of diagnostic accuracy for evidence-based practice. J Clin Epidemiol 62: 1045–1053.
29. Burnham KP, Anderson DR, Huyvaert KP (2011) AIC model selection and multimodel inference in behavioral ecology: some background, observations, and comparisons. Behav Ecol Sociobiol 65: 23–35.
30. Wagenmakers EJ and Farrell S (2004) AIC model selection using Akaike weights. Psychon Bull Rev 11: 192–196.
31. Moons KG, Kengne AP, Grobbee DE, Royston P, Vergouwe Y, et al. (2012) Risk prediction models: II. External validation, model updating, and impact assessment. Heart 98: 691–698.
32. Bleeker SE, Moll HA, Steyerberg EW, Donders AR, Derksen-Lubsen G, et al. (2003) External validation is necessary in prediction research: a clinical example. J Clin Epidemiol 56: 826–832.
33. Ludbrook J (2010) Confidence in Altman-Bland plots: a critical review of the method of differences. Clin Exp Pharmacol Physiol 37: 143–149.
34. Royston P, Altman DG, Sauerbrei W (2006) Dichotomizing continuous predictors in multiple regression: a bad idea. Stat Med 25: 127–141.
35. Bennett ND, Croke BFW, Guariso G, Guillaume JHA, Hamilton SH, et al. (2013) Characterising performance of environmental models. Environ Modell Softw 40: 1–20.
36. Madero M, Sarnak M (2011) Creatinine-based formulae for estimating glomerular filtration rate: is it time to change to chronic kidney disease epidemiology collaboration equation? Curr Opin Nephrol Hypertens 20: 622–630.
37. Silveiro SP, Araujo GN, Ferreira MN, Souza FD, Yamaguchi HM, et al. (2011) Chronic Kidney Disease Epidemiology Collaboration (CKD-EPI) equation pronouncedly underestimates glomerular filtration rate in type 2 diabetes. Diabetes care 34: 2353–2355.
38. Rognant N, Lemoine S, Laville M, Hadj-Aissa A, Dubourg L (2011) Performance of the chronic kidney disease epidemiology collaboration equation to estimate glomerular filtration rate in diabetic patients. Diabetes care 34: 1320–1322.
39. Kong X, Ma Y, Chen J, Luo Q, Yu X, et al. (2013) Evaluation of the Chronic Kidney Disease Epidemiology Collaboration equation for estimating glomerular filtration rate in the Chinese population. Nephrology, dialysis, transplantation 28: 641–651.
40. Ott NT (1975) A simple technique for estimating glomerular filtration rate with subcutaneous injection of (125I)Iothalamate. Mayo Clin Proc 50: 664–668.
41. Israelit AH, Long DL, White MG, Hull AR (1973) Measurement of glomerular filtration rate utilizing a single subcutaneous injection of 125I-iothalamate. Kidney Int 4: 346–349.
42. Tessitore N, Lo Schiavo C, Corgnati A, Previato G, Valvo E, et al. (1979) 125I-iothalamate and creatinine clearances in patients with chronic renal diseases. Nephron 24: 41–45.
43. Dai S-S, Yasuda Y, Zhang C-L, Horio M, Zuo L, et al. (2011) Evaluation of GFR measurement method as an explanation for differences among GFR estimation equations. Am J Kidney Dis 58: 496–498.
44. Chen L-I, Kuo M-C, Hwang S-J, Chen Y-W, Wu K-D, et al. (2011) Comparisons of technetium-99 m diethylenetriaminepentaacetic acid plasma clearance and renal dynamic imaging with inulin clearance. Am J Kidney Dis 58: 1043–1045.

Circulating Levels of Dimethylarginines, Chronic Kidney Disease and Long-Term Clinical Outcome in Non-ST-Elevation Myocardial Infarction

Viviana Cavalca[1,2]*, Fabrizio Veglia[1], Isabella Squellerio[1], Monica De Metrio[1], Mara Rubino[1], Benedetta Porro[1], Marco Moltrasio[1], Elena Tremoli[1,3], Giancarlo Marenzi[1]

1 Centro Cardiologico Monzino, I.R.C.C.S, Milan, Italy, **2** Dipartimento di Scienze Cliniche e di Comunità, Università degli Studi di Milano, Milan, Italy, **3** Dipartimento di Scienze Farmacologiche e Biomolecolari, Università degli Studi di Milano, Milan, Italy

Abstract

Background: Mechanisms linking chronic kidney disease (CKD) and adverse outcomes in acute coronary syndromes (ACS) are not fully understood. Among potential key players, reduced nitric oxide (NO) synthesis due to its endogenous inhibitors, asymmetric (ADMA) and symmetric (SDMA) dimethylarginine could be involved. We measured plasma concentration of arginine, ADMA and SDMA and investigated their relationship with CKD and long-term outcome in non-ST-elevation myocardial infarction (NSTEMI).

Methodology/Principal Findings: We prospectively measured arginine, ADMA, and SDMA at hospital admission in 104 NSTEMI patients. CKD was defined as an estimated glomerular filtration rate (eGFR) <60 ml/min/1.73 m^2. We considered a primary end point of combined cardiac death and re-infarction at a median follow-up of 21 months. In CKD (n = 33) and no-CKD (n = 71) patients, arginine and ADMA were similar, whereas SDMA was significantly higher in CKD patients (0.65 ± 0.23 vs. 0.42 ± 0.12 μmol/L; $P<0.0001$). Twenty-four (23%) patients had an adverse cardiac event during follow-up: 12 (36%) were CKD and 12 (17%) no-CKD patients (P = 0.02). When study population was stratified according to arginine, ADMA and SDMA median values, only SDMA (median 0.46 μmol/L) was associated with the primary end-point (P = 0.0016). In models adjusted for age, hemoglobin and left ventricular ejection fraction, the hazard ratio (HR) for CKD and SDMA were high (HR 2.93, interquartile range [IQR] 1.15–7.53; P = 0.02 and HR 6.80, IQR 2.09–22.2; P = 0.001, respectively) but, after mutual adjustment, only SDMA remained significantly associated with the primary end point (HR 5.73, IQR 1.55–21.2; P = 0.009).

Conclusions/Significance: In NSTEMI patients, elevated SDMA plasma levels are associated with CKD and worse long-term prognosis.

Editor: Claudio Moretti, S.G.Battista Hospital, Italy

Funding: No current external funding sources for this study.

Competing Interests: The authors have declared that no competing interests exist.

* E-mail: viviana.cavalca@unimi.it

Introduction

Growing evidence suggests that chronic kidney disease (CKD) is associated with increased cardiovascular risk. Indeed, patients with CKD have both traditional and non-traditional (related to the underlying uremic state) risk factors, and the combination of these favors the development of cardiovascular disease, contributes to progression of CKD, and, ultimately, perpetuates mortality risk [1,2]. The pervasive adverse influence of CKD has also been demonstrated in the setting of acute coronary syndromes (ACS). Among ACS patients, CKD doubles mortality rates and is third to cardiogenic shock and congestive heart failure as a predictor of mortality [3–7]. The mechanisms linking CKD and adverse outcomes in patients with ACS, however, are not fully understood. It is conceivable that the interplay among extensive co-morbidities, underutilization of known cardio-protective therapies, more frequent errors in dosing with excess toxicity from conventional therapies may explain part of their excessive risk, but other unidentified aspects related to the unique pathobiology of CKD are possibly involved [1,7–9]. Recognition of the mechanisms associated with increased risk of ACS patients with CKD is a critical challenge to better determine where to concentrate the efforts in future trials and to validate novel and effective therapies for these high-risk patients.

Among other potential key players contributing to the increased cardiovascular risk of CKD patients, dimethylarginines have recently received attention. Reduced nitric oxide (NO) synthesis due to increased levels of its circulating endogenous inhibitor, asymmetric dimethylarginine (ADMA), has been suggested to independently contribute to progression of CKD, to end-stage renal disease, and death [10,11]. Plasma concentrations of ADMA and of its isomer symmetric dimethylarginine (SDMA) are elevated in patients with CKD and in other cardiovascular risk-states such as hypertension, hypercholesterolemia, diabetes mellitus and chronic heart failure, and are associated with oxidative stress and endothelial dysfunction [12–18].

The role of these inhibitors of NO, as well as their relative levels in plasma, in ACS patients with CKD, are still unknown. Indeed, in the systemic, as well as in the coronary circulation, NO relaxes vascular smooth muscle to increase blood flow, and suppresses processes involved in vascular disease, including leukocyte adhesion and platelet aggregation [19,20]. All these effects might be particularly relevant in ACS, a complex disease in which coronary vasoconstriction and inflammatory and thrombotic processes represent major pathogenetic factors.

In this study, we measured plasma concentration of metabolites involved in the NO biosynthetic pathway, in particular arginine, ADMA and SDMA, and we investigated their relationship with renal function and long-term outcome of patients with ACS.

Materials and Methods

The Ethics Committee of the Centro Cardiologico Monzino approved the study, and all patients gave written, informed consent.

Study population

This prospective study was conducted at the Centro Cardiologico Monzino, University of Milan. All consecutive patients who were admitted to the Coronary Care Unit (CCU) for non-ST-elevation acute myocardial infarction (NSTEMI) between September 1, 2005 and October 24, 2007 were enrolled in the study. We included patients who presented within 24 hours of the onset of symptoms (characteristic chest pain with electrocardiographic ST-segment depression or T wave inversion, and increase in troponin I). We excluded patients receiving long-term peritoneal or hemodialysis treatment. In order to prevent potential misclassification of patients who might have developed acute kidney injury, we also excluded patients with ACS-associated hemodynamic (acute pulmonary edema, cardiogenic shock) or electrical (life-threatening ventricular arrhythmias, high-degree conduction disturbances) instability or other major clinical complications at hospital presentation. Patients with angina precipitated by anemia or other correctable factors, severe valvular heart disease, malignancies, and severe liver disease, were also excluded.

Study protocol

At hospital admission, before any pharmacologic therapy was started, venous blood samples were obtained for determination of arginine, ADMA and SDMA plasma concentrations. We also measured serum creatinine concentration in all patients at hospital admission. Glomerular filtration rate (eGFR) was estimated using the abbreviated Modification of Diet in Renal Disease (MDRD) equation [21]. Chronic kidney disease was categorized as an eGFR $\leq$60 ml/min per 1.73 m^2 [22].

The choice of pharmacologic therapy and interventional strategy for management of ACS was left to the discretion of the CCU cardiologists. In all cases, early coronary angiography (within 24 hours from hospital presentation) was performed, unless contraindicated.

After hospital discharge, all patients were followed-up for at least one year. During the follow-up, a combined end-point of cardiac death and re-infarction (primary end point of the study) was considered.

Clinical results were analyzed according to the presence (CKD group) or absence (no-CKD group) of CKD.

For comparison, we considered a historical sample of 20 healthy subjects (mean age 60, range 56–69 years) and of 10 CKD patients (Stage 3 in all cases) without ACS (mean age 65, range 47–73 years; eGFR 51±7 ml/min per 1.73 m^2) evaluated in our laboratory.

Blood sampling and biochemical measurements

Blood was collected from the antecubital vein into EDTA containing tubes and plasma samples were obtained after centrifugation (3000 g, 10 min. at 4°C). Aliquots of plasma were stored at −80°C until analysis. Arginine, ADMA and SDMA plasma concentrations were measured by liquid chromatography method, performed using an HPLC system (ESA Bioscences, Chelmford, MA, USA) equipped with fluorimetric detector FP-1520 (Jasco, Tokyo, Japan) [23]. Briefly, organic solid phase extraction onto Oasis MCX SPE cartridge (Waters Milford, MA, USA) and basic derivatization with ortho-Phthaldialdehyde were previously performed after adding MMA (0.2 μM) as internal standard. Fifty μL of the purified sample were loaded onto Onyx Monolythic C18 HPLC column (100×4.6 mm, Phenomenex, Torrance, CA, USA) eluted at 2 mL/min by 7% acetonitrile in phosphate buffer 25 mM pH 6.5. Fluorescence was measured at excitation and emission wavelengths of 340 and 455 nm, respectively.

Data were obtained after comparison with calibration curves using arginine, ADMA and SDMA pure standard solutions. The intra- and inter-CVs % obtained with standard samples were <5% for all the analytics considered. The limit of detection of arginine was 0.041 μmol/L; it was 0.025 μmol/L for both methylarginines.

Statistical analysis

Continuous variables are presented as mean±SD, and were compared using the *t*-test for independent samples. Variables not normally distributed are presented as median and interquartile ranges (IQR), and compared with the Wilcoxon rank-sum test. Categorical data were compared using the chi-square test or the Fisher exact test, as appropriate.

Pearson correlation analysis was used to examine the linear association between plasma arginine, ADMA, SDMA and eGFR.

Kaplan-Meier analysis was employed to generate time-to-event curves for the clinical end point (cardiac death and myocardial infarction), stratified according to values below or above medians of arginine, ADMA or SDMA. Multivariable-adjusted hazard ratios (HR) were computed by Cox proportional-hazard regression analysis.

All tests were two-tailed, and a P value of less than 0.05 was required for statistical significance. All calculations were computed with the aid of the SAS software package (Version 9.2 SAS Institute Inc, Cary, NC).

Results

A total of 104 consecutive patients with NSTEMI were included in this study. Of these, 33 (32%) had CKD (Stage 3 in 29 patients and Stage 4 in 4 patients) and 71 (68%) had normal renal function. The baseline demographic and clinical characteristics of ACS patients with and without CKD are shown in Table 1. Patients with CKD were older and more likely to be treated with diuretics. Moreover, they had significantly lower hemoglobin levels and higher high-sensitivity C-reactive protein (hs-CRP) values.

In the whole population, plasma arginine was lower than our reference values in healthy subjects (67.1±16.7 μmol/L vs. 92.2±17.5 μmol/L, respectively; P<0.0001), whereas ADMA (0.435±0.09 μmol/L vs. 0.461±0.11 μmol/L, respectively; P = 0.25) and SDMA (0.501±0.19 μmol/L vs. 0.457±0.11 μmol/L, respectively; P = 0.35) were similar. Arginine

Table 1. Baseline characteristics of the study patients.

	CKD group (n = 33)	no CKD group (n = 71)	P value
Clinical characteristics			
Age (yrs)	72±8	64±11	<0.001
Men, n (%)	22 (67%)	55 (77%)	0.24
Weight (kg)	74±13	76±13	0.46
Height (cm)	167±8	168±7	0.51
Smokers, n (%)	10 (30%)	24 (34%)	0.74
Diabetes mellitus, n (%)	11 (33%)	17 (24%)	0.31
Systemic hypertension, n (%)	19 (58%)	47 (66%)	0.39
Dyslipidemia, n (%)	19 (58%)	45 (63%)	0.57
Prior myocardial infarction, n (%)	8 (24%)	16 (23%)	0.84
Prior CABG, n (%)	5 (15%)	5 (7%)	0.28*
Prior PCI, n (%)	2 (6%)	7 (10%)	0.71*
Left ventricular ejection fraction, %	56±8	55±11	0.5
Medical therapy, n (%)	6 (18%)	8 (11%)	0.3
PCI, n (%)	22 (67%)	53 (75%)	0.39
CABG, n (%)	5 (15%)	10 (14%)	0.88
Medications at hospital presentation			
ACE inhibitor or ARB, n (%)	17 (52%)	30 (42%)	0.37
Aspirin, n (%)	23 (70%)	47 (66%)	0.72
Diuretics, n (%)	8 (24%)	7 (10%)	0.05
Statins, n (%)	12 (36%)	24 (34%)	0.79
Beta-blockers, n (%)	9 (27%)	19 (27%)	0.95
Calcium channel blockers, n (%)	8 (24%)	16 (23%)	0.84
Oral hypoglycemics, n (%)	10 (30%)	12 (17%)	0.12
Laboratory measures			
Serum creatinine (mg/dl)	1.37 (1.1–1.7)	0.98 (0.9–1.1)	NA
eGFR (ml/min/1.73 m^2)	48±9	79±12	NA
Hemoglobin (g/dl)	13±1.5	14±1.5	0.002
Total cholesterol (mg/dL)	188±46	199±38	0.2
LDL cholesterol (mg/dL)	109±45	122±35	0.11
HDL cholesterol (mg/dL)	46±10	48±11	0.37
Triglycerides (mg/dL)	120 (88–184)	113 (88–185)	0.97§
hs-CRP (mg/L)	5.7 (4.4–8.7)	3.8 (2.2–5.8)	0.05§
Arginine (μmol/L)	62±17	68±18	0.14
ADMA (μmol/L)	0.46±0.1	0.42±0.1	0.35
SDMA (μmol/L)	0.65±0.2	0.42±0.1	<0.001

*By Fisher exact test.
§by Wilcoxon Rank Sum Test.
ACE = angiotensin-converting enzyme; ARB = angiotensin II receptor blocker; CABG = coronary artery bypass graft surgery; CKD = chronic kidney disease; CRP = C-reactive protein; eGFR = estimated glomerular filtration rate; NA = not applicable; PCI = percutaneous coronary intervention.

and ADMA levels were not significantly different in CKD and no-CKD patients, whereas SDMA was significantly higher in CKD patients (Table 1). Figure 1 shows arginine, ADMA and SDMA values in healthy subjects, CKD controls, and in the two study groups. Arginine values were lower in CKD and ACS patients and ADMA levels were higher in CKD controls than in the other 3 groups. Finally, SDMA levels were higher in CKD patients than in patients with normal renal function.

Throughout the entire study population, both ADMA and SDMA were inversely correlated with eGFR, but this relationship was stronger for SDMA (Figure 2). No relationship, instead, was observed between arginine and eGFR ($R = 0.14$; $P = 0.16$). In addition, a significant correlation was observed between ADMA and SDMA levels ($R = 0.52$; $P < 0.0001$) and between SDMA and hs-CRP values ($R = 0.32$; $P = 0.018$).

No patient died during hospital stay; 3 patients died during the follow-up (median 21 months; IQR 7–33): 2 (6%) patients in CKD

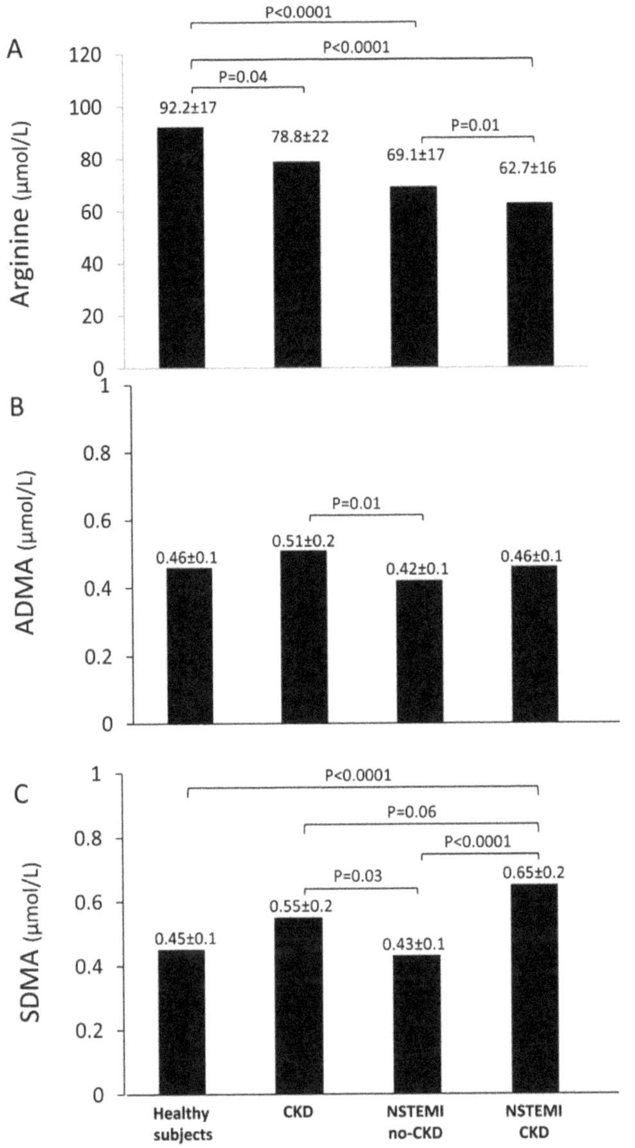

Figure 1. Arginine, ADMA and SDMA plasma levels. Arginine (panel A), asymmetric dimethylarginine (ADMA; panel B), and symmetric dimethylarginine (SDMA; panel C) plasma levels (mean±SD values) in healthy subjects (n = 20), in controls with chronic kidney disease (CKD; n = 10), and in NSTEMI patients without (n = 71) and with (n = 33) CKD.

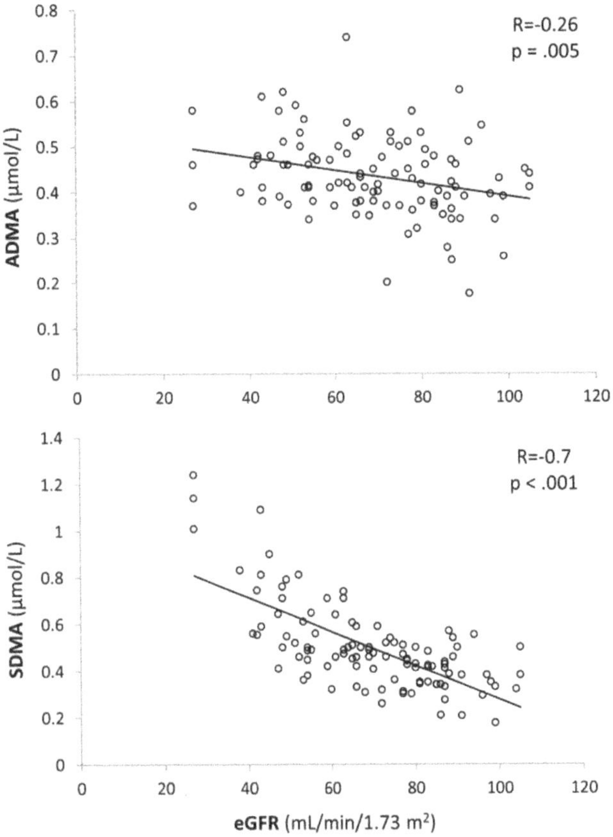

Figure 2. Relationships between NO synthesis inhibitors and renal function. Relationship between asymmetric (ADMA; upper panel) and symmetric (SDMA; lower panel) dimethylarginine plasma levels and estimated glomerular filtration rate (eGFR) in the study population.

group and 1 (1%) patient in no-CKD group. Overall, 24 (23%) patients reached the combined primary end-point of death and re-infarction during the follow-up: 12 (36%) patients in CKD group and 12 (17%) patients in no-CKD group (P = 0.02 in Kaplan-Meier analysis). Two (6%) and 14 (20%; P = 0.05) patients, respectively, underwent an elective percutaneous coronary procedure during the follow-up.

Figure 3 shows the Kaplan-Meier curves according to median arginine (68.1 µmol/L), ADMA (0.42 µmol/L), and SDMA (0.46 µmol/L) values stratification in the study population. Notably, a significantly different incidence in the combined end point of death and re-infarction was observed only for patients stratified by median SDMA levels. Similar results were obtained when the Kaplan-Meier curves were analyzed comparing the upper tertile of arginine (>74.8 µmol/L; P = 0.33), ADMA (>0.47 µmol/L; P = 0.10) and SDMA (>0.5 µmol/L; P = 0.003) with the lower two tertiles.

Table 2 reports the HRs for the primary end point obtained by different Cox models. In models adjusted only for age, hemoglobin and left ventricular ejection fraction, HR for CKD and SDMA were high but, after mutual adjustment, only SDMA remained significantly associated with the primary end point.

Discussion

The most significant finding of the present study is that plasma levels of SDMA, measured at hospital presentation, are elevated in NSTEMI patients with CKD, and are independent early predictors of the composite outcome of cardiac death and myocardial infarction.

Chronic kidney disease is present in a substantial proportion of patients with ACS and represents a potent and independent risk factor for short- and long-term adverse outcome [4–7,9]. The reasons for this close association, however, are not completely clear and cannot be entirely explained by the clustering of the traditional cardiovascular risk factors. Besides clinical and therapeutic differences, it is likely that peculiar characteristics of renal insufficiency may play a considerable role [1,24]. It has been hypothesized that the excessive risk associated with CKD can be attributed, at least in part, to endothelial dysfunction and reduced

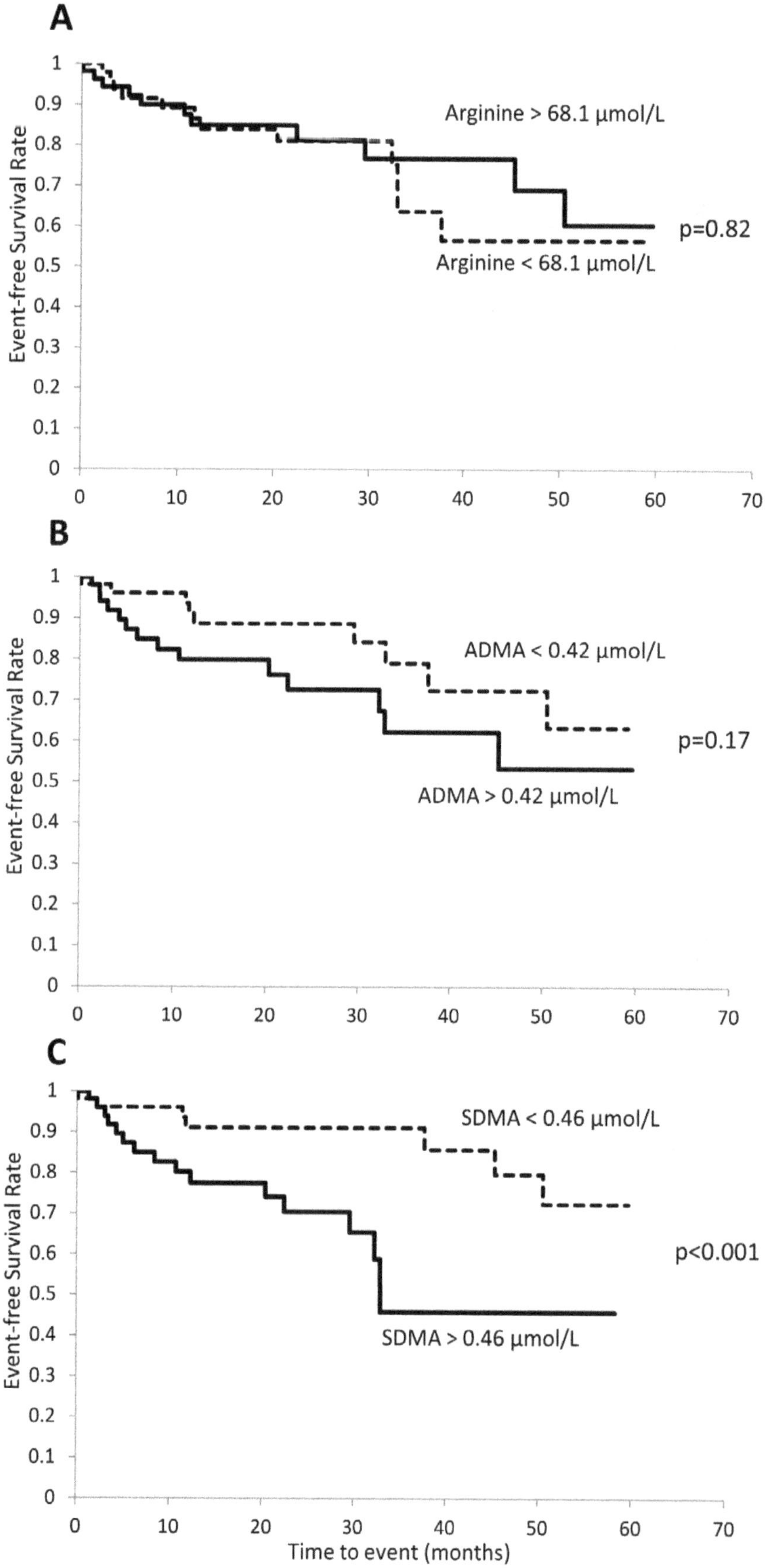

Figure 3. Kaplan-Meier survival analyses during follow-up. Composite outcomes of cardiac death and myocardial infarction according to concentrations of plasma arginine (panel A), asymmetric dimethylarginine (ADMA; panel B), and symmetric dimethylarginine (SDMA; panel C), divided by median levels. P values by log-rank test are shown.

Table 2. Cox regression analysis for the primary end point of the study (composite outcome of cardiac death and myocardial infarction).

Model	Variable	Adjusted HR	95% CI	P value
1	CKD	2.93	1.15–7.53	0.02
2	Arginine	0.95	0.37–2.42	0.91
3	ADMA	2.24	0.89–5.65	0.08
4	SDMA	6.80	2.09–22.2	0.001
5	Arginine	1.18	0.45–3.09	0.72
	CKD	3.04	1.16–7.97	0.02
6	ADMA	1.84	0.71–4.79	0.21
	CKD	2.52	0.96–6.64	0.06
7	SDMA	5.73	1.55–21.2	0.009
	CKD	1.35	0.49–3.71	0.55

Hazard ratios (HR) in models 1–4 are adjusted for age, hemoglobin and left ventricular ejection fraction; HRs in models 5–7 are also mutually adjusted. HRs for CKD are vs. no-CKD; for all other variables, HRs are for values above vs. below median.
ADMA = asymmetric dimethylarginine; CKD = chronic kidney disease; CI = confidence intervals; SDMA = symmetric dimethylarginine.

bioavailability of NO, a potential link between CKD and cardiovascular disease.

Elevated plasma concentrations of ADMA have been found in various clinical settings, ranging from critically ill patients admitted to the Intensive Care Unit [25] to patients with CKD [26] and end-stage renal disease [10], with stable coronary artery disease [27], and to those undergoing coronary angiography [28] and non-cardiac surgery [29]. In all these conditions, elevation of ADMA has been identified as an independent risk factor for future adverse cardiovascular events and death. It has been proposed that, by inhibiting NO synthesis, ADMA may contribute directly to endothelial dysfunction, depression of cardiac function, progression of chronic renal disease, and organ failure [12,30,31]. Recently, ADMA has also been measured in patients with ACS [32–34]. In a study by Cavusoglu et al. [33], plasma levels of ADMA were measured in a cohort of 182 men with ACS. The authors found that elevated plasma levels of ADMA were powerful and independent predictors of adverse cardiovascular outcomes. In particular, ACS patients who had the upper tertile of baseline ADMA had a significantly higher two-year mortality than those in the lower two tertiles combined (23.8% vs. 8.6%; $P = 0.004$).

In most previous studies, investigators focused mainly on ADMA and, until recently, little attention has been paid to the role of its structural isomer SDMA. To our knowledge, this is the first study evaluating the association between plasma levels of both dimethylarginines and long-term outcome in ACS. In our study, no increase in ADMA levels in plasma were found in comparison with healthy subjects, not even when the whole study group, as well as the two subsets of patients stratified according to the presence or absence of CKD, were considered. Moreover, no significant association between ADMA levels and clinical outcome was observed. Some important clinical (patients characteristics, type [STEMI vs. NSTEMI] and severity of ACS), methodological and analytical (ELISA vs. HPLC) differences among studies may explain the apparent inconsistency between our data and those previously published, regarding the capacity of ADMA to predict cardiac events in ACS [32–35].

Both dymethylarginines are physiologically present in plasma as a product of normal protein turnover. However, as SDMA is mainly eliminated by renal excretion, whereas ADMA is largely metabolized, it is not surprising to find a closer relationship between renal impairment and SDMA than with ADMA. The increase in SDMA observed in our study in CKD patients, as well as the good correlation found between SDMA and eGFR, are in agreement with a previous meta-analysis showing a strong correlation between SDMA and renal function [36]. As there is a high concentration of the ADMA degrading enzyme (DDAH) in the kidney, it is also conceivable that the decline in renal excretory function is paralleled by a reduction of DDAH activity (in the kidney). This, and the fact that about 10% of ADMA formed is also excreted by the kidneys, might explain why also ADMA is weakly related to parameters of renal function in some of the studies, including the present one.

When patients were stratified by median SDMA plasma concentration, a significant difference in long-term clinical outcome was found. Notably, SDMA was a stronger predictor of cardiac events, in particular re-infarction, than CKD, as defined according to GFR estimated by serum creatinine. The mechanism(s) linking SDMA and outcome, however, remains uncertain. Several mechanisms may potentially explain this association. First, SDMA might directly influence the outcome of ACS patients by participating to cause reduction in NO production and induction of endothelial dysfunction. Although SDMA has not been shown to directly affect NO synthase activity *in vitro* [37], we cannot exclude its influence on the production of NO in some clinical conditions characterized by its increase in plasma. Indeed, SDMA may have an indirect effect on NO synthesis, by inhibiting the y+ transporter that mediates the intracellular uptake of L-arginine and renal tubular arginine absorption [38,39]. These two mechanisms might indirectly inhibit NO synthesis by interfering with L-arginine uptake. Second, SDMA accumulation in the plasma due to reduced renal clearance might only reflect kidney dysfunction. Many studies have shown a good correlation between SDMA and established estimates of GFR in humans, as well as in animal models [40]. Based on these premises, SDMA fulfills all criteria for an ideal GFR marker, i.e. stable production rate, free glomerular filtration, and lack of tubular reabsorption [36]. On the other hand, estimates of GFR from serum creatinine may lack in necessary sensitivity due to considerable inter-individual variability in muscle mass, protein intake, age, and sex [41]. This limitation is even more critical in ACS, a clinical setting in which no renal baseline conditions are available and serum creatinine levels at hospital admission cannot be considered a true stable value because the occurrence of a transient hemodynamic impairment, which in turn results in the increase of serum creatinine in the plasma. Moreover, creatinine increase may lag far behind glomerular filtration changes, because of its delayed rise after renal injury, due to the slow variations in its metabolism and the exponential relationship existing between these two variables. Thus, it is likely that SDMA is able to more accurately reflect glomerular filtration than creatinine and its levels in plasma may better identify the "true" CKD patients with a worse prognosis. According to this hypothesis, the lower SDMA values in CKD controls than in NSTEMI patients with CKD, might be explained by the higher eGFR in the former than in the latter group (51 ± 7 and 48 ± 9 ml/min per 1.73 m^2, respectively). The list of mechanisms through which SDMA might directly contribute to unfavorable outcomes in ACS patients, however, is most likely not yet complete. In our study, SDMA levels in plasma were correlated with hs-CRP levels at hospital presentation, suggesting a possible role in promoting inflammatory response. A recent study has shown that SDMA is involved in the inflammatory process of CKD, by activating intracellular monocytic expression of interleukin 6 and tumor necrosis factor-alpha *in vitro*, whereas ADMA does not. This pro-inflammatory profile has been confirmed in a clinical study in which SDMA was associated with inflammatory markers [42]. Finally, a possible procoagulant state due to induction of tissue factor expression by peripheral monocytes, like that demonstrated for ADMA in ACS patients, cannot be excluded for SDMA [34].

Our data provide a basis for future studies which will investigate whether determination of SDMA, as well as its pharmacologic modulation, may help to guide care and improve outcomes of ACS patients. Irrespectively of its potential role in the pathophysiology of long-term adverse cardiac events, SDMA determination may have a considerable clinical usefulness in risk stratification of ACS patients. In particular, measurement of SDMA might allow for a more accurate and early recognition of CKD patients, who may require drug dose adjustments, renal prophylactic strategies, and targeted therapeutic interventions. Moreover, in these patients, long-term prognostic stratification may be more precise. Notably, in our study, we identified a potential cutoff value of SDMA of 0.46 µmol/L (median value) for risk classification.

Our study has some limitations. First, the size of the population is small and the findings need to be confirmed in larger studies. Similarly, the number of cardiac events is small, possibly due to the exclusion of high-risk patients from the study. Although this may represent an important limitation, the impossibility to differentiate between CKD and acute kidney injury on the bases of a single creatinine value measured at hospital admission, could have almost certainly lead to overestimate the number of patients with CKD. Nonetheless, the ADMA and SDMA levels in ACS patients developing acute kidney injury, as well as their possible association with short- and long-term outcomes, are not known and should be matter of future investigation. Second, being an observational study, our data do not unequivocally demonstrate that SDMA increase in plasma levels contributes to mortality and re-infarction. Further studies should investigate the relationship between SDMA increase and endothelial dysfunction, possibly evaluating endothelial-dependent vasodilatory response. Finally, we cannot exclude the possibility that some medications, taken by patients before hospital admission, may have influenced our results. Indeed, ADMA concentration has been shown to significantly decrease in ACS patients after a short-term medical therapy [32].

Conclusions

In NSTEMI patients, CKD is associated with increased SDMA plasma levels and worse long-term prognosis. Further studies are needed to establish whether the increased mortality risk of CKD patients is due to SDMA-induced impaired NO synthesis and whether pharmacologic modulation of SDMA may improve their outcomes.

Author Contributions

Conceived and designed the experiments: VC FV ET GM. Performed the experiments: IS BP. Analyzed the data: VC FV IS GM. Contributed reagents/materials/analysis tools: MD MR MM. Wrote the paper: VC FV BP ET GM.

References

1. Sarnak MJ, Levey AS, Schoolwerth AC, Coresh J, Culleton B, et al. (2003) Kidney disease as a risk factor for development of cardiovascular disease: a statement from the American Heart Association Councils on Kidney in Cardiovascular Disease, High Blood Pressure Research, Clinical Cardiology, and Epidemiology and Prevention. Hypertension 42: 1050–1065.
2. Go AS, Chertow GM, Fan D, McCullough CE, Hsu C (2004) Chronic kidney disease and the risk of death, cardiovascular events, and hospitalization. N Engl J Med 351: 1296–1305.
3. Herzog CA, Ma JZ, Collins AJ (1998) Poor-long-term survival after acute myocardial infarction among patients on long-term dialysis. N Engl J Med 339: 799–805.
4. Wright RS, Reeder GS, Herzog CA, Albright RC, Williams BA, et al. (2002) Acute myocardial infarction and renal dysfunction: a high-risk combination. Ann Intern Med 137: 563–570.
5. Shlipak MG, Heidenreich PA, Noguchi H, Chertow GM, Browner WS, et al. (2002) Association of renal insufficiency with treatment and outcomes after myocardial infarction in elderly patients. Ann Intern Med 137: 555–562.
6. Santopinto JJ, Fox KA, Goldberg RJ, Budaj A, Piñero G, et al. (2003) Creatinine clearance and adverse hospital outcomes in patients with acute coronary syndromes: findings from the global registry of acute coronary events (GRACE). Heart 89: 1003–1008.
7. Gibson CM, Dumaine RL, Gelfand EV, Murphy SA, Morrow DA, et al. (2004) Association of glomerular filtration rate on presentation with subsequent mortality in non-ST-segment elevation acute coronary syndrome; observations in 13307 patients in five TIMI trials. Eur Heart J 25: 1998–2005.
8. Szummer K, Lundman P, Jacobson SH, Schön S, Lindbäck J, et al. (2009) Influence of renal function on the effects of early revascularization in non-ST-elevation myocardial infarction: data from the Swedish Web-System for Enhancement and Development of Evidence-Based Care in Heart Disease Evaluated According to Recommended Therapies (SWEDEHEART). Circulation 120: 851–858.
9. Fox CS, Muntner P, Chen AY, Alexander KP, Roe MT, et al. (2010) Acute Coronary Treatment and Intervention Outcomes Network registry. Use of evidence-based therapies in short-term outcomes of ST-segment elevation myocardial infarction and non-ST-segment elevation myocardial infarction in patients with chronic kidney disease: a report from the National Cardiovascular Data Acute Coronary Treatment and Intervention Outcomes Network registry. Circulation 121: 357–365.
10. Zoccali C, Bode-Böger S, Mallamaci F, Benedetto F, Tripepi G, et al. (2001) Plasma concentration of asymmetrical dimethylarginine and mortality in patients with end-stage renal disease: a prospective study. Lancet 358: 2113–2117.
11. Ravani P, Tripepi G, Malberti F, Testa S, Mallamaci F, et al. (2005) Asymmetrical dimethylarginine predicts progression to dialysis and death in patients with chronic kidney disease: a competing risks modeling approach. J Am Soc Nephrol 16: 2449–2455.
12. Böger RH, Bode-Böger SM, Szuba A, Tsao PS, Chan JR, et al. (1998) Asymmetric dimethylarginine (ADMA): A novel risk factor for endothelial dysfunction—Its role in hypercholesterolemia. Circulation 98: 1842–1847.
13. Krzyzanowska K, Mittermayer F, Shnawa N, Hofer M, Schnabler J, et al. (2007) Asymmetrical dimethylarginine is related to renal function, chronic inflammation and macroangiopathy in patients with type 2 diabetes and albuminuria. Diabet Med 24: 81–86.
14. Lajer M, Tarnow L, Jorsal A, Teerlink T, Parving HH, et al. (2008). Plasma concentration of asymmetric dimethylarginine (ADMA) predicts cardiovascular morbidity and mortality in type 1 diabetic patients with diabetic nephropathy. Diabetes Care 31: 747–752.
15. Bode-Böger SM, Scalera F, Kielstein JT, Martens-Lobenhoffer J, Breithardt G, et al. (2006) Symmetrical dimethylarginine: a new combined parameter for renal function and extent of coronary artery disease. J Am Soc Nephrol 17:1128–1134.
16. Fleck C, Schweitzer F, Karge E, Busch M, Stein G (2003) Serum concentrations of asymmetric (ADMA) and symmetric (SDMA) dimethylarginine in patients with chronic kidney diseases. Clin Chim Acta 336:1–12.
17. Cighetti G, Fermo I, Aman CS, Ferraroni M, Secchi A, , et al. (2009) Dimethylarginines in complicated type 1 diabetes: roles of insulin, glucose, and oxidative stress. Free Radic Biol Med 47:307–311.
18. Wilson Tang WH, Tong W, Shrestha K, Wang Z, Levison BS, et al. (2008) Differential effects of arginine methylation on diastolic dysfunction and disease progression in patients with chronic systolic heart failure. Eur Heart J 29:2506–2511.
19. Moncada S, Palmer RMJ, Higgs EA (1991) Nitric oxide: physiology, pathophysiology and pharmacology. Pharmacol Rev 43: 109–143.
20. Radomski MW, Palmer RM, Moncada S (1987) Endogenous nitric oxide inhibits human platelet adhesion to vascular endothelium. Lancet 2: 1057–1058.
21. Levey AS, Bosch JP, Lewis JB, Greene T, Rogers N, et al. (1999) A more accurate method to estimate glomerular filtration rate from serum creatinine: a new prediction equation. Ann Intern Med 130: 461–470.
22. National Kidney Foundation (NKF) Kidney Disease Outcome Quality Initiative (K/DOQI) Advisory Board (2002) K/DOQI clinical practice guidelines for chronic kidney disease: evaluation, classification, and stratification. Am J Kidney Dis (Suppl. 1):S1–S246.
23. de Jong S, Teerlink T (2006) Analysis of asymmetric dimethylarginine in plasma by HPLC using a monolithic column. Anal Biochem 353: 287–289.

24. Marenzi G, Assanelli E, Bartorelli AL (2006) Management of acute coronary syndromes in patients with renal insufficiency. Current Cardiology Reviews 2: 11–16.
25. Nijveldt RJ, Teerlink T, Van Der Hoven B, Siroen MP, Kuik DJ, et al. (2003) Asymmetric dimethylarginine (ADMA) in critically ill patients: high plasma ADMA concentration is an independent risk factor of ICU mortality. Clin Nutr 22: 23–30.
26. Lu TM, Chung MY, Lin CC, Hsu CP, Lin SJ (2011) Asymmetric dimethylarginine and clinical outcomes in chronic kidney disease. Clin J Am Soc Nephrol 6: 1566–1572.
27. Lu TM, Ding YA, Lin SJ, Lee WS, Tai HC (2003) Plasma levels of asymmetrical dimethylarginine and adverse cardiovascular events after percutaneous coronary intervention. Eur Heart J 24: 1912–1919.
28. Lu TM, Chung MY, Lin MW, Hsu CP, Lin SJ (2011) Plasma asymmetric dimethylarginine predicts death and major adverse cardiovascular events in individuals referred for coronary angiography. Int J Cardiol 153: 135–140.
29. Maas R, Dentz L, Schwedhelm E, Thoms W, Kuss O, et al. (2007) Elevated plasma concentrations of the endogenous nitric oxide synthase inhibitor asymmetric dimethylarginine predict adverse events in patients undergoing noncardiac surgery. Crit Care Med 35: 1876–1881.
30. Achan V, Broadhead M, Malaki M, Whitley G, Leiper J, et al. (2003) Asymmetric dimethylarginine causes hypertension and cardiac dysfunction in humans and is actively metabolized by dimethylarginine dimethylaminohydrolase. Arterioscler Thromb Vasc Biol 23: 1455–1459.
31. Kielstein JT, Impraim B, Simmel S, Bode-Böger SM, Tsikas D, et al. (2004) Cardiovascular effects of systemic nitric oxide synthase inhibition with asymmetric dimethylarginine in humans. Circulation 109: 172–177.
32. Bae SW, Stühlinger MC, Yoo HS, Yu KH, Park HK, et al. (2005) Plasma asymmetric dimethylarginine concentrations in newly diagnosed patients with acute myocardial infarction or unstable angina pectoris during two weeks of medical treatment. Am J Cardiol 95: 729–733.
33. Cavusoglu E, Ruwende C, Chopra V, Poludasu S, Yanamadala S, et al. (2009) Relationship of baseline plasma ADMA levels to cardiovascular outcomes at 2 years in men with acute coronary syndrome referred for coronary angiography. Coron Artery Dis 20: 112–117.
34. Jiang DJ, Cao Y, Xin HY, Li XH, Luo ZQ, et al. (2009) Asymmetric dimethylarginine induces tissue factor expression in monocytes via NF-kappaB-dependent pathway: Role in acute coronary syndromes. Atherosclerosis 205: 554–560.
35. Meinitzer A, Puchinger M, Winklhofer-Roob BM, Rock E, Ribalta J, et al. (2007) Reference values for plasma concentrations of asymmetrical dimethylarginine (ADMA) and other arginine metabolites in men after validation of a chromatographic method. Clin Chim Acta 384: 141–148.
36. Kielstein JT, Salpeter SR, Bode-Boeger SM, Cooke JP, Fliser D (2006) Symmetric dimethylarginine (SDMA) as endogenous marker of renal function—a meta-analysis. Nephrol Dial Transplant 21: 2446–2451.
37. Vallance P, Leone A, Calver A, Collier J, Moncada S (1992) Accumulation of an endogenous inhibitor of nitric oxide synthesis in chronic renal failure. Lancet 339: 572–575.
38. Closs EI, Basha FZ, Habermeier A, Forstermann U (1997) Interference of L-arginine analogues with L-arginine transport mediated by the y carrier hCAT-2B. Nitric Oxide 1: 65–73.
39. Tojo A, Welch WJ, Bremer V, Kimoto M, Kimura K, et al. (1997) Colocalization of demethylating enzymes and NOS and functional effects of methylarginines in rat kidney. Kidney Int 52: 1593–1601.
40. Al Banchaabouchi M, Marescau B, Possemiers I, D'Hooge R, Levillain O, et al. (2000) NG, NG-dimethylarginine and NG, NG-dimethylarginine in renal insufficiency. Pflugers Arch 439: 524–531.
41. Shemesh O, Golbetz H, Kriss JP, Myers BD (1985) Limitations of creatinine as a filtration marker in glomerulopathic patients. Kidney Int 28: 830–838.
42. Schepers E, Barreto DV, Liabeuf S, Glorieux G, Eloot S, et al. (2011) Symmetric dimethylarginine as a proinflammatory agent in chronic kidney disease. Clin J Am Soc Nephrol 6: 2374–2383.

13

Indomethacin Reduces Glomerular and Tubular Damage Markers but not Renal Inflammation in Chronic Kidney Disease Patients

Martin H. de Borst[1]*, Ferdau L. Nauta[1], Liffert Vogt[2], Gozewijn D. Laverman[1], Ron T. Gansevoort[1], Gerjan Navis[1]

1 Division of Nephrology, Department of Internal Medicine, University Medical Center Groningen and University of Groningen, Groningen, the Netherlands, **2** Department of Nephrology, Academic Medical Center, Amsterdam, the Netherlands

Abstract

Under specific conditions non-steroidal anti-inflammatory drugs (NSAIDs) may be used to lower therapy-resistant proteinuria. The potentially beneficial anti-proteinuric, tubulo-protective, and anti-inflammatory effects of NSAIDs may be offset by an increased risk of (renal) side effects. We investigated the effect of indomethacin on urinary markers of glomerular and tubular damage and renal inflammation. We performed a post-hoc analysis of a prospective open-label crossover study in chronic kidney disease patients ($n = 12$) with mild renal function impairment and stable residual proteinuria of 4.7±4.1 g/d. After a wash-out period of six wks without any RAAS blocking agents or other therapy to lower proteinuria (untreated proteinuria (UP)), patients subsequently received indomethacin 75 mg BID for 4 wks (NSAID). Healthy subjects ($n = 10$) screened for kidney donation served as controls. Urine and plasma levels of total IgG, IgG4, KIM-1, beta-2-microglobulin, H-FABP, MCP-1 and NGAL were determined using ELISA. Following NSAID treatment, 24 h -urinary excretion of glomerular and proximal tubular damage markers was reduced in comparison with the period without anti-proteinuric treatment (total IgG: UP 131[38–513] vs NSAID 38[17–218] mg/24 h, $p<0.01$; IgG4: 50[16–68] vs 10[1–38] mg/24 h, $p<0.001$; beta-2-microglobulin: 200[55–404] vs 50[28–110] ug/24 h, $p = 0.03$; KIM-1: 9[5–14] vs 5[2–9] ug/24 h, $p = 0.01$). Fractional excretions of these damage markers were also reduced by NSAID. The distal tubular marker H-FABP showed a trend to reduction following NSAID treatment. Surprisingly, NSAID treatment did not reduce urinary excretion of the inflammation markers MCP-1 and NGAL, but did reduce plasma MCP-1 levels, resulting in an increased fractional MCP-1 excretion. In conclusion, the anti-proteinuric effect of indomethacin is associated with reduced urinary excretion of glomerular and tubular damage markers, but not with reduced excretion of renal inflammation markers. Future studies should address whether the short term glomerulo- and tubulo-protective effects as observed outweigh the possible side-effects of NSAID treatment on the long term.

Editor: Dominique Guerrot, Rouen University Hospital, France

Funding: The original study that served as the source of the current post-hoc analysis was supported by Merck & Company (grant MSGP 9661). Dr. De Borst is supported by personal development grants from the Dutch Kidney foundation (KJPB.08.07; http://www.nierstichting.nl) and the University Medical Center Groningen (Mandema stipend). The funders had no role in study design, data collection and analysis, decision to publish, or preparation of the manuscript.

Competing Interests: Part of the original study was supported by Merck & Company (grant MSGP 9661). This does not alter the authors' adherence to all the PLoS ONE policies on sharing data and materials.

* E-mail: m.h.de.borst@umcg.nl

Introduction

Reduction of proteinuria is a major therapy target to achieve long-term renoprotection in chronic kidney disease. To this end, blockade of the renin-angiotensin-aldosterone system (RAAS) ideally combined with a diuretic or dietary sodium restriction [1] is the cornerstone of current renoprotective therapy in chronic kidney disease [2,3]. Nevertheless, chronic kidney disease (CKD) progression persists in a considerable proportion of patients. Particularly in patients with high residual proteinuria despite RAAS blockade, there may be a place for alternative modes of antiproteinuric intervention, such as non-steroidal anti-inflammatory drugs (NSAIDs) [4].

Before the era of RAAS inhibitors, NSAIDs were well known for a distinct antiproteinuric effect. Their use in nephrotic syndrome was supported by retrospective data suggesting that NSAIDs may retard progression of renal function loss [5,6], although not all data are uniform [7].

Most renoprotective effects of NSAIDs are considered to be related to their effect on prostaglandin synthesis [8]. Prostaglandin inhibition reduces effective renal plasma flow (ERPF) and glomerular filtration rate (GFR), presumably resulting in a reduction of intraglomerular pressure, in turn leading to a reduction of proteinuria [9]. Moreover, through inhibition of prostaglandin synthesis, NSAIDs reduce inflammation, a determinant of renal and cardiovascular outcome in CKD [10,11]. Recent elegant studies implicated a central role for increased cyclooxygenase-2 (COX-2) expression in podocytes in the etiology of glomerular injury which could be reversed by COX-2 inhibition [12,13]. Beside these beneficial effects, however, NSAIDs also have side-effects in several organ systems including the gastrointestinal tract (e.g. peptic ulcers) and central nervous system side-effects. Also deleterious renal effects such as tubulointerstitial damage have been reported [14,15]. Since the presence of tubulointerstitial damage is a determinant of response to renoprotective therapy [11], this may negatively impact prognosis for CKD patients.

To further investigate the glomerular, tubular and anti-inflammatory effects of NSAIDs in CKD, we measured a panel of urinary renal damage markers representing different parts of the nephron in patients with overt proteinuria, before and after treatment with indomethacin. As a secondary aim we investigated whether pretreatment biomarker levels were associated with the anti-proteinuric response.

Materials and Methods

Ethics Statement

The study was approved by the medical ethics committee of the University of Groningen, and all participants provided written informed consent. All clinical investigations have been conducted according to the principles expressed in the Declaration of Helsinki.

Patients

This study is performed as a post-hoc analysis of a prospective open-label crossover study [16]. This study was performed in Caucasian patients ($n = 16$) who fulfilled the following inclusion criteria after a 6 week washout period without RAAS intervention: proteinuria >2 g/day, diastolic blood pressure <90 mmHg, creatinine clearance >30 mL/min and age 18–70 years. Blood and urine samples were available for 12 out of 16 patients due to biobank exhaustion: seven patients with non-diabetic nephropathy (membranous glomerulopathy ($n = 2$), primary focal segmental glomerular sclerosis (2), IgA nephropathy (2) and hypertensive nephropathy (1)), and five with (type 2) diabetic nephropathy. Diagnoses were established by kidney biopsy for all patients. The characteristics of these patients were similar to the original study population. Healthy subjects who were screened for kidney donation in our center were included as controls ($n = 10$).

Study Protocol

The detailed study protocol was published previously [16]. During an initial washout period, blood pressure was titrated with hydrochlorothiazide 12.5 mg QD combined with amlodipine or doxazosine if necessary; this regimen remained unchanged during the actual study. Following the washout period without anti-proteinuric treatment, urine and blood samples were collected. Subsequently patients were treated with indomethacin 75 mg BID (retard formula; Indocid® Merck & Co., Inc., Whitehouse Station, NJ, USA) for four weeks. At the end of this period a second set of urine and blood samples were collected.

Clinical Measurements

At each visit, after an overnight fast, blood was sampled, 24-h urine was collected and blood pressure was measured by an automatic device (Dinamap®, GE Healthcare, Waukesha, WI, USA). Twentyfour-hour urine was checked for collection errors using the equation previously formulated by Ix et al [17]. The mean arterial blood pressure (MAP) was calculated as 2/3× diastolic blood pressure +1/3× systolic blood pressure. The mean value of four readings after 15 min was used for analysis. Urinary protein was determined with the pyrogallol red-molybdate method. Serum creatinine, albumin and lipids were determined using an automated multi-analyzer (MEGA®, Merck, Darmstadt, Germany).

Measurement of Damage Markers

Aliquots from 24 h -urine were stored at −80°C until damage marker analysis. After thawing, all urine samples were vortexed and subsequently centrifuged (14.000 rpm). The supernatant was used for measurements. Samples were diluted to obtain optimal concentration for measurement. All urinary biomarkers were determined in one run. As glomerular damage markers we measured total IgG and IgG4, as markers of proximal tubular damage kidney injury molecule-1 (KIM-1) and beta-2-microglobulin (B2M), as markers of distal tubular damage heart-fatty acid binding protein (H-FABP), and as markers of inflammation neutrophil gelatinase associated lipocalin (NGAL), monocyte chemotactic protein-1 (MCP-1), as documented previously [18]. Urinary concentrations of total IgG, IgG4, NGAL, KIM-1, and H-FABP were measured by enzyme-linked immunosorbent assay. For KIM-1, B2M and NGAL, antibodies were obtained from R&D Systems (Minneapolis, MN, intra-assay CV 7.4%, 9.7% and 6.8%, respectively). H-FABP and total IgG, IgG-4 antibodies were obtained from Hytest (Turku, Finland, intra-assay CV 9.3%, 13.3% and 14.0%, respectively). All samples were measured in duplicate.

The 24-h excretion of renal damage markers was calculated by multiplying the urinary biomarker concentration with the total 24 h urine volume. Fractional excretion of renal damage markers was calculated as:

$$FE_{marker}(\%) = 100x([urine_{marker}] * [plasma_{creatinine}])/([plasma_{marker}] * [urine_{creatinine}])$$

Statistical Analyses

Data are expressed as median (interquartile range). Differences between healthy controls and CKD patients without anti-proteinuric treatment were analyzed by Mann Whitney non-parametric test. Differences between the study periods without anti-proteinuric treatment versus NSAID treatment, respectively, were analyzed by Wilcoxon paired non-parametric test. Associations between urinary biomarker excretion and proteinuria were studied using linear regression with proteinuria as an independent variable, and the individual renal damage markers as dependent variables. For these analyses, urinary biomarker excretions were logarithmically transformed. We also determined whether the change in biomarker excretion between the study period without anti-proteinuric treatment and NSAID (delta biomarker) was related to the anti-proteinuric response (delta proteinuria). Furthermore similar analysis were performed for the association between biomarker excretion during the period without anti-proteinuric therapy (i.e. before anti-proteinuric intervention) and the anti-proteinuric response, to evaluate which biomarker(s) would be able to predict the anti-proteinuric response. For all analyses, a two-sided $p<0.05$ was considered statistically significant.

All calculations and analyses were performed using SPSS 18.0 for Windows (SPSS Inc., Chicago, Illinois, USA).

Results

Baseline characteristics are given in Table 1. In CKD patients, proteinuria was reduced by NSAID treatment with a median of 51% (IQR 33–73%) compared with the study period without anti-proteinuric treatment ("untreated UP"; Figure 1A). CKD patients

Table 1. Baseline characteristics of proteinuric CKD patients and healthy controls.

	Healthy controls	CKD untreated	CKD+NSAID
n	10	12	12
Age (years)	57 (41–68)	56 (42–67)	56 (42–67)
Male sex (%)	70	69	69
Diabetes mellitus (n)	0	5*	5
Systolic blood pressure (mmHg)$	119 (105–151)	142 (125–179)*	148 (130–165)
Diastolic blood pressure (mmHg)$	70 (55–84)	81 (72–95)*	79 (74–85)
BMI (kg/m^2)	27 (23–29)	28 (23–38)	28 (25–34)
Body weight (kg)	87 (74–97)	89 (76–101)	88 (77–105)
Creatinine clearance (ml/min)	113 (59–187)	79 (30–155)*	70 (28–140)
Proteinuria (g/24 h)	0.0 (0.0–0.2)	3.3 (0.6–14.6)**	1.2 (0.7–2.5)##
UNaV (mmol/24 h)	219 (148–266)	213 (127–253)	173 (109–210)#
FE sodium (%)	0.9 (0.6–1.3)	1.5 (1.2–3.5)**	1.5 (1.1–2.9)

BMI, body mass index; UNaV, urinary sodium excretion; FE, fractional excretion.
*$p<0.05$, **$p<0.01$ CKD untreated vs healthy controls.
#$p<0.05$, ## $p<0.01$ CKD NSAID vs CKD untreated.
$Antihypertensive use remained stable during the study protocol.

had a significantly lower creatinine clearance compared to healthy controls. After four weeks of treatment with indomethacin, creatinine clearance showed a non-significant trend to further reduction (Figure 1B).

In parallel with proteinuria, 24-h urinary excretions of the glomerular damage markers total IgG and IgG4 were strongly increased in CKD patients as compared to healthy controls. Anti-proteinuric treatment with indomethacin reduced urinary total IgG and IgG4 excretion (Table 2). Plasma levels of total IgG and IgG4 were not affected by NSAID treatment (Table S1); therefore fractional excretion of these markers decreased significantly during treatment (Table 3). The glomerular charge selectivity index, calculated as the ratio of the fractional excretions of total IgG/IgG4, increased with NSAID treatment (untreated proteinuria: 6.98[1.24–16.8] vs NSAID 9.96[2.02–30.92], $p<0.05$).

The two proximal tubular markers KIM-1 and B2M were elevated in CKD patients during the study period without anti-proteinuric treatment, as compared to healthy controls, and reduced by NSAID treatment (Table 2). Fractional excretion of these markers was also significantly reduced by NSAID treatment (Table 3). Urinary excretion of the distal tubular marker H-FABP was elevated in untreated proteinuric patients when compared to healthy controls, and NSAID treatment resulted in a non-significant trend to reduced H-FABP excretion (Table 2) and a significant decline in plasma H-FABP levels (Table S1). Consequently the fractional excretion of H-FABP remained unchanged.

We subsequently investigated whether the anti-inflammatory drug indomethacin would affect renal inflammation, as reflected by urinary MCP-1 and NGAL excretion. Surprisingly, indomethacin did not reduce the 24 h -urinary excretions of MCP-1 or NGAL, both of which were higher in CKD patients than in healthy subjects (Table 2). In plasma, however, MCP-1 levels but not NGAL levels were reduced by indomethacin (Table S1). As a result, the fractional excretion of MCP1 increased (Table 3).

The relationship between urinary renal damage marker excretions and proteinuria was further investigated by regression analysis. Univariate analysis indicated that urinary excretions of total IgG (standardized beta.691, $p<.001$), IgG4 (standardized beta.642, $p<.001$), KIM-1 (standardized beta.662, $p<.001$), B2M (standardized beta.466, $p<.05$), and H-FABP (standardized beta.454, $p<.05$) were significantly associated with proteinuria. As expected, delta urinary total IgG excretion (with vs without antiproteinuric treatment, standardized beta.739, $p<.01$) and delta urinary IgG4 excretion (standardized beta.721, $p<.01$) were significantly associated with the anti-proteinuric response.

Finally we studied whether renal damage marker excretion during the period without anti-proteinuric treatment (i.e. before anti-proteinuric therapy) would be associated with the anti-proteinuric response to indomethacin. Interestingly, urinary excretion of KIM-1 (standardized beta −0.673, $p<0.05$) and MCP-1 (standardized beta −0.854, $p<0.001$) before anti-proteinuric treatment was inversely associated with the anti-proteinuric response. After adjustment for age and genderonly the association between MCP-1 and the anti-proteinuric response remained significant (standardized beta −0.662, $p<0.01$). A scatter plot illustrating the relationship between pre-treatment MCP-1 levels and the anti-proteinuric response is presented in Figure 2.

Discussion

RAAS blockade combined with volume restriction is the therapy of choice for most CKD patients, but the anti-proteinuric response to this regimen is often incomplete [19]. Therefore it is crucial to identify interventions that can serve as (adjunct) anti-proteinuric therapies. The main finding of the current study is that the anti-proteinuric effect of the NSAID indomethacin is accompanied by reduced urinary 24 h -excretion of glomerular and tubular damage markers. The 24 h -urinary excretion of inflammation markers, on the other hand, was not affected by NSAID treatment, and the fractional excretion of MCP-1 was even increased.

The reduced urinary excretion of glomerular damage markers total IgG and IgG4 is in line with the known anti-proteinuric effect of indomethacin, and may be related to prostaglandin inhibition affecting renal hemodynamics (i.e. vasoconstriction of the afferent arterioles). Furthermore, both 24 h -urinary excretion and fractional excretion of the proximal tubular damage markers were reduced following treatment with an NSAID, and the distal

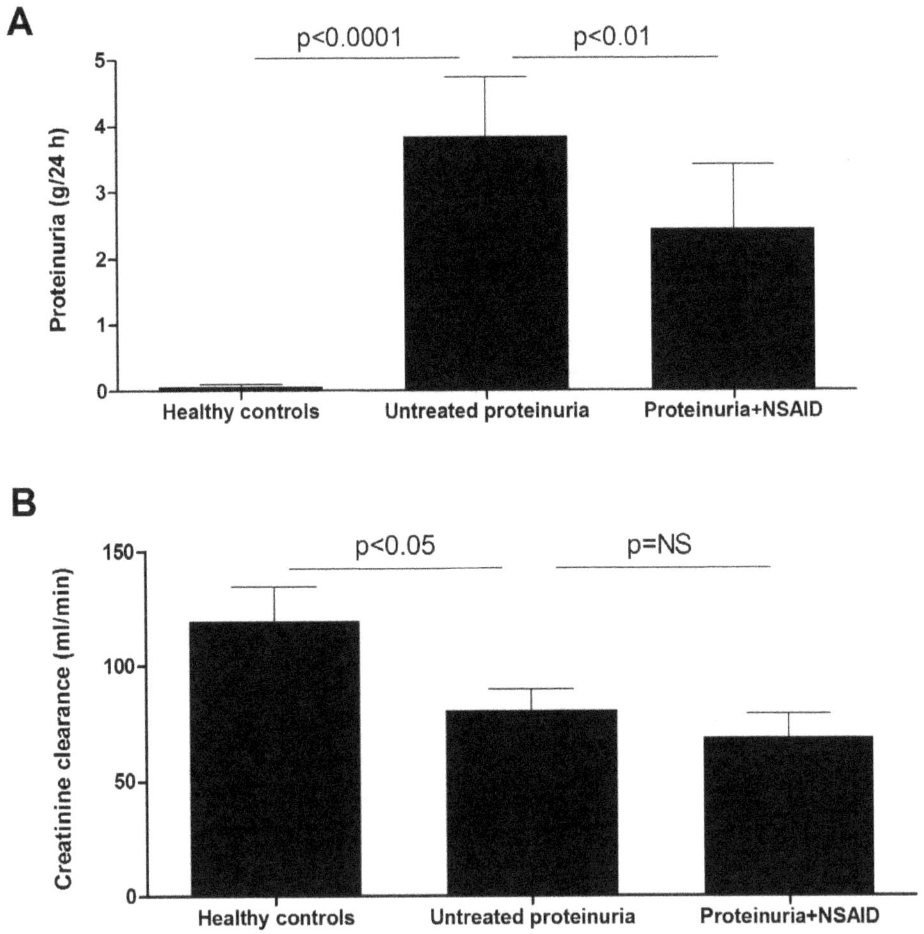

Figure 1. Proteinuria and creatinine clearance. A. Proteinuria was strongly increased in proteinuric CKD patients as compared to matched healthy controls. NSAID treatment significantly reduced proteinuria. B. Creatinine clearance was significantly lower in untreated CKD patients, whereas NSAID treatment did not significantly affect creatinine clearance. Horizontal lines indicate medians.

tubular marker H-FABP showed a trend to reduction. This suggests that NSAIDs may have protective effects, rather than toxic effects, on the tubular epithelium. Tubulotoxic effects may be seen in rare cases, but in our study on average signs of reduction of tubular damage are observed, probably secondary to the anti-proteinuric effect of NSAID treatment. This is in concert with previously observed tubulo-protective effects of RAAS-related anti-proteinuric therapy in both clinical cohorts [20] as well as preclinical studies, where also an association with protection against structural renal damage was observed [21,22]. In addition, direct protective (e.g. anti-apoptotic) effects as implicated by in vitro studies [15] may play a role. NSAID treatment did not significantly affect the distal tubular marker H-FABP, although a trend to reduction was observed. Much less is known about the effects of proteinuria on distal as compared to proximal tubular cells, although the distal tubule is considered less sensitive to the

Table 2. 24-h urinary excretion of renal damage markers in healthy controls, CKD patients after a period with no anti-proteinuric treatment (untreated UP), and after NSAID treatment.

Damage marker	Healthy controls	Untreated UP	P vs healthy	NSAID	P vs untreated UP
Total IgG (mg/24 h)	3.9 (2.9–5.6)	130.9 (37.8–513.4)	<0.001	38.1 (17.0–218.4)	<0.01
IgG4 (mg/24 h)	0.0 (0.0–0.1)	50.3 (16.4–68.3)	<0.001	10.2 (1.2–38.0)	<0.001
KIM-1 (μg/24 h)	2.3 (1.6–4.9)	8.9 (5.2–13.9)	0.004	4.6 (2.0–7.8)	0.01
B2M (μg/24 h)	56.3 (34.8–75.6)	199.5 (54.9–404.2)	0.03	47.8 (27.6–109.6)	0.03
H-FABP (μg/24 h)	0.0 (0.0–0.2)	28.4 (8.7–11.9)	<0.001	9.1 (1.2–89.9)	0.11
MCP-1 (μg/24 h)	0.8 (0.4–1.1)	1.8 (0.9–2.6)	0.01	1.8 (1.1–2.3)	0.88
NGAL (μg/24 h)	23.0 (15.1–29.4)	37.2 (29.2–89.9)	0.001	35.2 (26.8–89.9)	0.37

Table 3. Fractional excretion of damage markers in CKD patients after a period with no anti-proteinuric treatment, and after NSAID treatment.

Damage marker	Untreated UP	NSAID	P
Total IgG (%)	6.6×10^{-4} (0.9–14.3×10^{-4})	3.0×10^{-4} (0.7–8.0×10^{-4})	0.03
IgG4 (%)	1.25 (0.62–3.89)	0.31 (0.14–0.50)	0.004
KIM-1 (%)	4.70 (3.53–8.56)	3.16 (1.32–6.02)	0.03
B2M (%)	0.83 (0.19–11.13)	0.30 (0.14–2.83)	0.04
H-FABP (%)	24.9 (9.9–150.5)	22.7 (2.9–164.0)	0.72
MCP-1 (%)	5.61 (4.25–8.31)	13.23 (6.80–22.47)	0.006
NGAL (%)	1.60 (1.04–4.01)	1.73 (0.65–4.64)	0.40

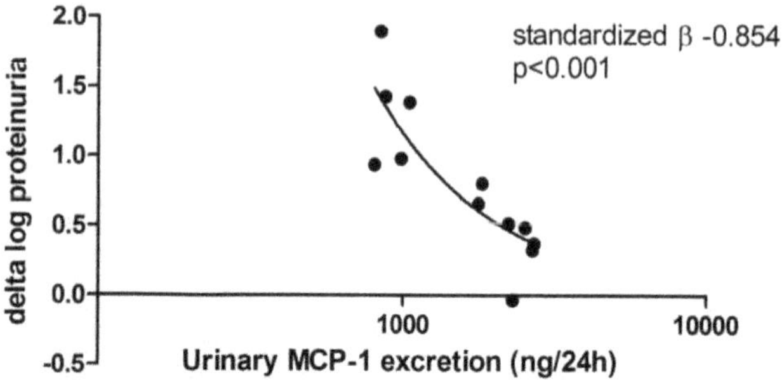

Figure 2. Pre-treatment urinary MCP-1 excretion and treatment response. Scatter plot indicating the relationship between the 24 h -urinary excretion of MCP-1 before start of anti-proteinuric therapy (i.e. NSAID) and the anti-proteinuric response (i.e. delta proteinuria without vs with NSAID). A negative association is present, suggesting that high baseline MCP-1 excretion is associated with poor anti-proteinuric response to therapy.

toxic effects of proteinuria. We recently reported that H-FABP is associated with albuminuria in diabetic subjects; moreover, H-FABP was the only damage marker from the investigated marker set that was significantly associated with eGFR after adjustment for albuminuria [18]. Future studies should address the relevance of H-FABP modulation by antiproteinuric therapy.

Surprisingly, NSAID treatment had no effect on the 24 h-urinary excretion of inflammation markers MCP-1 or NGAL. In contrast, fractional excretion of MCP-1 even increased following NSAID treatment. This was unexpected given the anti-inflammatory properties of this drug. On the other hand, the dissociation of renoprotective effects from anti-inflammatory effects of NSAIDs is in line with preclinical studies [15,23]. Furthermore, we recently found that in a cohort of CKD patients receiving an angiotensin receptor blocker in addition to an angiotensin converting enzyme inhibitor, urinary excretion of proximal tubular markers was reduced, but inflammatory markers did not change (*data submitted*). Our finding that the extent of pre-treatment renal inflammation is independently associated with the anti-proteinuric response is also in line with preclinical studies [11]. This finding may have two important implications. First, these data suggest that the renoprotective potential of NSAIDs may be limited by the absence of intra-renal anti-inflammatory effects (in spite of systemic anti-inflammatory effects as reflected by lower plasma MCP-1 and B2M levels). Second, these data suggest that the antiproteinuric, and potentially also the renoprotective effect of NSAIDs is limited to disease states with less intra-renal inflammation, for instance excluding the use of these drugs in immune-mediated renal disease.

Treatment with indomethacin induced a trend towards decreased creatinine clearance in our study, and although this reduction was relatively small, our study lacks power to exclude an effect on renal function. Previous studies demonstrated an anti-proteinuric response in the presence of a significant decline of GFR following NSAID treatment [24,25]. The limited decline in creatinine clearance in our study may also be explained by the sodium replete state of our population. Although dietary salt restriction is part of current best available renoprotective therapy, in clinical practice it is notoriously difficult to implement a persistent reduction in dietary salt intake, and in fact in most published studies, the salt intake of CKD patients is similar to that in the general population [26] [26]. In line, several landmark randomized controlled trials published over the last years have also not been performed against the background of dietary sodium restriction. In the setting of NSAID treatment, however, sodium restriction may increase the risk of a fall in GFR [4]. Of note, the antiproteinuric effect of NSAIDs has also been described to be blunted by sodium repletion at least in severely nephrotic patients [27]. The current anti-proteinuric efficacy of NSAID treatment despite high sodium intake is therefore remarkable, suggesting an optimal balance between efficacy and safety of NSAIDs under liberal sodium intake. Our findings also suggest that NSAID treatment increased charge selectivity, which is known to be reduced in nephrotic-range proteinuria [28].

NSAIDs are nowadays rarely considered for anti-proteinuric therapy in CKD. This is for the large part explained by the availability of RAAS blockers with a more favorable potential, whereas NSAIDs may have tubulotoxic effects. Also, the reduction of creatinine clearance observed in up to 20% of patients treated with NSAIDs [29,30], although reversible and presumably reflecting a beneficial renal hemodynamic effect (lowering of intraglomerular pressure), has raised concern against using these drugs in patients with CKD. In our study, none of the 24 h-excretions of renal damage markers increased following NSAID treatment as compared to the period without anti-proteinuric treatment. The decrease in creatinine clearance was small and did not reach statistical significance, perhaps due to the sodium-replete condition of our patients. The limited follow-up of our study does not allow to address longer term safety of NSAID therapy.

Our study has its limitations such as limited sample size and study duration, and the post-hoc design. Given the heterogeneity of the population with respect to the underlying type of renal disease, it may be surprising that significant reductions of glomerular and proximal tubular biomarkers were found. This suggests that irrespective of the underlying disease, one or more shared pathophysiologic pathways (including proteinuria) are reduced by NSAID treatment. The current findings cannot be extrapolated to patients with more severe renal disease, who may experience more side effects such as hyperkalemia or edema, or patients on background RAAS blockade. The latter category may not tolerate the combined regimen, and a previous study has questioned the additional efficacy of NSAID when give on top of maximum RAAS blockade as anti-proteinuric therapy [31]. Furthermore it would be of interest to study intra-individual changes of these biomarkers over time, and their prognostic value, in a longitudinal analysis. Nevertheless our data may provide a rationale to prescribe NSAIDs in patients with glomerular disease and proteinuria in whom immunosuppressive therapy and RAAS blockade are either ineffective or contra-indicated. Randomized controlled clinical trials investigating the long-term renoprotective (i.e. protective against loss of renal function) as well as cardiovascular effects of NSAIDs (as monotherapy or on top of RAAS blockade) are, however, warranted.

In conclusion, NSAID treatment is associated with a change in urinary biomarker profile that suggests glomerulo- and tubulo-protective effects along with reduction of proteinuria. Our findings, although they cannot be extrapolated to a setting of (maximally tolerated) background RAAS blockade with optimal volume depletion, suggest that under specific conditions NSAIDs may be used to reduce proteinuria as well as glomerular and tubular damage markers in CKD. This may be relevant given the prognostic importance of tubulointerstitial damage for the progression of renal function loss [32,33]. On the other hand no intra-renal anti-inflammatory effects of NSAID treatment could be demonstrated and renal inflammation, another important prognostic determinant of renal function loss [34], may even be increased by NSAID treatment. NSAID may thus be considered with caution as a non-hypotensive antiproteinuric therapy when RAAS blockade is not tolerated, e.g. due to hypotension. Whether NSAIDs, either as monotherapy or given on top of RAAS blockade, have the potential to modulate long term renal outcome remains to be proven.

Acknowledgments

The authors express their gratitude to Wim van Oeveren for facilitating the biomarker measurements.

Author Contributions

Conceived and designed the experiments: MHdB LV GDL. Performed the experiments: FLN LV. Analyzed the data: MHdB FLN. Contributed reagents/materials/analysis tools: FLN LV. Wrote the paper: MHdB FLN LV GDL RTG GN.

References

1. Vogt L, Waanders F, Boomsma F, de Zeeuw D, Navis G (2008) Effects of dietary sodium and hydrochlorothiazide on the antiproteinuric efficacy of losartan. J Am Soc Nephrol 19(5): 999–1007.
2. Ruggenenti P, Perna A, Gherardi G, Gaspari F, Benini R, et al. (1998) Renal function and requirement for dialysis in chronic nephropathy patients on long-term ramipril: REIN follow-up trial. gruppo italiano di studi epidemiologici in nefrologia (GISEN). ramipril efficacy in nephropathy. Lancet 352(9136): 1252–1256.
3. Maschio G, Alberti D, Janin G, Locatelli F, Mann JF, et al. (1996) Effect of the angiotensin-converting-enzyme inhibitor benazepril on the progression of chronic renal insufficiency. the angiotensin-converting-enzyme inhibition in progressive renal insufficiency study group. N Engl J Med 334(15): 939–945.
4. Vogt L, Laverman GD, Navis G (2010) Time for a comeback of NSAIDs in proteinuric chronic kidney disease? Neth J Med 68(12): 400–407.
5. Lagrue G, Laurent J, Belghiti D (1988) Renal survival in membranoproliferative glomerulonephritis (MPGN): Role of long-term treatment with non-steroid anti-inflammatory drugs (NSAID). Int Urol Nephrol 20(6): 669–677.
6. Vriesendorp R, Donker AJ, de Zeeuw D, de Jong PE, van der Hem GK, et al. (1986) Effects of nonsteroidal anti-inflammatory drugs on proteinuria. Am J Med 81(2B): 84–94.
7. Gansevoort RT, Heeg JE, Vriesendorp R, de Zeeuw D, de Jong PE (1992) Antiproteinuric drugs in patients with idiopathic membranous glomerulopathy. Nephrol Dial Transplant 7 Suppl 1: 91–96.
8. Vriesendorp R, de Zeeuw D, de Jong PE, Donker AJ, Pratt JJ, et al. (1986) Reduction of urinary protein and prostaglandin E2 excretion in the nephrotic syndrome by non-steroidal anti-inflammatory drugs. Clin Nephrol 25(2): 105–110.
9. Vriesendorp R, Donker AJ, de Zeeuw D, de Jong PE, van der Hem GK (1985) Antiproteinuric effect of naproxen and indomethacin. A double-blind crossover study. Am J Nephrol 5(4): 236–242.
10. Carrero JJ, Stenvinkel P (2009) Persistent inflammation as a catalyst for other risk factors in chronic kidney disease: A hypothesis proposal. Clin J Am Soc Nephrol 4 Suppl 1: S49–55.
11. Kramer AB, Laverman GD, van Goor H, Navis G (2003) Inter-individual differences in anti-proteinuric response to ACEi in established adriamycin nephrotic rats are predicted by pretreatment renal damage. J Pathol 201(1): 160–167.
12. Cheng HF, Wang CJ, Moeckel GW, Zhang MZ, McKanna JA, et al. (2002) Cyclooxygenase-2 inhibitor blocks expression of mediators of renal injury in a model of diabetes and hypertension. Kidney Int 62(3): 929–939.
13. Cheng H, Fan X, Moeckel GW, Harris RC (2011) Podocyte COX-2 exacerbates diabetic nephropathy by increasing podocyte (pro)renin receptor expression. J Am Soc Nephrol 22(7): 1240–1251.
14. John R, Herzenberg AM (2009) Renal toxicity of therapeutic drugs. J Clin Pathol 62(6): 505–515.
15. Sauvant C, Schneider R, Holzinger H, Renker S, Wanner C, et al. (2010) Indomethacin corrects alterations associated with ischemia/reperfusion in an in vitro proximal tubular model. Am J Nephrol 32(1): 57–65.
16. Vogt L, de Zeeuw D, Woittiez AJ, Navis G (2009) Selective cyclooxygenase-2 (COX-2) inhibition reduces proteinuria in renal patients. Nephrol Dial Transplant 24(4): 1182–1189.
17. Ix JH, Wassel CL, Stevens LA, Beck GJ, Froissart M, et al. (2011) Equations to estimate creatinine excretion rate: The CKD epidemiology collaboration. Clin J Am Soc Nephrol 6(1): 184–191.
18. Nauta FL, Boertien WE, Bakker SJ, van Goor H, van Oeveren W, et al. (2011) Glomerular and tubular damage markers are elevated in patients with diabetes. Diabetes Care 34(4): 975–981.
19. Slagman MC, Waanders F, Hemmelder MH, Woittiez AJ, Janssen WM, et al. (2011) Moderate dietary sodium restriction added to angiotensin converting enzyme inhibition compared with dual blockade in lowering proteinuria and blood pressure: Randomised controlled trial. BMJ 343: d4366.
20. Waanders F, Vaidya VS, van Goor H, Leuvenink H, Damman K, et al. (2009) Effect of renin-angiotensin-aldosterone system inhibition, dietary sodium restriction, and/or diuretics on urinary kidney injury molecule 1 excretion in nondiabetic proteinuric kidney disease: A post hoc analysis of a randomized controlled trial. Am J Kidney Dis 53(1): 16–25.
21. de Borst MH, van Timmeren MM, Vaidya VS, de Boer RA, van Dalen MB, et al (2007) Induction of kidney injury molecule-1 in homozygous Ren2 rats is attenuated by blockade of the renin-angiotensin system or p38 MAP kinase. Am J Physiol Renal Physiol 292(1): F313–20.
22. Kramer AB, van Timmeren MM, Schuurs TA, Vaidya VS, Bonventre JV, et al. (2009) Reduction of proteinuria in adriamycin-induced nephropathy is associated with reduction of renal kidney injury molecule (kim-1) over time. Am J Physiol Renal Physiol 296(5): F1136–45.
23. Schneider R, Meusel M, Renker S, Bauer C, Holzinger H, et al. (2009) Low-dose indomethacin after ischemic acute kidney injury prevents downregulation of Oat1/3 and improves renal outcome. Am J Physiol Renal Physiol 297(6): F1614–21.
24. Heeg JE, de Jong PE, Vriesendorp R, de Zeeuw D (1990) Additive antiproteinuric effect of the NSAID indomethacin and the ACE inhibitor lisinopril. Am J Nephrol 10 Suppl 1: 94–97.
25. Heeg JE, de Jong PE, de Zeeuw D (1991) Additive antiproteinuric effect of angiotensin-converting enzyme inhibition and non-steroidal anti-inflammatory drug therapy: A clue to the mechanism of action. Clin Sci (Lond) 81(3): 367–372.
26. Krikken JA, Laverman GD, Navis G (2009) Benefits of dietary sodium restriction in the management of chronic kidney disease. Curr Opin Nephrol Hypertens 18(6): 531–538.
27. Donker AJ, Brentjens JR, van der Hem GK, Arisz L (1978) Treatment of the nephrotic syndrome with indomethacin. Nephron 22(4–6): 374–381.
28. Guasch A, Deen WM, Myers BD (1993) Charge selectivity of the glomerular filtration barrier in healthy and nephrotic humans. J Clin Invest 92(5): 2274–2282.
29. Whelton A, Hamilton CW (1991) Nonsteroidal anti-inflammatory drugs: Effects on kidney function. J Clin Pharmacol 31(7): 588–598.
30. Whelton A, Lefkowith JL, West CR, Verburg KM (2006) Cardiorenal effects of celecoxib as compared with the nonsteroidal anti-inflammatory drugs diclofenac and ibuprofen. Kidney Int 70(8): 1495–1502.
31. Pisoni R, Ruggenenti P, Sangalli F, Lepre MS, Remuzzi A, et al. (2002) Effect of high dose ramipril with or without indomethacin on glomerular selectivity. Kidney Int 62(3): 1010–1019.

14

Circulating Endoglin Concentration is not Elevated in Chronic Kidney Disease

David M. Charytan[1]*, Alexander M. Helfand[1], Brian A. MacDonald[2], Angeles Cinelli[1], Raghu Kalluri[2], Elisabeth M. Zeisberg[2]

1 Renal Division, Department of Medicine, Brigham and Women's Hospital, Boston, Massachusetts, United States of America, **2** Division of Matrix Biology, Department of Medicine, Beth Israel Deaconess Medical Center, Boston, Massachusetts, United States of America

Abstract

Background: Soluble endoglin, a TGF-β receptor, plays a key role in cardiovascular physiology. Whether circulating concentrations of soluble endoglin are elevated in CKD or underlie the high risk of cardiovascular death associated with chronic kidney disease (CKD) is unknown.

Methods: Individuals with and without CKD were recruited at a single center. Estimated glomerular filtration rate (eGFR) was estimated using the modified MDRD study equation and the serum creatinine at the time of recruitment, and patients were assigned to specific CKD stage according to usual guidelines. Serum endoglin concentration was measured by ELISA and univariate and multivariable regression was used to analyze the association between eGFR or CKD stage and the concentration of soluble endoglin.

Results: Serum endoglin was measured in 216 patients including 118 with stage 3 or higher CKD and 9 individuals with end stage renal disease (ESRD). Serum endoglin concentration did not vary significantly with CKD stage (increase of 0.16 ng/mL per 1 stage increase in CKD, $P = 0.09$) or eGFR (decrease -0.06 ng/mL per 10 mL/min/1.73 m^2 increase in GFR, $P = 0.12$), and was not higher in individuals with ESRD than in individuals with preserved renal function (4.2 ± 1.1 and 4.3 ± 1.2 ng/mL, respectively). Endoglin concentration was also not significantly associated with urinary albumin excretion.

Conclusions: Renal function is not associated with the circulating concentration of soluble endoglin. Elevations in soluble endoglin concentration are unlikely to contribute to the progression of CKD or the predisposition of individuals with CKD to develop cardiovascular disease.

Editor: Aristidis S. Charonis, Biomedical Research Foundation of the Academy of Athens, Greece

Funding: Dr. Charytan was funded by an American Heart Association Scientist Development Grant, a Norman S. Coplon Grant from Satellite Health Care, and the Paul Teschan Research Fund. Dr. Zeisberg was funded by an American Heart Association Scientist Development Grant (SDG0735602T) and a Mentored Clinical Scientist Development Award (KO8CA129204) from the National Institutes of Health. Dr. Kalluri was funded by NIH DK 55001. The funders had no role in study design, data collection and analysis, decision to publish, or preparation of the manuscript.

Competing Interests: The authors have declared that no competing interests exist.

* E-mail: dcharytan@partners.org

Introduction

Angiogenesis plays a critical role in renal homeostasis, and emerging data have increasingly suggested that dysregulation of angiogenesis contributes to the progression of chronic kidney disease (CKD) and its associated complications[1,2,3,4,5,6,7,8,9]. Increases in the circulating levels of angiogenesis inhibitors may play an important role in the rarefaction of renal capillaries that accompanies uremia[8]. Similarly, a wealth of data has demonstrated that vascular endothelial growth factor (VEGF) signaling plays a critical role in the maintenance of normal glomerular function[1,5,7,10], and that inhibiting VEGF induces hypertension, proteinuria and significant pathologic changes within the glomerulus [6,7,10,11].

The auto-regulation of angiogenesis plays a similarly important role in cardiovascular homeostasis [12,13,14]. Inhibition of VEGF signaling, for example, induces interstitial inflammation and endothelial apoptosis in the heart [15,16], and in both animal models and human CKD uremia is accompanied by significant rarefaction of the myocardial microvasculature[12,13,17]. These observations suggest that circulating anti-angiogenic factors may contribute to the progression of CKD and that their concentrations are likely to be elevated in individuals with significant loss of glomerular filtration rate (GFR) or proteinuria. Furthermore, Elevations in the ambient level of circulating angiogenesis inhibitors in individuals with CKD would also provide a mechanistic explanation for the high risk of cardiovascular morbidity and mortality associated with CKD.

Although, two recent studies have demonstrated that soluble fms-like kinase (sFLT-1) concentration rises as GFR declines [18,19], it remains uncertain whether angiogenesis inhibitors are generally elevated in the setting of CKD or whether sFLT-1 is uniquely increased in this respect. In particular, it is unknown whether the concentration of soluble endoglin, a key angiogenesis inhibitor implicated in the pathogenesis of preeclampsia cardiovascular disease, hypertension and endothelial dysfunction [20,21,22,23], is correlated with GFR. Because endoglin appears to play key roles in the pathogenesis of renal and cardiovascular pathology, we hypothesized that elevations in the concentration of circulating endoglin in CKD could contribute to the progression of CKD and underlie the association of CKD and cardiovascular disease. We undertook this study in order to determine whether endoglin levels are higher in individuals with CKD compared to individuals with preserved renal function.

Methods

Ethics Statement

This research was approved by and conducted in accordance with the standards of the local institutional review committees of the Brigham & Women's Hospital and Beth Israel Deaconess Medical Center and the principles of the Declaration of Helsinki. All subjects involved in the research signed written informed consent forms prior to enrollment.

Subjects

Subjects with and without CKD between the ages of 18–80 years old were recruited from the cardiac catheterization lab and the outpatient nephrology clinics (including the general nephrology, stone, and renal transplant donor clinics) of Brigham and Women's Hospital. Individuals receiving anti-angiogenic or immunosuppressive therapy, those with active malignancy or acute coronary ischemia, a history of thoracic or abdominal radiation therapy, and individuals with acute kidney injury were excluded. Individuals undergoing angiography were additionally excluded if they had a history of prior coronary artery bypass surgery.

Clinical Data and Laboratories

Data on blood pressure, demographics and baseline clinical conditions were obtained by patient interview, supplemental chart review and a brief exam at the time of recruitment. Serum creatinine, albumin, and hemoglobin were measured on the day of enrollment in the hospital laboratory using standard clinical techniques. The most recent measurements of total cholesterol, urinary albumin and creatinine excretion within 6 months of recruitment were also collected. Estimated glomerular filtration rate (eGFR) was calculated using the modified MDRD equation [24]. Renal function was categorized using a modification of the National Kidney Foundation 5-stage system [25]. Because the MDRD equation is not precise in patients with preserved renal function, individuals with eGFR ≥90 mL/min/1.73 m^2 were combined into a single category ("preserved function/stage 1 CKD)—this category included all patient with eGFR≥90 mL/min/1.73 m^2. As a sensitivity analysis, we separately analyzed endoglin concentrations in those whose GFR was estimated to be within the normal range (eGFR ≥110 mL/min/1.73 m^2) [26] and in individuals who were seen as transplant donors or for renal stones (without concomitant CKD). Non-dialysis dependent stage 4 and 5 CKD were considered jointly, chronic dialysis patients were evaluated as a unique category.

Samples and Measurement of Endoglin

Serum was centrifuged within 15 minutes at 1000 g and stored at −80°C. Samples were batch analyzed for soluble endoglin concentration in a blinded fashion using ELISA kits from R&D systems. Intra and inter-assay coefficient of variations for the assay were 4.0 and 13.1%, respectively.

Statistical Analysis

Data are presented as mean±standard deviation (SD), n (%) or median (inter-quartile ratio, IQR). Differences in baseline characteristics such as demographic data, blood pressure and comorbid medical conditions across categories of renal function were compared using ANOVA or non-parametric trend tests for continuous data and Chi-Square tests of trend for count data. The Pearson correlation coefficient was used to measure correlation between continuous variables. The relationship between eGFR or categories of renal function and soluble endoglin was assessed using univariate linear regression and a series of 4 different multivariable regression models to correct for potential confounding. The primary comparison was performed using linear regression models with serum endoglin concentration as the dependent variable, renal function (either as a continuous or categorical variable) as the primary independent variable and with additional adjustment for age, sex, race, diabetes, hypertension, smoking, cholesterol, congestive heart failure, peripheral vascular disease, and obstructive lung disease and recruitment site (Model 1). An expanded linear regression model (Model 2) additionally adjusted for Hispanic ethnicity and serum albumin. Additional linear models including terms for interaction with diabetes and recruitment site (outpatient clinics vs. coronary catheterization lab) were performed as a pre-specified analysis. Two sensitivity analyses were performed in order to examine the robustness of our results and their sensitivity to modeling assumptions. In the first, the independent terms from Model 1 were used in an ordered categorical regression model using quartiles of endoglin as the outcome variable. Logistic regression models using the median value of endoglin as the cutoff were generated in an analogous fashion. Model fit was tested using graphical techniques, inspection of residual distribution, and tests of model specification. All analyses were performed in STATA 9.0 (Stata Corporation, College Station, TX). $P<0.05$ was considered significant for all analyses.

Results

Baseline Characteristics

As shown in Table 1 and Table 2, serum creatinine and eGFR were significantly different across categories of renal function: eGFR in preserved function/Stage 1 CKD 105.9±12.0 mg/dL, Stage 2 CKD 73.8±8.5, Stage 3 CKD 44.8±8.5, Stage 4/5 CKD 22.5±6.5, Dialysis , 8.9±2.1 ,P <0.001. Age increased across increasing categories of CKD, but was actually lower in individuals on dialysis (52.3±18.0 years) than in individuals with preserved renal function/stage 1 CKD (57.3±8.0). Among baseline comorbidities, only coronary artery disease (P = 0.003), peripheral vascular disease (P = 0.007), and diabetes (P = 0.01) demonstrated a significantly increasing frequency across categories of renal function. Congestive heart failure was more prevalent in individuals with more severe renal dysfunction, but this trend did not achieve significance (P = 0.07). Diastolic blood pressure increased from 74.0±12.9 in individuals with preserved function/Stage 1 CKD to 82.6±18.5 in individuals on dialysis (P = 0.02). Similar trends were observed with systolic blood pressure but were not significant.

Urinary albumin excretion was available for 66 patients. Logarithmically transformed albumin to creatinine ratio was 5.0± mg/G among those with preserved renal function, 4.0±2.3 in those with stage 2 CKD, and 4.1±2.0 mg/G in those with stage 3 CKD, and 5.1±1.5 in those with stage 4/5 CKD (P = 0.51).

Endoglin Concentration and Renal Function

Endoglin concentration did not vary significantly across categories of baseline renal function (**Figure 1**). Mean Endoglin concentration was 4.3±1.2 ng/mL among those with preserved renal function, 4.5±1.7 ng/mL in stage 2 CKD, 4.7±1.6 ng/mL

Table 1. Baseline Clinical Characteristics of the Study Population.

Characteristic	Preserved Function-Stage 1 CKD	Stage 2 CKD	Stage 3 CKD	Stage 4-5 CKD	Dialysis	P Value*
(Mean±S.D.)	(N = 30)	(N = 5)	(N = 92)	(N = 27)	(N = 9)	
Demographics						
Age, years	57.3 ±8.0	59.8 ±11.3	63.5±13.2	68.2±14.7	52.3±18.0	0.001
Male, n (%)	22 (73.3)	38 (65.5)	49 (53.3)	18 (66.7)	3 (33.3)	0.10
Race, n (%)						
Black	3 (10.0)	9 (15.8)	10 (11.2)	4 (15.4)	4 (44.4)	0.06
White	25 (83.3)	42 (73.7)	68 (76.4)	18 (69.2)	2 (22.2)	
Other	2 (6.7)	6 (10.5)	11 (12.4)	4 (15.4)	3 (33.3)	
Hispanic	2 (6.7)	6 (10.3)	15 (16.5)	6 (24.0)	2 (22.2)	0.31
Physical Exam						
Weight, kilogram	86.1±19.2	86.8 ±21.7	89.8±23.8	85.5±20.0	81.9±32.7	0.87
Systolic blood pressure, mm Hg	128.0±24.2	124.7±17.3	128.9±21.4	130.2±19.7	146.4±13.8	0.08
Diastolic blood pressure, mm Hg	74.0±12.9	70.7±11.2	67.8±11.9	70.8±20.9	82.6±18.5	0.02
Past Medical History, n (%)						
Coronary disease	13 (76.5)	17 (43.6)	20 (26.0)	10 (38.5)	3 (42.9)	0.003
Hypertension	23 (76.7)	42 (72.4)	72 (78.3)	25 (92.6)	9 (100.0)	0.13
Diabetes	9 (30.0)	20 (34.5)	45 (48.9)	19 (70.4)	5 (55.6)	0.01
Congestive heart failure	4 (13.3)	11 (19.0)	16 (17.4)	6 (22.2)	5 (55.6)	0.07
Obstructive lung disease	0 (0.0)	2 (3.5)	6 (6.5)	1 (3.7)	2 (22.2)	0.10
Peripheral vascular disease	2 (6.7)	3 (5.2)	8 (8.7)	8 (29.6)	2 (22.2)	0.007
Hyperlipidemia	21 (70..0)	42 (72.4)	62 (67.4)	19 (70.4)	6 (66.7)	0.98
Smoking	3 (13.0)	9 (17.0)	7 (8.1)	0 (0.0)	1 (12.5)	0.17
Cause of CKD						0.29
Diabetes	--	--	13 (14.1)	8 (29.6)	1 (11.1)	
Hypertension	--	--	17 (18.5)	2 (7.4)	2 (22.2)	
Other/Unknown	--	--	62 (67.4)	17 (63.0)	6 (66.7)	

S.D. = Standard deviation., I.Q.R. = Interquartile Range,
*ANOVA for normally distributed continuous variables, chi-square test for -parametric trend test for non-normally distributed continuous variables, and chi-squared tests for count variables.

in stage 3 CKD, 5.4±2.4 ng/mL in stage 4/5 CKD, and 4.2±1.1 ng/mL in individuals with ESRD, (P = 0.12). There was a non-significant (P = 0.09) trend consistent with an increase in endoglin across categories of CKD among the subgroup of subjects not on chronic dialysis. However, as shown in **Figure 2**, the correlation was weak (r = 0.12) and non-significant (P = 0.05). Within the preserved renal function/stage 1 CKD group, endoglin concentrations were not different in individuals with eGFR ≥110 mL/min/1.73 m^2 compared with eGFR 90-<110 mL/min (4.65±1.32 ng/mL vs. 4.09±1.09 ng/mL, P = 0.23). Endoglin concentration was also similar among individuals recruited as transplant donors/stone patients compared to subjects with eGFR≥90 recruited for other reasons (4.24±0.74 ng/mL vs. 4.27±1.21, P = 0.95). Endoglin concentration also did not vary across categories of renal function when eGFR>110 mL/min/1.73 m^2 (P = 0.16) or transplant donor/stone patient (P = 0.19) were considered as distinct categories of baseline renal function.

Although endoglin concentrations were marginally higher among individuals recruited from clinic (β = 0.67, P = 0.003, **Table 3**) than in individuals recruited from the catheterization lab, the association between endoglin concentration and class of renal function was qualitatively similar in both groups, and it was not significantly associated with CKD class, P = 0.45 and P = 0.43, respectively (**Table 4**). The association between endoglin and CKD was also non-significant when the analysis was restricted to women (P = 0.21) or to the subgroup of individuals with diabetes (P = 0.28). Among other baseline and demographic characteristics, only the presence of diabetes (β = 0.47, P = 0.04) was significantly associated with circulating endoglin concentration. Neither total cholesterol nor baseline hemoglobin concentration was associated with circulating endoglin concentration. Although endoglin concentrations were lower in individuals with serum albumin concentrations less than the median value of ≤4.3 gm/dL compared with individuals with albumin > 4.3 gm/dL (4.4±1.5 ng/mL vs. 4.9±2.0 ng/mL), the difference was not significant, P = 0.07.

To understand whether the apparent lack of an association between renal function and endoglin concentration was confounded by other characteristics, we constructed a series of multivariable regression models as shown in **Tables 5** and **6**. Adjusting for age, sex, race, diabetes, hypertension, smoking, cholesterol, congestive heart failure, peripheral vascular disease, obstructive lung disease, and recruitment site attenuated the association between baseline renal function and circulating

Table 2. Baseline Laboratory Characteristics of the Study Population.

Characteristic	Preserved Function-Stage 1 CKD	Stage 2 CKD	Stage 3 CKD	Stage 4-5 CKD	Dialysis	P Value*
(Mean±S.D.)	(N = 30)	(N = 5)	(N = 92)	(N = 27)	(N = 9)	
Labs						
Total cholesterol, mg/dL	160.6 ±32.9	160.4±42.9	166.6±41.6	147.2±40.6	147.4±42.9	0.42
Hemoglobin, g/dL	13.9±1.4	13.2±2.0	12.9±1.8	12.0±1.5	11.8±1.8	<0.001
Creatinine, mg/dL	0.8±0.1	1.0±0.2	1.6±0.4	3.3±2.0	7.1±3.4	<0.001
Blood urea nitrogen, mg/dL	14.5±3.8	20.2±5.8	30.3±10.7	55.6±28.5	42.1±12.9	<0.001
Estimated GFR, mL/min/1.73 m^2	105.9±12.0	73.8±8.5	44.8±8.5	22.2±6.5	8.9±2.9	<0.001
Albumin, gm/dL	4.1±0.4	4.2±0.3	4.3±0.4	4.1±0.4	3.6±0.5	<0.001
Albumin:creatinine ratio, mg/G, median (IQR)[1]	0.0 (152.3)	20.7 (433.0)	53.8 (216)	90.4 (184.1)		0.37
Log albumin:creatinine, mg/G[1]	5.0	4.0±2.3	4.1±2.0	5.1±1.5		0.51

S.D. = Standard deviation., I.Q.R. = Interquartile Range,
*ANOVA for normally distributed continuous variables, chi-square test for -parametric trend test for non-normally distributed continuous variables, and chi-squared tests for count variables. [1]N = 66: Preserved renal function n = 1, Stage 2 CKD n = 10, Stage 3 CKD n = 44, Stage 4/5 CKD n = 11.

endoglin concentration. No significant associations between renal function and endoglin concentration were observed regardless of whether renal function was analyzed as a continuous (eGFR) or categorical (CKD class) predictor. Results were qualitatively similar after additional adjustment for Hispanic ethnicity and serum albumin concentration, and the association between renal function and endoglin concentration remained non-significant ($P \geq 0.42$) regardless of whether endoglin concentration was analyzed as a continuous or categorical outcome variable. There was no evidence for a significant interaction between renal function and diabetes or renal function and recruitment site in any of the models (Linear Model $P_{interaction} = 0.53$ and 0.17 for interactions between eGFR and diabetes and GFR and recruitment site, respectively).

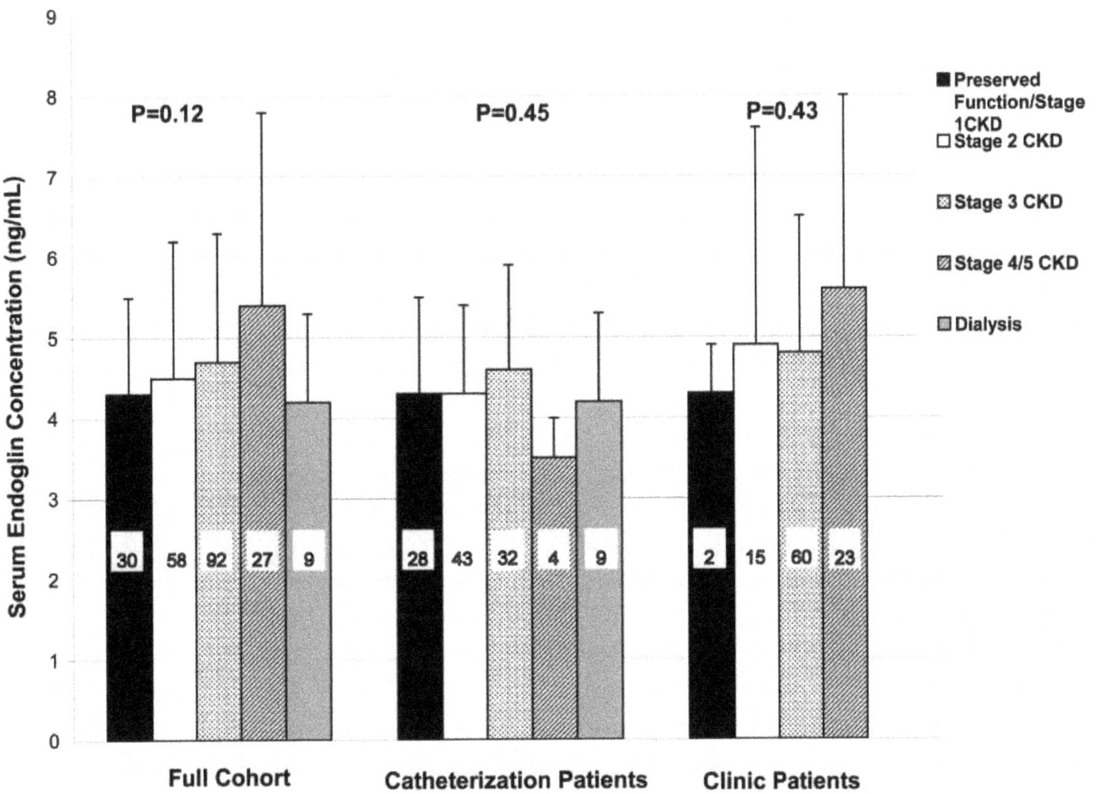

Figure 1. Endoglin concentration according to CKD class. Number of patients for each category is listed within the corresponding bar.

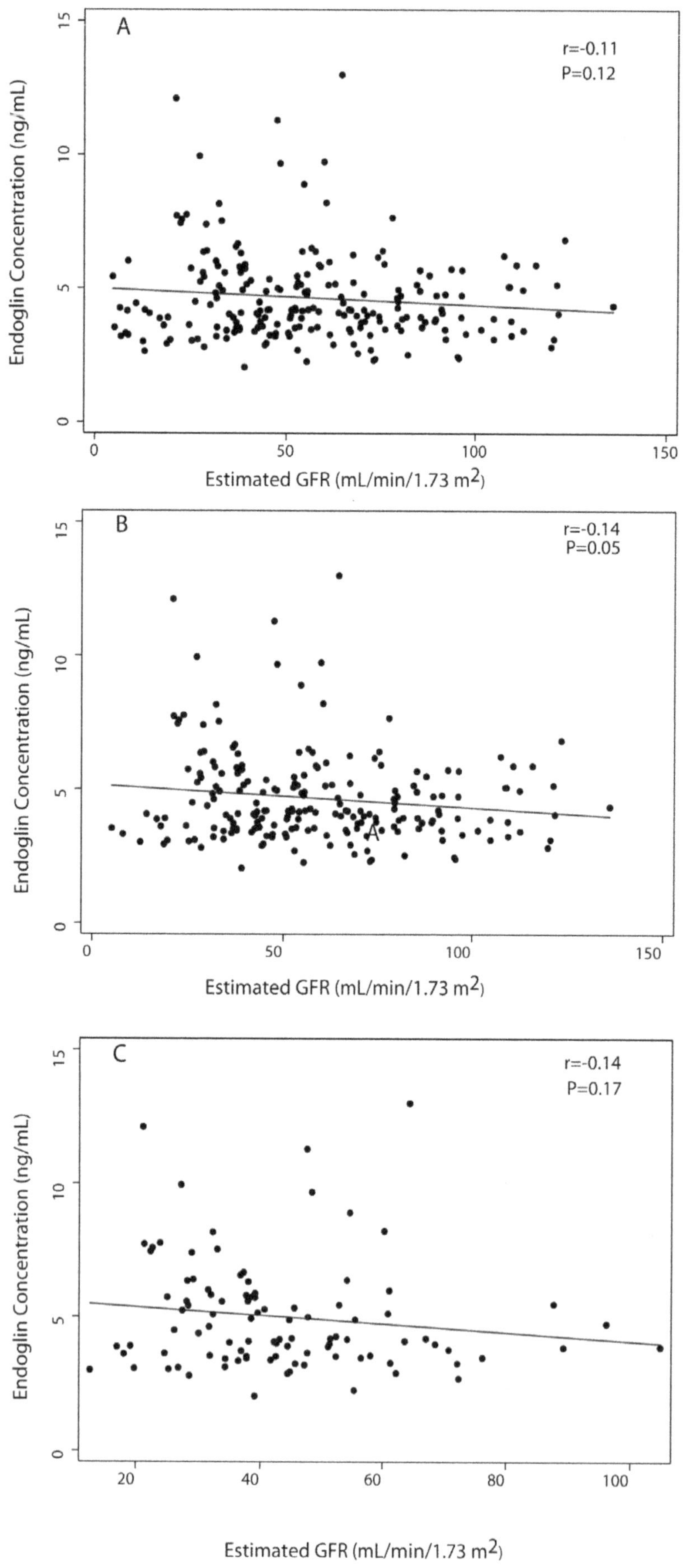
A
r=-0.11
P=0.12
Endoglin Concentration (ng/mL)
0
5
10
15
0
50
100
150
Estimated GFR (mL/min/1.73 m2)
B
r=-0.14
P=0.05
Endoglin Concentration (ng/mL)
0
5
10
15
0
50
100
150
Estimated GFR (mL/min/1.73 m2)
C
r=-0.14
P=0.17
Endoglin Concentration (ng/mL)
0
5
10
15
20
40
60
80
100
Estimated GFR (mL/min/1.73 m2)

Figure 2. Scatter plots of endoglin concentration vs. estimated glomerular filtration rate. a) All comers b) Dialysis patients excluded c) Patients recruited in clinic.

Results were qualitatively similar when eGFR was analyzed as a restricted cubic spline, and were not suggestive of an association between renal function and endoglin concentration (**Figure S1**).

Endoglin Concentration and Albuminuria

Urinary albumin concentrations were higher among individuals with higher circulating endoglin concentrations (**Figure 3**). However, this correlation was weak and did not achieve statistical significance ($r = 0.13$, $P = 0.30$).

Table 3. Univariate Associations of Clinical Characteristics with Endoglin Concentration.

Characteristic	Unadjusted *B* (95% CI)	P Value
Demographics		
Age		
≤40 years	Reference	Reference
40-60 years	-0.15	0.76
>60 years	-0.47	0.32
Male, n (%)	0.27	0.25
Black Race (vs. other race)	0.48	0.15
Hispanic	-0.41	0.21
Recruitment site, (clinic vs. cardiac catheterization lab)	0.67	0.003
Physical Exam		
Weight, kilogram, >88.6 vs. ≤88.6 Kg	0.31	0.31
Systolic blood pressure, per 10 mm Hg	0.01	0.37
Diastolic blood pressure, per quintile	0.12	0.15
Past Medical History		
Coronary disease	-0.11	0.71
Hypertension	0.13	0.64
Diabetes	0.47	0.04
Congestive heart failure	0.16	0.58
Obstructive lung disease	-0.15	0.78
Peripheral vascular disease	0.25	0.50
Hyperlipidemia	-0.12	0.64
Smoking	0.10	0.80
Cause of CKD		
Diabetes	1.35	0.001
Hypertension	1.27	0.002
Other/Unknown	Reference	Reference
Labs		
Total cholesterol, > 158 vs. ≤158 mg/dL	-0.27	0.37
Hemoglobin, >13 vs. ≤13 g/dL	0.29	0.23
Albumin, >4.3 vs. ≤4.3 g/dL	0.50	0.07

mg = milligram. G = gram. dL = deciliter. Kg = kilogram. CKD = Chronic Kidney Disease.

Discussion

Changes in the regulation of angiogenesis appears to be a key factor in the pathogenesis of CKD and cardiovascular disease [1,2,3,4,5,6,7,27,28]. This suggests that increased concentrations of angiogenesis inhibitors may partly explain the markedly increased risk of developing and dying from cardiovascular disease in individuals with CKD. Endoglin, an ancillary TGF-β receptor, is a key player in angiogenesis, nitric oxide coupling and heart development that plays an important regulatory role in both renal and cardiovascular disease [20,29,30,31]. We therefore hypothesized that an increase in soluble endoglin concentration as GFR declines might contribute to the progression of CKD or play a mechanistic role in the association of CKD with increased risks of developing and dying from cardiovascular disease.

In this study, we analyzed 216 individuals with various degrees of renal dysfunction and were unable to confirm an association between CKD and increases in the concentration of soluble endoglin. We found, in fact, that patients with ESRD, the most severe form of renal dysfunction, had on average the lowest circulating concentration of soluble of endoglin. Renal protein excretion, another indicator of renal disease, was also not associated with circulating endoglin concentration in the subset of patients in whom albuminuria was measured. Our data thus suggest that an elevation in the baseline concentration of soluble endoglin with progressive CKD is unlikely to play a causative role in the progression of CKD or the association of CKD with cardiovascular disease. They further suggest that, despite its well described role in the pathogenesis of preeclampsia [20], elevation in the baseline concentration of soluble endoglin is unlikely to underlie the increased risk of preeclampsia associated with CKD.

Experimental studies have consistently demonstrated that both glomerular and renal interstitial endoglin expression increase dramatically following induction of either acute or chronic renal dysfunction, regardless of the mechanism of renal injury [32,33,34,35]. Similarly, a single human study demonstrated

Table 4. Univariate Associations of Renal Function with Endoglin Concentration.

Characteristic	Unadjusted *B* (95% CI)	P Value
Renal Function		
Estimated GFR (per 10/mL/min/1.73m^2)	-0.06	0.12
CKD Class (per 1 category change)*	0.16	0.09
CKD Category	--	--
Preserved Renal function/Stage 1 CKD	Reference	Reference
Stage 2 CKD	0.18 (-0.56, 0.92)	0.63
Stage 3 CKD	0.46 (-0.23, 1.15)	0.19
Stage 4-5 CKD	1.03 (0.15, 1.90)	0.02
Dialysis	-0.10	0.89

GFR = glomerular filtration rate CKD Classes include normal/stage 1 CKD, stage 2 CKD, stage 3 CKD, stage 4/5 CKD, and dialysis.

Table 5. Adjusted Association of Glomerular Filtration Rate with Endoglin Concentration.

Model	Measure of Association (95% CI) per 10 mL/min/1.73 m²	Significance
Linear Regression	**β**	**P Value**
Model 1	0.01 (-0.09, 0.11)	0.81
Model 2	-0.01 (-0.10, 0.09)	.91
Categorical Regressions	**Odds Ratio**	**P Value**
Ordered logistic regression	1.01 (0.91, .13)	0.85
Logistic regression	0.99 (0.87, 1.13)	0.90

Categorical models and linear Model 1 adjusted for age, sex, race, diabetes, hypertension, smoking, cholesterol, congestive heart failure, peripheral vascular disease, obstructive lung disease and recruitment site. Model 2 additionally adjusted for Hispanic ethnicity and serum albumin. CI = confidence intervals. CKD = chronic kidney disease.

increased tissue expression of endoglin in the renal interstitium of diseased compared with healthy human kidneys [36]. The absence of an increase in soluble endoglin in our study suggests that the increases in tissue concentrations of endoglin following renal injury are not accompanied by concomitant release of cellular endoglin into the circulation.

To the best of our knowledge, ours is the first study to analyze the association of circulating endoglin concentration with renal function. The apparent lack of an association between either GFR or proteinuria and circulating endoglin concentration is surprising. Although our study was not designed to explore the mechanisms controlling the synthesis of endoglin, a low rate of release of membrane bound endoglin into the circulation as well as a differential regulation of the production of the soluble and membrane forms of endoglin may explain these contrasting findings.

Our findings are also notable in light of recent studies demonstrating an inverse correlation between eGFR and sFLT-1 and a direct correlation between sFLT-1 and proteinuria [18,37]. These findings suggested the possibility that a universal,

Table 6. Adjusted Association of CKD Stage with Endoglin Concentration.

Model	Measure of Association (95% CI) per 10 mL/min/1.73 m²	Significance
Linear Regression	**β**	**P Value**
Model 1		
Preserved Renal function/Stage 1 CKD	Reference	Reference
Stage 2 CKD	-0.04 (-0.82, 0.74)	0.93
Stage 3 CKD	-0.04 (-0.89, 0.81)	0.93
Stage 4-5 CKD	0.34 (-0.73, 1.40)	0.54
Dialysis	-0.08 (-1.48, 1.31)	0.91
Model 2		
Preserved Renal function/Stage 1 CKD	Reference	Reference
Stage 2 CKD	-0.00 (-0.77, 0.76)	0.99
Stage 3 CKD	-0.07 (-0.91, 0.76)	0.86
Stage 4-5 CKD	0.43 (-0.63, 1.49)	0.42
Dialysis	0.39 (-0.98, 1.77)	0.57
Categorical Regressions	**Odds Ratio**	**P Value**
Ordered logistic regression		
Preserved Renal function/Stage 1 CKD	Reference	Reference
Stage 2 CKD	1.05 (0.45, 2.45)	0.91
Stage 3 CKD	1.20 (0.48, 3.00)	0.70
Stage 4–5 CKD	1.28 (0.39, 4.24)	0.68
Dialysis	1.09 (0.24, 4.99)	0.92
Logistic regression		
Preserved Renal function/Stage 1 CKD	Reference	Reference
Stage 2 CKD	0.74 (0.28, 2.00)	0.54
Stage 3 CKD	0.96 (0.33, 2.78)	0.93
Stage 4–5 CKD	0.91 (0.23, 3.55)	0.89
Dialysis	1.78 (0.30, 10.58)	0.53

Categorical models and linear Model 1 adjusted for age, sex, race, diabetes, hypertension, smoking, cholesterol, congestive heart failure, peripheral vascular disease, obstructive lung disease and recruitment site. Model 2 additionally adjusted for Hispanic ethnicity and serum albumin. CI = confidence intervals. CKD = chronic kidney disease.

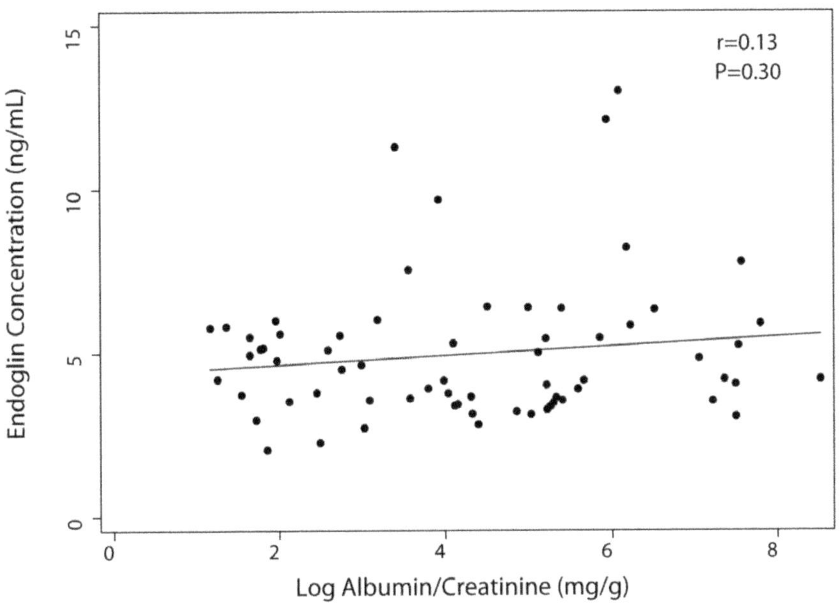

Figure 3. Association of endoglin concentration and urinary albumin excretion. Scatter plot of endoglin concentration vs. microalbumin to creatinine ratio.

synchronous increase in the concentration of angiogenesis inhibitors might occur in CKD and predispose individuals with CKD to cardiovascular disease and preeclampsia. The present study, however, suggests a more complex biology with disparate associations between renal function and the various pro and anti-angiogenic factors.

Endoglin plays an important role in embryonic heart development [31,38] and is also involved in post-embryonic maintenance of normal cardiovascular function. Endoglin expression on coronary artery endothelial cells appears to modulate the effects of angiotensin 2 on vascular remodeling [39], and it helps regulate vascular reactivity via improved coupling of eNOS activity [30,40]. The expression of the soluble form is negatively regulated by heme-oxygenase-1 [41], which itself plays a key role in cellular responses to oxidative stress and ischemia-reperfusion injury [42]. Finally, in more general terms, studies of both plaque angiogenesis [14] and myocardial angiogenesis [12,13] have strongly implicated angiogenesis-related factors (such as endoglin) as important players in cardiovascular pathophysiology.

On the basis of this evidence, important effects on cardiovascular homeostasis would be expected if renal injury induced changes in circulating endoglin concentrations comparable to the changes observed in intra-renal tissue levels. To our knowledge, however, the hypothesis that changes in soluble endoglin concentration partly underlie the high incidence of cardiovascular morbidity and mortality in individuals with CKD has not been previously investigated. The absence of significant increases in soluble endoglin levels in the setting of CKD in the current study, suggests that (despite the theoretical attractiveness of our initial hypothesis) that soluble endoglin is not an important factor in the etiology in the enhanced atherosclerosis and cardiovascular disease that accompanies CKD.

It should be noted, that when individuals with the most severe forms of CKD—those with ESRD—were excluded, our data was more suggestive of a trend towards increasing endoglin concentration with declining GFR. However, even within this subgroup, the differences across categories of CKD were small and did not achieve statistical significance. Nevertheless, additional studies including larger numbers of individuals with both ESRD and pre-dialysis CKD are needed to clarify the behavior of endoglin in the most advanced stages of CKD.

Other limitations of our study should be recognized. We were unable to measure GFR directly and thus estimated GFR on the basis of serum creatinine level at the time of recruitment. GFR estimating equations are susceptible to inaccuracy, and we cannot rule out the possibility that CKD status was misclassified in some cases. Such misclassification is unlikely to explain our findings since we excluded patients with overt acute kidney injury, recruited many patients from a renal clinic (in which individuals generally have overt/well-established CKD), and because endoglin concentrations were lowest in the group with ESRD in whom estimation of GFR was not needed to classify the CKD status. Another issue is that the numbers of individuals with ESRD and severely reduced GFR was small. Additional studies including larger number of patients with advanced renal disease are warranted to confirm our findings.

It should also be noted that our patients were recruited from 2 different settings within a single hospital. The single-center nature of our study may limit the generalizability of our findings to other populations with CKD, and our findings merit confirmation in populations from other centers. Soluble endoglin levels collected within a single, uniform setting within our center would likely have been more homogenous. However, our approach has the advantage of being generalizable to a fuller spectrum of CKD patients and presentations than would have been possible had we recruited patients at only a single site within the institution. Additionally, although absolute levels were somewhat different between the two subgroups, the relative change across categories of CKD was similar regardless of subgroup, and our findings were unchanged when recruitment site was included as a co-factor in multivariable analyses.

In conclusion, soluble endoglin has been implicated in the pathogenesis of renal and cardiovascular disease. To understand whether increases in the concentration of soluble endoglin underlie the strong associations of CKD with increased risks of developing cardiovascular death, we analyzed soluble endoglin concentrations in a large cohort of individuals with and without CKD and found no association between eGFR or urinary albumin excretion and soluble endoglin levels. Our findings suggest that increases in the baseline levels of soluble endoglin in individuals with CKD are unlikely to contribute to the progression of CKD or to explain CKD-associated cardiovascular disease.

Acknowledgments

We would like to acknowledge the patients who contributed their time and samples to this project.

Author Contributions

Conceived and designed the experiments: DMC BAM RK EMZ. Performed the experiments: DMC BAM AMH AC EMZ. Analyzed the data: DMC BAM AMH AC BAC RK EMZ. Contributed reagents/materials/analysis tools: RK EMZ DMC. Wrote the paper: DMC AMH BAM AC RK EMZ.

References

1. Eremina V, Sood M, Haigh J, Nagy A, Lajoie G, et al. (2003) Glomerular-specific alterations of VEGF-A expression lead to distinct congenital and acquired renal diseases. J Clin Invest 111: 707–716.
2. Ly J, Alexander M, Quaggin SE (2004) A podocentric view of nephrology. Curr Opin Nephrol Hypertens 13: 299–305.
3. Cui S, Li C, Ema M, Weinstein J, Quaggin SE (2005) Rapid isolation of glomeruli coupled with gene expression profiling identifies downstream targets in Pod1 knockout mice. J Am Soc Nephrol 16: 3247–3255.
4. Eremina V, Cui S, Gerber H, Ferrara N, Haigh J, et al. (2006) Vascular endothelial growth factor a signaling in the podocyte-endothelial compartment is required for mesangial cell migration and survival. J Am Soc Nephrol 17: 724–735.
5. Eremina V, Baelde HJ, Quaggin SE (2007) Role of the VEGF--a signaling pathway in the glomerulus: evidence for crosstalk between components of the glomerular filtration barrier. Nephron Physiol 106: 32–37.
6. Eremina V, Jefferson JA, Kowalewska J, Hochster H, Haas M, et al. (2008) VEGF inhibition and renal thrombotic microangiopathy. N Engl J Med 358: 1129–1136.
7. Sison K, Eremina V, Baelde H, Min W, Hirashima M, et al. (2010) Glomerular structure and function require paracrine, not autocrine, VEGF-VEGFR-2 signaling. J Am Soc Nephrol 21: 1691–1701.
8. Matsumoto Y, Ueda S, Yamagishi S, Matsuguma K, Shibata R, et al. (2007) Dimethylarginine dimethylaminohydrolase prevents progression of renal dysfunction by inhibiting loss of peritubular capillaries and tubulointerstitial fibrosis in a rat model of chronic kidney disease. J Am Soc Nephrol 18: 1525–1533.
9. Amann K, Tyralla K, Gross ML, Schwarz U, Tornig J, et al. (2003) Cardiomyocyte loss in experimental renal failure: prevention by ramipril. Kidney Int 63: 1708–1713.
10. Maynard SE, Min JY, Merchan J, Lim KH, Li J, et al. (2003) Excess placental soluble fms-like tyrosine kinase 1 (sFlt1) may contribute to endothelial dysfunction, hypertension, and proteinuria in preeclampsia. J Clin Invest 111: 649–658.
11. Sugimoto H, Hamano Y, Charytan D, Cosgrove D, Kieran M, et al. (2003) Neutralization of circulating vascular endothelial growth factor (VEGF) by anti-VEGF antibodies and soluble VEGF receptor 1 (sFlt-1) induces proteinuria. J Biol Chem 278: 12605–12608.
12. Amann K, Wiest G, Zimmer G, Gretz N, Ritz E, et al. (1992) Reduced capillary density in the myocardium of uremic rats--a stereological study. Kidney Int 42: 1079–1085.
13. Amann K, Kronenberg G, Gehlen F, Wessels S, Orth S, et al. (1998) Cardiac remodelling in experimental renal failure--an immunohistochemical study. Nephrol Dial Transplant 13: 1958–1966.
14. Finn AV, Jain RK (2010) Coronary plaque neovascularization and hemorrhage: a potential target for plaque stabilization? JACC Cardiovasc Imaging 3: 41–44.
15. Tang J, Wang J, Kong X, Yang J, Guo L, et al. (2009) Vascular endothelial growth factor promotes cardiac stem cell migration via the PI3K/Akt pathway. Exp Cell Res 315: 3521–3531.
16. Park CW, Kim HW, Lim JH, Yoo KD, Chung S, et al. (2009) Vascular endothelial growth factor inhibition by dRK6 causes endothelial apoptosis, fibrosis, and inflammation in the heart via the Akt/eNOS axis in db/db mice. Diabetes 58: 2666–2676.
17. Amann K, Breitbach M, Ritz E, Mall G (1998) Myocyte/capillary mismatch in the heart of uremic patients. J Am Soc Nephrol 9: 1018–1022.
18. Di Marco GS, Reuter S, Hillebrand U, Amler S, Konig M, et al. (2009) The soluble VEGF receptor sFlt1 contributes to endothelial dysfunction in CKD. J Am Soc Nephrol 20: 2235–2245.
19. Onoue K, Uemura S, Takeda Y, Somekawa S, Iwama H, et al. (2009) Reduction of circulating soluble fms-like tyrosine kinase-1 plays a significant role in renal dysfunction-associated aggravation of atherosclerosis. Circulation 120: 2470–2477.
20. Venkatesha S, Toporsian M, Lam C, Hanai J, Mammoto T, et al. (2006) Soluble endoglin contributes to the pathogenesis of preeclampsia. Nat Med 12: 642–649.
21. Blazquez-Medela AM, Garcia-Ortiz L, Gomez-Marcos MA, Recio-Rodriguez JI, Sanchez-Rodriguez A, et al. (2010) Increased plasma soluble endoglin levels as an indicator of cardiovascular alterations in hypertensive and diabetic patients. BMC Med 8: 86.
22. Ikemoto T, Hojo Y, Kondo H, Takahashi N, Hirose M, et al. (2011) Plasma endoglin as a marker to predict cardiovascular events in patients with chronic coronary artery diseases. Heart Vessels.
23. Mohsenin V, Urbano F (2011) Circulating antiangiogenic proteins in obstructive sleep apnea and hypertension. Respir Med 105: 801–807.
24. Levey AS, Coresh J, Greene T, Stevens LA, Zhang YL, et al. (2006) Using standardized serum creatinine values in the modification of diet in renal disease study equation for estimating glomerular filtration rate. Ann Intern Med 145: 247–254.
25. Eknoyan G, Hostetter T, Bakris GL, Hebert L, Levey AS, et al. (2003) Proteinuria and other markers of chronic kidney disease: a position statement of the national kidney foundation (NKF) and the national institute of diabetes and digestive and kidney diseases (NIDDK). Am J Kidney Dis 42: 617–622.
26. Sun X, Chen Y, Chen X, Wang J, Xi C, et al. (2009) Change of glomerular filtration rate in healthy adults with aging. Nephrology (Carlton) 14: 506–513.
27. Jeansson M, Gawlik A, Anderson G, Li C, Kerjaschki D, et al. (2011) Angiopoietin-1 is essential in mouse vasculature during development and in response to injury. J Clin Invest 121: 2278–2289.
28. Kappers MH, van Esch JH, Sleijfer S, Danser AH, van den Meiracker AH (2009) Cardiovascular and renal toxicity during angiogenesis inhibition: clinical and mechanistic aspects. J Hypertens 27: 2297–2309.
29. Levine RJ, Lam C, Qian C, Yu KF, Maynard SE, et al. (2006) Soluble endoglin and other circulating antiangiogenic factors in preeclampsia. N Engl J Med 355: 992–1005.
30. Toporsian M, Gros R, Kabir MG, Vera S, Govindaraju K, et al. (2005) A role for endoglin in coupling eNOS activity and regulating vascular tone revealed in hereditary hemorrhagic telangiectasia. Circ Res 96: 684–692.
31. Arthur HM, Ure J, Smith AJ, Renforth G, Wilson DI, et al. (2000) Endoglin, an ancillary TGFbeta receptor, is required for extraembryonic angiogenesis and plays a key role in heart development. Dev Biol 217: 42–53.
32. Rodriguez-Pena A, Prieto M, Duwel A, Rivas JV, Eleno N, et al. (2001) Up-regulation of endoglin, a TGF-beta-binding protein, in rats with experimental renal fibrosis induced by renal mass reduction. Nephrol Dial Transplant 16 Suppl 1: 34–39.
33. Rodriguez-Pena A, Eleno N, Duwell A, Arevalo M, Perez-Barriocanal F, et al. (2002) Endoglin upregulation during experimental renal interstitial fibrosis in mice. Hypertension 40: 713–720.
34. Prieto M, Rodriguez-Pena AB, Duwel A, Rivas JV, Docherty N, et al. (2005) Temporal changes in renal endoglin and TGF-beta1 expression following ureteral obstruction in rats. J Physiol Biochem 61: 457–467.
35. Prieto M, Rodriguez-Pena A, Arevalo M, Rivas JV, Duwel A, et al. (2005) Effect of the Long-Term Treatment with Trandolapril on Endoglin Expression in Rats with Experimental Renal Fibrosis Induced by Renal Mass Reduction. Kidney Blood Press Res 28: 32–40.
36. Roy-Chaudhury P, Simpson JG, Power DA (1997) Endoglin, a transforming growth factor-beta-binding protein, is upregulated in chronic progressive renal disease. Exp Nephrol 5: 55–60.
37. Kim NH, Oh JH, Seo JA, Lee KW, Kim SG, et al. (2005) Vascular endothelial growth factor (VEGF) and soluble VEGF receptor FLT-1 in diabetic nephropathy. Kidney Int 67: 167–177.
38. Vincent EB, Runyan RB, Weeks DL (1998) Production of the transforming growth factor-beta binding protein endoglin is regulated during chick heart development. Dev Dyn 213: 237–247.
39. Li D, Chen H, Mehta JL (2001) Angiotensin II via activation of type 1 receptor upregulates expression of endoglin in human coronary artery endothelial cells. Hypertension 38: 1062–1067.
40. Jerkic M, Rivas-Elena JV, Prieto M, Carron R, Sanz-Rodriguez F, et al. (2004) Endoglin regulates nitric oxide-dependent vasodilatation. Faseb J 18: 609–611.
41. Cudmore M, Ahmad S, Al-Ani B, Fujisawa T, Coxall H, et al. (2007) Negative regulation of soluble Flt-1 and soluble endoglin release by heme oxygenase-1. Circulation 115: 1789–1797.
42. Kim YM, Pae HO, Park JE, Lee YC, Woo JM, et al. (2011) Heme oxygenase in the regulation of vascular biology: from molecular mechanisms to therapeutic opportunities. Antioxid Redox Signal 14: 137–167.

Beneficial Effects on Arterial Stiffness and Pulse-Wave Reflection of Combined Enalapril and Candesartan in Chronic Kidney Disease

Marie Frimodt-Møller[1]*, Anne-Lise Kamper[1], Svend Strandgaard[2], Svend Kreiner[3], Arne Høj Nielsen[2]

1 Departments of Nephrology, Rigshospitalet, University of Copenhagen, Copenhagen, Denmark, **2** Herlev Hospital, Copenhagen, Denmark, **3** Department of Biostatistics, University of Copenhagen, Copenhagen, Denmark

Abstract

Background: Cardiovascular disease (CVD) is highly prevalent in patients with chronic kidney disease (CKD). Inhibition of the renin-angiotensinsystem (RAS) in hypertension causes differential effects on central and brachial blood pressure (BP), which has been translated into improved outcome. The objective was to examine if a more complete inhibition of RAS by combining an angiotensin converting enzyme inhibitor (ACEI) and an angiotensin receptor antagonist (ARB) compared to monotherapy has an additive effect on central BP and pulse-wave velocity (PWV), which are known markers of CVD.

Methods: Sixty-seven CKD patients (mean GFR 30, range 13–59 ml/min/1.73 m^2) participated in an open randomized study of 16 weeks of monotherapy with either enalapril or candesartan followed by 8 weeks of dual blockade aiming at a total dose of 16 mg candesartan and 20 mg enalapril o.d. Pulse-wave measurements were performed at week 0, 8, 16 and 24 by the SphygmoCor device.

Results: Significant additive BP independent reductions were found after dual blockade in aortic PWV (−0.3 m/s, $P<0.05$) and in augmentation index (−2%, $P<0.01$) compared to monotherapy. Furthermore pulse pressure amplification was improved ($P<0.05$) and central systolic BP reduced (−6 mmHg, $P<0.01$).

Conclusions: Dual blockade of the RAS resulted in an additive BP independent reduction in pulse-wave reflection and arterial stiffness compared to monotherapy in CKD patients.

Trial Registration: Clinical trial.gov NCT00235287

Editor: Robert Clarke, University of Oxford, United Kingdom

Funding: This work is funded by the Danish Kidney Association (Nyreforeningen), the Danish Society of Nephrology, The Danish Heart Association, the Research Council of Herlev Hospital, the Foundations of Augustinus, Hørslev, Aase and Ejnar Danielsen and Aase Bay, Denmark. The funders had no role in study design, data collection and analysis, decision to publish, or preparation of the manuscript.

Competing Interests: The authors have declared that no competing interests exist.

* E-mail: mariefm@dadlnet.dk.

Introduction

Markers of arterial stiffness such as aortic pulse-wave velocity (PWV) and central blood pressure (BP) are known independent predictors of cardiovascular morbidity and mortality in chronic kidney disease (CKD) [1–3]. Inhibition of the renin-angiotensinsystem (RAS) with an angiotensin converting enzyme inhibitor (ACEI) or an angiotensin receptor blocker (ARB) has been shown to afford cardio-renal protection beyond the BP lowering effects [4–8]. This may be due to preferential lowering of the central BP by the RAS blockers compared to other antihypertensives [9,10]. Central BP, which is markedly influenced by vascular stiffness, has been found to be a better predictor of cardiovascular outcome than the conventional brachial BP [11–13]. Treatment with combinations of ACEI and ARB in full doses would expectedly lead to a more complete blockade of the RAS than can be obtained with either drug group. Such dual blockade has been demonstrated to have beneficial effects on arterial wave reflection and PWV in resistant hypertension [14,15]. Surprisingly, in the recent ONTARGET study no beneficial effect of dual blockade on cardio-renal outcome was found in high risk cardiovascular patients [16]. Furthermore, in another recent observational study dual blockade did not reduce cardiovascular death in chronic hemodialysis patients [17].

In the present study it was investigated for the first time whether in CKD patients dual RAS blockade has an additive effect on central pressure waves and arterial stiffness evaluated by pulse-wave analysis (PWA) and PWV respectively, compared to mono RAS blockade, and whether these effects if present are BP independent.

Methods

The protocol for this trial and supporting CONSORT checklist are available as supporting information; see Checklist S1 and Protocol S1.

Study Population

Sixty-seven patients, all Caucasians, from the outpatient nephrology clinic, Herlev University Hospital, 52 men and 15 women, mean age 60 (range 31–75) were enrolled in this open randomised cross-over trial from September 2005 to September 2009. All patients gave informed consent and the study was approved by the Ethical Committee of Copenhagen County. The authors adhered to the Declaration of Helsinki and the study was monitored by the Good Clinical Practice (GCP) unit at Copenhagen University Hospitals, and was registered by EudraCT number 2005-001568-29 and in the public trial registry: www.clinicaltrials.gov, registration number NCT00235287.

The eligibility criteria for patients entering the study were predialysis CKD with plasma creatinine between 150 and 350 μmol/l, plasma potassium below 5.6 mmol/l, systolic BP above 109 mmHg and age between 18 and 75 years. Patients with congestive heart failure (NYHA III-IV), chronic liver insufficiency, amputation of a limb or the presence of cardiac arrhythmia or a pacemaker were not included. None of the patients were to be treated with immunosuppressives, non-steroidal anti-inflammatory drugs, aldosterone antagonists or dual RAS blockade at the entry of the study.

Seventy-two per cent of the patients were treated with ACEI or ARB before enrolment and thus were known RAS blockade tolerant. Additionally, most were treated with furosemide and non ACEI/ARB antihypertensive therapy, which were continued during the trial. Demographic data and renal diagnoses are shown in table 1.

Study Protocol

In order to ensure close balance of the numbers in each group at any time during the trial, block randomization was used [18]. In every block of 10 participants five would be allocated to each arm of the trial.

Table 1. Demographic data of the studied patients.

	total N = 67 (%)
Gender (f/m)	15/52 (22/78)
Age (years)	60±6
Previous cardiovascular events	16 (24)
Smoking	9 (13)
Diabetes mellitus	14 (21)
Kidney disease	
Nephrosclerosis	6 (9)
Polycystic kidney disease	11 (16)
Diabetic nephropathy	2 (3)
Chronic glomerulonephritis	6 (9)
Unknown	37 (55)
Other	5 (7)
Pre-trial antihypertensive treatment	
ACE-inhibitior	22 (33)
Angiotensin receptor blocker	26 (39)
No RAS-blocking agents	19 (28)
Beta-blocker	26 (39)
Diuretics	43 (64)
Calcium-channel-blocker	39 (58)

Mono therapy period. *Randomization of patients treated with either an ACEI or an ARB prior to the study* was carried out by drawing a closed envelope; to ensure that half of the patients had enalapril for the first 16 weeks and the other half had candesartan the first 16 weeks.

Randomization of patients not treated with an ACEI or ARB prior to the study was likewise carried out by drawing an envelope from a bag to ensure that half of the patients had enalapril in the first 8 weeks and candesartan in the following 8 weeks and the other half of the patients had candesartan in the first 8 weeks and enalapril in the following 8 weeks. By this means, tolerance to either drug was demonstrated in the patients not previously treated with RAS blockers before dual blockade.

In either of the four randomized patient groups, doses were increased gradually over a period of 8 weeks from enalapril 5 mg to 20 mg, and from candesartan 4 mg to 16 mg, given once daily. All randomisations were carried out by the GCP-trained nurse staff members of the outpatient clinic without any conflict of interest in the trial. A flowchart of the randomized patients in the study is found in figure 1.

Dual blockade period. *All patients:* After 16 weeks of monotherapy with either enalapril or candesartan, the complementary drug was added in incremental doses over a period of 5 weeks, aiming at reaching a combination of enalapril 20 mg and candesartan 16 mg and maintaining this full dose dual blockade for an additionally 3 weeks. The therapeutic goal was a systolic/diastolic BP of 130/80 mmHg or below according to the K/DOQI-guidelines [19]. Additional antihypertensive treatment was simultaneously reduced, discontinued or added as needed.

During the 24 weeks study period, 10 control visits were planned: 4 visits in the laboratory, at which pulse-wave measurements were done and blood samples drawn, at the beginning of the trial and after 8, 16 and 24 weeks; 6 'clinical control'-visits in the outpatient clinic, at which BP was measured and blood samples drawn. All the visits were planned with an interval of 2–3 weeks throughout the study, so that 2 'clinical control'-visits were placed between two pulse-wave measurements. Glomerular filtration rate (GFR) was estimated at the first and last visit in the trial by the plasma clearance of ^{51}Cr-EDTA as described below. Urinary albumin excretion/24 h was measured at each of the four visits of pulse-wave measurements.

Measurements of pulse-wave analysis and pulse-wave velocity. Measurements of PWA and PWV were performed using the SphygmoCor© device [20] (version 7.0, Atcor Medical, Sydney, Australia). All measurements were performed in the morning in the supine position after a minimum of 10 min rest in a quiet, temperature-controlled room. Patients were requested to be fasting and abstain from tea, coffee and smoking for 8 h and from alcohol for 24 h. Diabetic patients were allowed a light meal before examination. Study and other morning medication were to be taken 2 hours before measurements. The method of PWA and PWV measurement has been described in detail elsewhere [21]. Briefly, PWA was done with the use of a validated general transfer function [22]. The central pressure waveform was estimated based on radial pressure waveform recordings, calibrated to a brachial BP on the same arm. PWV was calculated based on the pulse transit time divided by the travel distance. The PWV of the 'aortic' segment (aortic PWV) was recorded between the femoral and carotid artery and the PWV of the 'brachial' segment (brachial PWV) was recorded between the radial and carotid artery. When determining the aortic PWV, the distance from the carotid recording site to the suprasternal notch was subtracted from the distance between the femoral recording site to the suprasternal notch [23]. When determining the brachial PWV, the distance

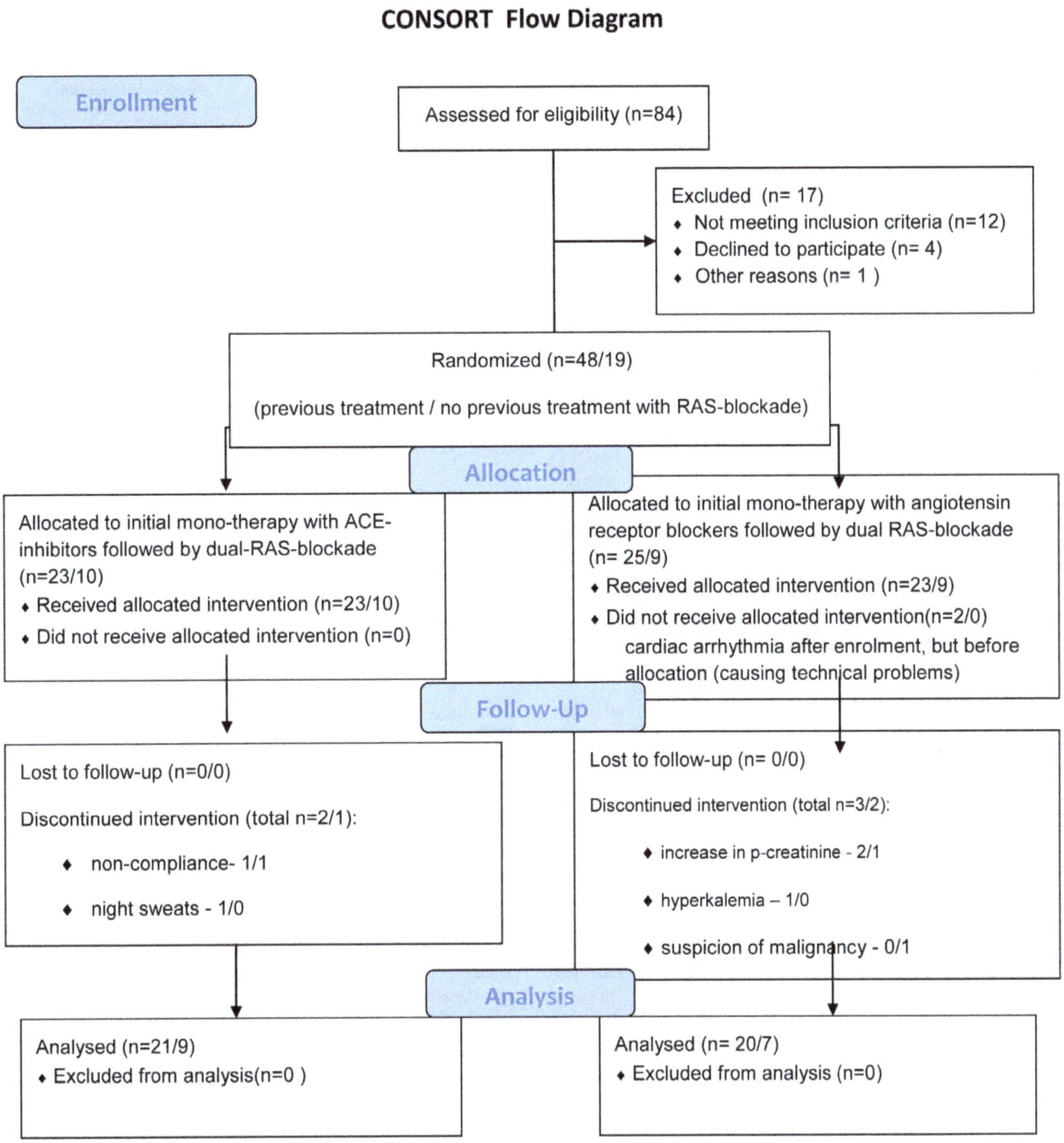

Figure 1. CONSORT Flowchart of the randomization in the study.

from the carotid-suprasternal notch was subtracted from the distance between the radial-suprasternal notch.

The quality demands of PWA and PWV were followed as suggested by the manufacturer. This included visually acceptable pulse-wave recordings with variations in pulse height, diastole and pulse length ≤5% and the mean pulse height ≥80 mV as expressed by a quality index (%) provided by the software. A quality index ≥80% was accepted. In case of PWV, the time difference between the ECG-signal and the signal from the recording sites should have a SD ≤10% of the mean value. All measurements of PWA and PWV were made in duplicate.

Management of hyperkalemia, excess rise in plasma creatinine and hypotension have been described in details elsewhere [24].

BP Measurement and Clinical Chemistry

The brachial BP used for calibration of PWA and all other brachial BPs were measured by use of a mercury sphygmomanometer after at least 10 min of supine rest. The mean of the last two out of three BP measurements were averaged and used for analysis. Plasma creatinine was analyzed using reagents from Vitros Chemistry 5.1, which are compatible with the IDMS method (isotope dilution mass spectrometry). Plasma potassium

Table 2. Effects of dual RAS blockade on pulse-wave measurements and kidney function.

Intervention N = 57	start ACE-I/ARB	ACE-I/ARB	start dual blockade	end dual blockade
Brachial systolic BP (mmHg)	142±19	131±16	131±17	124±17***
Brachial diastolic BP (mmHg)	82±11	78±10	77±11	75±11 NS
Brachial PP(mmHg)	60±18	53±13	54±16	50±15 NS
Central systolic BP (mmHg)	133±20	122±17	121±17	115±19**
Central diastolic BP(mmHg)	82±12	79±10	77±10	75±11 NS
Central PP(mmHg)	49±17	42±14	42±15	38±14 NS
TR (msec)	146±14	145±15	147±14	146±16 NS
Aix@HR75 (%)	21±10	20±11	19±10	17±13**
Brachial PWV (m/s)	9.9±1.4	9.6±1.7	9.5±1.3	9.5±1.7 NS
Aortic PWV (m/s)	9.6±2.8	9.2±2.5	9.0±2.7	8.7±2.8*
Heart rate (bpm)	62±11	62±11	61±11	61±10 NS
ED (ms)	337±28	335±28	335±29	331±27 NS
P-creatinine (μmol/l)	216±57	228±70	232±67	239±78*
P-urea (mmol/l)	14±5	15±7	15±7	17±7***
P-potassium (mmol/l)	4.4±0.5	4.6±0.4	4.6±0.5	4.6±0.5 NS
GFR (Cr-EDTA, ml/min/1.73 m^2)	**29.8 (13–60.1)**			**23.9 (10–64)*** **
U-albumin excret. (μmol/24 h)	**2.4 (0.1–31.5)**	**2.3 (0.1–53.3)**	**1.5 (1.1–1.8)**	**0.9 (0.1–49.9)** NS

Blood pressure (BP), pulse pressure (PP), Time to Reflection (TR), heart rate adjusted Augmentation Index (AIx@HR75), Pulse-wave velocity (PWV), Ejection Duration (ED). P-value refers to statistical comparison between the end and start of dual blockade except for GFR which refers to comparison between start and end of study. *P<0.05, **P<0.01, ***P<0.001, NS = non-significant. Data in bold is geometric means with ranges in brackets.

and other clinical chemistry parameters were measured using standard methods.

^{51}Cr-EDTA Clearance

Plasma clearance was calculated on the basis of plasma activity in four blood samples drawn at 20-min intervals in the fourth hour after injection [25]. In case of an expected GFR <21 ml/min, blood samples were drawn at 5 and 24 h after injection of ^{51}Cr-EDTA [26].

Arterial Hemodynamics

The pulse-wave is composed of an initial pulse-wave generated by left ventricular ejection and its reflection from the periphery. AIx@HR75 defined as the difference between the first and second systolic peaks expressed as a percentage of the pulse pressure adjusted to a heart rate of 75 beats/min- was taken to represent measures of arterial wave reflection [21]. Time to reflection (TR) was defined as the total travel time of the pulse-wave to the periphery and its return. Aortic PWV and brachial PWV are measures of central and muscular arterial stiffness, respectively [21] and were the pre-specified primary outcome measures. Pulse pressure (PP) amplification was calculated as the ratio of brachial PP/central PP [27]. Furthermore the following parameters were registered: central and brachial systolic and diastolic BP, left ventricular ejection duration (ED) and heart rate, which were the secondary outcome measures in addition to AIx@HR75, TR and PP-amplification.

Statistics

The sample size was calculated using a two-sided paired sample t-test based on variations from previous data [28]. Twenty patients were needed without previous treatment with RAS-blockade, with previous treatment with ACE-I and with previous treatment with ARB, respectively. This sample size would give a 99% chance of detecting a difference of 1 m/s in aortic PWV and 80% in brachial PWV with an alpha-level of 5%.

The two groups with or without prior RAS-blockade were then randomized to four different treatment groups, which were compared for differences in demographic characteristics by analysis of variance. As no differences were found between groups demographic data are shown for all patients together. The effects of dual therapy and monotherapy on pulse-wave measurements were analyzed by general linear models for repeated measurements. As no differences were found between the four treatment arms data were pooled and further analyzed in total. We aimed to evaluate the effects of dual blockade on pulse-wave measurements and therefore based the statistical analysis on the 57 patients who completed dual blockade.

The effects of treatment on kidney function were evaluated by use of Student's t-test for dependent data. During the analyses of repeated measurements, AIx@HR75, aortic PWV and brachial PWV were adjusted for diastolic BP, gender and age. Furthermore AIx@HR75 was adjusted for body-height, aortic PWV, TR and ED in a similar way, like the PP-amplification ratio which was adjusted for heart rate and body-height. Data are presented as mean ± standard deviation (SD) unless otherwise stated. Due to skewed distribution urine albumin excretion and GFR were log-transformed before analysis and the geometrical mean presented with range in brackets. A P-value <0.05 was considered significant. Data were analyzed by use of a statistical computer program (SPSS, version 17).

Results

Of the 67 randomized patients, 57 completed the trial. All pulse-wave measurements were within our quality standard as described in the methods section. The mean quality index was 95±6%.

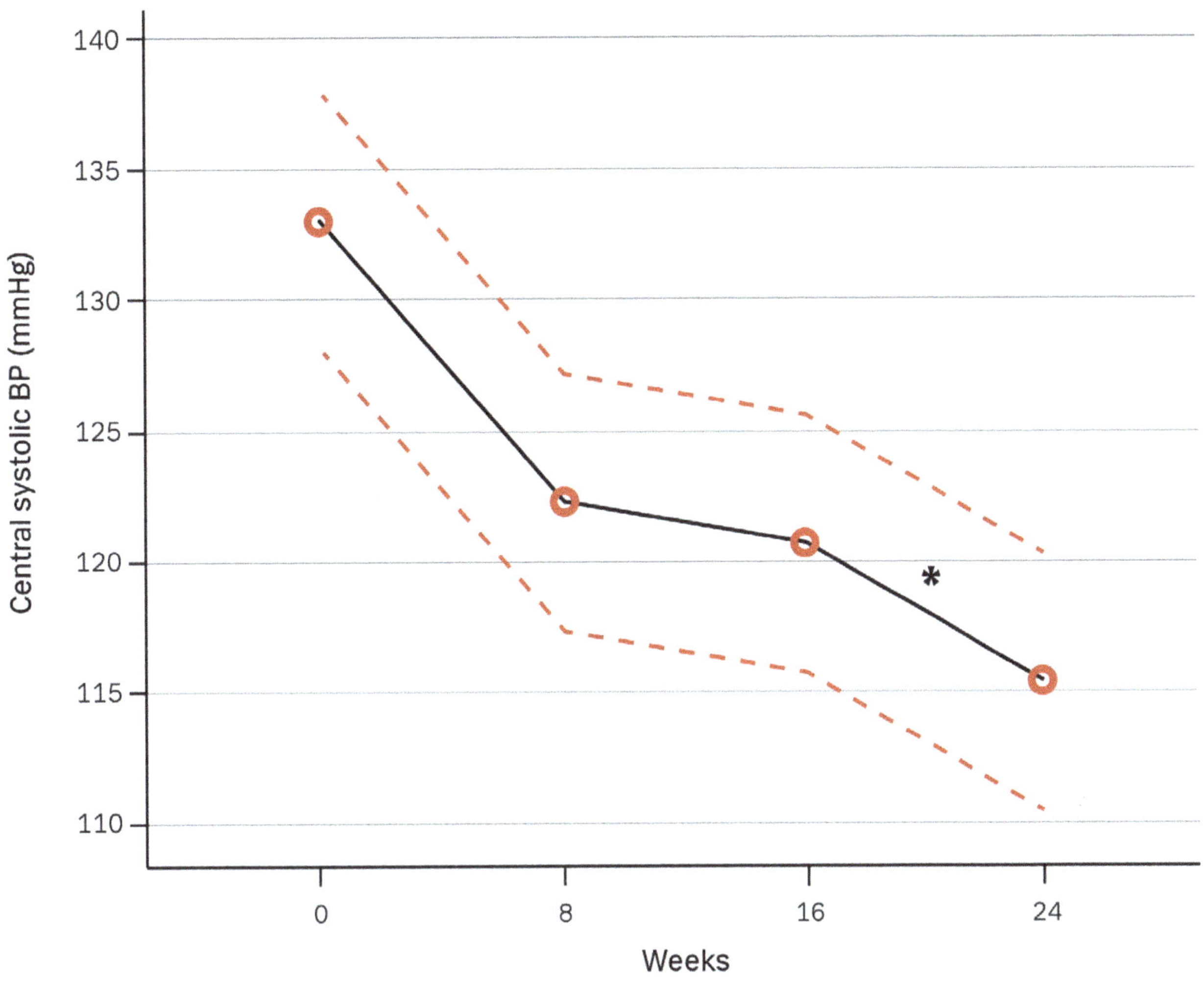

Figure 2. The effect of dual blockade compared to mono blockade on central systolic blood pressure with 95% confidence intervals as dotted lines. The number of measurement indicates 1. for baseline (mix of patients with and without previous treatment with either ACEI/ARB), 2. after 8 weeks of mono blockade with either ACEI/ARB, 3. after further 8 weeks of mono blockade and 4. after 8 weeks of dual blockade. * P<0.01.

Pooling of Randomization Groups

No differences were found between randomization groups in demographic data or baseline-values of pulse-wave measurements and clinical chemistry parameters. No differences were detected between treatment arms in the response of dual- versus mono-RAS blockade. These data are therefore presented as pooled data (table 1 and 2). Treatment with ACEI, ARB or the absence of RAS-blocking treatment prior to the trial, did not influence the response of dual RAS therapy versus mono-therapy for any of the parameters.

Blood Pressures

The effects of mono- and dual RAS-blockade on pulse-wave measurements and on kidney function are presented in table 2. Brachial and central systolic BP (figure 2) decreased significantly after start of combination treatment compared to monotherapy, but no further change was seen in brachial and central diastolic BP. Even though neither central nor brachial pulse pressure (PP) achieved a significant reduction, a significant increase (P = 0.02) on PP amplification was seen as illustrated in figure 3. This PP amplification changed from 1.26 at study entry to 1.30 and 1.30 after 8 and 16 weeks of monotherapy respectively and increased to 1.34 after dual blockade without any influence of height or heart rate.

Pulse-wave Velocity and Augmentation Index

A significant additive reduction was observed in aortic PWV of 0.3 m/s after combined treatment compared to monotherapy corresponding to a difference of 3%. This was independent of diastolic BP, age and gender. No significant change was detected in brachial PWV (table 2). The heart rate adjusted augmentation index.

(AIx@HR75) decreased significantly during dual blockade versus monotherapy by 2% corresponding to a proportional difference of 11%. This was independent of diastolic BP, age, body-height and gender (figure 4). This change in AIx@HR75 was related to the change in brachial PWV (P = 0.009) and not related to changes in Time to reflection (TR), Ejection duration (ED) or aortic PWV. No additive change was seen in TR, heart rate or ED during dual-blockade.

Change in Clinical Chemistry Parameters

There was a further increase in p-creatinine and p-urea after dual blockade compared to mono-blockade (table 2). No additive

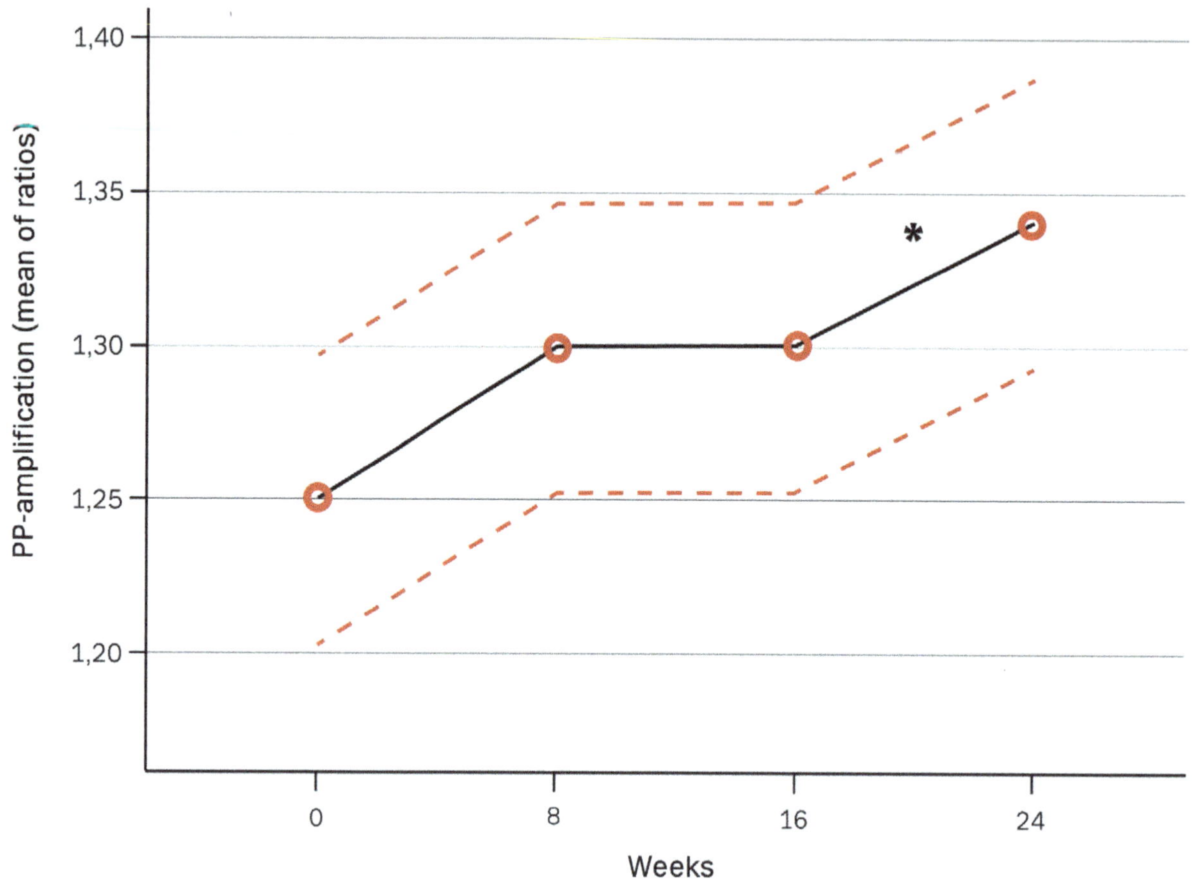

Figure 3. The effect of dual blockade compared with mono blockade on pulse-pressure-amplification with 95% confidence intervals as dotted lines. The number of measurement indicates 1. for baseline (mix of patients with and without previous treatment with either ACEI/ARB), 2. after 8 weeks of mono blockade with either ACEI/ARB, 3. after further 8 weeks of mono blockade and 4. after 8 weeks of dual blockade. * P<0.05.

effects were seen in p-potassium or urinary albumin excretion. There was a significant reduction seen in glomerular filtration rate (GFR) after dual blockade compared to baseline.

Tolerance and Other Medication

Thirty-three (49%) of the patients failed to tolerate full dual blockade with enalapril and candesartan, and had to be given lower doses of one or both of the drugs, or in 10 cases withdrawn from the study [24]. Hence, 34 (51%) of the patients tolerated the full dual blockade. Eight patients were withdrawn during mono-therapy: 2 due to early technical difficulties with the pulse wave measurements, 3 due to adverse reactions (unacceptable increase in p-creatinine, intractable rise in p-potassium or night sweats), one patient due to suspicion of malignancy early in the trial and 2 patients due to non-compliance. Two patients were withdrawn during dual-therapy, both because of unacceptable increases in p-creatinine. There were no differences in other antihypertensive medicine between the mono-therapy and dual-therapy period. Notably, the frequency of increasing or prescribing diuretics due to hyperkalemia was the same for the two periods.

Transient hyperkalemia was frequently seen as previously described [24], but was evenly distributed between the two treatment regimens.

Discussion

The main finding of this study is the BP independent reduction in arterial stiffness and pulse-wave reflection after combined treatment with enalapril and candesartan compared to monotherapy in patients with CKD. Furthermore pressure amplification was increased during dual blockade compared to monotherapy.

Aortic PWV is considered a direct measure of arterial stiffness [21] and is a strong independent predictor of all-cause and cardiovascular mortality and events in patients with ESRD [1,29] and CKD [3]. We found a significant reduction in aortic PWV of 0.3 m/s during dual blockade independent of BP and corrected for age and gender. In contrast no significant change was seen in brachial PWV.

Pulse-waves are in most studies analyzed by three parameters: central PP, central systolic BP and AIx [21] of which all have shown independent predicting value of all-cause mortality in ESRD [2,30]. In one study, for each increase of AIx of 10%, the relative mortality risk was increased by 1,51 [2]. We found a modest but significant reduction in the heart rate adjusted AIx (AIx@HR75) of 2% after dual blockade compared to a reduction during mono-blockade of 2% as well. Even after adjustment for known determinants of AIx as diastolic BP, height, gender and age [21,31] the reduction in AIx@HR75 was still significant. This reduction in AIx@HR75 was related to the change in brachial

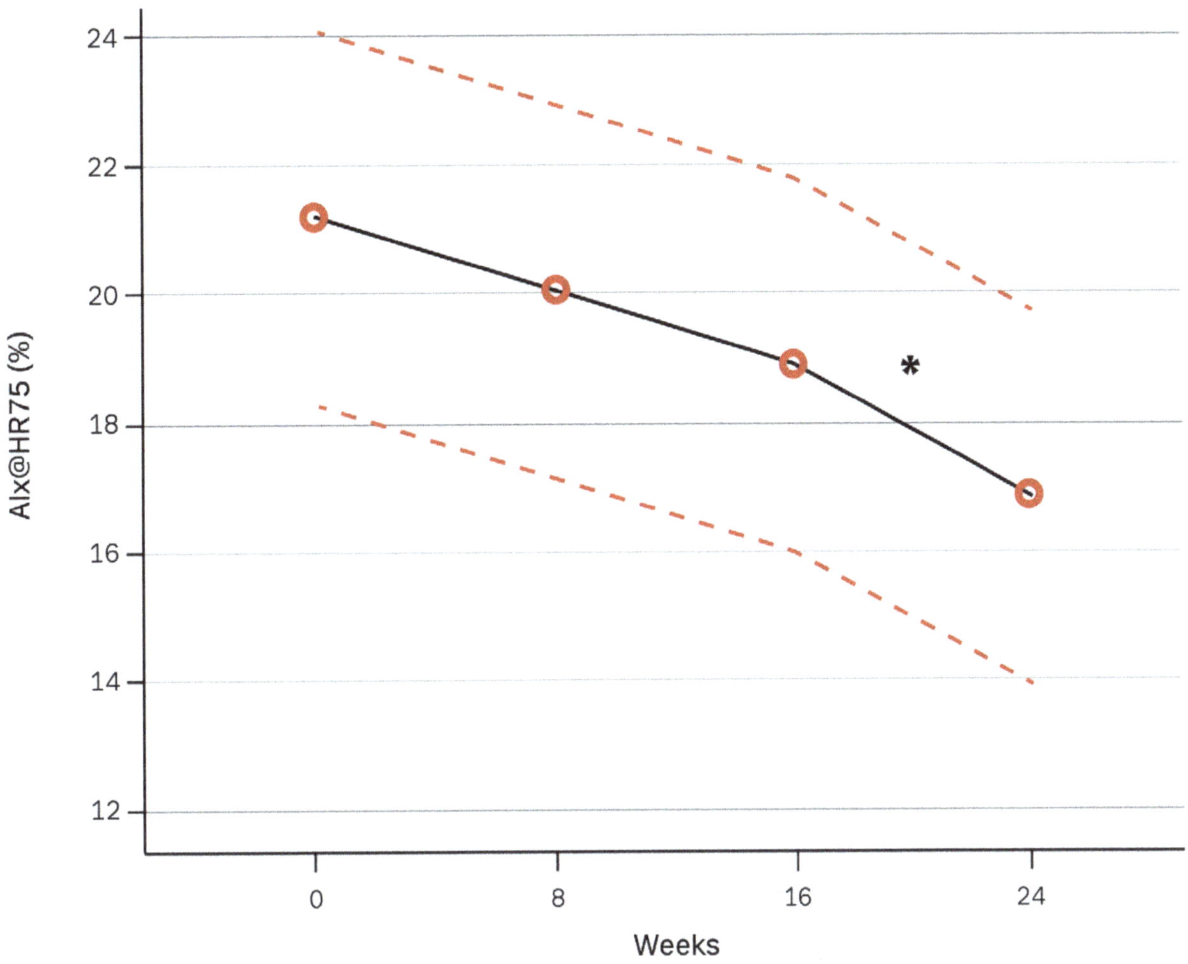

Figure 4. The effect of dual blockade compared with mono blockade on heart rate adjusted Augmentation Index (AIx@HR75) with 95% confidence intervals as dotted lines. The number of measurement indicates 1. for baseline (mix of patients with and without previous treatment with either ACEI/ARB), 2. after 8 weeks of mono blockade with either ACEI/ARB, 3. after further 8 weeks of mono blockade and 4. after 8 weeks of dual blockade. * $P<0.01$.

PWV even though this change did not achieve statistical significance. This indicates that the reduction in the intensity of wave-reflection was the principal mechanism of the change in AIx@HR75 caused by a dilatation of medium-sized muscular arteries and thereby a reduced brachial PWV. This relationship has been emphasized by others [32].

Dual blockade significantly reduced brachial and central systolic BP on average by 7 and 6 mmHg respectively on top of a decrease during monotherapy of 11 and 12 mmHg respectively. A significant increase in PP-amplification was seen (figure 3), indicating a larger effect of dual blockade on central BP than on brachial BP. This was despite the lack of proven significant changes in central or brachial PP which were most likely caused by a statistical error type II due to a limited number of patients. A lower pressure amplification indicates a higher left ventricular afterload because of higher central PP [33]. Thus the reduction of PP amplification has prospectively been shown to be a strong independent predictor of all-cause and CV mortality in ESRD and superior to central PP [30]. RAS-blocking agents have previously been shown to cause increased pressure amplification. London et al. reported an increase in amplification ratio from 1.0 to 1.13 after treatment with perindopril in patients with ESRD for 12 months [34]. In hypertensive patients Dhakam et al. found an increase in PP amplification ratio from 1.38 to 1.42 after treatment with eprosartan for 6 weeks [35]. In our study, 8 weeks of dual blockade increased amplification ratio from 1.30 to 1.34.

No previous studies have been conducted on the effects of dual blockade on pulse-wave measurements in CKD patients. A study of 18 hypertensive patients with normal renal function treated with ACEI showed that add on valsartan reduced central BP more than brachial BP. A significant reduction in AIx of 13% was found after 2 weeks [14]. In contrast, the same group observed no further change in amplification in another study of 12 hypertensive patients with normal renal function, comparing the effects of valsartan, captopril and their combination [36]. Significant reductions of both the central and brachial BP were found, but to the same extent. Like us, they observed a BP independent additive reduction of AIx and aortic PWV during combination therapy compared to monotherapy. In a third study in 31 hypertensive patients with normal renal function, combining valsartan and perindopril did also further reduce PWV but without correction for BP [15].

Our patients had moderate to advanced CKD (stage 3–5) where inhibition of RAS can be a challenge due to loss of kidney function [37] and hyperkalemia [38]. Ten patients were withdrawn from the study including two during the dual blockade period. Patients were closely monitored and incidences such as hyperkalemia and unacceptable increases in p-creatinine [39] were carefully managed. Thus the full dose study medication of RAS blockers was reduced in 42% of the patients. We have previously reported on the feasibility of dual blockade in the first 47 patients of the study [24].

Reduction of BP is known to reduce arterial stiffness [32]. The fact that the decrease in aortic PWV and AIx@HR75 was independent of BP suggests that the decrease in arterial stiffness was caused by the direct effect of the drug on the vascular wall. The common feature of ACEI and ARB appears to be their dilating capacity on especially peripheral muscular arteries and their ability to reduce wave-reflections, as expressed by AIx [32]. Combination of ACEI and ARB might produce a more complete inhibition of RAS and enhance bradykinin accumulation resulting in increased endothelial NO production. Furthermore ANGII is known to cause cardiovascular remodelling and vascular hypertrophy, and it therefore seems likely that the action on vascular wall includes chronic inverse remodelling of the small arteries leading to improved viscoelastic properties. Because of the relatively short period of treatment in our study, the additive beneficial effects of dual blockade are probably caused by functional changes, but due to the BP independent findings structural changes cannot be excluded.

Study Limitations

The cross-over design allowed for comparisons within the same patient. It would, however have been valuable with a control group treated with ACEI/ARB monotherapy parallel to the dual treatment period to rule out the time factor as a confounder. The period of dual blockade was deliberately not randomized, because of the crucial need for a cautious dose titration in each monotherapy before start of dual blockade in these vulnerable patients, which necessitated the placement of the dual blockade treatment period in the end of the trial.

There was no statistical difference between randomization arms, which allowed for analysis of data pooled together. We cannot though, exclude the possibility that inter-group differences did exist, but were not found due to small numbers in each randomization group. However, we consider, that by pooling data more powerful results were achieved.

Conclusion

In CKD patients, combined RAS blockade with enalapril and candesartan caused additive significant BP independent reductions in aortic PWV and AIx@HR75 compared to mono-therapy. Likewise, central systolic BP was reduced and PP-amplification was increased during dualblockade. As these are all independent predictors of cardiovascular mortality in CKD patients, the beneficial effects of dual RAS blockade found in this study might lead to a favorable effect on cardiovascular outcomes in CKD patients beyond that achieved by monotherapy.

Acknowledgments

We thank the staff of the Nephrology outpatient clinic, Department of Clinical Physiology and Nuclear Medicine at Herlev Hospital, the GCP-unit at Copenhagen University Hospital and all the patients who have participated in the study.

Author Contributions

Conceived and designed the experiments: MFM ALK SS SK AHN. Performed the experiments: MFM. Analyzed the data: MFM SK. Contributed reagents/materials/analysis tools: MFM ALK SS SK AHN. Wrote the paper: MFM ALK SS SK AHN.

References

1. Blacher J, Guerin AP, Pannier B, Marchais SJ, Safar ME, et al. (1999) Impact of aortic stiffness on survival in end-stage renal disease. Circulation 99: 2434–2439.
2. London GM, Blacher J, Pannier B, Guerin AP, Marchais SJ, et al. (2001) Arterial wave reflections and survival in end-stage renal failure. Hypertension 38: 434–438.
3. Covic A, Haydar AA, Bhamra-Ariza P, Gusbeth-Tatomir P, Goldsmith DJ (2005) Aortic pulse wave velocity and arterial wave reflections predict the extent and severity of coronary artery disease in chronic kidney disease patients. J Nephrol 18: 388–396.
4. Yusuf S, Sleight P, Pogue J, Bosch J, Davies R, et al. (2000) Effects of an angiotensin-converting-enzyme inhibitor, ramipril, on cardiovascular events in high-risk patients. The Heart Outcomes Prevention Evaluation Study Investigators. N Engl J Med 342: 145–153.
5. Brenner BM, Cooper ME, de ZD, Keane WF, Mitch WE, et al. (2001) Effects of losartan on renal and cardiovascular outcomes in patients with type 2 diabetes and nephropathy. N Engl J Med 345: 861–869.
6. Sleight P, Yusuf S, Pogue J, Tsuyuki R, Diaz R, et al. (2001) Blood-pressure reduction and cardiovascular risk in HOPE study. Lancet 358: 2130–2131.
7. Poulter NR, Wedel H, Dahlof B, Sever PS, Beevers DG, et al. (2005) Role of blood pressure and other variables in the differential cardiovascular event rates noted in the Anglo-Scandinavian Cardiac Outcomes Trial-Blood Pressure Lowering Arm (ASCOT-BPLA). Lancet 366: 907–913.
8. Dahlof B, Devereux RB, Kjeldsen SE, Julius S, Beevers G, et al. (2002) Cardiovascular morbidity and mortality in the Losartan Intervention For Endpoint reduction in hypertension study (LIFE): a randomised trial against atenolol. Lancet 359: 995–1003.
9. Williams B, Lacy PS, Thom SM, Cruickshank K, Stanton A, et al. (2006) Differential impact of blood pressure-lowering drugs on central aortic pressure and clinical outcomes: principal results of the Conduit Artery Function Evaluation (CAFE) study. Circulation 113: 1213–1225.
10. Hirata K, Vlachopoulos C, Adji A, O'Rourke MF (2005) Benefits from angiotensin-converting enzyme inhibitor 'beyond blood pressure lowering': beyond blood pressure or beyond the brachial artery? J Hypertens 23: 551–556.
11. Wang KL, Cheng HM, Chuang SY, Spurgeon HA, Ting CT, et al. (2009) Central or peripheral systolic or pulse pressure: which best relates to target organs and future mortality? J Hypertens 27: 461–467.
12. Roman MJ, Devereux RB, Kizer JR, Lee ET, Galloway JM, et al. (2007) Central pressure more strongly relates to vascular disease and outcome than does brachial pressure: the Strong Heart Study. Hypertension 50: 197–203.
13. Pini R, Cavallini MC, Palmieri V, Marchionni N, Di BM, et al. (2008) Central but not brachial blood pressure predicts cardiovascular events in an unselected geriatric population: the ICARe Dicomano Study. J Am Coll Cardiol 51: 2432–2439.
14. Mahmud A, Feely J (2000) Favourable effects on arterial wave reflection and pulse pressure amplification of adding angiotensin II receptor blockade in resistant hypertension. J Hum Hypertens 14: 541–546.
15. Anan F, Takahashi N, Ooie T, Yufu K, Hara M, et al. (2005) Effects of valsartan and perindopril combination therapy on left ventricular hypertrophy and aortic arterial stiffness in patients with essential hypertension. Eur J Clin Pharmacol 61: 353–359.
16. Yusuf S, Teo KK, Pogue J, Dyal L, Copland I, et al. (2008) Telmisartan, ramipril, or both in patients at high risk for vascular events. N Engl J Med 358: 1547–1559.
17. Chan KE, Ikizler TA, Gamboa JL, Yu C, Hakim RM, et al. (2011) Combined angiotensin-converting enzyme inhibition and receptor blockade associate with increased risk of cardiovascular death in hemodialysis patients. Kidney Int 80: 978–985.
18. Altman DG, Schulz KF, Moher D, Egger M, Davidoff F, et al. (2001) The revised CONSORT statement for reporting randomized trials: explanation and elaboration. Ann Intern Med 134: 663–694.

19. National Kidney Foundation (2002) K/DOQI clinical practice guidelines for chronic kidney disease: evaluation, classification, and stratification. Am J Kidney Dis 39: S1–266.
20. Pauca AL, O'Rourke MF, Kon ND (2001) Prospective evaluation of a method for estimating ascending aortic pressure from the radial artery pressure waveform. Hypertension 38: 932–937.
21. Laurent S, Cockcroft J, Van BL, Boutouyrie P, Giannattasio C, et al. (2006) Expert consensus document on arterial stiffness: methodological issues and clinical applications. Eur Heart J 27: 2588–2605.
22. Gallagher D, Adji A, O'Rourke MF (2004) Validation of the transfer function technique for generating central from peripheral upper limb pressure waveform. Am J Hypertens 17: 1059–1067.
23. Weber T, Ammer M, Rammer M, Adji A, O'rourke MF, et al. (2009) Noninvasive determination of carotid-femoral pulse wave velocity depends critically on assessment of travel distance: a comparison with invasive measurement. J Hypertens 27: 1624–1630.
24. Frimodt-Moller M, Nielsen AH, Strandgaard S, Kamper AL (2009) Feasibility of combined treatment with enalapril and candesartan in advanced chronic kidney disease. Nephrol Dial Transplant.
25. Brochner-Mortensen J (1972) A simple method for the determination of glomerular filtration rate. Scand J Clin Lab Invest 30: 271–274.
26. Brochner-Mortensen J, Freund LG (1981) Reliability of routine clearance methods for assessment of glomerular filtration rate in advanced renal insufficiency. Scand J Clin Lab Invest 41: 91–97.
27. Avolio AP, Van Bortel LM, Boutouyrie P, Cockcroft JR, McEniery CM, et al. (2009) Role of pulse pressure amplification in arterial hypertension: experts' opinion and review of the data. Hypertension 54: 375–383.
28. Frimodt-Moller M, Nielsen AH, Kamper AL, Strandgaard S (2006) Pulse-wave morphology and pulse-wave velocity in healthy human volunteers: examination conditions. Scand J Clin Lab Invest 66: 385–394.
29. Pannier B, Guerin AP, Marchais SJ, Safar ME, London GM (2005) Stiffness of capacitive and conduit arteries: prognostic significance for end-stage renal disease patients. Hypertension 45: 592–596.
30. Safar ME, Blacher J, Pannier B, Guerin AP, Marchais SJ, et al. (2002) Central pulse pressure and mortality in end-stage renal disease. Hypertension 39: 735–738.
31. Lemogoum D, Flores G, Van den Abeele W, Ciarka A, Leeman M, et al. (2004) Validity of pulse pressure and augmentation index as surrogate measures of arterial stiffness during beta-adrenergic stimulation. J Hypertens 22: 511–517.
32. Nichols WW, Denardo SJ, Wilkinson IB, McEniery CM, Cockcroft J, et al. (2008) Effects of arterial stiffness, pulse wave velocity, and wave reflections on the central aortic pressure waveform. J Clin Hypertens (Greenwich) 10: 295–303.
33. Protogerou AD, Papaioannou TG, Lekakis JP, Blacher J, Safar ME (2009) The effect of antihypertensive drugs on central blood pressure beyond peripheral blood pressure. Part I: (Patho)-physiology, rationale and perspective on pulse pressure amplification. Curr Pharm Des 15: 267–271.
34. London GM, Pannier B, Guerin AP, Marchais SJ, Safar ME, et al (1994) Cardiac hypertrophy, aortic compliance, peripheral resistance, and wave reflection in end-stage renal disease: Comparative effects of ACE inhibition and calcium channel blockade. Circulation 90: 2786–2796.
35. Dhakam Z, McEniery CM, Yasmin Cockcroft JR, Brown MJ, et al. (2006) Atenolol and eprosartan: differential effects on central blood pressure and aortic pulse wave velocity. Am J Hypertens 19: 214–219.
36. Mahmud A, Feely J (2002) Reduction in arterial stiffness with angiotensin II antagonist is comparable with and additive to ACE inhibition. Am J Hypertens 15: 321–325.
37. Kamper AL, Thomsen HS, Nielsen SL, Strandgaard S (1990) Initial effect of enalapril on kidney function in patients with moderate to severe chronic nephropathy. Scand J Urol Nephrol 24: 69–73.
38. Palmer BF (2004) Managing Hyperkalemia Caused by Inhibitors of the Renin-Angiotensin-Aldosterone System. N Engl J Med 351: 585–592.
39. Bakris GL, Weir MR (2000) Angiotensin-converting enzyme inhibitor-associated elevations in serum creatinine: is this a cause for concern? Arch Intern Med 160: 685–693.

16

Prevalence and Risk Factors Associated to Chronic Kidney Disease in HIV-Infected Patients on HAART and Undetectable Viral Load in Brazil

Andréia M. Menezes[1], Jorge Torelly Jr[1], Lúcia Real[1], Mônica Bay[2], Julia Poeta[1], Eduardo Sprinz[1,2]*

1 Faculdade de Medicina, Universidade Federal do Rio Grande do Sul, Porto Alegre, Rio Grande do Sul, Brazil, **2** Hospital de Clínicas de Porto Alegre, Porto Alegre, Rio Grande do Sul, Brazil

Abstract

Background: To determine the prevalence and associated factors with chronic kidney disease (CKD) in a cohort of HIV-positive individuals with undetectable viral load on HAART.

Methods: From March, 2009 to September 2009, 213 individuals between 18-70 years, period on HAART $\geq$12 months, viral load $<$ 50 copies/mm^3, and CD4 $\geq$ 200 cells/mm^3, were consecutively enrolled at the outpatient clinic of Hospital de Clínicas, Porto Alegre, Brazil. Exclusion criteria were obesity, malnourishment, amputee, paraplegic, previous history of renal disease, pregnancy and hepatic insufficiency. Renal function was determined by estimated glomerular filtration rate (eGFR) assessed by the modification of diet in renal disease. CKD was defined as an eGFR less or equal than 60 ml/min/1.73 m^2, for a period of at least 3 months. Poisson regression was used to determine factors associated with CKD.

Results: CKD was diagnosed in 8.4% of the population, and after adjustment, the risk factors were hypertension (RR = 3.88, 95%CI, 1.84 - 8.16), time on HAART (RR = 1.15, 95%CI,1.03–1.27) and tenofovir exposure (RR = 2.25, 95%CI, 1.04–4.95). Higher weight (RR = ,0.88 95%CI, 0.82–0.96) was associated to normal function.

Conclusions: CKD was a common finding in this cohort of patients and was related to hypertension, time on HAART and tenofovir exposure. We suggest a more frequent monitoring of renal function, especially for those with risk factors to early identify renal impairment.

Editor: Esper Georges Kallas, University of Sao Paulo, Brazil

Funding: This work was partially supported by Fundo de incentivo a Pesquisa do Hospital de Clínicas de Porto Alegre (FIPE), Center for Reseach Support (CAPES/REUNI) and National Research Council (CNPq) of Brazil. The funders had no role in study design, data collection and analysis, decision to publish, or preparation of the manuscript.

Competing Interests: The authors have declared that no competing interests exist.

* E-mail: eduardo.sprinz@gmail.com.br

Introduction

The advances of antiretroviral therapy (HAART) had turned HIV/AIDS into a chronic disease [1–5]. As a consequence of living longer, individuals might present complications not only related to the virus, but also related to the treatment itself and ageing process [1–4]. These complications might be related to heart, lung, hepatic or renal diseases, for instance, which could be associated to a higher mortality [2,3].

In this scenario, kidney disease has been increasingly reported, with a prevalence of chronic kidney disease (CKD), varying from 4.7% to 7.6% according to several studies [5–8]. Risks that have already been associated include the "traditional" factors related to ageing, diabetes mellitus (DM) and hypertension [5,6]. Besides that, other features such as the virus itself and some of the antiretrovirals (ARVs) currently used, such as indinavir (IDV) and tenofovir (TDF) have already been linked with nephrotoxicity in these individuals [5,7,8].

The first stage of renal impairment is silent and only detectable through laboratory analysis [9]. Although the most used biomarker for renal dysfunction diagnosis, the measurement of serum creatinine has limitations, such as the relatively low sensitivity, which underestimates the underlying renal status, and therefore, its values could be in the "normal range", even after the loss of 50–60% of the glomerular filtration rate (GFR) [9,10]. Although not clearly validated to HIV-infected individuals, equations adjusting for muscle mass, age, weight, ethnicity and sex, provide a more sensitive estimation of the true renal function, and have been used in general population (eGFR)[11,12]. Currently, the most common formulas to estimate the GFR are Modification of Diet in Renal Disease formula (MDRD) [13,14], Cockcroft-Galt (CG) [14,15] and Chronic Kidney Disease Epidemiology Collaboration (CKD-epi) [16].

The objectives of our study were to describe the prevalence of CKD and to determine the risk factors associated to the development of renal disease in a cohort of HIV infected individuals on HAART, undetectable viral load, and not severely immunosupressed (CD4 count $>$ 200 cells/mm3), which would better resemble the general population, in Brazil.

Materials and Methods

Population

Two hundred fifty five patients attended in the HIV/AIDS outpatient clinic at Hospital de Clínicas, Porto Alegre, Brazil, were consecutively enrolled from March, 2009 through September, 2009. To be included, patients needed to be on HAART and undetectable viral load (<50 copies/ml) for a period equal or greater than 12 months, CD4 counts higher than 200 cells/mm3 and age between 18 and 70 years. Patients were excluded if were obese or malnourishment [17,18] due to the MDRD equation; amputee and paraplegic (with decreased muscle mass), previous history of kidney disease; present history of hepatitis B or C infection (confirmed by a positive polymerase chain reaction) or hepatic insufficiency; and, pregnant women.

Methods

Data were collected at the moment of the appointment and included demographic variables (ethnicity, height, weight, BMI, sex and age); diagnosis of DM (according to "The American Diabetes Association")[19], use of antidiabetic agents; hypertension (according to the Joint National Comittee 7 [20]); a complete history of HAART; use of drugs for prophylaxis against opportunistic infections; CD4 cell counts (cells/mm^3, measured by flow cytometry); plasma HIV-RNA level (copies/ml, measured by b-DNA; HIV-1 RNA 3.0 assay, with limit of detection of 50 copies/ml); serum creatinine (mg/dl, measured by Jaffé; calibrated method by isotope dilution mass spectrometry - IDMS); date of HIV diagnosis and other comorbidities.

The biochemical data was measured in the same laboratory. The main outcome of interest in our study was to eGFR assessed by two measurements, at least, three months apart utilizing the MDRD in its simplified version (which considers serum creatinine concentration, age, sex and ethnicity) and CKD-epi equations. CKD was defined as an eGFR less or equal than 60 ml/min per 1.73 m^2 or the presence of proteinuria independent of eGFR in both estimations.

Renal function was classified in five stages depending on the level of eGFR, as proposed by the Kidney Disease Outcomes Quality Initiative (KDOQI): normal, GFR equal or higher 90 ml/min per 1.73 m^2; mild decrease, GFR between 60–89 ml/min per 1.73 m^2 or presence of proteinuria with normal eGFR; moderate decrease, GFR between 30-59 ml/min per 1.73 m^2; severe decrease, GFR between 15–29 ml/min per 1.73 m^2; and, renal failure or dialysis, GFR less than 15 ml/min per 1.73 m^2 [12].

The study was approved by the Research and Ethic Committee of Hospital de Clinicas and all patients signed the informed consent.

Statistical analysis

Statistical analysis included descriptive (mean and standard deviation), univariate and multivariate analysis. Absolute and relative frequencies were utilized for continuous and categorical variables respectively.

To evaluate the association between CKD and categorical variables Chi-square test or Fisher exact were applied as required. Independent T test or one way ANOVA were used to compare means; in case of asymmetry Mann Whitney test or Kruskal-Wallis test were used. Variables significantly associated with renal impairment in univariate analysis ($p<0.05$) were included in the multivariate model. Those significant in the multivariate model ($p<0.1$) were included in the final model. Poisson Regression was used to determine the factors associated with CKD in an univariate analysis and in a multivariate model. Pearson coefficient and Bland-Altman graph were used to evaluate the correlation and the concordance between the two equations to eGFR (MDRD and CKD-epi). A p value of less than 0.05 was considered significant. Analysis was performed using the statistical package for the social sciences (SPSS) version 17.0 (SPSS Inc., Chicago, Illinois, USA).

Sample size

The sample size calculation was based on a prevalence of at least 4% of CKD in that population with a confidence level of 95%. A sample size of at least 198 individuals was needed to be representative of the 2,050 individuals on HAART in our site to have a power of 80%

Results

From the initial 255 included patients, there were 42 losses (16.5%): 28 due to incomplete laboratory data; 13 withdrew the informed consent; and, one additional patient died after signing the consent. The characteristics and clinical variables of the remained 213 patients are shown in Table 1. One hundred and ten patients were men (51.6%), 174 were euro-descendants (81.7%) and mean age was 45.6 years old, BMI was 24.75±4.05; mean time on HAART was 7.7±4.7 years, mean CD4+ count was 568±269 cells/mm^3, and mean nadir CD4 count was 169±137 cells/mm^3. The prevalence of hypertension and DM was 20.7% (n = 44) and 14.1% (n = 30), respectively. There was no statistical difference between ethnicity characteristics (data not shown).

There was a significant correlation between the CKD-epi and MDRD equations (Pearson coefficient = 0.9; $p<0.001$; Bland-Altman graph analysis p = 0.296; 95% IC -4.14–3.34, Figure 1). The mean eGFR was 98.04±30.35 ml/min/1.73 m2 for MDRD and 96.37±24.46 ml/min/1.73 m2 for CKD-epi (Table 2 shows the eGFR by MDRD equation of the cohort).

The factors significantly associated with CKD in the univariate models (table 3) were: hypertension, DM, time after HIV diagnosis, older age, body weight, time on HAART, TDF and ritonavir (RTV) exposure (100 mg/day). After adjustment by the multivariate analysis (table 3), hypertension (RR = 3.88, 95% CI

Table 1. Main demographic characteristics (data are presented as mean ± standard deviation or percentage).

	N = 213 (%)
Age (years)	45.6±11,5
Men	110 (51.6 %)
Ethnicity	
Euro-descendants	174 (81.7%)
Creatinine (mg/dl)	0.89±0.32
Urea (mg/dl)	35.44 ±13.34
eGFR[a] (ml/mim)	98.04±30.35
CD4 (cells/mm^3)	569.81±269
Hypertension	44 (20.7%)
Diabetes Mellitus	30 (14.1%)
Time on HAART[b] (years)	7.8±4.8

[a]Estimated glomerular filtration rate,
[b]Antiretroviral therapy

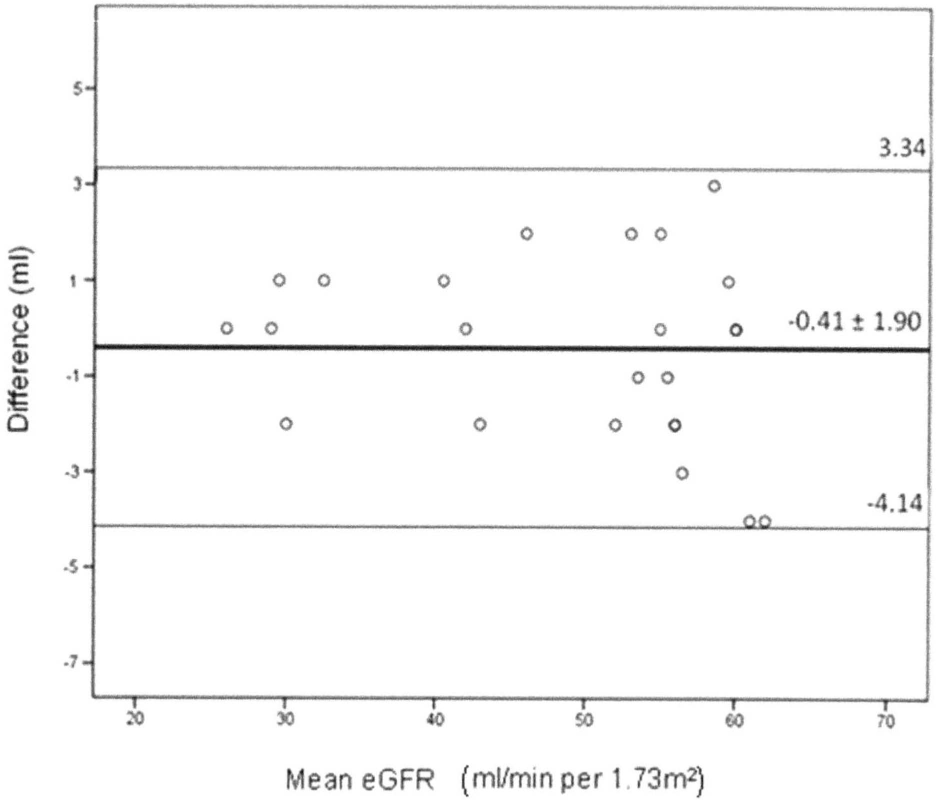

Figure 1. Bland-Altman graph comparing MDRD and CKD-epi in individuals with chronic kidney disease. There was a concordance in eGFR between the MDRD and CKD-epi equations in individuals with chronic kidney disease (the mean difference was 0.41±1.90 ml). eGFR = estimated glomerular filtration rate; MDRD = modified diet in renal disease; CKD-epi = chronic kidney disease epidemiology.

1.84–8.16, p=<0.001), time on HAART (RR=1.15, 95% CI 1.03–1.27, p= 0.011), and TDF exposure (RR=2.25, 95% CI 1.04–4.95, p=0.038) remained significantly associated to CKD. Higher weight (RR=0.89, 95% CI 0.82–0.96, p=0.005) was significantly associated to a normal kidney function.

Discussion

Our study examined the prevalence of CKD and its associated factors among HIV infected individuals on HAART for at least one year and undetectable viral load (which is a quite clinically stable population). The prevalence of CKD was 8.4%, which is quite close, albeit higher, to the ones reported by other studies that vary from 4.7% to 7.6% [21–26]. Although somehow expected, this finding was worrisome for us, as it is estimated that about 5% of the general Brazilian population older than 60 years is expected to have CKD, whereas our cohort had a greater prevalence with CKD with a mean age almost 15 years younger (mean age was 45.6 years) [27,28]. Likewise, as we selected HIV "healthy" patients (undetectable viral load and CD4 > 200 cells/3) and without previous renal disease we were anticipating a lower prevalence of CKD.

Table 2. Prevalence of alteration in the renal function according to Kidney Disease Outcomes Quality Initiative – KDOQI [12], assessed by the modification of diet in renal disease.

Rena Function	eGFR[a] (ml/min/1.73m²)	Our findings
		N=213 (%)
Normal	> or equal 90	127 (59.6)
Mild Reduction	60–89	68 (31.9)
Moderate Reduction	30–59	15 (7)
Severe Reduction	15–29	3 (1.4)
Renal failure or dialysis	<15	0

[a]Estimated Glomerular filtration rate

The factors associated were: hypertension, time on HAART and TDF use. As expected, hypertension was found to be a major risk factor associated with CKD (RR= 3.88, 95% CI 1.84–8.16)), which is in accordance to other studies [5,6–8,22,24]. The risk was slightly higher than the other studies, which varied from 1.68% to 3.8% [5,6,8].

Another unique finding was that time on antiretroviral therapy was significantly associated with CKD. In our study, there was a 15% increased prevalence of CKD per year of additional exposure to ARVs (RR= 1.15, 95% CI 1.03–1.27). This could be explained by the fact that prolonged use of HAART could be associated with greater long term renal toxicity, meaning the more exposition leading to higher toxicity.

Adverse effects of the exposure to individuals ARVs were demonstrated by other studies which described the cumulative association of TDF, ATV, indinavir and RTV to the development of CKD [6,8]. In our study, the only antiretroviral that was independently associated to CKD, was TDF (RR=2.25, 95% CI 1.04–4.95). Our findings were somewhat

Table 3. Risk factors associated to alteration in the renal function (eGFR < 60 ml/min per 1.73 m^2 by MDRD); univariate and multivariate analysis.

	Univariate analysis			Multivariate analysis		
	RR	95% CI	P	RR	95% CI	p
Euro-descendants	5.15	0.78–37.03	0.103			
Men	1.06	0.50–2.26	0.864			
Use of atazanavir	2.03	0.87–4.70	0.098			
Use of tenofovir	**2.49**	**1.18–5.22**	**0.016**	**2.25**	**1.04–4.95**	**0,038**
Use of ritonavir (100mg)	3.88	1.66–9.03	0.02			
Use of ritonavir (200mg)	1.94	0.67–5.59	0.23			
Hypertension	**5.37**	**2.56–11.21**	**<0.001**	**3.88**	**1.84–8.16**	**<0.001**
Diabetes Mellitus	1.26	1.13–2.37	0.026			
Older age (years)	1.069	1.04–1.10	<0.001			
Time on HAART (years)	**1.14**	**1.06–1.23**	**<0.001**	**1.15**	**1.03–1.27**	**0.011**
Body weight (Kg)	**0.92**	**0.86–0.97**	**0.038**	**0.89**	**0.82–0.96**	**0.005**
Time of diagnosis of HIV	0.910	0.68–1.9	0.031	1.07	0.98–1.17	0.11
CD4 (cells/mm^3)	1.0	0.99–1.01	0.97			

CKD defined as confirmed (persisting for ≤ 3 months) decrease in eGFR to 60 ml/min per 1.73m^2 by MDRD or the presence of proteinuria independent of eGFR. CI, confidence interval; RR, risk ratio; eGFR, estimated glomerular filtration rate. All variables significant in univariate analyses (P<0.05) were included in multivariate model. All variables with P<0.1 in the multivariate analysis (data not shown) were included in the final model

higher than what have been found in other studies which varied from 1.5 to 2.18 higher chance of renal disease [5,6,8]. We did not have enough patients on indinavir (only 2) to find any association. Perhaps with a larger sample we could come across major findings regarding ritonavir use and, consequently, atazanavir, as it is the antiretroviral used along with 100 mg of ritonavir daily.

An important finding was related to the body weight (RR = 0.89, 95% CI 0.82–0.96, which was significantly associated as a protection factor. To our knowledge, this is the first study that found this association. Individuals with lower body weight were at greater risk of having CKD. Despite it is known that weight may play an important function in drug metabolism, once it can influence the bioavailability and pharmacokinetics of ARVs [29], there is still limited data about the effect of weight in HAART. Perhaps this should be a window of opportunity to individualize ARVs dosage and minimize toxicity.

The study has several limitations that should be considered when interpreting the results. Although all studies estimate the GFR in HIV individuals, this could be not accurate enough to allow a firm conclusion of kidney function. MDRD equation, generally more accurate and utilized [11,13], might not be fully applicable to specific populations. Limited data suggests that MDRD may underestimate GFR in individuals with normal renal function [11,13,16] and therefore have led to an overestimation of renal impairment. We suggest that there is a need of an individualized equation to estimate the GFR in each population. Likely, due to constraints of MDRD, we excluded malnourished and obese patients, which could have better contributed to some of our findings. Secondly, our sample size might have limited our findings as it may have not been large enough to detect all CKD risk factors in this population, such as age and DM. Thirdly, this is a cross sectional study and therefore we can only draw association of events and not establish temporal sequence. Lastly, although we tried to minimize HIV infection and its co-morbidities, selecting individuals with CD4 counts greater than 200 cells/mm^3 and at least one year with undetectable viral load, it is not possible to exclude any influence of HIV infection and related diseases or other nephrotoxic medications in the prevalence of renal impairment [5].

In summary, according to our findings, in HIV population which would most resemble the general population, hypertension, time on HAART, and exposure to tenofovir were associated with a higher prevalence of CKD. On the other hand, individuals with higher body weight appeared to be "protected" from chronic kidney disease. We suggest that an equation to eGFR should be routinely applied to better identify decrease in renal function, and should be performed at the moment of HIV diagnosis and later at regular intervals, depending on the associated risk factors. Further studies are necessary to confirm risks associated to renal disease in HIV-infected individuals.

Author Contributions

Conceived and designed the experiments: ES AMM. Performed the experiments: ES AMM. Analyzed the data: ES AMM. Contributed reagents/materials/analysis tools: ES AMM LR JP JT MB. Wrote the paper: ES AMM LR JP JT MB. Data collection: ES AMM LR JP JT MB.

References

1. Wyatt CM, Winston JA, Malvestutto CD, Fishbein DA, Barash I, et al. (2007) Chronic kidney disease in HIV infection: an urban epidemic. AIDS 21: 2101–2103.
2. Palella FJ Jr., Baker RK, Moorman AC, Chmiel JS, Wood KC, et al. (2006) Mortality in the highly active antiretroviral therapy era: Changing causes of death and disease in the HIV outpatient study. J Acquir Immune Defic Syndr 43: 27–34.
3. Michaels SH, Clark R, Kissinger P (1998) Declining morbidity and mortality among patients with advanced human immunodeficiency virus infection. N Engl J Med 339: 405–406.

4. Gardner LI, Klein RS, Szczech LA, Phelps RM, Tashima K, et al. (2003) Rates and risk factors for condition-specific hospitalizations in HIV-infected and uninfected women. J Acquir Immune Defic Syndr 34: 320–330.
5. Mocroft A, Kirk O, Gatell J, Reiss P, Gargalianos P, et al. (2007) Chronic renal failure among HIV-1-infected patients. AIDS 21: 1119–1127.
6. Crum-Cianflone N, Ganesan A, Teneza-Mora N, Riddle M, Medina S, et al. (2010) Prevalence and Factors Associated with Renal Dysfunction Among HIV-Infected Patients. AIDS Patient Care STDS 24: 353–360.
7. Barrios A, Garcia-Benayas T, Gonzalez-Lahoz J, Sorianon V (2004) Tenofovir-related nephrotoxicity in HIV-infected patients. AIDS 18: 960–963.
8. Mocroft A, Kirk O, Reiss P, De Wit S, Sedlacek D, et al. (2010) Estimated glomerular filtration rate, chronic kidney disease and antiretroviral drug use in HIV-positive patients. AIDS 24: 1667–1678.
9. Perrone RD, Madias NE, Levey AS (1992) Serum creatinine as an index of renal function: new insights into old concepts. Clin Chem 38: 1933–1953.
10. Shemesh O, Golbetz H, Kriss JP, Myers BD (1985) Limitations of creatinine as a filtration marker in glomerulopathic patients. Kidney Int 28: 830–838.
11. Levey AS, Bosch JP, Lewis JB, Greene T, Rogers N, et al. (1999) A more accurate method to estimate glomerular filtration rate from serum creatinine: a new prediction equation Modification of diet in renal disease study group. Ann Intern Med 130: 461–470.
12. K/DOQI: National Kidney Foundation (2002) K/DOQI clinical practice guidelines for chronic kidney disease: evaluation, classification, and stratification. Am J Kidney Dis 39 (2 Suppl 1): S1–S266.
13. Stevens LA, Levey AS (2005) Measurement of kidney function. Med Clin Am 89: 457–473.
14. Stöhr W, Walker AS, Munderi P, Tugume S, Gilks CF, et al. (2008) Estimating glomerular filtration rate in HIV-infected adults in Africa: comparison of Cockcroft-Gault and Modification of Diet in Renal Disease formulae. Antivir Ther 13: 761–770.
15. Cockcroft DW, Gault MH (1976) Prediction of creatinine clearance from serum creatinine. Nephron16: 31–41.
16. Soares AA, Eyff TF, Campani RB, Ritter L, Weinert LS, et al. (2010) Performance of the CKD Epidemiology Collaboration (CKD-EPI) and the Modification of Diet in Renal Disease (MDRD) Study Equations in Healthy South Brazilians. Am J Kidney Dis 55: 1162–1163.
17. World Health Organization (WHO) (2011) Global database on body mass index. Available: http://apps.who.int/bmi/index.jsp?introPage=intro_3.html Accessed 2010 Dec 15.
18. Report of a WHO Expert Committee (1995) Physical status: the use and interpretation of anthropometry. World Health Organ Tech Rep Ser 854: 1–452.
19. American Diabetes Association (2010) Diagnosis and classification of diabetes mellitus. Diabetes Care 33 (Suppl 1):S62-S69. Erratum in: Diabetes Care 2010; 33: 57.
20. Chobanian AV, Bakris GL, Black HR, Cushman WC, Green LA, et al. (2003) The Seventh Report of the Joint National Committee on Prevention, Detection, Evaluation, and Treatment of High Blood Pressure: the JNC 7 report. JAMA 289:2560-2572. Erratum in: JAMA 2003; 290-197.
21. Déti EK, Thiébaut R, Bonnet F, Lawson-Ayayi S, Dupon M, et al. (2010) Prevalence and factors associated with renal impairment in HIV-infected patients, ANRS C03 Aquitaine Cohort, France. HIV Med 11: 308–317.
22. Overton ET, Nurutdinova D, Freeman J, Seyfried W, Mondy KE (2009) Factors associated with renal dysfunction within an urban HIV-infected cohort in the era of highly active antiretroviral therapy. HIV Med 10: 343–350.
23. Lucas GM, Lau B, Atta MG, Fine DM, Keruly J, et al. (2008) Chronic kidney disease incidence and progression to end-stage renal disease, in HIV-infected individuals: a tale of two races. J Infect Dis 197: 1548–1557.
24. Sorlí ML, Guelar A, Montero M, González A, Rodriguez E, et al. (2008) Chronic kidney disease prevalence and risk factors among HIV-infected patients. J Acquir Immune Defic Syndr 48: 506–508.
25. Gupta SK, Mamlin BW, Johnson CS, Dollins MD, Topf JM, et al. (2004) Prevalence of proteinuria and the development of chronic kidney disease in HIV-infected patients. Clin Nephrol 61: 1–6.
26. Cheung CY, Wong KM, Lee MP, Liu YL, Kwok H, et al. (2007) Prevalence of chronic kidney disease in Chinese HIV-infected patients. Nephrol Dial Transplant 22: 3186–3190.
27. Romão Júnior JE (2004) Doença Renal Crônica: Definição, Epidemiologia e Classificação. J Bras Nefrol 26: 1–3.
28. Lugon JR (2009) Chronic Kidney Disease in Brazil: A Public Health Problem. J Bras Nefrol 31: 2–5.
29. Tozzi V (2010) Pharmacogenetics of antiretrovirals. Antiviral Res 85: 190–200.

17

Angiopoietin-2 is Associated with Albuminuria and Microinflammation in Chronic Kidney Disease

Fan-Chi Chang[1,2,3], Tai-Shuan Lai[1,4], Chih-Kang Chiang[1], Yung-Ming Chen[1], Ming-Shiou Wu[1], Tzong-Shinn Chu[1,2]*, Kwan-Dun Wu[1], Shuei-Liong Lin[1,3]

1 Renal Division, Department of Medicine, National Taiwan University Hospital, Taipei, Taiwan, **2** Department of Internal Medicine, National Taiwan University Hospital Chu-Tung Branch, Hsin-Chu County, Taiwan, **3** Graduate Institutes of Physiology, College of Medicine, National Taiwan University, Taipei, Taiwan, **4** Department of Internal Medicine, National Taiwan University Hospital Bei-Hu Branch, Taipei, Taiwan

Abstract

Although cardiovascular disease (CVD) is the leading cause of mortality in patients with chronic kidney disease (CKD), the pathophysiology is not thoroughly understood. Given that elevated albuminuria or circulating angiopoietin-2 associates with CVD and mortality in CKD patients, we were intrigued by the relationship between albuminuria and angiopoietin-2. A total of 416 patients with CKD stages 3 to 5 were stratified by urine albumin-creatinine ratio as normoalbuminuria (<30 mg/g), microalbuminuria (30–300 mg/g), or macroalbuminuria (>300 mg/g). The levels of plasma angiopoietin-2 and vascular endothelial growth factor (VEGF) increased, and soluble Tie-2 decreased in the subgroups of albuminuria; whereas angiopoietin-1 did not change. Linear regression showed a positive correlation between urine albumin-creatinine ratio (ACR) and plasma angiopoietin-2 (correlation coefficient $r = 0.301$, 95% confidence interval 0.211–0.386, $P < 0.0001$), but not between ACR and VEGF or soluble Tie-2. Multivariate linear regression analysis showed that plasma angiopoietin-2 was independently associated with ACR ($P = 0.025$). Furthermore, plasma angiopoietin-2 was positively correlated with high sensitive C-reactive protein ($r = 0.114$, 95% confidence interval 0.018–0.208, $P = 0.020$). In conclusion, plasma angiopoietin-2 was associated with albuminuria and markers of systemic microinflammation in CKD patients. Although previous evidence has shown that angiopoietin-2 destabilizes vasculature and induces inflammation in different scenarios, further study will be required to delineate the role of angiopoietin-2 in albuminuria and microinflammation in CKD patients.

Editor: Jeremy Stuart Duffield, University of Washington, United States of America

Funding: This study was supported by the National Science Council (99-2628-B-002-013, S.L.L., 101-2321-B-002-060, S.L.L.) (http://web1.nsc.gov.tw/), and Mrs. Hsiu-Chin Lee Kidney Research Foundation. The funders had no role in study design, data collection and analysis, decision to publish, or preparation of the manuscript.

Competing Interests: The authors have declared that no competing interests exist.

* E-mail: tschu@ntu.edu.tw

Introduction

It is well established that chronic kidney disease (CKD) is an independent risk factor of cardiovascular disease (CVD). Patients with CKD are more likely to die of CVD than to enter dialysis. High prevalence of traditional Framingham risk factors in CKD patients undoubtedly leads to high cardiovascular events. Nevertheless, the non-traditional risk factors more precisely elucidate the CKD-related elements.

Albuminuria is one of the manifestations in renal glomerular disease. Moreover, it is also indicative of endothelial damage and vascular disease in diverse populations. Evidence has shown that albuminuria is an independent predictor of cardiovascular events in both CKD and non-CKD patients [1,2,3,4,5,6]. Moreover, systemic microinflammation also infers the increased cardiovascular morbidity and mortality [7,8,9]. Although albuminuria and microinflammation explain the complex interplay in CKD, the effectors mediating the cross talk between CKD and CVD are still not confirmative.

Angiopoietin-1 (Ang-1) and angiopoietin-2 (Ang-2) are ligands of the Tie-2 receptor, the second class of vascular specific receptor tyrosine kinases in vascular development. The Ang/Tie-2 system regulates the quiescent and activated endothelial phenotype in a unique and nonredundant fashion [10]. Ang-1-mediated Tie-2 activation is required to maintain the quiescent resting endothelium [11,12]. Ang-1 functions are antagonized by Ang-2. Ang-2 destabilizes the quiescent endothelium and primes it to respond to exogenous stimuli, thereby modulate the activities of inflammatory (tumor necrosis factor-α, TNF-α) and angiogenic (vascular endothelial growth factor, VEGF) cytokines [10,13]. Concomitant occurrence of Ang-2 and other stimuli, such as TNF-α or VEGF, will promote endothelial cell proliferation, facilitate angiogenesis and induce inflammation. In the absence of VEGF, the endothelium switches back to the resting state, resulting in endothelial cell apoptosis and vascular regression. Elevated plasma Ang-2 has been shown in diseases with systemic inflammation including diabetes mellitus, hypertension, congestive heart failure, acute coronary syndrome, peripheral artery disease, critical illness, CKD and end-stage renal disease (ESRD) [14,15,16,17,18,19,20]. Notably, previous studies have shown that circulating Ang-2 levels are associated with CVD and predict the long-term mortality in CKD patients [20,21,22].

Given that elevated albuminuria and circulating Ang-2 predict CVD and mortality in CKD, we were intrigued by the relationship between albuminuria and Ang-2. In this cross-sectional study, we

Table 1. Clinical characteristics of the patients[a].

Albuminuria[b]	All (n = 416)	normoalbuminuria (n = 70)	microalbuminuria (n = 132)	macroalbuminuria (n = 214)	P[c]
Age (yr)	63.0 (54.0–71.0)	68.0 (56.0–73.0)	65.5 (55.0–71.0)	59.0 (50.8–71.0)**	0.005
Men [%, (n)]	63.5 (264)	78.6 (55)	62.1 (82)*	59.3 (127)*	0.014
Diabetes [%, (n)]	39.2 (163)	34.3 (24)	26.5 (35)	48.6 (104)*	<0.0001
Hypertension [%, (n)]	86.8 (361)	87.1 (61)	81.1 (107)	90.2 (193)	0.051
Smoker [%, (n)]	11.1 (46)	10.0 (7)	9.8 (13)	12.1 (26)	0.765
Dyslipidemia [%, (n)]	30.0 (125)	24.3 (17)	28.0 (37)	33.2 (71)	0.307
BMI (kg/m^2)	24.4 (22.0–27.0)	24.7 (22.5–26.7)	24.0 (21.2–27.1)	24.4 (22.2–27.1)	0.334
eGFR (mL/min/1.73 m^2)	27.3 (14.4–41.0)	42.0 (34.4–51.5)	29.5 (18.0–41.7)**	20.3 (10.6–34.1)**	<0.0001
Creatinine (mg/dL)	2.3 (1.7–4.2)	1.6 (1.4–2.0)	2.1 (1.6–3.6)**	3.0 (2.0–5.1)**	<0.0001
Albumin (g/dL)	4.5 (4.2–4.7)	4.6 (4.5–4.8)	4.6 (4.3–4.8)*	4.4 (4.1–4.6)**	<0.0001
Calcium (mmol/L)	2.32 (2.26–2.42)	2.38 (2.30–2.48)	2.34 (2.27–2.42)*	2.30 (2.23–2.39)**	<0.0001
Phosphate (mg/dL)	3.8 (3.3–4.5)	3.3 (3.0–3.6)	3.7 (3.3–4.2)**	4.2 (3.6–4.9)**	<0.0001
Urine albumin-creatinine ratio (mg/g)	332.8 (59.4–794.5)	14.7 (8.6–19.6)	105.6 (58.6–178.3)**	762.5 (537.2–1205.8)**	<0.0001
Hemoglobin (g/dL)	11.5 (9.9–13.5)	13.3 (11.4–14.4)	11.9 (9.7–13.6)*	11.1 (9.4–12.9)**	<0.0001
hsCRP (mg/dL)	0.120 (0.063–0.260)	0.110 (0.070–0.313)	0.130 (0.070–0.280)	0.120 (0.060–0.210)	0.392
iPTH	92.1 (51.2–176.0)	64.0 (41.9–86.6)	84.3 (50.1–147.8)*	119.0 (58.0–273.3)**	<0.0001
Uric acid (mg/dL)	8.2 (7.1–9.4)	7.5 (6.3–8.9)	7.8 (6.8–9.2)	8.5 (7.5–9.5)*	<0.0001
Ferritin	173.0 (103.0–282.8)	183.0 (104.3–324.5)	157.0 (100.3–268.3)	185.0 (104.5–283.8)	0.478

Note:
[a]Continuous and categorical variables were expressed as median (interquartile range) and percentage (number) respectively.
[b]Patients were stratified based on albuminuria (urine albumin-creatinine ratio) as normoalbuminuria (<30 mg/g), microalbuminuria (30–300 mg/g), macroalbuminuria (>300 mg/g).
[c]Chi-Square test in categorical variables, Kruskall-Wallis test in continuous variables.
*P<0.05 compared with normoalbuminuria group (Chi-Square test in categorical variables, Mann-Whitney U test in continuous variables).
**P<0.0001 compared with normoalbuminuria group (Chi-Square test in categorical variables, Mann-Whitney U test in continuous variables).
Abbreviations: BMI, body mass index; eGFR, estimated glomerular filtration rate; Calcium phosphate product, Calcium x Phosphate x 4; hsCRP, high sensitivity C-reactive protein; iPTH, intact parathyroid hormone.

aimed to define the relationship between plasma Ang-2 levels and albuminuria in patients with CKD stage 3 to 5.

Materials and Methods

Study Population

A cross-sectional study was performed in a single tertiary medical center in Taiwan from December 2006 to December 2007. Patients aged more than 18 years old from the outpatient clinic with CKD were eligible for inclusion. CKD was defined by either kidney damage or GFR criteria for at least 3 months [23]. We used the four-variable equation of the Modification of Diet in Renal Disease (MDRD) Study to estimate the GFR (eGFR) [24]. The urine albumin-creatinine ratio (ACR) was measured by dividing the urine albumin to creatinine concentration. Proteinuria based on ACR was defined as normoalbuminuria (<30 mg/g), microalbuminuria (30–300 mg/g), or macroalbuminuria (>300 mg/g). We excluded patients with current infection, malignancy, pregnancy, who had already received a kidney transplant or were receiving maintenance dialysis. All patients were maintained on their regular medication. The study was approved by the institutional review board of National Taiwan University Hospital (201105023RC) and registered. Written informed consent was obtained from all participants.

Ascertainment of Covariates

Patients were classified as hypertensive if systolic blood pressure ≥140 mmHg, diastolic blood pressure ≥90 mmHg, or with antihypertensive drugs use. Diabetes was defined by history and blood glucose values (using the American Diabetes Association criteria), oral hypoglycemic medication, or insulin use. The clinical definition of dyslipidemia was fasting total cholesterol ≥200 mg/dL, low-density lipoprotein ≥130 mg/dL, triglyceride ≥200 mg/dL, or lipid-lowering medication.

Blood and Urine Samplings

Fasting blood samples were collected in the morning. Blood samples were taken by antecubital venopuncture in the sitting position after resting for more than 5 minutes. The blood samples were collected into EDTA vacutainers and placed on ice immediately. Within 30 minutes of collection, samples were centrifuged at 3000 rpm (1000 g) and 4°C for 15 minutes. After overnight fasting, a random morning urine sample was collected for measurement of creatinine and albumin. The additional first-void specimens were collected after 3 months to confirm the presence of albuminuria. Plasma and urine were kept frozen in aliquots. Complete blood cell count and all biochemical analyses were performed in the Department of Laboratory Medicine, National Taiwan University Hospital.

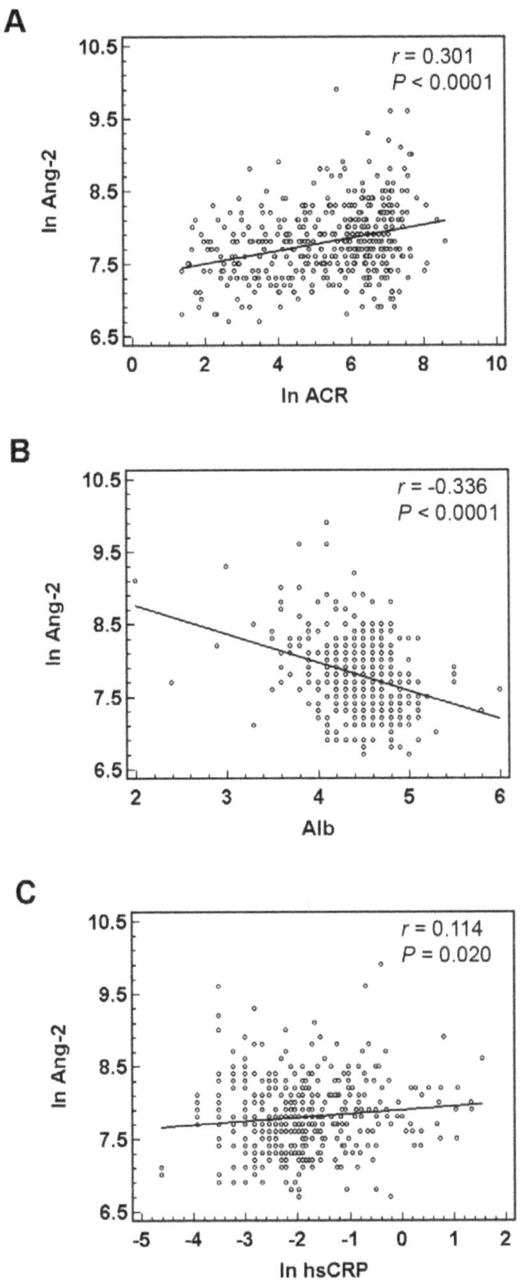

Figure 1. Plasma angiopoietin-2 was correlated with malnutrition, inflammation, and albuminuria. Univariate regression analysis showed the linear correlation of plasma angiopoietin-2 (Ang-2) with urine albumin-creatinine ratio (ACR) (A), high sensitive C-reactive protein (hsCRP) (B), and serum albumin (C). The levels of plasma Ang-2, ACR and hsCRP were expressed as natural logarithm (ln); r, Pearson correlation coefficient.

Enzyme-linked Immunosorbent Assay

Plasma Ang-1, Ang-2, VEGF and soluble Tie-2 (sTie-2) were measured in duplicate using commercial enzyme-linked immunosorbent assays (R&D System) according to the instructions of the manufacturer. The sensitivities of Ang-1, Ang-2, VEGF, and sTie-2 assays were 1.36, 1.20, 1.61, and 1.00 pg/mL, respectively. Intraassay coefficients of variation of Ang-1, Ang-2, VEGF, and sTie-2 were 2.1%, 1.3%, 1.6%, and 0.8%, respectively. Interassay coefficients of variance of Ang-1, Ang-2, VEGF, and sTie-2 were 1.8%, 2.0%, 2.1%, and 9.3%, respectively.

Statistical Analysis

Since the continuous baseline variables, including angiotrophic growth factors, were not normally distributed, differences between these variables among albuminuric status were analyzed using Kruskall-Wallis test. Differences in categorical variables were compared using the chi square test. To examine the correlations between Ang-2 and albumin, uric acid, high sensitive C-reactive protein (hsCRP) and ACR, Ang-2 was log-transformed. Pearson correlation coefficients were computed.

The Shapiro-Wilk test was used to test normality. Logarithmic transformation was made for variables when needed. A linear regression model was used to assess the relationship between Ang-2 and albuminuria. We first computed the univariate regression analysis and then generated several multivariable models. First, we adjusted for age and gender in model 1. Second, we further adjusted for all traditional and nontraditional risk factors for albuminuria, including diabetes, hypertension, dyslipidemia, mean brachial systolic blood pressure, eGFR levels, calcium phosphate product, hemoglobin, hsCRP, and medications in use. Estimated glomerular filtration rate was treated as a continuous variable. Medications included angiotensin converting enzyme (ACE) inhibitors or angiotensin II receptor blockers (ARBs), statins, calcium channel blocker, β-blocker, pentoxifylline. Each of them was treated as a categorical variable. Finally, we used the stepwise regression method to select variables. All statistical analyses were performed with STATA, version 9 (Stata Corp., College Station, Texas, USA).

Results

Clinical Characteristics of Patients

Total 416 participants with CKD stage 3 to 5 (average age 63 yr; 63.5% men) were analyzed (Table 1). We stratified patients into three groups according to the urine ACR level. Of all patients, 51.4% have macroalbuminuria (n = 214), 31.7% microalbuminuria (n = 132) and 16.8% are normoalbuminuria (n = 70). There is significant elevation of serum creatinine, phosphate and intact parathyroid hormone in patients with macroalbuminuria (P<0.0001). Likewise, anemia is more severe in the microalbuminuria and macroalbuminuria group (P= 0.001 and P<0.0001, respectively). Elevated uric acid and decreased albumin level were evident in patients with macroalbuminuria (P= 0.001 and P<0.0001) but not microalbuminuria group. Inflammatory biomarkers, including hsCRP and ferritin, did not vary with albuminuria.

Plasma Levels of Angiotrophic Growth Factors

Although there was no difference in the plasma levels of Ang-1 in the subgroups of albuminuria (P= 0.355, Table 2), plasma levels of Ang-2 were higher in the subgroups (P<0.0001, Table 2) and showed a positive correlation with ACR (correlation coefficient r= 0.301, 95% CI 0.211–0.386, P<0.0001, Fig. 1A). Although the plasma levels of VEGF were also higher in the subgroups of albuminuria (P= 0.001, Table 2), linear regression revealed no correlation between ACR and VEGF. Likewise, even though the plasma levels of sTie-2 were lower in the subgroups of albuminuria (P= 0.011, Table 2), there was no linear correlation with ACR.

We further analyzed the relationship between angiotrophic growth factors and eGFR. Linear regression analysis revealed an inverse correlation between Ang-2 levels and eGFR (r= -0.245, P<0.0001). The endogenous Ang-2 antagonist, sTie-2, was

Table 2. Plasma levels of angiotrophic growth factors.

Albuminuria	All (n = 416)	normoalbuminuria (n = 70)	microalbuminuria (n = 132)	macroalbuminuria (n = 214)	P
Ang-1 (pg/mL)	6636.3 (2850.0–11690.4)	6784.8 (2286.6–12698.2)	5707.3 (2779.4–10754.1)	6821.9 (2905.9–13082.5)	0.355
Ang-2 (pg/mL)	2355.1 (1726.3–3287.1)	1863.2 (1434.5–2448.7)	2252.3 (1679.7–2964.6)*	2580.2 (2000.7–3775.6)**	<0.0001
VEGF (pg/mL)	126.5 (69.7–215.0)	92.7 (33.9–174.9)	105.6 (60.7–195.3)	139.5 (81.0–237.7)*	0.001
sTie-2 (pg/mL)	12.4 (10.2–14.6)	13.6 (11.7–15.2)	11.8 (10.1–14.4)*	12.4 (10.2–14.3)*	0.011

Note: Data expressed as median (interquartile range).
*$P<0.05$ compared with normoalbuminuria group (Chi-Square test in categorical variables, Mann-Whitney U test in continuous variables).
**$P<0.0001$ compared with normoalbuminuria group (Chi-Square test in categorical variables, Mann-Whitney U test in continuous variables).
Abbreviations: Ang-1, angiopoietin-1; Ang-2, angiopoietin-2; VEGF, vascular endothelial growth factor; sTie-2, soluble Tie-2 receptor.

positively correlated with eGFR ($r = 0.186$, $P<0.0001$). Additional analyses of Ang-1 and VEGF only revealed weak association with eGFR ($P = 0.031$ for Ang-1, $P = 0.182$ for VEGF).

Plasma Ang-2 Associated with Markers of Systemic Microinflammation

Since Ang-2 sensitizes endothelial cells and has a crucial role in the induction of inflammation [10], markers representative of microinflammation were assessed. In the measurements of hsCRP, 78.8% and 56.7% of our patients were >0.05 mg/dL and >0.1 mg/dL respectively. We confirmed the association between the plasma levels of Ang-2 and hsCRP ($r = 0.114$, 95% CI 0.018–0.208, $P = 0.020$, Fig. 1B). Blood uric acid and ferritin level were also positively correlated with plasma levels of Ang-2 ($r = 0.171$, 95% CI 0.076–0.263, $P = 0.001$ for uric acid, and $r = 0.129$, 95% CI 0.033–0.222, $P = 0.009$ for ferritin). On the contrary, the levels of serum albumin and hemoglobin showed an inverse correlation with Ang-2 ($r = -0.336$, 95% CI -0.412– -0.248, $P<0.0001$, Fig. 1C; $r = -0.322$, 95% CI -0.406– -0.233, $P<0.0001$). Among all patients, there were 10.8% with albumin <4 g/dL and 39.1% with hemoglobin <11 g/dL.

Plasma Ang-2 Associated with Albuminuria Independently

To delineate the association between Ang-2 and ACR, linear regression analyses adjusted for potential confounding factors was performed (Table 3). ACR was log-transformed and treated as the outcome variable. Univariate regression analysis revealed significant association between Ang-2 and ACR ($P<0.001$). After multivariate adjustment, Ang-2 still revealed independent association with ACR ($P = 0.026$). Age, diabetes, mean systolic blood pressure, eGFR and medication in use were further selected in the stepwise regression analysis. We confirmed the independent association between plasma levels of Ang-2 and ACR ($P = 0.025$; with 1 pg/mL increment of Ang-2 increased ACR by 1 mg/g after exponentiation).

Discussion

This is the first study that demonstrates the association of plasma Ang-2 with albuminuria and microinflammation in patients with CKD stages 3 to 5. Among the angiogenic growth factors, only Ang-2 shows the positive correlation with albuminuria and hsCRP. We also report inverse correlation between eGFR and plasma Ang-2 levels in moderate to severe CKD patients.

Table 3. Multivariate-adjusted linear regression analyses of albumin-creatinine ratio and angiopoietin-2[a].

	Albuminuria (ACR)		
	Regression Coefficient β (10^{-4})	P	95% Confidence Interval
Univariate			
Ang-2	2.292	<0.001	1.452–3.132
Multivariate			
Model 1[b]	2.354	<0.001	1.518–3.191
Model 2[c]	0.921	0.026	0.113–1.730
Model 3[d]	0.902	0.025	0.113–1.692

Note:
[a]Albuminuria (ACR) was natural logarithm transformed.
[b]Model 1: Ang-2+age+gender.
[c]Model 2: Model 1+traditional risk (hypertension, diabetes, dyslipidemia, mean brachial SBP, eGFR) +nontraditional risk (Calcium phosphate product, hemoglobin, high sensitive C reactive protein, medication including ACE inhibitor, ARB, statin, calcium channel blocker, β-blocker, pentoxifylline).
[d]Model 3: stepwise regression method for variables in model 2.
Abbreviations: ACR, urine albumin-creatinine ratio; SBP, systolic blood pressure; ACE inhibitor, angiotensin-converting enzyme inhibitor; ARB, angiotensin II receptor blocker.

We demonstrated the independent association of plasma Ang-2 with albuminuria in CKD patients. The magnitude of albuminuria is associated with not only increased risk of CVD in general population, but also mortality and ESRD in diverse CKD populations [6,25]. Several hypotheses have been postulated in translating albuminuria to high cardiovascular risk in CKD [6]. However, the exact mechanism is still obscure. David S et al have reported that increased circulating Ang-2 is associated with CVD and mortality in CKD and dialysis patients [20,21,22]. In our CKD patients, plasma levels of Ang-2 were still associated with higher albuminuria after we adjusted for possible confounders, including blood pressure and eGFR. The association between plasma Ang-2 levels and albuminuria might suggest the role of Ang-2 in linking CVD in CKD. It is recognized that CVD increases since the early CKD stage without markedly increased uremic toxins or asymmetric dimethylarginine (ADMA) [2,26,27,28]. Although we cannot demonstrate the causal relationship in this observational study, these observations suggest the crucial role of endothelial damage in the pathogenesis.

We also found the positive correlation between plasma Ang-2 and inflammatory markers in our CKD patients. CKD is recognized as a disease with persistent and low-grade inflammation. Altered cytokine milieu and acute-phase protein, including interleukin-6, TNF-α, and CRP may directly mediate the initiation and progression of CKD complications [9]. Among them, CRP truly reflects a status of microinflammation and increased cardiovascular events [7]. Nevertheless, the functional role of CRP is still an issue of dilemma [29,30,31,32,33]. In acute inflammation, CRP responds rapidly with wide dynamic range, but direct toxic effect does not appear. In addition to the endothelial effect, Ang-2 has complex effects on inflammatory responses [10,34]. Noteworthily, there was no correlation between hsCRP and albuminuria in our CKD patients, which might suggest the more promising role of Ang-2 in the endothelial damage and inflammatory induction in CKD.

The mechanism linking endothelial dysfunction, albuminuria and CVD is that endothelial dysfunction leads to increased vascular permeability and glomerular albumin leakage [1]. Increased endothelial Ang-2 secretion is stimulated by exogenous stimuli such as hypoxia, angiotensin II, TNF-α, and reactive oxygen species (ROS) [35]; all of them are common features of CKD and glomerular albuminuria. Mice with podocyte-specific expression of Ang-2 displayed endothelial cell apoptosis and albuminuria [36]. Sustained increases in plasma Ang-2 by conditional expression in liver promoted the remodeling of coronary arteries and reduced the density of endocardial vessels [37]. It is reasonable to propose that endothelial damage in general and glomerular vasculature may lead to endothelial Ang-2 secretion in CKD patients. Elevated Ang-2 might further increase glomerular albuminuria through endothelial damage. However, it is still not clear whether the plasma Ang-2 levels are good indicators of tissue effects in CKD.

There were several limitations in this cross-sectional study. We could only demonstrated the association between Ang-2 and symbolized markers (of microinflammation and vascular injury). In proposing that Ang-2 connects albuminuria to cardiovascular event, we need to investigate the relationship between albuminuria and Ang-2 in early-stage CKD and control group with endothelial dysfunction (such as hypertension or diabetes mellitus). Prospective studies based on Ang-2 stratification are necessary to study the renal and cardiovascular prognosis in CKD. Besides, the mechanisms attributable to increased systemic Ang-2 are not clearly recognized. A delicate animal model is necessary to investigate the exact origin and the causal relationship between Ang-2 and albuminuria in CKD.

In conclusion, plasma Ang-2 was associated with albuminuria and microinflammation in patients with CKD stage 3 to 5. Ang-2 might be a novel non-traditional cardiovascular risk factor in CKD patients. We need further study to identify its role in translating the systemic cardiovascular effect of albuminuria.

Acknowledgments

Thanks to Dr. Wen-Chih Chiang, Vin-Cent Wu, Tze-Wah Kao, Chung-Jen Yen for recruiting patients and valuable discussion, Mr. Kuo-Tong Huang for technical assistance.

Author Contributions

Conceived and designed the experiments: F-CC T-SC S-LL. Performed the experiments: F-CC C-KC. Analyzed the data: F-CC T-SL. Contributed reagents/materials/analysis tools: T-SL C-KC Y-MC M-SW T-SC K-DW S-LL. Wrote the paper: F-CC T-SC S-LL.

References

1. Hillege HL, Fidler V, Diercks GF, van Gilst WH, de Zeeuw D, et al. (2002) Urinary albumin excretion predicts cardiovascular and noncardiovascular mortality in general population. Circulation 106: 1777–1782.
2. Arnlov J, Evans JC, Meigs JB, Wang TJ, Fox CS, et al. (2005) Low-grade albuminuria and incidence of cardiovascular disease events in nonhypertensive and nondiabetic individuals: the Framingham Heart Study. Circulation 112: 969–975.
3. Cirillo M, Laurenzi M, Panarelli P, Mancini M, Zanchetti A, et al. (2004) Relation of urinary albumin excretion to coronary heart disease and low renal function: role of blood pressure. Kidney Int 65: 2290–2297.
4. Brenner BM, Cooper ME, de Zeeuw D, Keane WF, Mitch WE, et al. (2001) Effects of losartan on renal and cardiovascular outcomes in patients with type 2 diabetes and nephropathy. N Engl J Med 345: 861–869.
5. de Zeeuw D, Remuzzi G, Parving HH, Keane WF, Zhang Z, et al. (2004) Albuminuria, a therapeutic target for cardiovascular protection in type 2 diabetic patients with nephropathy. Circulation 110: 921–927.
6. Stehouwer CD, Smulders YM (2006) Microalbuminuria and risk for cardiovascular disease: Analysis of potential mechanisms. J Am Soc Nephrol 17: 2106–2111.
7. Libby P, Ridker PM, Maseri A (2002) Inflammation and atherosclerosis. Circulation 105: 1135–1143.
8. Yeun JY, Levine RA, Mantadilok V, Kaysen GA (2000) C-Reactive protein predicts all-cause and cardiovascular mortality in hemodialysis patients. Am J Kidney Dis 35: 469–476.
9. Stenvinkel P, Ketteler M, Johnson RJ, Lindholm B, Pecoits-Filho R, et al. (2005) IL-10, IL-6, and TNF-alpha: central factors in the altered cytokine network of uremia–the good, the bad, and the ugly. Kidney Int 67: 1216–1233.
10. Fiedler U, Reiss Y, Scharpfenecker M, Grunow V, Koidl S, et al. (2006) Angiopoietin-2 sensitizes endothelial cells to TNF-alpha and has a crucial role in the induction of inflammation. Nat Med 12: 235–239.
11. Kim I, Kim HG, So JN, Kim JH, Kwak HJ, et al. (2000) Angiopoietin-1 regulates endothelial cell survival through the phosphatidylinositol 3′-kinase/Akt signal transduction pathway. Circ Res 86: 24–29.
12. Thurston G, Rudge JS, Ioffe E, Zhou H, Ross L, et al. (2000) Angiopoietin-1 protects the adult vasculature against plasma leakage. Nat Med 6: 460–463.
13. Maisonpierre PC, Suri C, Jones PF, Bartunkova S, Wiegand S, et al. (1997) Angiopoietin-2, a natural antagonist for Tie2 that disrupts in vivo angiogenesis. Science 277: 55–60.
14. Lim HS, Blann AD, Chong AY, Freestone B, Lip GY (2004) Plasma vascular endothelial growth factor, angiopoietin-1, and angiopoietin-2 in diabetes: implications for cardiovascular risk and effects of multifactorial intervention. Diabetes Care 27: 2918–2924.
15. Nadar SK, Blann A, Beevers DG, Lip GY (2005) Abnormal angiopoietins 1&2, angiopoietin receptor Tie-2 and vascular endothelial growth factor levels in hypertension: relationship to target organ damage [a sub-study of the Anglo-Scandinavian Cardiac Outcomes Trial (ASCOT)]. J Intern Med 258: 336–343.
16. Chong AY, Caine GJ, Freestone B, Blann AD, Lip GY (2004) Plasma angiopoietin-1, angiopoietin-2, and angiopoietin receptor tie-2 levels in congestive heart failure. J Am Coll Cardiol 43: 423–428.
17. Lee KW, Lip GY, Blann AD (2004) Plasma angiopoietin-1, angiopoietin-2, angiopoietin receptor tie-2, and vascular endothelial growth factor levels in acute coronary syndromes. Circulation 110: 2355–2360.
18. Kontos CD, Findley CM, Mitchell RG, Duscha BD, Annex BH (2008) Plasma levels of soluble Tie2 and vascular endothelial growth factor distinguish critical

limb ischemia from intermittent claudication in patients with peripheral arterial disease. J Am Coll Cardiol 52: 387–393.
19. Orfanos SE, Kotanidou A, Glynos C, Athanasiou C, Tsigkos S, et al. (2007) Angiopoietin-2 is increased in severe sepsis: Correlation with inflammatory mediators. Crit Care Med 35: 199–206.
20. David S, Kumpers P, Hellpap J, Horn R, Leitolf H, et al. (2009) Angiopoietin 2 and cardiovascular disease in dialysis and kidney transplantation. Am J Kidney Dis 53: 770–778.
21. David S, Kumpers P, Lukasz A, Fliser D, Martens-Lobenhoffer J, et al. (2010) Circulating angiopoietin-2 levels increase with progress of chronic kidney disease. Nephrol Dial Transplant 25: 2571–2576.
22. David S, John SG, Jefferies HJ, Sigrist MK, Kumpers P, et al. (2012) Angiopoietin-2 levels predict mortality in CKD patients. Nephrol Dial Transplant 27: 1867–1872.
23. National Kidney Foundation (2002) K/DOQI clinical practice guidelines for chronic kidney disease: evaluation, classification, and stratification. Am J Kidney Dis 39: S1–266.
24. Levey AS, Bosch JP, Lewis JB, Greene T, Rogers N, et al. (1999) A more accurate method to estimate glomerular filtration rate from serum creatinine: a new prediction equation. Modification of Diet in Renal Disease Study Group. Ann Intern Med 130: 461–470.
25. Astor BC, Matsushita K, Gansevoort RT, van der Velde M, Woodward M, et al. (2011) Lower estimated glomerular filtration rate and higher albuminuria are associated with mortality and end-stage renal disease. A collaborative meta-analysis of kidney disease population cohorts. Kidney Int 79: 1331–1340.
26. Kielstein JT, Zoccali C (2005) Asymmetric dimethylarginine: a cardiovascular risk factor and a uremic toxin coming of age? Am J Kidney Dis 46: 186–202.
27. Klausen K, Borch-Johnsen K, Feldt-Rasmussen B, Jensen G, Clausen P, et al. (2004) Very low levels of microalbuminuria are associated with increased risk of coronary heart disease and death independently of renal function, hypertension, and diabetes. Circulation 110: 32–35.
28. Watts GF, Herrmann S, Dogra GK, Playford DA, Best JD, et al. (2001) Vascular function of the peripheral circulation in patients with nephrosis. Kidney Int 60: 182–189.
29. Kaplan MH, Volanakis JE (1974) Interaction of C-reactive protein complexes with the complement system. I. Consumption of human complement associated with the reaction of C-reactive protein with pneumococcal C-polysaccharide and with the choline phosphatides, lecithin and sphingomyelin. J Immunol 112: 2135–2147.
30. Pasceri V, Cheng JS, Willerson JT, Yeh ET (2001) Modulation of C-reactive protein-mediated monocyte chemoattractant protein-1 induction in human endothelial cells by anti-atherosclerosis drugs. Circulation 103: 2531–2534.
31. Zhang R, Zhang YY, Huang XR, Wu Y, Chung AC, et al. (2010) C-reactive protein promotes cardiac fibrosis and inflammation in angiotensin II-induced hypertensive cardiac disease. Hypertension 55: 953–960.
32. Paul A, Ko KW, Li L, Yechoor V, McCrory MA, et al. (2004) C-reactive protein accelerates the progression of atherosclerosis in apolipoprotein E-deficient mice. Circulation 109: 647–655.
33. Tennent GA, Hutchinson WL, Kahan MC, Hirschfield GM, Gallimore JR, et al. (2008) Transgenic human CRP is not pro-atherogenic, pro-atherothrombotic or pro-inflammatory in apoE−/− mice. Atherosclerosis 196: 248–255.
34. Lemieux C, Maliba R, Favier J, Theoret JF, Merhi Y, et al. (2005) Angiopoietins can directly activate endothelial cells and neutrophils to promote proinflammatory responses. Blood 105: 1523–1530.
35. Fiedler U, Augustin HG (2006) Angiopoietins: a link between angiogenesis and inflammation. Trends Immunol 27: 552–558.
36. Davis B, Dei Cas A, Long DA, White KE, Hayward A, et al. (2007) Podocyte-specific expression of angiopoietin-2 causes proteinuria and apoptosis of glomerular endothelia. J Am Soc Nephrol 18: 2320–2329.
37. Bureau W, Van Slyke P, Jones J, Han RN, Ward NL, et al. (2006) Chronic systemic delivery of angiopoietin-2 reveals a possible independent angiogenic effect. Am J Physiol Heart Circ Physiol 291: H948–956.

18

Chronic Kidney Disease is Characterized by "Double Trouble" Higher Pulse Pressure plus Night-Time Systolic Blood Pressure and More Severe Cardiac Damage

Massimiliano Fedecostante[1]*, Francesco Spannella[1], Giovanna Cola[2], Emma Espinosa[1], Paolo Dessì-Fulgheri[1], Riccardo Sarzani[1]

1 Internal Medicine and Geriatrics and "Hypertension Excellence Centre" of the European Society of Hypertension, Department of Clinical and Molecular Sciences, University "Politecnica delle Marche", Italian National Research Centre on Aging "U. Sestilli", IRCCS-INRCA, Ancona, Italy, **2** Cardiology Clinic, Department of Cardiovascular Sciences, University "Politecnica delle Marche", "Ospedali Riuniti", Ancona, Italy

Abstract

Background: Hypertension plays a key role in chronic kidney disease (CKD), but CKD itself affects the blood pressure (BP) profile. The aim of this study was to assess the association of BP profile with CKD and the presence of cardiac organ damage.

Methods: We studied 1805 patients, referred to our Hypertension Centre, in whom ABPM, blood tests, and echocardiography were clinically indicated. The glomerular filtration rate was estimated (eGFR) using the MDRD equation and CKD was defined as eGFR<60 mL/min/1.73 m^2. Cardiac organ damage was evaluated by echocardiography.

Results: Among patients with CKD there were higher systolic blood pressure (SBP) during the night-time, greater prevalence of non-dippers (OR: 1.8) and increased pulse pressure (PP) during 24-hour period, daytime and night-time (all p<0.001). Patients with CKD had a greater LVM/h$^{2.7}$ index, and a higher prevalence of left ventricular hypertrophy and diastolic dysfunction (all p<0.001). Nocturnal SBP and PP correlated more strongly with cardiac organ damage (p<0.001). Patients with CKD had a greater Treatment Intensity Score (p<0.001) in the absence of a significantly greater BP control.

Conclusions: CKD patients have an altered night-time pressure profile and higher PP that translate into a more severe cardiac organ damage. In spite of a greater intensity of treatment in most patients with CKD, BP control was similar to patients without CKD. Our findings indicate the need of a better antihypertensive therapy in CKD, better selected drugs, dosages and posology to provide optimal coverage of 24 hours and night-time BP.

Editor: Partha Mukhopadhyay, National Institutes of Health, United States of America

Funding: The authors have no support or funding to report.

Competing Interests: The authors have declared that no competing interests exist.

* E-mail: mfedek@gmail.com

Introduction

Chronic kidney disease (CKD) is a major health problem and its prevalence is increasing worldwide [1]. A GFR lower than 60 mL/min/1.73 m^2 for 3 months indicates CKD, regardless of the presence or absence of kidney damage [2]. More than 10% of the adult population of U.S. has some degree of renal impairment and almost half of these subjects (5–6%) are affected by a significant reduction of renal function (GFR <60 ml/min/1.73 m^2) [3]. Data available from many European Countries are similar regarding prevalence and incidence of CKD [4] whereas only limited data concerning the prevalence of CKD in Italy have been published [5].

High blood pressure (BP) can be either a cause or a consequence of CKD [2]. Considering also the role of BP in diabetes, high BP is believed to be the leading cause of end-stage renal disease (ESRD). Every year, high BP causes more than 25,000 new cases of kidney failure in the United States [6]. A recent study shows that even pre-hypertension is significantly associated with an increased risk of CKD and it can be considered one of the relevant causes of CKD in the general population because of its high frequency [7]. In any case, when CKD is established BP increases. The results of Modification of Diet in Renal Disease (MDRD) study confirmed previous reports indicating that, in renal disease, hypertension is determined by the level of renal function [8].

Moreover, CKD is strongly associated with inadequate BP control. Many individuals with CKD are hypertensive and receive medications for controlling BP. However, the majority of these patients seem to be undertreated. Optimizing blood pressure treatment in this high-risk population can have a great potential in decreasing renal disease incidence and cardiovascular mortality [9].

Several studies reported that patients with an altered circadian blood pressure pattern, as non-dippers, have a higher risk of major cardiovascular events compared with patients with a normal pressure pattern [10–13].

Patients with CKD may have a non-dipping BP pattern. The explanation for this is not clear, but many factors have been proposed (e.g. defective natriuresis during daytime and increased blood pressure/natriuresis during the night) [14,15].

To date, to the best of our knowledge, there is little data available, especially for the Italian population, regarding the interrelationships between estimated glomerular filtration rate (eGFR), BP values and patterns (dipper, non-dipper) and echocardiographic parameters. Therefore, the rationale of our study was to investigate the associations between eGFR, BP values and patterns and echocardiographic parameters, to see how CKD and BP values and patterns may correlate with the presence of a cardiac organ damage.

The main aim of our study was to assess 24-h BP values and patterns and their relationship with eGFR and cardiac damage, in a population referred to a single "Hypertension Excellence Centre" for BP evaluation, in the hope to improve the clinical management of these patients in the absence of similar published data.

Materials and Methods

All participants have given their informed written consent and clinical investigations have been conducted according to the principles expressed in the Declaration of Helsinki. This study was approved by the local institutional ethics committee (Comitato di Bioetica, Ospedali Riuniti, Ancona). We studied outpatients referred to our Hypertension Centre for BP related problems Inclusion criteria were: clinical indication to undergo ABPM, plasma creatinine measurement and echocardiography. Main exclusion criteria were: age<18 years, low-quality of pressure monitoring (rate of artifacts >25% and/or recording duration less than 20 continuous hours and/or <2 record per hour at daytime and 1 record per hour at night-time), and unreliable data regarding anti-hypertensive treatment. After exclusions, 1805 patients were studied; eGFR was estimated using the MDRD study equation [8] taking into account the dosage of creatinine by the Jaffé reaction.

CKD was defined as the presence of confirmed eGFR <60 ml/min/1.73 m^2 in patients having the clinical indication to at least two creatinine determinations, the second one obtained 3 to 6 months after the first one (n = 962, 53.5% of the studied population, 100% of patients with eGFR <60 ml/min/1.73 m^2). No significant differences in creatinine/eGFR were found between the two time points (assessed by paired t-Test), supporting the notion that 15% of our patients truly had CKD.

CKD stages were defined according to the international classification of National Kidney Foundation [2]. For each subject 24-h BP, daytime BP (defined as the BP values from 6 a.m. to 10 p.m.), night-time BP (defined as the BP values from 10 p.m. to 6 a.m) and pulse pressure (PP) [defined as systolic blood pressure (SBP) - diastolic blood pressure (DBP)] were evaluated. Daytime and night-time periods were defined based on a questionnaire, in which patients were asked about their sleeping behavior. Among patients under anti-hypertensive treatment, those with mean 24-h BP <130/80 mmHg, mean daytime BP <135/85 mmHg, and mean night-time BP <120/70 mmHg were defined as controlled hypertensive. Among untreated patients we labeled not-hypertensive those patients with mean 24-h BP <130/80 mmHg, mean daytime BP <135/85 mmHg, and mean night-time BP <120/70 mmHg [16]. We considered dippers those patients with a change in mean awake SBP to sleep SBP equal to or grater than 10%. We considered as night-to-day ratio the ratio between medium night-time and daytime values recorded performing ABPM. Night-to-day ratios were multiplied by 100, expressing night-time BP as a percentage of a daytime level. A ratio of 100% or higher indicated the absence of a BP fall at night [17]. After evaluating drug therapy adherence by MMAS [18] a treatment intensity score (TIS) was calculated to compare many different drug associations. As previously reported [19], the recorded daily dose taken by the patients was divided by the maximum recommended daily dose to obtain a proportional dose (called "intensity") for that medication. The maximum recommended daily doses set by the Italian National Drug Agency (AIFA) were used for calculations. For completeness, dual-class drugs were separated into their components, and intensity was calculated separately for each chemical compound. The sum of all the different values was recorded as the TIS.

Statistical analysis

Data were analyzed with the Statistical Package for Social Science version 13 (SPSS Inc. Chicago, Illinois, USA). A value of $p<0.05$ was defined as statistically significant. Quantitative variables were checked for normality. Normally distributed continuous variables were described as a mean ± standard deviation (SD). The unpaired t-test and ANOVA (for multiple comparisons) were used to compare normally distributed quantitative variables with Bonferroni correction for multiple comparisons. The χ^2 test was used to analyze the differences between the categorical variables. Logistic and linear regression analysis and ANCOVA were used to create adjusted models.

Results

General characteristics of the population with reliable ABPM and drug therapy are shown in Table 1. We studied 1805 patients: 1012 men (56.1%) and 793 women (43.9%). There were 1535 (85.0%) patients with eGFR ≥60 ml/min/1.73 m^2 and 270 (15.0%) CKD patients. Hypertension was present in 1680 (93.1%) patients; 1194 (71.1%) were on drug treatment: 311 (26.0%) were controlled, 883 (74.0%) were not controlled. CKD stages are shown in Table 2. Only 10 patients (3.7%) of CKD subgroup had stages 4–5 (eGFR <30 ml/min/1.73 m^2). Among the CKD patients 264 (almost all: 97.8%) were hypertensives, 218 (82.6%) were currently drug-treated, but only 63 (28.9%) had controlled BP.

CKD and BP values

As shown in Figure 1. Panel A-Panel B, 24-h and daytime SBP did not differ significantly between patients with or without CKD, but CKD patients had higher night-time SBP (127.6±17.6 vs. 123.4±15.2 mmHg; $p<0.001$; Figure 1. Panel C). On the contrary, lower 24 hours (75.6±10.4 vs. 80.6±10.6 mmHg; Figure 1. Panel A), daytime (77.9±10.8 vs. 83.7±10.9 mmHg; Figure 1. Panel B), and night-time (69.8±10.3 vs. 73.0±10.9 mmHg; Figure 1. Panel C) DBP were found in CKD where PP was higher in 24 hours (57.5±13.3 vs.

Table 1. General characteristics of 1805 patients studied with ABPM, echocardiography, and eGFR.

	eGFR ≥ 60 ml/min/1.73 m^2	CKD	P
Age (years ± SD)	53.6±13.2	66.2±11.4	**<0.001**
BMI (Kg/m^2 ± SD)	27.4±4.4	27.7±4.7	n.s.
eGFR	79.0±12.3	51.2±8.9	**<0.001**

Table 2. Prevalence of CKD stages.

eGFR (ml/min/ 1.73 m²)	Mean ± Sd.	95% CI	n°	%
45≤eGFR<60	54.9±4.2	54.4–55.5	215	79.6%
30≤eGFR<45	39.3±3.7	38.1–40.4	45	16.7%
eGFR<30	24.2±5.3	20.4–28.1	10	3.7%

50.8±9.8 mmHg), daytime (57.6±13.5 vs. 51.0±10.0 mmHg) and night-time (57.7±14.0 vs. 50.3±10.3 mmHg) periods (all p<0.001) (Figure 2). These results were confirmed within worsening CKD stages (Figure 3 panel A–D), after adjustment for age and TIS, and in the linear regression model (Table 3): a significant relationship between the 24-h pressure profile and CKD was found only for nocturnal pressure values and for daytime, night-time and 24-h PP.

CKD, dipping pattern, and night-to-day ratio

Along with higher night-time SBP, patients with CKD showed higher prevalence of non-dipping pattern (72.6% vs. 59.4%; OR: 1.8, CI: 1.36–2.41; p<0.001) (Figure 4) and CKD was an independent risk factor for non- dipping pattern even after adjusting for sex, age, BMI, and TIS in a logistic regression model (Table 4). Patients with CKD also showed a linear association between eGFR reduction and night-to-day ratio ($\beta = -0.123$; p<0.001), another index of altered nocturnal BP.

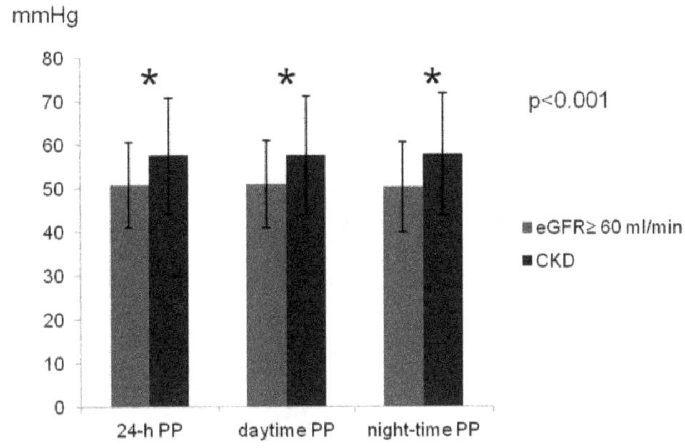

Figure 2. Difference in PP between patients with CKD and the rest of the population.

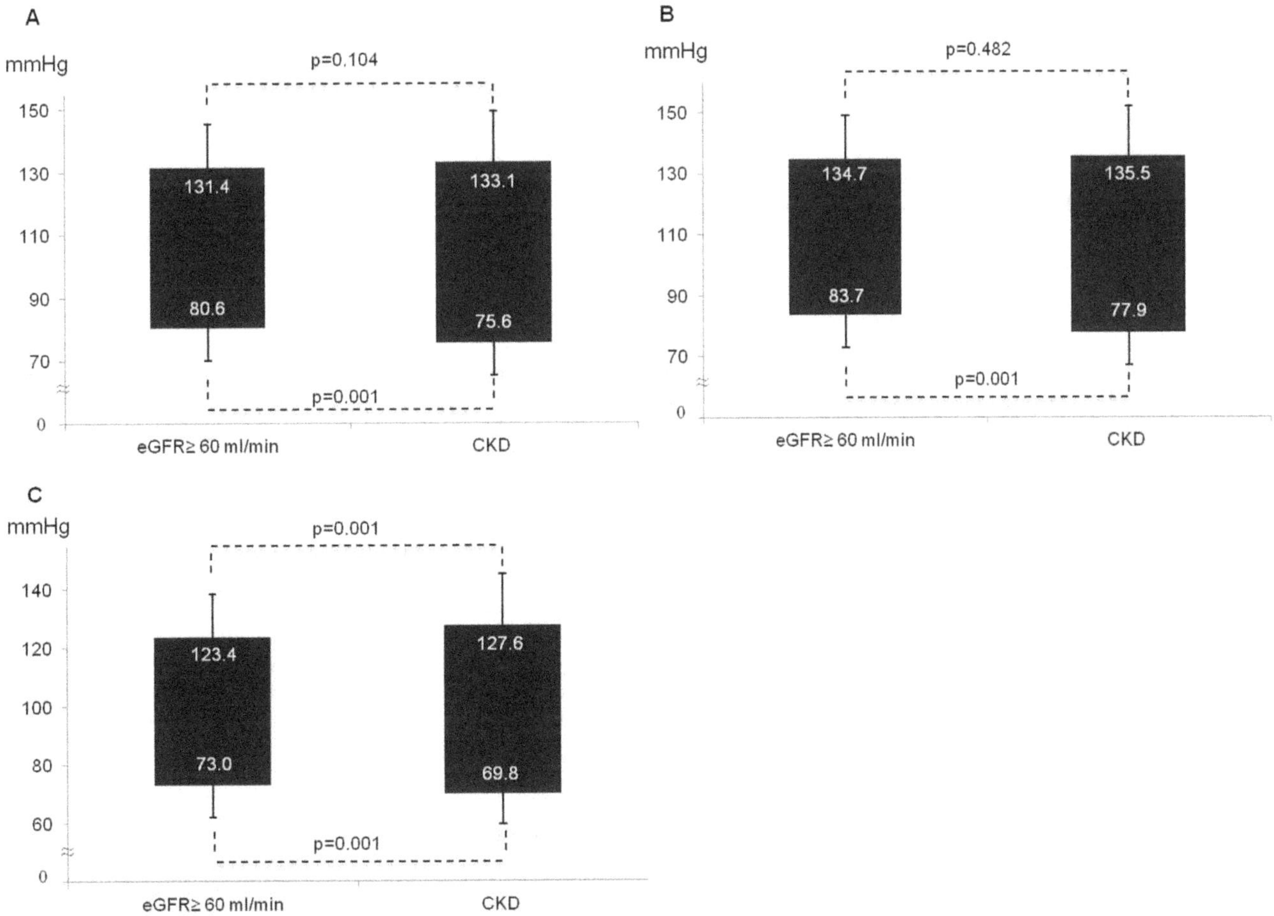

Figure 1. ABPM values in CKD patients vs. the rest of the population. Panel A. Difference in 24-h BP between patients with CKD and the rest of the population. Panel B. Difference in daytime BP between patients with CKD and the rest of the population. Panel C. Difference in night-time BP between patients with CKD and the rest of the population.

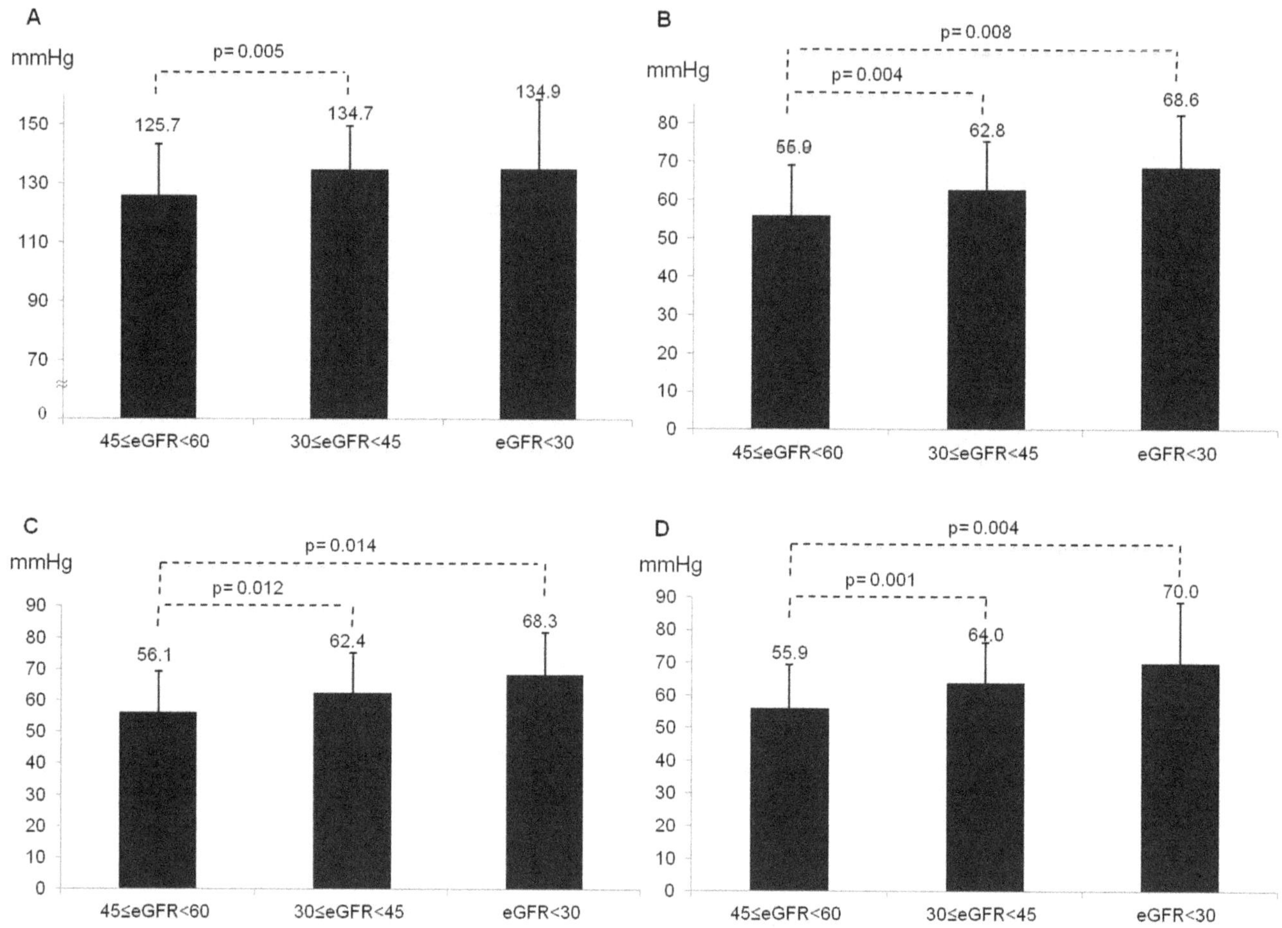

Figure 3. Correlation between ABPM values and CKD stages. Panel A. Difference in night-time BP between CKD stages. Panel B. Difference in 24 h PP between CKD stages. Panel C. Difference in daytime PP between CKD stages. Panel D. Difference in night-time PP between CKD stages.

CKD, BP values and patterns and cardiac damage

Considering the association with cardiac organ damage, patients with CKD had greater LVM/$h^{2.7}$ (60.9±21.9 vs. 51.8±13.1 g/$m^{2.7}$, $p<0.001$) and higher prevalence of left ventricular hypertrophy (79.0% vs. 61.4%, OR 2.48 CI:1.58–3.56; $p<0.001$) (Figure 5 Panel A–B). Indeed, linear regression model showed that night-time SBP as well as 24-h, daytime and night-time PP were independently associated with LVM/$h^{2.7}$ after adjusting for age, sex, BMI, TIS and the presence/absence of CKD (Tables 5, 6, 7, 8). A higher prevalence of an index of diastolic dysfunction that was available in all patients, was also found in patients with CKD (E/A ratio <1: 79.3% vs. 54.5%, OR 3.2 CI:1.97–5.18; $p<0.001$).

Table 3. Correlation between ABPM parameters and eGFR assessed by linear regression.

	B	P
24-h SBP	−0.019	0.413
24-h DBP	0.172	**<0.001**
Daytime SBP	0.007	0.765
Daytime DBP	0.192	**<0.001**
Night-time SBP	−0.066	**0.005**
Night-time DBP	0.118	**<0.001**
24-h PP	−0.197	**<0.001**
Daytime PP	−0.186	**<0.001**
Night-time PP	−0.205	**<0.001**

CKD and BP control

Patients with CKD had a greater TIS (1.56±0.91 vs. 1.19±0.72; $p<0.001$) without significantly better BP control but, on the contrary, a tendency toward worse control (25.4% vs. 28.9%; p = n.s.). Among hypertensive patients treated but with BP not controlled, there was a significantly higher percentage (87.3%) of CKD with uncontrolled night-time SBP; OR = 2.4 (CI:1.11–5.33; p = 0.022). Isolated uncontrolled night-time SBP were also increased in CKD (prevalence 20.6%) vs patients with eGFR ≥ 60 ml/min/1.73 m^2 (12.9%; p = 0.012) OR = 1.7 (CI:1.12–2.74).

Discussion

We studied a large patient population with clinical indication to perform ABPM, lab test for plasma creatinine and echocardiography. The main findings in patients with CKD were an altered SBP profile at night-time (higher BP and a more frequent non dipper-pattern) and a higher PP which depends also on a significantly lower DBP. Higher SBP values in patients with

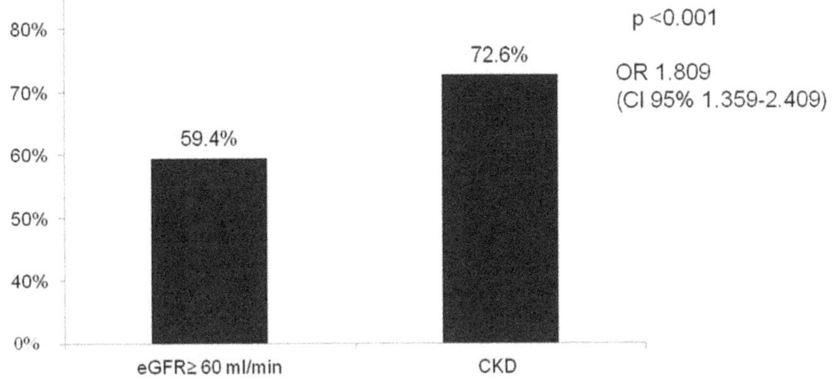

Figure 4. Prevalence of non dipping pattern in CKD.

CKD could be merely due to the higher prevalence of hypertension in these patients, as well as to a higher prevalence of severe hypertension in CKD. However, 24-hours and daytime pressures were not different between patients with and without CKD. Only night-time SBP and the dipper pattern were altered, leading to the hypothesis of a direct influence of CKD on nocturnal blood pressure profile. Impaired natriuresis in daytime may increase nocturnal SBP in order to compensate the diminished natriuresis with pressure natriuresis. Fujii et al [20] showed that the circadian rhythm of natriuresis is disturbed in patients with a non-dipper type of essential hypertension, in whom BP was usually sodium sensitive [21,22]. Since the sodium sensitivity of blood pressure is considered to be caused by reduced GFR and/or increased tubular reabsorption of sodium [23,24], such disarrangement may be clearly recognized in CKD in which renal function is deteriorated. In line with these findings, Fukuda et al [25] showed that, in the impaired renal function characterizing glomerulopathy, the nocturnal dipping of blood pressure is lost, resulting in enhanced urinary sodium and protein excretion during night-time. An important role seems to be played by the autonomic nervous system, since renal denervation has resulted in improvement of the nocturnal blood pressure profile in patients with moderate to severe CKD, leading to a reduction in night-to-day ratio and a restoration of the physiological circadian BP rhythm [26].

In our study, the association between non-dipping pattern and CKD was independent of age, sex, BMI and TIS, highlighting a direct influence of CKD on circadian pressure profile. The rise in differential pressures and the reduction in DBP were independent of age and TIS; in patients with CKD, this could be due to an increase in arterial stiffness. Increased atherosclerosis and arteriosclerosis, as well as the metabolic alteration present in CKD with secondary calcifications of the intima and media layers of the artery wall, are likely contributors to this process [27]. This is probably of great relevance in the population with CKD as the patients with CKD are likely to be older (in our study the medium age of CKD patients was 66.2±11.4). Franklin et al [28] demonstrated that, from age 60 and above, DBP was negatively related to coronary heart disease (CHD) risk, when considered together with SBP, and PP emerged as the best predictor. The increased CHD risk due to isolated systolic hypertension may depend not only on the elevated peak of SBP reached in the aorta (ie, increased afterload) but also on the low DBP (ie, potentially favoring a decreased coronary blood flow) [29]. In patients older than 60, with central and peripheral PPs approximating each other, PP becomes the dominant predictor of CHD risk, incorporating both the positive predictive role of SBP and the negative predictive role of DBP. In this way CKD worsens the age-related arterial stiffness and potentiates its effects. Our data overall strongly support the concept that once CKD appears and worsens, some aspects of blood pressure worsen too, as a consequence of CKD implications. These BP aspects (higher night-time BP, more non-dippers and higher PP) are known as important cardiovascular risk factors [30–32] and they translate in greater severity of cardiac damage in CKD.

Our patients with CKD had a higher prevalence of both myocardial hypertrophy and diastolic dysfunction, suggesting that the higher PP and the night-time SBP significantly increased the heart load. Linear regression analysis revealed a strong association between nocturnal blood pressure, PP and cardiac organ damage. CKD itself was also independently associated with cardiac damage, suggesting that other factors (such as CKD-related metabolic alterations) in addition to BP are involved in the higher prevalence of cardiac damage and cardiovascular risk in these patients. Ad-hoc designed studies will be needed to investigate the association between metabolic alterations in CKD and cardiac damage, relevant aspects that were not the focus of our present work. Despite greater intensity of treatment in CKD, BP control is similar in the overall distribution. However, during night-time, there is a higher percentage of subjects with poor nocturnal control in CKD, a finding enlightened only by ABPM. Because of the lack of recognized pressure target for ABPM, we had to use arbitrary cut offs to define BP control, referring to the values in the range of normotension for ABPM in general population. Notwithstanding, according to initial evidences [33], ABPM target pressure values in patients with CKD should be lower than the one we considered.

Table 4. CKD is an indipendent risk factor for non dipping pattern after adjusting for sex, age, BMI, and TIS (logistic regression).

	OR	95% CI	P
Sex (male vs female)	0.855	0.659–1.109	n.s.
Age	1.013	1.002–1.023	**0.016**
TIS*	1.072	0.916–1.255	n.s.
BMI	1.055	1.024–1.087	**<0.001**
CKD (CKD vs eGFR≥60)	1.803	1.200–2.707	**0.005**

*TIS = Treatment Intensity Score.

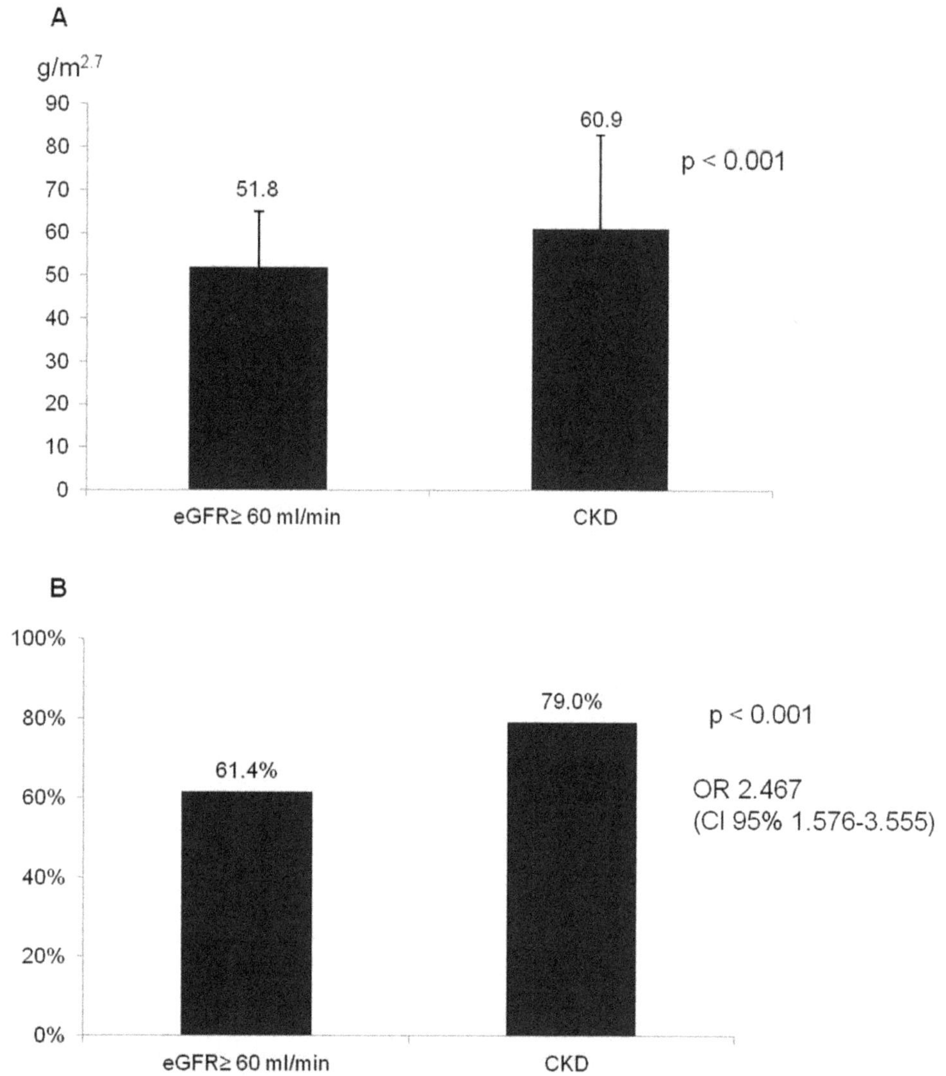

Figure 5. CKD and cardiac damage. Panel A. Difference in left ventricular mass/$h^{2.7}$ between patients with CKD and the rest of the population. Panel B. Prevalence of ventricular hypertrophy in patients with CKD vs the rest of the population.

Conclusions

Our "real-life patient" data are relevant for clinicians that often evaluate BP-related clinical problems on the basis of a single plasma creatinine value in the initial evaluation of outpatients. Our study shows that patients with a reduced eGFR (<60 ml/min/1.73 m^2) had an altered 24-hour BP profile, especially at

Table 5. Night-time SBP associated with LVM/$h^{2.7}$ in a linear regression model.

	B	p
AGE	**0.262**	**<0.001**
SEX	0.074	**0.005**
CKD	0.098	**<0.001**
Night-time SBP	**0.200**	**<0.001**
TIS*	0.092	**0.001**
BMI	**0.358**	**<0.001**

BMI and age were also two other important independent factors for LVM/$h^{2.7}$.
*TIS = Treatment Intensity Score.

Table 6. 24-h PP associated with LVM/$h^{2.7}$ in a linear regression model.

	B	p
AGE	**0.217**	**<0.001**
SEX	0.097	**<0.001**
CKD	0.097	**0.001**
24-h PP	**0.173**	**<0.001**
TIS*	0.082	**0.003**
BMI	**0.351**	**<0.001**

BMI and age were also two other important independent factors for LVM/$h^{2.7}$.
*TIS = Treatment Intensity Score.

Table 7. Daytime PP associated with LVM/h$^{2.7}$ in a linear regression model.

	B	p
AGE	**0.219**	**<0.001**
SEX	0.096	**<0.001**
CKD	0.099	**<0.001**
Daytime PP	**0.169**	**<0.001**
TIS*	0.082	**0.003**
BMI	**0.353**	**<0.001**

BMI and age were also two other important independent factors for LVM/h$^{2.7}$.
*TIS = Treatment Intensity Score.

Table 8. Night-time PP associated with LVM/h$^{2.7}$ in a linear regression model.

	B	p
AGE	**0.218**	**<0.001**
SEX	0.097	**0.001**
CKD	0.094	**0.001**
Night-time PP	**0.170**	**<0.001**
TIS*	0.084	**0.002**
BMI	**0.347**	**<0.001**

BMI and age were also two other important independent factors for LVM/h$^{2.7}$.
*TIS = Treatment Intensity Score.

night-time. Higher night-time SBP, a more frequent non-dipper pattern and higher PP are related with more severe cardiac organ damage.

Hypertension is the main cause of CKD and an accurate measurement of BP is the critical first step for the proper management of hypertensive patients. Our data highlight the fundamental role of ABPM in optimizing antihypertensive therapy when eGFR is low. The altered night-time BP pattern in CKD suggests the need of improving BP therapy in these subjects, by choosing drugs, dosages and timing to cover the 24 hour period, taking at least one drug at bedtime, and using effective diuretics. ABPM should be the preferred method in the clinical management of patients with CKD as well as in clinical studies.

Study limits

The main limitation of our study is the use of post-hoc analysis of consecutive ABPM recordings that were performed for usual clinical reasons (including/excluding hypertension diagnosis, verify the BP control in treated hypertensive patients). Although a selection of patients was unavoidable (e.g. the three "inclusion criteria": ABPM, creatinine and echocardiography), patient selection was based only on the best clinical practice for the management of arterial hypertension.

Overall, our analysis is based on one creatinine/eGFR and this is certainly a limitation. Nevertheless, our data fit in the context of current literature because most of the data available have been obtained with a similar approach. Our "real-life patient" data are relevant for clinicians that make their decisions most often on the basis of a single creatinine determination during the initial evaluation of "stable" outpatients coming for BP related problems. Moreover, patients having the clinical indication for at least two creatinine determinations, had the second one taken 3 to 6 months apart. There were no significant differences in creatinine values/eGFR between the two time points, supporting the notion that 15% of our patients truly had CKD.

Our study is based on "real-life" clinical practice, and we have not been able to include all potential causes of non-dipping pattern in the statistical adjustments (e.g. presence of obstructive sleep apnoea documented by cardio-pulmonary monitoring), a limitation similar to other studies that investigated the relationship between lower eGFR and ABPM patterns. Moreover, we didn't study some CKD biochemical factors (e.g. regarding Ca, P metabolism) and their role in influencing the association between CKD, BP profile and cardiac damage. This was because some metabolic parameters of CKD are not routinely assessed when patients are referred for BP evaluation in a cardiovascular setting. However, the overall night-time results (night-time SBP, night-time PP, non dipping pattern) and increased 24 h PP in our large population, even after statistical adjustments, strongly indicate an altered pattern of night-time BP in CKD patients, with a negative impact on the heart and therefore with important clinical implications.

Author Contributions

Conceived and designed the experiments: RS MF. Performed the experiments: MF FS. Analyzed the data: MF FS. Contributed reagents/materials/analysis tools: GC. Wrote the paper: MF FS. Reviewed the manuscript: PDF EE RS.

References

1. (2000) U.S. Renal Data System, USRDS 2000 Annual Data Report, National Institutes of Health, National Institute of Diabetes and Digestive and Kidney Diseases, Bethesda, MD, June 2000. National Institutes of Health, National Institute of Diabetes and Digestive and Kidney Diseases, Bethesda, MD, June 2000.
2. National Kidney Foundation. (2002) K/DOQI Clinical Practice Guidelines for Chronic Kidney Disease: Evaluation, Classification and Stratification. Am J Kidney Dis 39 (suppl 1): S1–S266.
3. Coresh J, Selvin E, Stevens LA, Manzi J, Kusek JW, et al. (2007) Prevalence of Chronic Kidney Disease in the USA. JAMA 298: 2038–2047.
4. Meguid El Nahas A, Bello AK. (2005) Chronic Kidney Disease: the global challenge. Lancet 365: 331–340.
5. De Nicola L, Donfrancesco C, Minutolo R, Lo Noce C, De Curtis A, et al. (2011) Epidemiologia della malattia renale cronica in Italia: stato dell'arte e contributo dello studio CARHES. G Ital Nefrol 28: 401–407.
6. (2007) U.S. Renal Data System, USRDS 2007 Annual Data Report: Atlas of Chronic Kidney Disease and End-Stage Renal Disease in the United States, National Institutes of Health, National Institute of Diabetes and Digestive and Kidney Diseases, Bethesda, MD, 2007.
7. Kanno A, Kikuya M, Ohkubo T, Hashimoto T, Satoh M, et al. (2012) Pre-hypertension as a significant predictor of chronic kidney disease in a general population: the Ohasama Study. Nephrol Dial Transplant 27: 3218–3223.
8. Buckalew VM Jr, Berg RL, Wang SR, Porush JG, Rauch S, et al. (1996) Prevalence of hypertension in 1,795 subjects with chronic renal disease: the modification of diet in renal disease study baseline cohort. Modification of Diet in Renal Disease Study Group. Am J Kidney Dis 28: 811–821.
9. Coresh J, Wei GL, McQuillan G, Brancati FL, Levey AS, et al. (2001) Prevalence of high blood pressure and elevated serum creatinine level in the United States: findings from the third National Health and Nutrition Examination Survey (1988–1994). Arch Intern Med 161: 1207–1216.
10. Ohkubo T, Hozawa A, Yamaguchi J, Kikuya M, Ohmori K, et al. (2002) Prognostic significance of the nocturnal decline in blood pressure in individuals with and without high 24-h blood pressure: the Ohasama study. J Hypertens 20: 2183–2189.
11. O'Brien E, Sheridan J, O'Malley K. (1988) Dippers and non-dippers. Lancet 13; 2(8607): 397.
12. Verdecchia P, Porcellati C, Schillaci G, Borgioni C, Ciucci A, et al. (1994) Ambulatory blood pressure. An independent predictor of prognosis in essential hypertension. Hypertension 24(6): 793–801.

13. Khattar RS, Senior R, Lahiri A. (2001) Prognostic value of direct, continuous ambulatory blood pressure monitoring in essential hypertension. J Clin Hypertens 3(2): 90–8.
14. Agarwal R, Light RP, Billset JE, Hummel LA. (2009) Nocturia, Nocturnal Activity, and Non dipping. Hypertension 54: 646–651.
15. Andersen MJ, Agarwal R. (2005) Etiology and management of hypertension in chronic kidney disease. Med Clin North Am 89: 525–547.
16. Mancia G, De Backer G, Dominiczak A, Cifkova R, Fagard R, et al. (2007) 2007 Guidelines for the management of arterial hypertension: The Task Force for the Management of Arterial Hypertension of the European Society of Hypertension (ESH) and of the European Society of Cardiology (ESC). Eur Heart J 28: 1462–1536.
17. Staessen JA, Bieniaszewski L, O'Brien E, Gosse P, Hayashi H, et al. (1997) Nocturnal blood pressure fall on ambulatory monitoring in a large international database. The "Ad Hoc' Working Group. Hypertension 29: 30–39.
18. Morisky DE, Ang A, Krousel-Wood M, Ward HJ. (2008) Predictive validity of a medication adherence measure in an outpatient setting. J Clin Hypertens (Greenwich) 10: 348–354.
19. Bailey KR, Grossardt BR, Graves JW. (2008) Novel use of Kaplan-Meier methods to explain age and gender differences in hypertension control rates. Hypertension 51: 841–847.
20. Fujii T, Uzu T, Nishimura M, Takeji M, Kuroda S, et al. (1999) Circadian rhythm of natriuresis is disturbed in non-dipper type of essential hypertension. Am J Kidney Dis 33: 29–35.
21. Uzu T, Kazembe FS, Ishikawa K, Nakamura S, Inenaga T, et al. (1996) High sodium sensitivity implicates nocturnal hypertension in essential hypertension. Hypertension 28: 139–142.
22. Uzu T, Ishikawa K, Fujii T, Nakamura S, Inenaga T, et al. (1997) Sodium restriction shifts circadian rhythm of blood pressure from non dipper to dipper in essential hypertension. Circulation 96: 1859–1862.
23. Kimura G, Brenner BM (1995) The renal basis for salt sensitivity in hypertension. In: Hypertension: Pathophysiology, Diagnosis and Management, ed. Laragh JH, Brenner BM. Raven Press: New York. pp. 1569–1588.
24. Kimura G, Brenner BM. (1997) Implications of linear pressure-natriuresis relationship and importance of sodium sensitivity in hypertension. J Hypertens 15: 1055–1061.
25. Fukuda M, Munemura M, Usami T, Nakao N, Takeuchi O, et al. (2004) Nocturnal blood pressure is elevated with natriuresis and proteinuria as renal function deteriorates in nephropathy. Kidney Int 65: 621–625.
26. Hering D, Mahfoud F, Walton AS, Krum H, Lambert GW, et al. (2012) Renal Denervation in Moderate to Severe CKD. J Am Soc Nephrol 23: 1250–1257.
27. Toussaint ND, Lau KK, Strauss BJ, Polkinghorne KR, Kerr PG. (2008) Associations between vascular calcification, arterial stiffness and bone mineral density in chronic kidney disease. Nephrol Dial Transplant 23: 586–593.
28. Franklin SS, Larson MG, Khan SA, Wong ND, Leip EP, et al. (2001) Does the relation of blood pressure to coronary heart disease risk change with aging? The Framingham Heart Study. Circulation 103: 1245–1249.
29. Nichols WW, O'Rourke MF (1998) McDonald's Blood Flow in Arteries: Theoretical, Experimental and Clinical Principles 4th ed. Edward Arnold, Hodder Headline Group: London.
30. Sega R, Facchetti R, Bombelli M, Cesana G, Corrao G, et al. (2005) Prognostic value of ambulatory and home blood pressures compared with office blood pressure in the general population: Follow-up results from the Pressioni Arteriose Monitorate e Loro Associazioni (PAMELA) study. Circulation 111: 1777–1783.
31. Fagard RH, Thijs L, Staessen JA, Clement DL, De Buyzere ML, et al. (2009) Night-day blood pressure ratio and dipping pattern as predictors of death and cardiovascular events in hypertension. J Hum Hypertens 23: 645–653.
32. Hansen TW, Li Y, Boggia J, Thijs L, Richart T, et al. (2011) Predictive Role of the Nighttime Blood Pressure. Hypertension 57: 3–10.
33. Head GA, McGrath BP, Mihailidou AS, Nelson MR, Schlaich MP, et al. (2012) Ambulatory blood pressure monitoring in Australia: 2011 consensus position statement. J Hypertens 30: 253–266.

19

Prevalence of Anemia in Chronic Kidney Disease in the United States

Melissa E. Stauffer[1]*, Tao Fan[2]

1 SCRIBCO, Effort, Pennsylvania, United States of America, 2 Merck & Co., Inc., Whitehouse Station, New Jersey, United States of America

Abstract

Anemia is one of the many complications of chronic kidney disease (CKD). However, the current prevalence of anemia in CKD patients in the United States is not known. Data from the National Health and Nutrition Examination Survey (NHANES) in 2007–2008 and 2009–2010 were used to determine the prevalence of anemia in subjects with CKD. The analysis was limited to adults aged >18 who participated in both the interview and exam components of the survey. Three outcomes were assessed: the prevalence of CKD, the prevalence of anemia in subjects with CKD, and the self-reported treatment of anemia. CKD was classified into 5 stages based on the glomerular filtration rate and evidence of kidney damage, in accordance with the guidelines of the National Kidney Foundation. Anemia was defined as serum hemoglobin levels ≤12 g/dL in women and ≤13 g/dL in men. We found that an estimated 14.0% of the US adult population had CKD in 2007–2010. Anemia was twice as prevalent in people with CKD (15.4%) as in the general population (7.6%). The prevalence of anemia increased with stage of CKD, from 8.4% at stage 1 to 53.4% at stage 5. A total of 22.8% of CKD patients with anemia reported being treated for anemia within the previous 3 months–14.6% of patients at CKD stages 1–2 and 26.4% of patients at stages 3–4. These results update our knowledge of the prevalence and treatment of anemia in CKD in the United States.

Editor: Ivan Cruz Moura, Institut national de la santé et de la recherche médicale (INSERM), France

Funding: This study was funded by Merck & Co., Inc. Web site: http://www.merck.com/index.html. The funders had no role in study design, data collection and analysis, decision to publish, or preparation of the manuscript.

Competing Interests: The authors have the following interests. This study was funded by Merck & Co., Inc., the employer of Tao Fan. Melissa Stauffer received remuneration from SCRIBCO to perform the work described in this manuscript. There are no patents, products in development or marketed products to declare. This does not alter our adherence to all the PLOS ONE policies on sharing data and materials, as detailed online in the guide for authors.

* E-mail: melstauff@charter.net

Introduction

The kidneys function as filters of the blood, removing waste products and controlling the balance of fluid and electrolytes. Filtration occurs via bundles of capillaries called glomeruli (singular, glomerulus). A reduction in the glomerular filtration rate (GFR) to <60 mL/min/1.73 m^2 indicates chronic kidney disease (CKD), as do structural or functional renal abnormalities, which may be present in people with normal GFR [1]. Cross-sectional estimates of the prevalence of CKD in the United States range from 1.5% to 15.6% [2].

One of the lesser known functions of the kidneys is the production of erythropoietin, a signaling molecule that stimulates red blood cell production, in response to decreased oxygen levels in the blood. Any disruption of this process, e.g., secondary to a functional abnormality due to CKD, has the potential to produce anemia, a condition in which the number of circulating red blood cells, and therefore the level of hemoglobin, is lower than normal [3].

Other possible causes of anemia in CKD include iron deficiency, inflammation, and the accumulation of uremic toxins [3,4]. Thus, the abnormal composition of blood or urine is an additional indicator of kidney damage.

Anemia in CKD is associated with cognitive impairment, sleep disturbances, CKD progression, cardiovascular comorbidities, and higher mortality [3,5–7]. Direct healthcare costs are higher in CKD patients with anemia than in those without [7], and quality of life issues (e.g., fatigue, reduced productivity) are common [3,5]. The prevalence of anemia (with or without CKD) increases with age [8,9], which means that, as the US population ages, the number of people affected by anemia in CKD will also increase.

Available population-based determinations of the prevalence of anemia in CKD are becoming dated, with many studies referring back to the National Health and Nutrition Examination Survey (NHANES) III, which ended in 1994 [8,10–12]. The most recent studies include NHANES data up to 2006 [8,13], but one was limited to adults over age 64 with advanced CKD [13] and the other used a GFR classification not directly comparable to that of most other studies [8]. This analysis assessed the prevalence of anemia in CKD in the adult (>18 years of age) US population during 2007–2010 using the GFR categories specified by the National Kidney Foundation.

Methods

Study Design and Data Source

This was an analysis of cross-sectional data from the NHANES in 2007–2008 and 2009–2010. The NHANES is a biennial national survey that assesses the physical health of the non-institutionalized civilian population in the United States (www.cdc.gov/nchs/nhanes.htm). It is carried out and overseen by the National Center for Health Statistics, whose institutional review board approves each survey cycle.

Study Sample

The study sample comprised adult subjects aged >18 years who participated in both the interview and examination components of NHANES. Participants provided written informed consent at the time of the survey.

Study Variables

Glomerular filtration rate (GFR) was calculated using the formula $GFR = 175 \times (S_{Cr})^{-1.154} \times (age)^{-0.203} \times (0.742$ if female) $\times (1.210$ if African American), where S_{Cr} is serum creatinine in mg/dL and age is expressed in years [14]. GFR units are mL/min/1.73 m^2. CKD was classified into five stages defined by the GFR and/or evidence of kidney damage, as recommended by the National Kidney Foundation [14] and shown in Table 1. Evidence of kidney damage was derived from the presence of albuminuria, which is defined as a urinary albumin-to-creatinine ratio (ACR) ≥30 mg/g [14]. The NHANES 2009–2010 data set provided a variable for the urinary ACR (URDACT), but the 2007–2008 data set did not. Therefore, the urinary ACR was calculated for both survey periods from the variables for urinary albumin and creatinine as follows: ACR (mg/g) = urinary albumin (mg/dL)/urinary creatinine (g/dL). Stage of CKD was not calculated if data for either GFR or ACR were missing, except when GFR values alone indicated CKD of stages 3–5. Anemia was defined as serum hemoglobin levels ≤12 g/dL in women and ≤13 g/dL in men, as recommended by the National Anemia Action Council and the World Health Organization [15,16].

Statistical Analysis

All analyses were performed in Stata MP v. 12.1 (StataCorp, College Station, TX). Four-year sample weights were calculated for the combined survey cycles as described in the NHANES analytic guidelines [17]. The sample weights were applied to calculate the proportions of subjects with CKD, anemia, and treatment for anemia. Standard errors obtained by Taylor series linearization were used to obtain 95% confidence intervals. Each outcome was determined for all subjects and by stage of CKD. The 'subpopulation' option in Stata was used for analyses of subgroups. Subjects with no calculated stage of CKD (N = 977; 8.1%) were classified as not having CKD. The prevalence of anemia was determined in all subjects and then separately in subjects with and without CKD. Treatment for anemia was assessed only in subjects with anemia (and CKD). Prevalence values were converted to projections of the respective numbers in the US population based on the 2000 US census.

Table 1. Classification of stage of chronic kidney disease.

Stage	Criteria
1	GFR ≥90 plus evidence of kidney damage
2	GFR 60–89 plus evidence of kidney damage
3	GFR 30–59
4	GFR 15–29
5	GFR <15

Stages of CKD were defined in accordance with the recommendations of the National Kidney Foundation. [14].

Results

Participants

A total of 12,077 adults participated in the interview and examination components of the NHANES surveys in 2007–2008 and 2009–2010.

Prevalence of CKD

The prevalence of CKD was 14.0% (Table 2). This represents an estimated 31.4 million people in the US population. About half (48.4%) of the people with CKD were at stage 3. A similar proportion (46.9%) was in stages 1–2 combined. Only 4.7% were in stages 4–5.

Prevalence of Anemia in CKD

The prevalence of anemia in the combined survey population, regardless of CKD, was 7.6% (result not shown). The prevalence of anemia was 15.4% in people with CKD (Table 3). This represents an estimated 4.8 million people. The prevalence of anemia increased with stage of CKD, from 8.4% at stage 1 to 53.4% at stage 5. The prevalence of anemia in people without CKD was 6.3%.

Treatment of Anemia

A total of 22.8% of CKD patients with anemia reported being treated for it (Table 4). Treatment frequencies were similar at stages 1 and 2 (12.1% and 16.2%; P = 0.57; weighted mean 14.6%) and stages 3 and 4 (26.5% and 20.7%; P = 0.76; weighted mean 26.4%).

Discussion

In our analysis of NHANES data from 2007–2010, an estimated 14.0% of the US population had CKD. There are several indications that this value represents a slightly increasing prevalence of CKD in the United States. The first is a comparison with an analysis of the NHANES III (1988–1994), in which the prevalence of CKD was 11.0% [18]. Secondly, the unweighted prevalence of CKD in the NHANES 1999–2004 surveys was reported to be 16.8% [19], slightly lower than the unweighted prevalence in the current study (17.6%). Thirdly, Coresh et al. reported prevalence values of 9.4–13.1% for stages 1–4 of CKD in various analyses covering NHANES III through 2004 [20,21]. Our analysis of stages 1–4 in years 2007–2010 yielded an estimated prevalence of 13.9%. Finally, reports on the Kidney Early Evaluation Program (KEEP) cohort of patients at high risk for CKD indicate that 15.6% of the cohort had GFRs corresponding to CKD stages 3–5 in 2000–2001 [22], whereas 16.8% met this criterion over the period 2000–2009 [23].

In our analysis, anemia was estimated to be present in 15.4% of people with any stage of CKD. The prevalence of anemia increased with stage of CKD, from 8.4% at stage 1 to 53.4% at stage 5. A similar trend has been reported by several other authors [11,24,25], consistent with the known pathogenesis of CKD (i.e., that erythropoietin production decreases as kidney function worsens). Fishbane et al. found high rates of iron deficiency in adult men (57.8 to 58.8%) and women (69.9 to 72.8%) with CKD stages 3–5 in the NHANES III and 1999–2004 surveys [12], indicating that anemia in higher stage CKD may have multiple causes.

Other studies of the prevalence of anemia in CKD focused on older adults (>64 years of age). According to Stevens et al., 29.9% of KEEP 2000–08 participants and 19.9% of NHANES 1999–2006 subjects in CKD stages 3–5 and over age 64 had comorbid

Table 2. Prevalence of chronic kidney disease.

	N	Weighted percentage (95% CI)	95% CI	Projected number in US
With CKD	2,125	14.0	13.2–15.0	31.4×10^6
Stage 1	507	3.1	2.7–3.6	6.8×10^6
Stage 2	489	3.4	2.9–3.9	7.4×10^6
Stage 3	1,028	7.0	6.2–7.9	16×10^6
Stage 4	70	0.4	0.3–0.5	0.9×10^6
Stage 5	31	0.1	0.1–0.2	0.3×10^6
Without CKD	9,952	86.0	85.0–86.9	190×10^6

Percentages reflect the prevalence of each stage of CKD, survey weighted to the US population. The analysis was limited to subjects aged >18 with data from both the exam and interview components of the survey (N = 12,077).

anemia, defined as hemoglobin levels <13.5 g/dL for men and <12 g/dL for women [13]. For comparison, the prevalence of anemia in stage 3–5 CKD patients aged >64 in the 2007–2010 NHANES surveys was 24.4%. A higher prevalence of anemia (64.9%; defined as hemoglobin <13 g/dL for men, <12 g/dL for women) was observed in US nursing home residents aged >64 with CKD stages 3–5 [25].

Treatments for anemia include iron supplementation and erythropoietin stimulating agents. Reported treatment rates are typically low (10–15%), regardless of the source of data. In an analysis of the National Ambulatory Medical Care Survey (1996–2002), just 10% of outpatient visits for anemia management in CKD resulted in prescription of medication for anemia [26]. In an online survey conducted in 2006, just 15% of 376 family medicine and internal medicine trainees in the United States reported that they would initiate treatment for anemia in CKD at hemoglobin levels <11 g/dL [27]. In our analysis of NHANES 2007–2010, 22.8% of CKD patients with anemia reported being treated for anemia within the previous 3 months.

Insight into the usual timing and types of treatments received (at least among older men) can be gleaned from a study of the Veterans Health Administration database by Lawler et al. [28]. Among 89,000 patients with anemia and CKD (96.7% male, median age 77.5), 7.1% initiated erythropoietin stimulating agents within a year of diagnosis of anemia, while 30.8% initiated iron therapy and 16.5% used blood transfusions in the same time span. The median time to erythropoietin stimulating agent initiation was 138 days.

Table 3. Prevalence of anemia.

	N	Weighted percentage	95% CI	Projected number in US
With CKD	410	15.4	13.1–18.2	4.8×10^6
Stage 1	57	8.4	5.5–12.4	0.6×10^6
Stage 2	68	12.2	9.2–16.0	0.9×10^6
Stage 3	231	17.4	13.7–21.8	2.7×10^6
Stage 4	37	50.3	37.2–63.4	0.5×10^6
Stage 5	17	53.4	34.1–71.7	0.2×10^6
Without CKD	729	6.3	5.3–7.4	11×10^6

The percentages reflect the prevalence of anemia, survey weighted to the US population. The analysis by stage of CKD was limited to subjects with CKD as defined in the Methods section (N = 2,125); data for anemia were missing for a total of 7 CKD patients (<1%), all in stages 1–3. Prevalence of anemia in subjects without CKD was determined in 9,269 subjects with non-missing data on anemia status.

CKD prevalence values can vary markedly depending on how GFR is estimated [23,29]. We chose to use the definitions of CKD and GFR established by the National Kidney Foundation to maximize the comparability of our results with previous NHANES and other studies that used these same definitions. We note that a new method for estimating GFR has been shown to be slightly more accurate in classifying patients by stage of CKD [23]. In addition, hemoglobin levels may vary not only by sex but also by age, pregnancy, altitude and smoking status [30]. We used the definitions of anemia given by the National Anemia Action Council and the World Health Organization for simplicity, but did not account for the variables listed above. Our analysis of treatment for anemia was limited by the fact that NHANES data on the various treatments for anemia (e.g., ESAs, iron) were sparse.

Several elements of the study design may have skewed our estimation of the prevalence of CKD. First, inclusion of subject with missing data on GFR and/or ACR likely resulted in underestimation of the full number of people with CKD. On the other hand, albuminuria was assessed with a single spot urine test in NHANES and may have been a temporary condition, resulting in overestimation of the number of subjects at CKD stages 1–2. Lastly, as described in other NHANES-based analyses of CKD, "nonparticipation rates caused by illness relating to having a very low GFR are expected to be particularly high in [stage 5], severely

Table 4. Self-reported treatment of anemia in chronic kidney disease.

Stage of CKD	N	Weighted percentage	95% CI
1	8	12.1	5.4–25.0
2	9	16.2	7.0–33.3
3	59	26.5	21.2–32.6
4	8	20.7	8.8–41.2
5	6	43.0	17.1–73.4
Total	90	22.8	18.5–27.7

The weighted percentages reflect the frequency of treatment of anemia among people within each stage of CKD, survey weighted to the US population. The analysis was limited to subjects with anemia (N = 410).

downwardly biasing these prevalence estimates" [18].

In summary, CKD prevalence appears to be increasing in the US adult population. In 2007–2010, anemia was present in approximately 15% of CKD patients and was more frequent at higher stages of CKD. Relatively few CKD patients with anemia were being treated for anemia.

Acknowledgments

The authors thank Lauren Weisenfluh, MPH, of SCRIBCO for medical writing assistance; Alan Morrison, PhD, of SCRIBCO for critical review of the manuscript; and Mari Palta, PhD, of the University of Wisconsin-Madison for advice on the analytical methods.

Author Contributions

Conceived and designed the experiments: TF MS. Analyzed the data: MS. Wrote the paper: MS.

References

1. National Kidney Foundation (2002) K/DOQI Clinical Practice Guidelines for Chronic Kidney Disease: Evaluation, Classification and Stratification. Am J Kidney Dis 39: S1–S266.
2. Zhang QL, Rothenbacher D (2008) Prevalence of chronic kidney disease in population-based studies: systematic review. BMC Public Health 8: 117.
3. Smith RE, Jr. (2010) The clinical and economic burden of anemia. Am J Manag Care 16 Suppl Issues: S59–66.
4. National Kidney Foundation (2006) KDOQI Clinical Practice Guidelines and Clinical Practice Recommendations for Anemia in Chronic Kidney Disease. Am J Kidney Dis 47: S11–145.
5. Mehdi U, Toto RD (2009) Anemia, diabetes, and chronic kidney disease. Diabetes Care 32: 1320–1326.
6. Herzog CA, Muster HA, Li S, Collins AJ (2004) Impact of congestive heart failure, chronic kidney disease, and anemia on survival in the Medicare population. J Card Fail 10: 467–472.
7. van Nooten FE, Green J, Brown R, Finkelstein FO, Wish J (2010) Burden of illness for patients with non-dialysis chronic kidney disease and anemia in the United States: review of the literature. J Med Econ 13: 241–256.
8. Bowling CB, Inker LA, Gutierrez OM, Allman RM, Warnock DG, et al. (2011) Age-specific associations of reduced estimated glomerular filtration rate with concurrent chronic kidney disease complications. Clin J Am Soc Nephrol 6: 2822–2828.
9. Nissenson AR, Wade S, Goodnough T, Knight K, Dubois RW (2005) Economic burden of anemia in an insured population. J Manag Care Pharm 11: 565–574.
10. Hsu CY, McCulloch CE, Curhan GC (2002) Epidemiology of anemia associated with chronic renal insufficiency among adults in the United States: results from the Third National Health and Nutrition Examination Survey. J Am Soc Nephrol 13: 504–510.
11. Clase CM, Kiberd BA, Garg AX (2007) Relationship between glomerular filtration rate and the prevalence of metabolic abnormalities: results from the Third National Health and Nutrition Examination Survey (NHANES III). Nephron Clin Pract 105: c178–184.
12. Fishbane S, Pollack S, Feldman HI, Joffe MM (2009) Iron indices in chronic kidney disease in the National Health and Nutritional Examination Survey 1988–2004. Clin J Am Soc Nephrol 4: 57–61.
13. Stevens LA, Li S, Wang C, Huang C, Becker BN, et al. (2010) Prevalence of CKD and comorbid illness in elderly patients in the United States: results from the Kidney Early Evaluation Program (KEEP). Am J Kidney Dis 55: S23–33.
14. National Kidney Foundation. Frequently Asked Questions about GFR Estimates. http://www.kidney.org/professionals/kls/pdf/12-10-4004_KBB_FAQs_AboutGFR-1.pdf. Accessed August 1, 2012.
15. National Anemia Action Council. Anemia & Kidney Disease. http://www.anemia.org/patients/information-handouts/kidney-disease/?handout = kidney-disease%2F. Accessed August 1, 2012.
16. World Health Organization (2001) Iron Deficiency Anaemia: Assessment, Prevention, and Control. Geneva, Switzerland. Available at: http://www.who.int/nutrition/publications/micronutrients/anaemia_iron_deficiency/WHO_NHD_01.3/en/index.html.
17. Centers for Disease Control and Prevention. (2012) National Health and Nutrition Examination Survey Analytic and Reporting Guidelines. http://www.cdc.gov/nchs/nhanes/nhanes2003-2004/analytical_guidelines.htm. Accessed October 18, 2012.
18. Coresh J, Astor BC, Greene T, Eknoyan G, Levey AS (2003) Prevalence of chronic kidney disease and decreased kidney function in the adult US population: Third National Health and Nutrition Examination Survey. Am J Kidney Dis 41: 1–12.
19. Centers for Disease Control and Prevention (2007) Prevalence of Chronic Kidney Disease and Associated Risk Factors – United States, 1999–2004. Morbidity and Mortality Weekly Report 58: 161–165.
20. Coresh J, Byrd-Holt D, Astor BC, Briggs JP, Eggers PW, et al. (2005) Chronic kidney disease awareness, prevalence, and trends among U.S. adults, 1999 to 2000. J Am Soc Nephrol 16: 180–188.
21. Coresh J, Selvin E, Stevens LA, Manzi J, Kusek JW, et al. (2007) Prevalence of chronic kidney disease in the United States. JAMA 298: 2038–2047.
22. Brown WW, Peters RM, Ohmit SE, Keane WF, Collins A, et al. (2003) Early detection of kidney disease in community settings: the Kidney Early Evaluation Program (KEEP). Am J Kidney Dis 42: 22–35.
23. Stevens LA, Li S, Kurella Tamura M, Chen SC, Vassalotti JA, et al. (2011) Comparison of the CKD Epidemiology Collaboration (CKD-EPI) and Modification of Diet in Renal Disease (MDRD) study equations: risk factors for and complications of CKD and mortality in the Kidney Early Evaluation Program (KEEP). Am J Kidney Dis 57: S9–16.
24. Moossavi S, Freedman BI (2009) Treating anemia with erythropoiesis-stimulating agents: effects on quality of life. Arch Intern Med 169: 1100–1101.
25. Robinson B, Artz AS, Culleton B, Critchlow C, Sciarra A, et al. (2007) Prevalence of anemia in the nursing home: contribution of chronic kidney disease. J Am Geriatr Soc 55: 1566–1570.
26. Rasu RS, Manley HJ, Crawford T, Balkrishnan R (2007) Undertreatment of anemia in patients with chronic kidney disease in the United States: analysis of national outpatient survey data. Clin Ther 29: 1524–1534.
27. Lenz O, Fornoni A (2006) Chronic kidney disease care delivered by US family medicine and internal medicine trainees: results from an online survey. BMC Med 4: 30.
28. Lawler EV, Gagnon DR, Fink J, Seliger S, Fonda J, et al. (2010) Initiation of anaemia management in patients with chronic kidney disease not on dialysis in the Veterans Health Administration. Nephrol Dial Transplant 25: 2237–2244.
29. Snyder JJ, Foley RN, Collins AJ (2009) Prevalence of CKD in the United States: a sensitivity analysis using the National Health and Nutrition Examination Survey (NHANES) 1999–2004. Am J Kidney Dis 53: 218–228.
30. Agarwal AK (2006) Practical approach to the diagnosis and treatment of anemia associated with CKD in elderly. J Am Med Dir Assoc 7: S7–S12; quiz S17–21.

20

^{1}H NMR-Based Metabolite Profiling of Plasma in a Rat Model of Chronic Kidney Disease

Ju-Ae Kim[1,2], Hyo-Jung Choi[3], Yong-Kook Kwon[1,4], Do Hyun Ryu[2], Tae-Hwan Kwon[3]*, Geum-Sook Hwang[1,4]*

1 Integrated Metabolomics Research Group, Seoul Center, Korea Basic Science Institute, Seoul, Korea, 2 Department of Chemistry, Sungkyunkwan University, Suwon, Korea, 3 Department of Biochemistry and Cell Biology, School of Medicine, Kyungpook National University, Taegu, Korea, 4 Graduate School of Analytical Science and Technology, Chungnam University, Daejeon, Korea

Abstract

Chronic kidney disease (CKD) is characterized by the gradual loss of the kidney function to excrete wastes and fluids from the blood. ^{1}H NMR-based metabolomics was exploited to investigate the altered metabolic pattern in rats with CKD induced by surgical reduction of the renal mass (i.e., 5/6 nephrectomy (5/6 Nx)), particularly for identifying specific metabolic biomarkers associated with early of CKD. Plasma metabolite profiling was performed in CKD rats (at 4- or 8-weeks after 5/6 Nx) compared to sham-operated rats. Principle components analysis (PCA), partial least squares-discriminant analysis (PLS-DA) and orthogonal partial least squares-discriminant analysis (OPLS-DA) score plots showed a significant separation between the groups. The resulting metabolic profiles demonstrated significantly increased plasma levels of organic anions, including citrate, β-hydroxybutyrate, lactate, acetate, acetoacetate, and formate in CKD. Moreover, levels of alanine, glutamine, and glutamate were significantly higher. These changes were likely to be associated with complicated metabolic acidosis in CKD for counteracting systemic metabolic acidosis or increased protein catabolism from muscle. In contrast, levels of VLDL/LDL $(CH_2)_n$ and N-acetylglycoproteins were decreased. Taken together, the observed changes of plasma metabolite profiles in CKD rats provide insights into the disturbed metabolism in early phase of CKD, in particular for the altered metabolism of acid-base and/or amino acids.

Editor: Leighton R. James, University of Florida, United States of America

Funding: This study was supported by the National Research Foundation of Korea (NRF) funded by the Ministry of Science, ICT & Future Planning, Korea (2010-0019393, 2010-0019394, 2013R1A1A2007266, and 2013M3A9B6046418); the Korea Healthcare Technology R&D Project, Ministry of Health & Welfare, Korea (A111345), Korea Basic Science Institute (T33409), the Creative Allied Project (CAP), and Kyungpook National University Research Fund, 2012. The funders had no role in study design, data collection and analysis, decision to publish, or preparation of the manuscript.

Competing Interests: The authors have declared that no competing interests exist.

* E-mail: gshwang@kbsi.re.kr (GSH); thkwon@knu.ac.kr (THK)

Introduction

Kidney is an organ which metabolizes a large number of substrates. Systemic metabolic disorder complicated in chronic kidney disease (CKD) is likely due to decreased renal function and altered metabolic activity of the kidney. These changes include disturbance of acid-base, water and electrolyte homeostasis, altered metabolism of glucose, amino acid, and lipid, accumulation of uremic toxins, and partial breakdown of endocrine function [1,2,3]. In particular, 3kidney plays a key role in the regulation of systemic acid–base balance by filtering blood and handling of acids and buffers. This includes the synthesis and secretion of ammonia, the excretion of titratable acids and free hydrogen ions, and the reabsorption and regeneration of bicarbonate (HCO_3^-) in the renal tubular epithelial cells [4].

In healthy individuals, systemic acid–base balance is maintained by the actions of both kidneys and lungs. When glomerular filtration rate (GFR) decreases in CKD, the balance is severely disturbed [5,6], and metabolic acidosis could be complicated due to both decreased net acid excretion and impaired regeneration of bicarbonate [7]. In human patients, acid–base disorders caused by CKD are associated with a number of clinical manifestations, e.g., nausea and vomiting, electrolyte disturbances, increased susceptibility to cardiovascular events, activation of muscle proteolysis, and protein degradation [5,8]. Moreover, animals with CKD induced by partial nephrectomy demonstrate that metabolic acidosis is associated with increased ammoniagenesis and activation of alternative complement pathway leading to tubulointerstitial inflammation and renal damage [9,10]. Importantly, a recent study demonstrated that bicarbonate supplementation to correct metabolic acidosis in CKD patients slows the disease progression and improves nutritional status [11].

^{1}H nuclear magnetic resonance (NMR) spectroscopy, a nondestructive chemical technique, provides detailed information on molecular structure, both for pure compounds and complex mixtures, as well as information on absolute or relative concentration of metabolites [12,13]. The successful application of ^{1}H NMR spectroscopy to plasma, urine, and other biofluids for studying altered metabolism in disease conditions has recently been established, and several important metabolites have been discovered as novel biomarkers for predicting the courses of diseases, such as diabetes mellitus or cardiovascular disease [13,14,15,16,17,18]. In particular, we have recently demonstrated altered metabolic profiling in serum from human CKD patients with peritoneal dialysis or hemodialysis [12] and in the kidneys and urine from rats with lithium-induced nephrogenic diabetes insipidus [13]. Moreover, we did an integrated analysis of the transcriptome and metabolome in the kidney collecting duct cells, revealing that decreased extracellular osmolality is associated with decreased levels of organic osmolytes, glucose, intermediates of citric acid cycle, and branched chain amino acids [19]. In the present study, it is hypothesized that systemic metabolism, including metabolism of acid-base or amino acids, could be affected by renal failure and hence we aimed to identify specific metabolic biomarkers associated with early stage of CKD. The differences in the plasma levels of metabolites were investigated between rats with CKD induced by 5/6 nephrectomy (4- and 8-weeks) and corresponding sham-operated control rats by exploiting high resolution ^{1}H NMR spectroscopy coupled with multivariate statistical analysis.

Materials and Methods

CKD animal model (4- and 8-weeks after 5/6 nephrectomy in rats)

Pathogen-free male Sprague-Dawley (SD) rats (180–200 g) were obtained from Charles River (Orient Bio, Seongnam, Korea). The animal protocols were approved by the Animal Care and Use Committee of the Kyungpook National University, Korea. Experimental CKD was induced by the excision of about two-thirds of right kidney and left total nephrectomy using the so-called excision remnant kidney model, as we previously demonstrated [20,21]. Rats were anesthetized under enflurane inhalation. During surgery, they were placed on heated tables to maintain the rectal temperature at 37–38°C. Right kidney was exposed through right flank incision, gently dissected free from the adrenal gland, and approximately two-thirds of the right kidney, including the upper and lower poles, was excised. One week later, the rats were again anesthetized with enflurane inhalation, and left kidney was removed through left flank incision after dissecting it free from the adrenal gland. As a control group, rats were subjected to the sham operation identical to that used for the CKD rats except that their kidneys and poles were not removed. Both 5/6 nephrectomized CKD rats and sham-operated control rats were monitored for either 4- or 8-weeks.

Table 1. Changes of renal functions.

Parameter	Sham −4 wk	CKD −4 wk	Sham −8 wk	CKD −8 wk
n	10	10	12	12
BW (g)	435±8.2	390±7.9*	504±8.6	478±12.7
RK wt (g)	1.6±0.1	1.3±0.1*	1.6±0.1	2.2 ±0.2*
p-osm (mosm/KgH_2O)	299± 0.4	306±1.2*	297±0.7	307±1.5*
p-Na^+ (mmol/L)	136±0.4	135±0.9	136±0.2	136±0.3
p-K^+ (mmol/L)	3.8±0.1	4.2±0.1*	3.7±0.0	4.3±0.1*
p- urea nitrogen (mmol/L)	6.0±0.2	15.2±2.1*	5.7±0.1	16.2±1.2*
p-Creat (μmol/L)	19.4±1.2	49.8±5.6*	21.4±1.3	59.7±3.9*

n, number of rats; BW, body weight; RK, right kidney in sham-operated control rats and remnant kidney in CKD rats; p-osm, plasma osmolality; p-Na, plasma sodium, p-K, plasma potassium, p-urea nitrogen, plasma urea nitrogen; p-Creat, plasma creatinine. *$P<0.05$.

Plasma sample preparation

Plasma samples from the CKD rats and sham-operated rats at 4 weeks (CKD, n = 10; Sham, n = 10) or 8 weeks (CKD, n = 12; Sham, n = 12) were obtained after collecting venous blood from inferior vena cava in heparinized tubes (BD Vacutainer, Franklin Lakes, NJ). The plasma samples were stored at −80°C until NMR analysis. Before NMR analysis, the frozen plasma samples were thawed at room temperature and centrifuged (10 min at 13,000 rpm, 4°C). Next, 200 μL of the supernatant was mixed with 400 μL of saline buffer solution (10% D_2O and 0.9% NaN_3) in 5 mm NMR tubes for analysis [12,15].

^{1}H NMR spectroscopy

^{1}H NMR spectra were acquired on a VNMRS 600-MHz NMR spectrometer at 25°C using a triple resonance 5 mm HCN salt-tolerant cold probe (Agilent Technologies Inc., Santa Clara, CA). The Carr-Purcell-Meiboom-Gill (CPMG) spin-echo pulse sequence (RD-90°-[τ-180°-τ] n-ACQ). A total T_2 relaxation time of 60 ms was used to attenuate broad signals from proteins and lipoproteins. The ^{1}H NMR spectrum was collected with a spectral width of 6720.4 Hz, relaxation delay of 2.0 s, and acquisition time of 4.0 s. Water solvent signal was suppressed by weak irradiating pulse on water peak during saturation delay. Free induction decay (FID) was acquired into 32,000 data points and the FID acquisitions were accumulated 128 times to increase signal-to-noise ratio. FIDs were weighted by an exponential function with a 0.3-Hz line broadening factor prior to Fourier transformation. All acquired NMR spectra were phase- and baseline-corrected, then referenced to the doublet at 1.32 ppm.

Data processing of the NMR spectra and multivariate statistical analysis

All NMR spectra were phased and baseline-corrected using AMIX software (version 3.9.4; Bruker Biospin GmbH, Rheinstetten, Germany). Each ^{1}H NMR spectrum from plasma collected 4 and 8 weeks after surgery was segmented into equal widths (0.005 ppm), corresponding to regions 0–9 ppm. The spectral data were normalized to the total spectral area. The data files were imported into MATLAB (R2008a; Mathworks, Natick, MA) and all spectra were aligned using the correlation-optimized warping method. The resulting data sets were then imported into SIMCA-P+ version 12.0 (Umetrics, Umea, Sweden), and all data were Pareto-scaled for multivariate statistical analysis. Principal components analysis (PCA), an unsupervised pattern recognition method, was performed to examine the intrinsic variation in the data set. To maximize the separation between samples, partial least-squares discriminant analysis (PLSDA), was applied. Permutation test was performed to check overfitting of the PLS-DA models. The PLS-DA models were validated using jackknife cross-validation [22]. Next, orthogonal partial least squares-discriminant analysis (OPLS-DA) was used to maximize covariance between the measured data (peak intensities from the NMR spectra) and the response variable (predictive classifications). The OPLS-DA color-coded coefficient loading plot was then used, which showed metabolites contributing to the separation between the CKD and sham-operated rats. The qualities of the models were described using R^2 and Q^2 values. R^2, which indicates the goodness of fit, is defined as the proportion of variance in the data explained by the model. Q^2, which indicates predictability, is defined as the

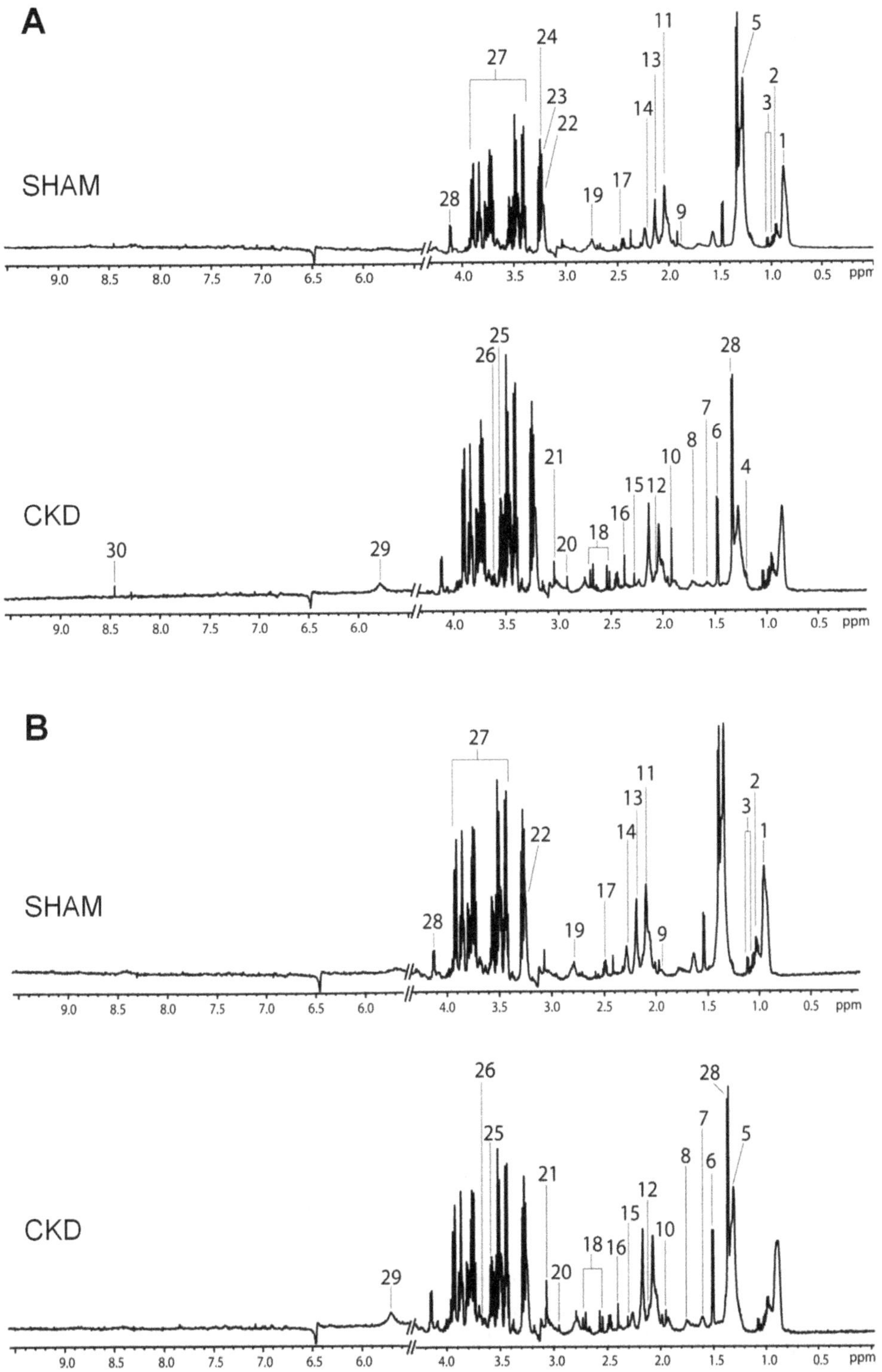

Figure 1. Representative 600 MHz ^{1}H nuclear magnetic resonance (NMR) spectra of plasma obtained from 5/6 nephrectomized CKD rats and sham-operated control rats at 4 weeks (A) or 8 weeks (B) after 5/6 nephrectomy and sham operation. 1, VLDL/LDL CH_3; 2, Leucine/Isoleucine; 3, Valine; 4, β-hydroxybutyrate; 5, VLDL/LDL $(CH_2)_n$; 6, Alanine; 7, Lipid $CH_2CH_2C=O$; 8, Lipid $CH_2CH_2C=C$; 9, Arginine; 10, Acetate; 11, N-acetylglycoproteins; 12, Glutamine; 13, Methionine; 14, Lipid $CH_2C=O$; 15, Acetoacetate; 16, Pyruvate; 17, Glutamate/Glutamine; 18, Citrate; 19, Dimethylamine (DMA); 20, Trimethylamine (TMA); 21, Creatinine; 22, Choline; 23, Trimethylamine-N-oxide (TMAO); 24, O-phosphocholine; 25, Myo-inositol; 26, Glycine; 27, Glucose/Maltose; 28, Lactate; 29, Urea; and 30, Formate. CKD, chronic kidney disease.

proportion of variance in the data predictable by the model [14]. A non-overlapping ^{1}H signal from each metabolite was used to calculate the integral area and the identified metabolites were quantified by relative peak intensity [23]. Resonant frequencies of each metabolite were referred from library of Chenomx NMR Sutie 7.1(Chenomx, Edomonton, Canada) and previous studies

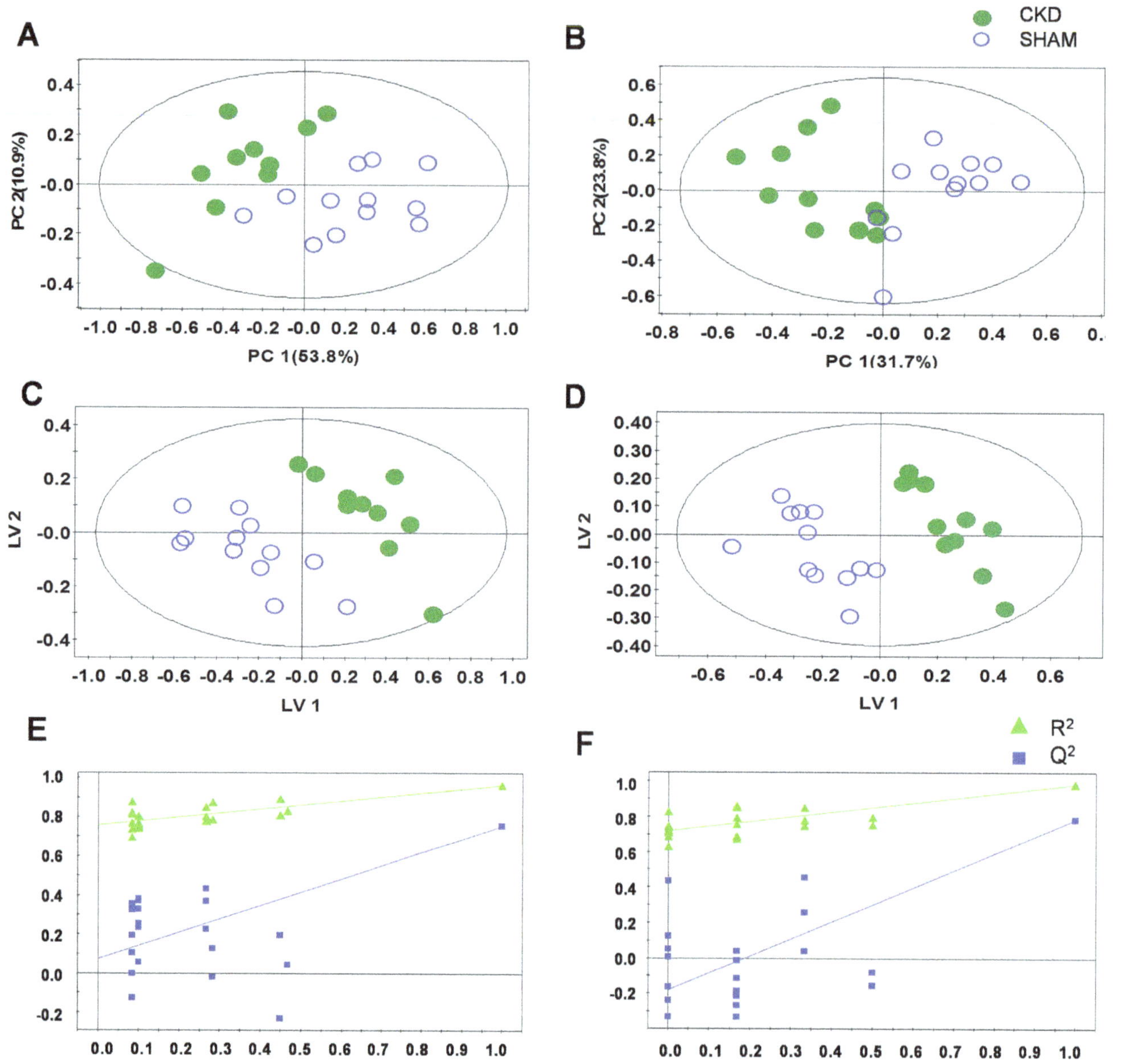

Figure 2. Principal component analysis (PCA), partial least squares-discriminant analysis (PLS-DA) score scatter plots and permutation tests of PLS-DA obtained from the ^{1}H NMR spectra of plasma at 4 weeks (A, C, E) or 8 weeks (B, D, F) after 5/6 nephrectomy and sham operation, demonstrating a clear differentiation between the two groups. CKD, chronic kidney disease.

[12,15,24,25,26]. The Mann–Whitney test and Welch' t-test were performed to compare metabolite levels between the two groups. Statistical analyses were performed using Prism version 5 for Windows (GraphPad Software, San Diego, CA).

Results

CKD induced by 5/6 nephrectomy in rats

As shown in Table 1, CKD rats exhibited significantly decreased renal functions. The levels of plasma creatinine in CKD rats at 4 weeks (49.8±5.6 μmol/L, n = 10, P<0.05) and 8 weeks (59.7±3.9 μmol/L, n = 12, P<0.05) were significantly higher than their corresponding sham-operated control rats. Moreover, plasma urea nitrogen levels in CKD rats at 4 weeks (15.2±2.1 mmol/L, n = 10, P<0.05) and 8 weeks (16.2±1.2 mmol/L, n = 12, P<0.05) were significantly increased (Table 1). In addition, CKD rats had higher plasma osmolality and plasma potassium levels, whereas plasma sodium concentrations were unchanged (Table 1). The weight of remnant kidneys in CKD was significantly lower at 4 weeks (1.3±0.1 g, n = 10, P<0.05) than that of their corresponding sham-operated control rats (right kidney: 1. 6±0.1 g, n = 10, Table 1). In contrast, at 8 weeks the weight of remnant kidneys was significantly higher (2.2±0.2 g, n = 12, P<0.05) than their corresponding sham-operated control rats (right kidney: 1.6±0.1 g, n = 12, Table 1), indicating that the remnant kidneys in CKD were significantly hypertrophied.

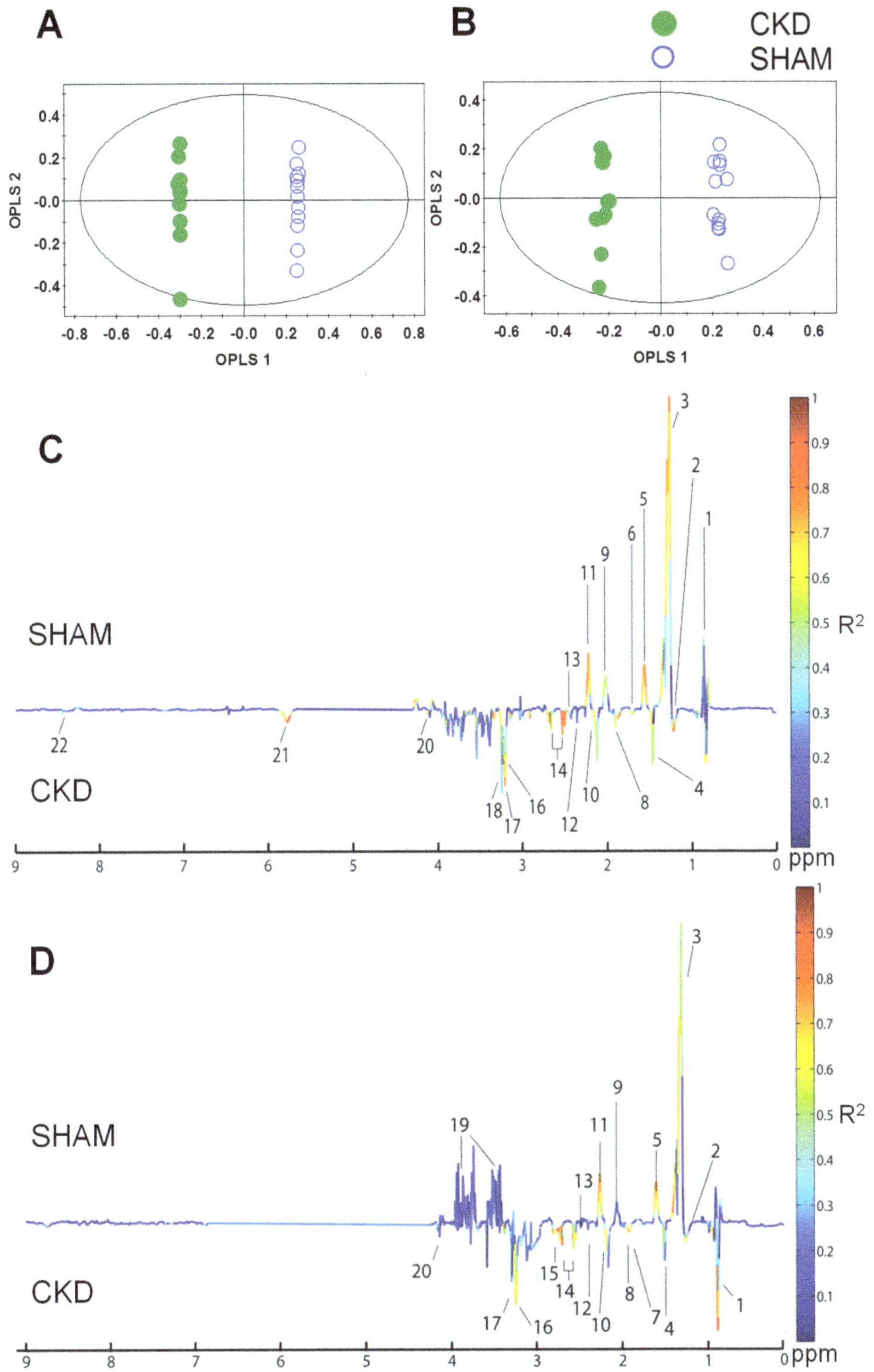

Figure 3. Orthogonal partial least-squares discriminant analysis (OPLS-DA) score and coefficient loading plots derived from the ^1H NMR spectra derived from plasma at 4 weeks (A, C) or 8 weeks (B, D) after 5/6 nephrectomy and sham operation. The OPLS-DA coefficient loading plot shows a significant difference in the metabolite levels between the two groups. 1, VLDL/LDL CH_3; 2, β-hydroxybutyrate; 3, VLDL/LDL $(CH_2)_n$; 4, Alanine; 5, Lipid $CH_2CH_2C=O$; 6, Lipid $CH_2CH_2C=C$; 7, Arginine; 8, Acetate; 9, N-acetylglycoproteins; 10, Methionine; 11, Lipid $CH_2C=O$; 12, Acetoacetate; 13, Glutamine/Glutamate; 14, Citrate; 15, Trimethylamine (TMA); 16, Choline; 17, Trimethylamine-N-oxide (TMAO); 18, O-phosphocholine; 19, Glucose/Maltose; 20, Lactate; 21, Urea; and 22, Formate. CKD, chronic kidney disease.

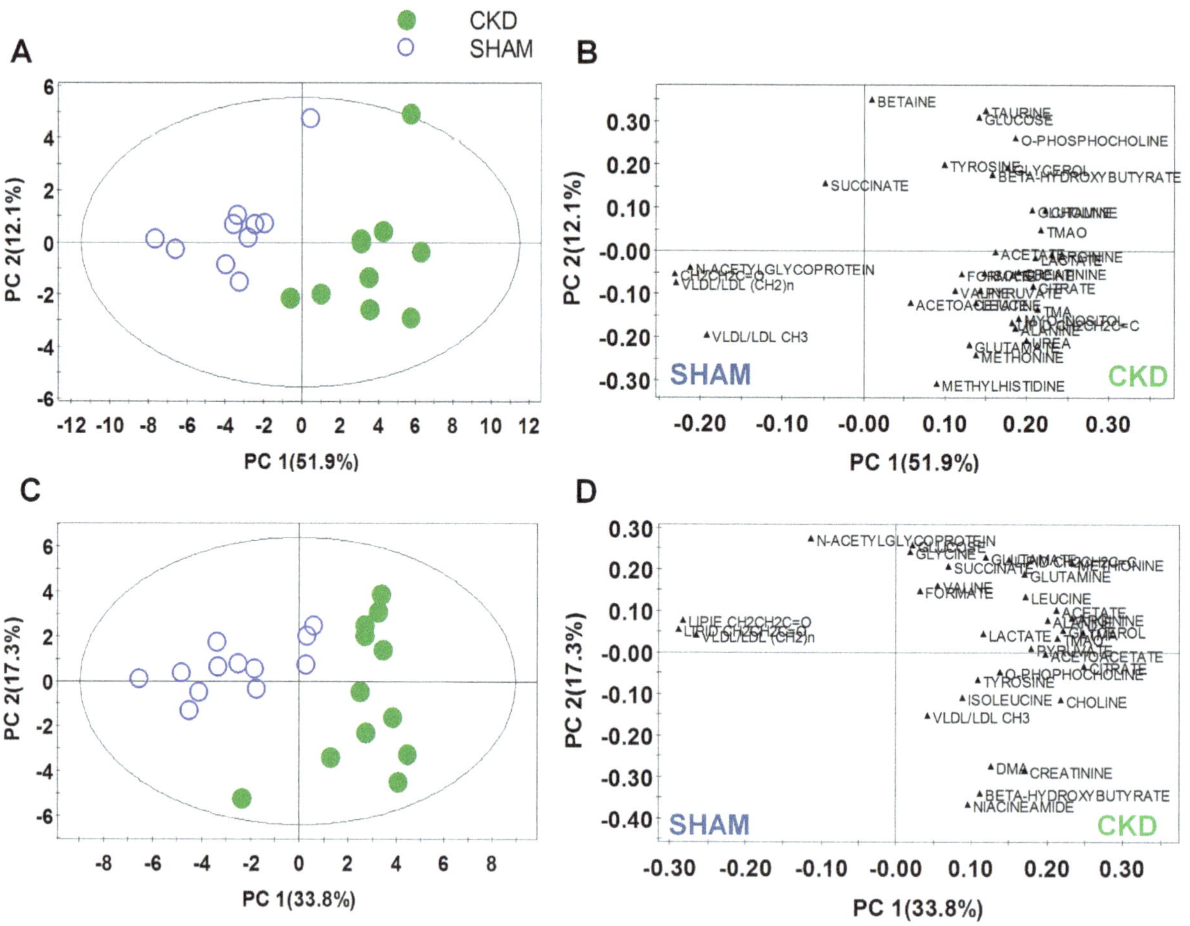

Figure 4. PCA score scatter and loading plots of metabolites quantification through targeted profiling of plasma at 4 weeks (A, B) and 8 (C, D), respectively. The loading plots were produced from the score plots which showed a significant differentiation between the two groups. CKD, chronic kidney disease.

^{1}H NMR spectroscopic analysis of plasma

The plasma metabolites were investigated using ^{1}H NMR spectroscopy coupled with multivariate data analysis to identify the metabolic characteristics of early stage of CKD. ^{1}H NMR (600 MHz) spectra of plasma samples obtained from sham-operated and CKD rats over 4 or 8 weeks are shown in Figure 1A and B. The spectral resonance of each metabolite was assigned on the basis of the 600-MHz library in Chenomx NMR suite 7.1 (Chenomx) and previous studies. Ambiguous peaks due to overlap or slight shifts were confirmed by spiking samples with the respective standard compounds. The plasma ^{1}H NMR spectra contained a number of metabolites, including VLDL/LDL CH_3, leucine, isoleucine, valine, β-hydroxybutyrate, VLDL/LDL $(CH_2)_n$, alanine, lipid $CH_2CH_2C=O$, lipid $CH_2CH_2C=C$, arginine, acetate, *N*-acetylglycoproteins, glutamine, methionine, lipid $CH_2C=O$, acetoacetate, pyruvate, glutamate, citrate, dimethylamine (DMA), trimethylamine (TMA), creatinine, choline, TMA-N-oxide (TMAO), *O*-phosphocholine, myo-inositol, glycine, glucose, lactate, urea, and formate. Those metabolites showing the greatest difference between the CKD and sham-operated groups were VLDL/LDL CH_3, β-hydroxybutyrate, VLDL/LDL $(CH_2)_n$, alanine, acetate, glutamine, methionine, acetoacetate, citrate, TMA, creatinine, lactate, and formate.

Multivariate pattern recognition analysis

To examine intrinsic variations between the two plasma data sets, PCA was initially performed using ^{1}H NMR data [14]. As shown in Figure 2, the score plots for those samples collected at 4 weeks (Figure 2A: $R^2X=0.722$, $Q^2=0.562$) and 8 weeks (Figure 2B: $R^2X=0.672$, $Q^2=0.493$) were distinct between the CKD and sham-operated groups. Next, PLS-DA was employed, and it also indicated a clear difference, with increasing predictability of the separation between the two groups at 4 weeks (Figure 2C: $R^2X=0.769$, $R^2Y=0.997$, $Q^2=0.924$) and 8 weeks (Figure 2D: $R^2X=0.464$, $R^2Y=0.982$, $Q^2=0.782$). The PLS-DA models were validated using jackknife cross-validation. The accuracy of PLS-DA model for 4 weeks CKD models was 95% with 5 latent variables (LVs). The accuracy of PLS-DA models for 8 weeks CKD models was 100% with 3 LVs. The permutation tests of PLS-DA models showed that our models were not overfitted (Figures 2E and 2F). Next, to minimize the possible contribution of intergroup variability and to further improve the separation between the two groups, OPLS-DA was applied [15]. As shown in Figure 3, the score plots for 4 weeks (Figure 3A: $R^2X=0.769$, $R^2Y=0.997$, $Q^2=0.845$) and 8 weeks (Figure 3B: $R^2X=0.728$, $R^2Y=0.996$, $Q^2=0.899$) were clearly different between the CKD and sham-operated rats. The model parameters for explained variation, R^2, and predictive capability, Q^2, were calculated to assess the significance of the differences and were

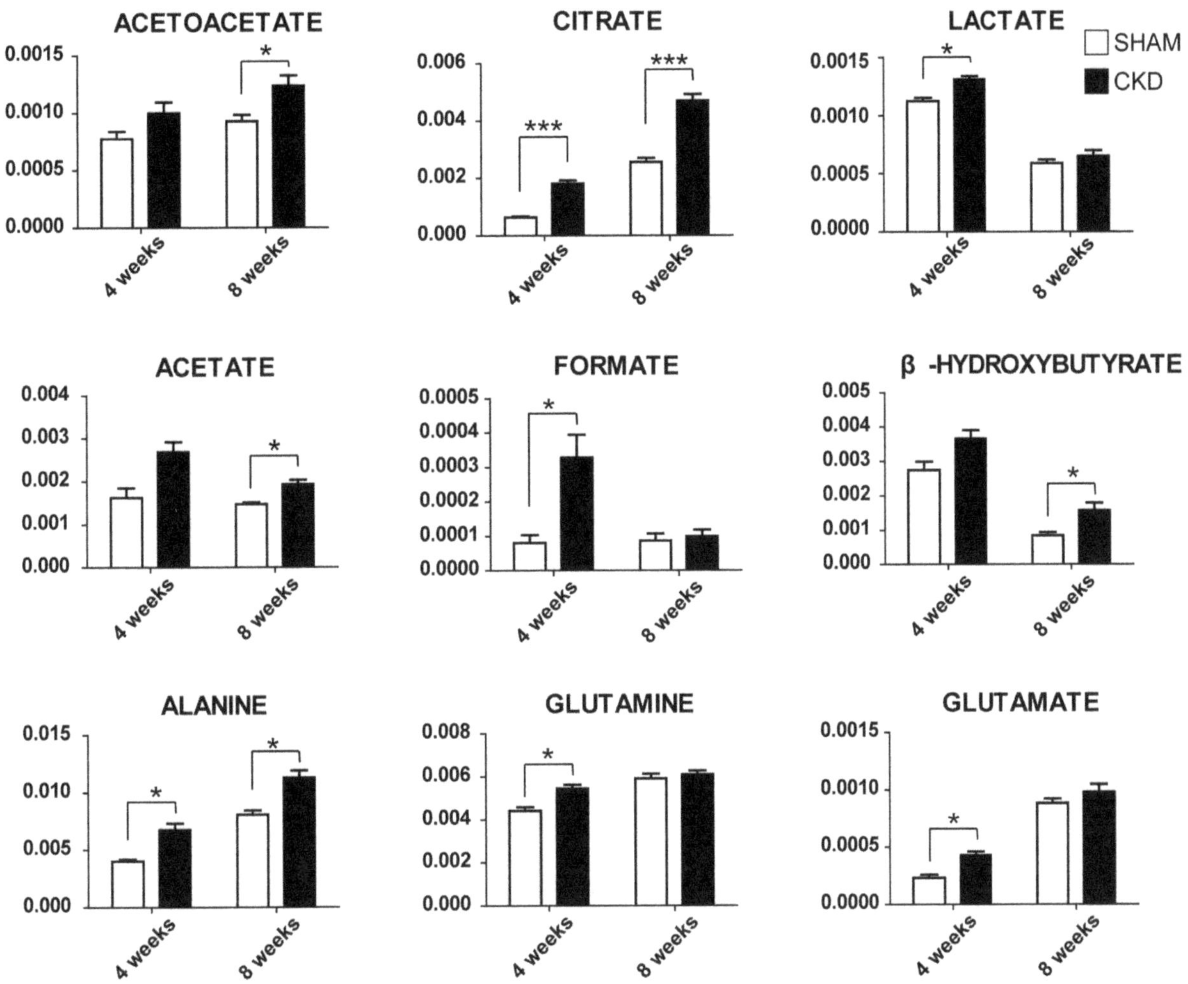

Figure 5. Quantification of changes of plasma metabolites in rats with CKD at 4 weeks and 8 weeks after 5/6 nephrectomy, respectively. *, **, *** indicate bonferroni corrected $P<0.05$, <0.01, and <0.001, respectively.

substantially high in plasma, indicating that the disease model of CKD was well established. Compared with the PCA model, our PLS-DA and OPLS-DA models indicated improved predictability, with increased Q^2 values. In terms of monitoring time, although the value of Q^2 did not exhibit a sharp difference, better separation between the two groups was seen at 4 weeks than at 8 weeks. An OPLS-DA coefficient plot, coded by color, was constructed to investigate the underlying variables contributing to the differentiation between the two groups. In the plot, negative peaks indicate higher metabolite levels in the plasma of the CKD rats compared to the sham-operated rats, while positive peaks indicate higher metabolite levels in the plasma of the sham-operated control rats.

As shown in the OPLS-DA coefficient loading plot (Figure 3), the CKD groups at 4 weeks (Figure 3C) and 8 weeks (Figure 3D) after 5/6 nephrectomy were characterized by elevated levels of β-hydroxybutyrate, lactate, alanine, acetate, acetoacetate, methionine, glutamine, glutamate, citrate, TMA, choline, phosphocholine, TMAO, urea, and formate, and by decreased levels of VLDL/LDL $(CH_2)_n$ and *N*-acetylglycoproteins, compared to the sham-operated control rats. In particular, the metabolites VLDL/LDL CH_3, VLDL/LDL $(CH_2)_n$, lipid $CH_2CH_2C=O$, *N*-acetylglycoproteins, lipid $CH_2C=O$, β-hydroxybutyrate, alanine, acetate, citrate, TMAO, and urea showed greater differences between the groups than the other metabolites, regardless of whether their levels were increased or decreased. These data indicate an altered metabolic pattern between the two groups, as well as the identities of the metabolites responsible for the observed differences.

Quantitative analysis of the metabolites

NMR spectroscopy is a highly quantitative technique that can be used to accurately determine metabolite concentration, because integral area of metabolite peak is directly proportional to the metabolite concentration. A spectral peak from each metabolite was used to calculate the integral area and the identified metabolites were quantified by peak intensity. The metabolites were identified according to previous reports and the 600-MHz library from the Chenomx 7.1 NMR suite; several metabolites are displayed in Table 2. Differences in the levels of the relatively quantified plasma metabolites between the CKD and sham-operated groups were compared using multivariate analysis. PCA score plots derived from the quantification of plasma metabolites at 4 (Figure 4A; $R^2X=0.72$, $Q^2=0.39$) and 8 weeks (Figure 4C; $R^2X=0.723$, $Q^2=0.279$) show clear separation. In the same manner as global profiling, better separation of the two groups was shown at 4 weeks compared to 8 weeks based on the value of Q^2. To identify the metabolites responsible for the differentiation

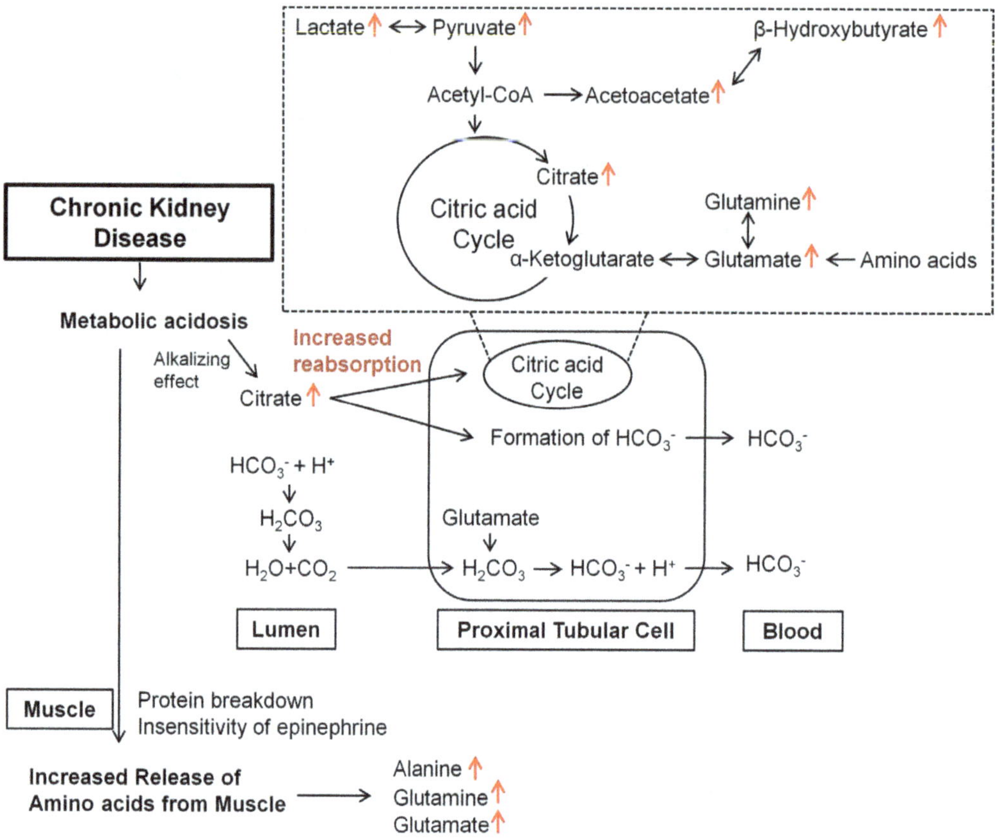

Figure 6. A diagram for the changes in plasma metabolites in CKD. The metabolite profiles of plasma in rats with CKD showed significantly increased levels of lactate, pyruvate, acetoacetate, β-hydroxybutyrate, glutamine, glutamate, and citrate. Metabolic acidosis is commonly complicated in CKD, due to both decreased net acid excretion and impaired regeneration of bicarbonate. This could change the citrate reabsorption in renal tubular cells, which metabolism generates HCO_3^- ions producing an alkalinizing effect. Moreover, increased protein breakdown and insensitivity to epinephrine in muscle in CKD could induce the increases of alanine, glutamate, and glutamine in plasma.

between the two groups in the PCA score plots, PCA loading scatter plots were generated (Figure 4B, 4 weeks; Figure 4D, 8 weeks) through targeted profiling. Notably, on the basis of our quantitative data, most of the identified metabolites were substantially higher in the CKD rats than in the sham-operated rats. β-Hydroxybutyrate, lactate, alanine, acetate, acetoacetate, methionine, pyruvate, glutamine, glutamate, citrate, TMA, choline, *O*-phosphocholine, TMAO, creatinine, formate, and urea (4 weeks only) were elevated in the plasma of the CKD rats. In contrast, VLDL/LDL $(CH_2)_n$, lipid $CH_2CH_2C=O$, and *N*-acetylglycoproteins were decreased in the rats with CKD. These results are consistent with the above OPLS-DA color-coded loading plots (Figure 3C and D). Those metabolites that differed markedly between the CKD and sham-operated groups were β-hydroxybutyrate, alanine, lipid $CH_2CH_2C=O$, acetate, acetoacetate, methionine, glutamate, citrate, TMA, TMAO, urea (4 weeks only), and formate. To determine whether the differences between the CKD and sham-operated groups were significant, the Mann–Whitney test and Welch's t-test were performed after the Shapiro–Wilk normality test. The p-value from Mann-Witney test and Welch's t-test were adjusted by bonferroni correction for multiple comparisons. Those metabolites that were significantly different between the two groups are summarized in Table 2; the ratios of the relative metabolite concentrations in the CKD *vs*. the sham-operated group were shown in Table 2. In particular, significant increases in organic acids, including β-hydroxybutyrate, lactate, acetate, acetoacetate, citrate, and formate, and muscle-related amino acids were identified (Figure 5) and metabolic pathway related to the alteration of plasma metabolites in CKD was presented in Figure 6.

Discussion

We investigated the changes of plasma metabolites in CKD using ^{1}H NMR-based metabolite profiling approach to understand the systemic disturbance of metabolism associated with the early stage of CKD. The metabolite profiles of plasma from rats with CKD showed significantly increased levels of organic acids, including citrate, β-hydroxybutyrate, lactate, acetate, acetoacetate, and formate, accompanied by increased alanine and glutamine levels.

In the present study, the levels of various metabolites in plasma were rapidly measured using the metabolite profiling procedure and thereafter the differences in the levels of plasma metabolites were compared using multivariate analysis, e.g., PCA-DA and OPLS-DA. The metabolic profiling and multivariate pattern recognition approach we have used herein allow us to observe simultaneously a wide range of metabolites which concentrations could be changed under the progression of CKD. Since metabolites can be regulated *via* a number of metabolic pathways, investigation of the whole feature of metabolites rather than several selected metabolites enables us to understand the underlying pathophysiological status of CKD more comprehen-

Table 2. ^{1}H chemical shift and relative concentrations of metabolites observed in plasma from CKD and sham-operated groups.

Metabolite	Chemical chifts (δ 1H p.p.m)	Fold change ratio CKD/SHAM	
		4 weeks	8 weeks
VLDL/LDL CH_3	0.36 (m), 0.86 (m)	0.853	1.077
Isoleucine	0.94 (t), 1.03 (d), 1.46 (m), 3.66 (d),	1.090	1.094
Leucine	0.94 (t), 0.99 (d), 1.70 (m), 3.72 (m)	1.156	1.076
Valine	1.00 (d), 10.3(d)	1.201	0.957
β-hydroxybutyrate	1.12 (d), 2.3 (dd), 2.4 (dd), 4.1 (m)	1.329	1.857 *
VLDL/LDL $(CH_2)_n$	1.25 (m)	0.55**	0.745*
Lactate	1.32(d), 4.13 (m)	1.164*	1.102
Alanine	1.48 (d), 3.81 (q)	1.689*	1.395*
Lipid $CH_2CH_2C=O$	1.56 (br)	1.296	1.124
Arginine	1.63–171 (m), 1.91 (m), 323 (t)	1.366**	1.471
Lipid $CH_2CH_2C=C$	1.7 (br)	0.335**	0.428**
Acetate	1.91 (s)	1.649	1.314*
N-acetylglycoproteins	2.04 (s)	0.844*	0.947
Glutamate	2.06 (m), 2.41 (m), 3.76 (m)	1.848*	1.109
Glutamine	2.12 (m), 2.44 (m), 3.76 (m)	1.231*	1.031
Methionine	2.15 (s), 2.16 (m), 2.65 (dd), 3.87(m)	1.953	1.199
Acetoacetate	2.26 (s), 3.49(s)	1.290	1.332*
Pyruvate	2.4 (s)	1.320	1.168
Dimethylanine	2.50 (s)	0.950	1.228*
Citrate	2.54 (d), 2.69 (d)	2.846***	1.834***
Trimethylamine	2.9 (s)	1.759***	1.379**
Creatinine	3.04 (s), 4.05 (s)	1.645	1.382
Choline	3.19 (s), 3.50 (m), 4.07 (m)	1.224**	1.104
Glucose	3.23 (t), 3.40–3.48 (m), 4.64 (d), 5.23 (d)	1.083	0.924
Trimethylamine-N-oxide	3.27 (s)	1.338*	1.148
O-phosphocholine	3.3 (s), 4.21(t), 3.61 (t)	1.157	1.034
Urea	5.8 (br)	3.748**	4 weeks only
Tyrosine	6.88(d),7.18(d)	1.220	1.213
Formate	8.45 (s)	4.049*	1.214

Letters in parentheses denote the peak multiplicities: s, singlet; d, double; t, triplet; dd, doublet of doublet; m, multiplets and br, broad; The fold change ratio indicates the ratio of relative concentrations between CKD and sham-operated groups; Statistical analysis was performed by Mann-Whitney test and Welch's t-test to assess the statistical significance between CKD vs. sham-operated groups; *, **, *** indicate bonferroni corrected $P<0.05$, <0.01, and <0.001, respectively.

sively. In this point, the current study differs from the previous reports and provides the significance of the observations.

In particular, plasma organic acids levels were significantly higher in rats with CKD. As the conjugate base of an acid, organic anions (e.g., citrate, β-hydroxybutyrate, lactate, acetate, acetoacetate, and formate) are potential bases, because they are readily metabolized HCO_3^-. Generally, renal contribution to acid–base homeostasis involves the regulated reabsorption of filtered HCO_3^- ions and the regeneration of sufficient HCO_3^- ions to neutralize the acid load. The kidneys also regulate alkaline compounds, including organic anions, to maintain the acid–base balance [4]. In the kidneys, HCO_3^- is freely filtered in the glomerulus and the proximal tubule reabsorbs approximately 80% of the filtered HCO_3^- and creates new HCO_3^- by secreting H^+ ions into its lumen through a Na^+/H^+ exchanger, and transporting HCO_3^- ions *via* the basolateral Na^+/HCO_3^- co-transporter [27,28,29]. The secreted H^+ ions react with filtered HCO_3^- to form carbonic acid (H_2CO_3), which dissociates to CO_2 and H_2O. These substances then enter the cell, forming H_2CO_3. The H_2CO_3 is converted into H^+ and HCO_3^- intracellularly, thereby regenerating protons for the secretion into the lumen and the reabsorption of HCO_3^- into the blood [4,5,30,31,32]. Next, the thick ascending limb of the loop of Henle reabsorbs 10–15% of the filtered HCO_3^- that has escaped from the proximal tubule and then the distal tubule and collecting duct reabsorb nearly all of the remaining HCO_3^- [4,31,33,34,35].

In CKD, reduced net acid excretion and/or impaired reabsorption and regeneration of HCO_3^- could result in systemic metabolic acidosis, due to the decreased glomerular filtration rates and the number of functioning nephrons. This was previously confirmed in CRF rats induced by 5/6 nephrectomy, demonstrating that blood pH and $[HCO_3^-]$ levels were significantly decreased [36]. In this study, blood pH or $[HCO_3^-]$ levels were not measured. However, CRF rats exhibited significantly increased blood urea nitrogen (BUN), creatinine, and potassium levels, compared with sham operated control rats. The finding indicated that renal function was significantly deteriorated and metabolic acidosis was likely to be associated with 5/6 nephrectomy.

Citrate is an important metabolic substrate in the kidneys and the most prevalent of the organic anions, accounting for about 10% of the energy production [37]. We demonstrated that citrate levels were significantly increased in plasma of rats with CKD. Citrate has three carboxyl groups, and consequently the metabolism of one citrate molecule generates three HCO_3^- ions producing an alkalinizing effect [37,38]. Therefore, retention of citrate and other organic anions by the kidneys is beneficial for counteracting metabolic acidosis, while increased excretion is beneficial for attenuating metabolic alkalosis [32]. Citrate is freely filtered by the glomerulus and up to 99% of the filtered load is reabsorbed in the proximal tubule *via* the apical membrane Na^+/citrate co-transporter [38]. Metabolic acidosis increases renal citrate reabsorption and decreases urinary excretion. Consistent with this, Brennan *et al.* [39] demonstrated that decreasing the luminal pH caused an increase in citrate reabsorption, while increasing the luminal pH resulted in a fall in citrate reabsorption. During metabolic acidosis, therefore, the changes in blood pH could be minimized partly by the changes in renal citrate transport and metabolism, which are brought about by an adaptive increase in the activity of the Na^+/citrate co-transporter [40]. The change of protein abundance of Na^+/citrate co-transporter in the kidneys of rats with CKD needs to be determined.

We also demonstrated that rats with CKD exhibited elevated levels of alanine, glutamine, and glutamate. Alanine and glutamine are the prime precursors in hepatic and renal gluconeogenesis, respectively, accounting for two-thirds of the total amino acids released from the muscle [41,42,43]. Previous studies demonstrated that metabolic acidosis induced by CKD was associated with higher levels of alanine, glutamine, and glutamate in blood, possibly due to abnormal nitrogen utilization and accelerated net protein breakdown stimulated by muscle proteolysis [44,45]. In addition, insensitivity to epinephrine affects the increases of alanine and glutamine in patients with CKD. Epinephrine is known to decrease the release and formation of alanine and glutamine by inhibiting the conversion of precursor amino acids to alanine and glutamine, and by reducing the rate of amino acid transport out of muscle cells [42]. Hence, the insensitivity to epinephrine observed in uremia, in turn, increases alanine and glutamine release from muscle [46].

In summary, we demonstrated the comprehensive systemic feature of metabolic disorders in the plasma in rats with CKD by exploiting ^{1}H NMR-based metabolomic approaches combined with multivariate analyses. The metabolite profiles of plasma from rats with CKD demonstrated significantly increased levels of organic acids, alanine and glutamine levels. The observed changes of metabolites are likely to be clinically relevant to the well-known disturbed metabolism in early phase of CKD, in particular altered metabolism of acid-base and/or amino acids. However, since this study focused on 5/6 nephrectomy model, i.e. a surgical resection model of renal mass, further studies are needed to understand whether the observed changes in plasma metabolites are generally applicable to the CKD, irrespective of the underlying causes, e.g., diabetic kidney diseases or immune-mediated CKD.

Author Contributions

Conceived and designed the experiments: THK GSH. Performed the experiments: JAK HJC. Analyzed the data: JAK HJC YKK DHR. Contributed reagents/materials/analysis tools: DHR THK GSH. Wrote the paper: JAK HJC YKK THK GSH.

References

1. Bouby N, Hassler C, Parvy P, Bankir L (1993) Renal synthesis of arginine in chronic renal failure: in vivo and in vitro studies in rats with 5/6 nephrectomy. Kidney Int 44: 676–676.
2. RJ A, editor (2000) The kidney.6th: W.B. WB saunders Co. 455–519 p.
3. Zhao YY, Liu J, Cheng XL, Bai X, Lin RC (2011) Urinary metabonomics study on biochemical changes in an experimental model of chronic renal failure by adenine based on UPLC Q-TOF/MS. Clin Chim Acta 413:642–649.
4. Weiner ID, Verlander JW, Wingo CS (2011) Renal acidification mechanisms. Core Concepts in the Disorders of Fluid, Electrolytes and Acid-Base Balance: 203–233.
5. Kraut JA, Kurtz I (2005) Metabolic acidosis of CKD: diagnosis, clinical characteristics, and treatment. Am J Kidney Dis 45: 978–993.
6. Roderick P, Willis N, Blakeley S, Jones C, Tomson C (2007) Correction of chronic metabolic acidosis for chronic kidney disease patients. Cochrane Database Syst Rev 1:CD001890.
7. Kovesdy CP, Anderson JE, Kalantar-Zadeh K (2009) Association of serum bicarbonate levels with mortality in patients with non-dialysis-dependent CKD. Nephrol Dial Transplant 24: 1232–1237.
8. Charles JC, Heilman RL (2005) Metabolic acidosis. Hospital Physician 41: 37–42.
9. Adeva MM, Souto G (2011) Diet-induced metabolic acidosis. Clin Nutr 30: 416–421.
10. Farber M, Szwed J, Dowell A, Strawbridge R (1976) The acute effects of respiratory and metabolic acidosis on renal function in the dog. Clin Sci Mol Med 50: 165–169.
11. de Brito-Ashurst I, Varagunam M, Raftery MJ, Yaqoob MM (2009) Bicarbonate supplementation slows progression of CKD and improves nutritional status. JASN 20: 2075–2084.
12. Choi J-Y, Yoon YJ, Choi H-J, Park S-H, Kim C-D, et al. (2011) Dialysis modality-dependent changes in serum metabolites: accumulation of inosine and hypoxanthine in patients on haemodialysis. Nephrol Dial Transplant 26: 1304–1313.
13. Hwang GS, Yang JY, Ryu DH, Kwon TH (2010) Metabolic profiling of kidney and urine in rats with lithium-induced nephrogenic diabetes insipidus by ^{1}H-NMR-based metabonomics. Am J Physiol Renal Physiol 298: F461–F470.
14. Jang ZH, Chung HC, Ahn YG, Kwon YK, Kim JS, et al. (2012) Metabolic profiling of an alcoholic fatty liver in zebrafish (Danio rerio). Mol BioSyst 8:2001–2009.
15. Jung JY, Lee HS, Kang DG, Kim NS, Cha MH, et al. (2011) ^{1}H-NMR-based metabolomics study of cerebral infarction. Stroke 42: 1282–1288.
16. Kirschenlohr HL, Griffin JL, Clarke SC, Rhydwen R, Grace AA, et al. (2006) Proton NMR analysis of plasma is a weak predictor of coronary artery disease. Nat Med 12: 705–710.
17. Schicho R, Shaykhutdinov R, Ngo J, Nazyrova A, Schneider C, et al. (2012) Quantitative Metabolomic Profiling of Serum, Plasma, and Urine by ^{1}H NMR Spectroscopy Discriminates between Patients with Inflammatory Bowel Disease and Healthy Individuals. J Proteome Res 11: 3344–3357.
18. Kim CD, Kim EY, Yoo H, Lee JW, Ryu DH, et al. (2010) Metabonomic analysis of serum metabolites in kidney transplant recipients with cyclosporine A- or tacrolimus-based immunosuppression. Transplantation 90: 748–756.
19. Choi H-J, Yoon Y-J, Kwon Y-K, Lee Y-J, Chae S, et al. (2012) Patterns of Gene and Metabolite Define the Effects of Extracellular Osmolality on Kidney Collecting Duct. J Proteome Res 11: 3816–3828.
20. Kwon TH, Frøkiaer J, Fernández-Llama P, Maunsbach AB, Knepper MA, et al. (1999) Altered expression of Na transporters NHE-3, NaPi-II, Na-K-ATPase, BSC-1, and TSC in CRF rat kidneys. Am J Physiol Renal Physiol 277: F257–F270.
21. Kwon TH, Frøkiaer J, Knepper MA, Nielsen S (1998) Reduced AQP1,-2, and-3 levels in kidneys of rats with CRF induced by surgical reduction in renal mass. Am J Physiol Renal Physiol 275: F724–F741.
22. Efron B, Gong G (1983) A leisurely look at the bootstrap, the jackknife, and cross-validation. Am Stat 37: 36–48.
23. Somashekar BS, Amin AG, Tripathi P, MacKinnon N, Rithner CD, et al. (2012) Metabolomic signatures in guinea pigs infected with epidemic-associated W-Beijing strains of Mycobacterium tuberculosis. J Proteome Res 11: 4873–4884.
24. Hong YS, Ahn YT, Park JC, Lee JH, Lee H, et al. (2010) ^{1} H NMR-based metabonomic assessment of probiotic effects in a colitis mouse model. Arch Pharm Res 33: 1091–1101.
25. Shin JH, Yang JY, Jeon BY, Yoon YJ, Cho SN, et al. (2011) 1H NMR-based metabolomic profiling in mice infected with Mycobacterium tuberculosis. J Proteome Res 10: 2238–2247.
26. Soininen P, Kangas AJ, Würtz P, Tukiainen T, Tynkkynen T, et al. (2009) High-throughput serum NMR metabonomics for cost-effective holistic studies on systemic metabolism. Analyst 134: 1781–1785.
27. Alpern R (1990) Cell mechanisms of proximal tubule acidification. Physiol Rev 70: 79–114.

28. Boron WF, Boulpaep EL (1983) Intracellular pH regulation in the renal proximal tubule of the salamander. Basolateral HCO_3-transport. J Gen Physiol 81: 53–94.
29. Romero MF, Hediger MA, Boulpaep EL, Boron WF (1997) Expression cloning and characterization of a renal electrogenic Na+/HCO3− cotransporter. Nature 387: 409–413.
30. Boron WF (2006) Acid-base transport by the renal proximal tubule. JASN 17: 2368–2382.
31. Laing CM, Toye AM, Capasso G, Unwin RJ (2005) Renal tubular acidosis: developments in our understanding of the molecular basis. Int J Biochem Cell Biol 37: 1151–1161.
32. Hamm LL (1990) Renal handling of citrate. Kidney Int 38: 728–735.
33. Choi I, Aalkjaer C, Boulpaep EL, Boron WF (2000) An electroneutral sodium/bicarbonate cotransporter NBCn1 and associated sodium channel. Nature 405: 571–575.
34. Kwon TH, Fulton C, Wang W, Kurtz I, Frøkiaer J, et al. (2002) Chronic metabolic acidosis upregulates rat kidney Na-HCO3- cotransporters NBCn1 and NBC3 but not NBC1. Am J Physiol Renal Physiol 282: F341–F351.
35. Vorum H, Kwon TH, Fulton C, Simonsen B, Choi I, et al. (2000) Immunolocalization of electroneutral Na-HCO3− cotransporter in rat kidney. Am J Physiol Renal Physiol 279: F901–F909.
36. Maddox DA, Horn JF, Famiano FC, Gennari FJ (1986) Load dependence of proximal tubular fluid and bicarbonate reabsorption in the remnant kidney of the Munich-Wistar rat. J Clin Invest 77: 1639–1649.
37. Tanner GA, Tanner JA (2000) Citrate therapy for polycystic kidney disease in rats. Kidney Int 58: 1859–1869.
38. Alpern RJ (1995) Trade-offs in the adaptation to acidosis. Kidney Int 47: 1205–1215.
39. Brennan S, Hering-Smith K, Hamm L (1988) Effect of pH on citrate reabsorption in the proximal convoluted tubule. Am J Physiol Renal Physiol 255: F301–F306.
40. Jenkins AD, Dousa TP, Smith LH (1985) Transport of citrate across renal brush border membrane: effects of dietary acid and alkali loading. Am J Physiol Renal Physiol 249: F590–F595.
41. Condon J, Asatoor A (1971) Amino acid metabolism in uraemic patients. Clin Chim Acta 32: 333–337.
42. Garber A, Karl I, Kipnis D (1976) Alanine and glutamine synthesis and release from skeletal muscle. I. Glycolysis and amino acid release. J Biol Chem 251: 826–835.
43. Garber AJ (1978) Skeletal muscle protein and amino acid metabolism in experimental chronic uremia in the rat: accelerated alanine and glutamine formation and release. J Clin Invest 62: 623–632.
44. May R, Kelly R, Mitch W (1986) Metabolic acidosis stimulates protein degradation in rat muscle by a glucocorticoid-dependent mechanism. J Clin Invest 77: 614–621.
45. May R, Kelly R, Mitch W (1987) Mechanisms for defects in muscle protein metabolism in rats with chronic uremia. Influence of metabolic acidosis. J Clin Invest 79: 1099–1103.
46. Garber AJ (1978) The regulation of skeletal muscle alanine and glutamine formation and release in experimental chronic uremia in the rat: subsensitivity of adenylate cyclase and amino acid release to epinephrine and serotonin. J Clin Invest 62: 633–641.

21

An Estimation of the Prevalence and Progression of Chronic Kidney Disease in a Rural Diabetic Cambodian Population

Bernadette Thomas[1]*, Maurits van Pelt[2], Rajnish Mehrotra[1], Cassianne Robinson-Cohen[3], James LoGerfo[4]

1 Division of Nephrology, Department of Medicine, University of Washington, Seattle, Washington, United States of America, **2** MoPoTsyo Patient Information Centre, Phnom Penh, Cambodia, **3** Kidney Research Institute, University of Washington, Seattle, Washington, United States of America, **4** Department of Medicine, University of Washington, Seattle, Washington, United States of America

Abstract

Background: To date, there are no known estimates of the prevalence of chronic kidney disease within Cambodia, the vast majority of whose citizens live in rural areas with limited access to renal replacement therapy.

Methods: Observational analysis of patients from the Takeo province in Cambodia who presented to MoPoTsyo, a non-governmental organization, for screening and management of diabetes mellitus between 2010 and 2012 (n = 402; 75% females). Estimated glomerular filtration rate (eGFR) was calculated using the CKD-Epi equation.

Results: On average, women were younger, with a higher percentage of hypercholesterolemia but also high-density lipoprotein level. Men had a higher serum creatinine level (1.31 mg/dl) than that of women (1.13 mg/dl) at 95% CI. More than half of all screened patients had a reduced eGFR; **60%** (95% CI 55%, 65%) had an eGFR<60 ml/min/1.73 m^2; **54%** (49%, 59%) had an eGFR 30–60 ml/min/1.73 m^2, and **5.7%** (3.4%, 8.0%) with eGFR 15–30 ml/min/1.73 m^2. Women had a greater prevalence of **stage 3** CKD (57% women vs. 47% men) and **stage 4** CKD (7.0% vs. 2.0%). The adjusted odds ratio for females compared to males having an eGFR <60 ml/min/1.73 m^2 was **3.19** (95% CI 1.78, 5.43; p value<0.001). Thirty-two percent of patients lost ≥5 ml/min/1.73 m2 eGFR during median follow-up time of 433 days (IQR 462 days) days.

Conclusions: Over one-half of Cambodians with diabetes mellitus had reduced eGFR, implying a point-prevalence of chronic kidney disease of 1.2% in among adult Cambodians within the country. This high burden of kidney disease in a society that lacks universal access to renal replacement therapy underscores the importance of early diagnosis – a largely unmet need in Cambodia.

Editor: Cordula M. Stover, University of Leicester, United Kingdom

Funding: Bernadette Thomas was supported by grant #5F32DK093167-02. The funders had no role in study design, data collection and analysis, decision to publish, or preparation of the manuscript.

Competing Interests: Maurits van Pelt is director of the non-profit organization MoPoTsyo. None of the other authors of this manuscript claim any affiliations requiring disclosures for this research. This does not alter the authors' adherence to all the PLOS ONE policies on sharing data and materials.

* E-mail: bathomas@uw.edu

Introduction

The projected rise in global rates of diabetes mellitus and hypertension portend increasing rates of associated diseases such as chronic kidney disease (CKD) [1–6]. Resource-limited countries lacking the ability to offer renal replacement therapy for end-stage renal disease (ESRD) face the significant challenge of early kidney disease detection to allow for timely intervention to retard disease progression [1,2,6,7]. Yet in many regions of the world, little data exist estimating the prevalence of CKD [8–11].

The south-east Asian kingdom of Cambodia lies bordered between Vietnam, Thailand, Laos, and the Gulf of Thailand. In 2010, the country population was totaled to be 14.1 million, with a life expectancy of 64.6 years for men and 70.1 years for women.[12] The World Health Organization lists Cambodia as a low-income country, with about 80% of its inhabitants living in rural settings. It is estimated that about 46% of all deaths in the country are secondary to non-communicable diseases [12].

In 2010, a national cross-sectional STEPS survey was performed in Cambodia estimating the prevalence of non-communicable diseases, allowing for the first-ever estimation of conditions that increase the risk for CKD. According to study results, about one in every ten respondents had hypertension and 2.9% of individuals were diagnosed with diabetes mellitus [13]. The prevalence of both hypertension and diabetes were significantly more common in the urban than in the rural areas. The results of the study also described the relationship between gender and chronic conditions. Hypertension was more frequent in men, but women had a higher prevalence of elevated total cholesterol and obesity [13].

These data raise concern for a large undetected burden of kidney disease in the country. However, to date no estimates on the prevalence of reduced renal function – either in the population-at-large or in high-risk sub-groups with diabetes and/or hypertension – have been made from anywhere in Cambodia. In order to bridge this gap in our knowledge, we undertook this analysis to develop the first-ever estimates of the prevalence of reduced glomerular filtration rate (GFR) in a screened cohort of individuals with diabetes mellitus from a rural community in Cambodia with a specific focus on gender differences in the prevalence of diabetic CKD.

Materials and Methods

This analysis was exempt from review by the Institutional Review Board of the University of Washington as it describes results of data collected for program evaluation.

This population-based analysis of renal function in adults from the Takeo province of southern Cambodia was performed using screening data gathered between 2010 and 2012 by the non-profit organization MoPoTsyo.

Data Source

MoPoTsyo is a Cambodian organization founded in 2004 to screen inhabitants of resource-limited regions for diabetes mellitus and hypertension [14]. The organization uses a peer-education network system to achieve its objectives of education, screening, and treatment for chronic diseases [14]. Analysis of data from Takeo province was selected due to the completeness of data over a two-year period. All patients included in this analysis had an existing diagnosis of diabetes mellitus at time of entry into MoPoTsyo, or were diagnosed to be diabetic by this non-governmental organization.

Data Collection

Individuals from the community were invited to present for screening or evaluation of previously diagnosed diabetes mellitus. Initial screening and data-gathering was performed by Cambodian peer educators trained by MoPoTsyo. The initial evaluation involved collection of demographic, lifestyle and diet information, exercise habits, height, weight, waist, and hip circumference, and current medications. The height and weight data were used to calculate the body mass index (BMI; kg/m^2). A fasting sample of blood was drawn for the measurement of baseline serum creatinine, cholesterol, and liver function measurements. Patients without a pre-existing diagnosis of hypertension were diagnosed to be hypertensive if their initial blood pressure was greater than 130/80 mmHg.

A total of 440 individuals with diabetes mellitus presented for the initial screening. However, data on eGFR were unavailable for 38 individuals, yielding an analytic cohort of 402 patients. Medication data were available for 366 of the 402 patients included in this analysis. A total of 398 individuals had eGFR re-evaluated after a median of 433 days (interquartile range 462 days).

Laboratory measurement

Serum creatinine was measured using the kinetic rate Jaffe method, and was aligned using isotope dilution mass-spectrometry (IDMS). Estimated GFR (eGFR) was calculated using the CKD-Epi equation based on measured serum creatinine. The CKD-Epi equation was chosen as it has been assessed to be more accurate than the Modification of Diet in Renal Disease (MDRD) equation in both high and low risk CKD populations [15].

Patients were grouped into stages of CKD, as defined by the National Kidney Foundation Kidney Disease Outcomes Quality Initiative (KDOQI): stage 3, eGFR, 30–60 ml/min/1.73 m^2; stage 4, 15–30 mlmin/1.73 m^2, and stage 5, <15 ml/min/1.73 m^2 or undergoing renal replacement therapy.

Statistical Analysis

Patients' age, BMI, waist circumference, waist-to-hip ratio, blood pressure, total cholesterol, and medication use are presented as mean values with 95% confidence intervals, stratified by gender (Tables 1, 2). Student's t-tests and Chi-square tests were performed to determine the significance of difference, by gender, evaluate of continuous and categorical characteristics, respectively, as listed in Tables 1 and 2. Hypercholesterolemia was defined as a serum total cholesterol level ≥240 mg/dl [16]. Uncontrolled hypertension was defined as a blood pressure recording ≥140/90 mmHg.

Blood pressure and blood sugar were assessed by MoPoTsyo staff who were trained to take these measurements using automated sphygmomanometers and handheld glucometers.

Change of renal function over time was assessed by calculating the mean percentage of patients who lost between 5–10, 10–15, and >15 ml/min/1.73 m^2 of eGFR between initial screening and follow-up (Figure 1). Statistical significance for outcome stratified by gender were determined using chi square analyses, with significance being interpreted as a p value<0.05.

Logistic regression was performed to examine the association between gender and reduced eGFR as defined by an eGFR ≤60 mmin/1.73 m^2. Unadjusted and adjusted results for available Framingham risk factors of age, BMI, blood pressure, total cholesterol, and high-density (HDL) cholesterol we calculated.

All analyses were performed using a licensed version of Stata 12.1. Values were considered statistically significant at the $\alpha = 0.05$ level.

Results

Patient characteristics and biological profile

The majority of patients that presented for screening were female. On average, women were younger and had higher total cholesterol levels, but also slightly higher HDL cholesterol (see Table 1, 2). There was no significant difference in mean blood pressure or BMI measurements between genders (Table 2).

Women were more likely to be taking or be prescribed treatment for high blood pressure, diabetes, or hypercholesterolemia at time of screening than men (Table 2).

Table 1. Patient demographics.

	Male	Female	Total
	100	302	402
Age, years*	56.1 (53.9, 58.2)	53.6 (52.4, 54.7)	54.2 (53.2, 55.1)
Body Mass Index (kg/m^2)	23.7 (23.0, 24.4)	23.2 (22.8, 23.6)	23.3 (23.0, 23.7)
Waist circumference (cm)	85.5 (83.4, 87.6)	83.4 (82.2, 84.6)	83.9 (82.9, 85.0)
Waist-Hip Ratio	0.9 (0.9, 0.9)	0.9 (0.9, 0.9)	0.9 (0.9, 0.9)

Results indicate mean values unless otherwise indicated.
Parentheses indicate 95% confidence intervals.
*indicates a statistically significant association with gender (p value<0.05).

Table 2. Disease and medication history.

	Male	Female	Total
	100	402	302
Diabetes Mellitus			
Time since diagnosis (years, mean)	4.8 (4.2, 5.3)	5.0 (4.7, 5.3)	4.95 (4.7, 5.2)
Fasting blood glucose (mg/dl; mean)	187.8 (174.5, 201.1)	191.6 (183.2, 199.9)	190.6 (183.5, 197.7)
Post-prandial glucose (mg/dl; mean)	284.2 (261.9, 306.4)	284.8 (273.4, 296.2)	284.7 (274.5, 294.8)
Blood Pressure (mmHg), mean			
Systolic (mmHg)[a]	132 (127, 137)	133 (130, 136)	133 (130, 135)
Diastolic (mmHg)[a]	83 (80, 85)	84 (83, 85)	84 (82, 85)
Established diagnosis of Hypertension (mean)*	13	23	20
Cholesterol (mg/dl) mean			
Total cholesterol [b]	169 (158, 181)	168 (161, 176)	169 (162, 175)
HDL* [c]	41 (38, 45)	46 (44, 49)	45 (43, 47)
Hypercholesterolemia %	7	12	10.7
Triglycerides	243 (214.4, 272.8)	270.1 (251.4, 288.9)	263.5 (247.7, 279.4)
Medications [d] (mean)			
Ace inhibitor	42.4 (36.3, 48.4)	44.2 (34.5, 53.9)	42.8 (37.7, 47.9)
Diabetic medications	74 (65, 83)	85 (80, 89)	82 (78, 86)

Abbreviation: HDL, high density lipoprotein.
Results indicate mean values unless otherwise indicated.
Parentheses indicate 95% confidence intervals.
*indicates a statistically significant association with gender (p value<0.05).
[a]missing: 1 male, 1 female; [b] missing: 3 male, 16 female; [c] missing: 19 male, 67 female; [d] among 366 patients.

Estimated glomerular filtration rate

On average, men had higher serum creatinine than women. While only 1.7% of women had serum creatinine >2 mg/dl, 7% of men had a serum creatinine value greater than 2 mg/dl (Table 3; (p-value<0.05).

A total of 60% (N) of patients had an eGFR less than 60 ml/min/1.73 m^2. Women had a higher CKD prevalence per category of CKD for both stages 4 and 5, though this difference was not statistically significant (Table 4).

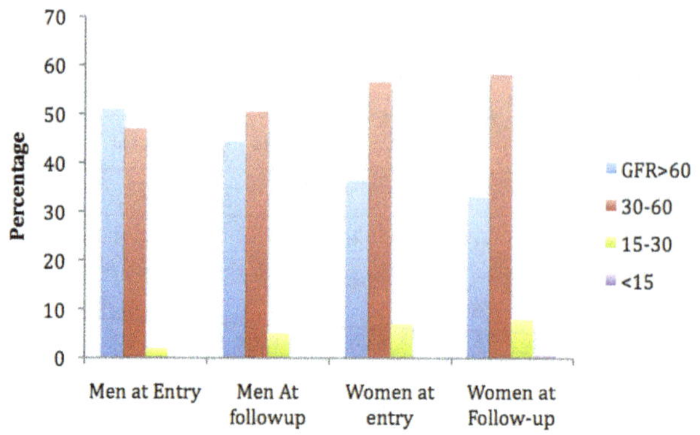

Figure 1. Renal function at entry and follow-up stratified by gender.

Table 3. Creatinine in patients at entry.

Creatinine (mg/dl)	Male	Female	Total
	n = 100	n = 302	n = 401
< = 1mg/dl*	16 (9, 23)	48 (42, 53)	39.8 (35, 45)
1–2 mg/dl*	77 (69, 85)	51 (45, 56)	57 (52, 62)
2–3 mg/dl*	7 (2, 12)	1.3 (0.03, 2.6)	3 (1, 4)
>3mg/dl	0.0 (0.0, 0.0)	0.3 (−0.3, 1.0)	0.2 (−0.2, 0.7)

Results indicate percentages.
Parentheses indicate 95% confidence intervals.
*indicates a statistically significant association with gender (p value<0.05).

Renal Function at Follow-Up

Upon follow-up, (20) 20.2% of men and (50) 16.7% of women with eGFR >60 ml/min/1.73 m^2 at baseline were determined to have an eGFR of <60 ml/min/m^2 (Tables 4 and 5, Figure 1).

Gender and CKD Progression

Of the 398 patients who had a second creatinine reading taken within a median of 433 days, 32% of patients lost ≥5 ml/min/m^2 of eGFR, 24% lost greater than 10 ml/min/m^2, and 13% lost greater than 15 ml/min/m^2. The difference between women (32.6%, 95% CI: 0.27, 0.38) and men (31.3%; 95% CI 0.22, 0.41)

Table 4. Estimated glomerular filtration rate in patients at entry.

GFR[a] (ml/min/ 1.73m^2)	Male	Female	Total
	n = 100	n = 302	n = 402
>60*	51 (41, 61)	36 (31, 42)	40 (35, 45)
30–60	47 (37, 57)	57 (51, 62)	54 (49, 59)
15–30	2 (0, 5)	7 (4, 10)	6 (3, 8)
<15	0.0	0.0	0.0

Abbreviation: GFR, glomerular filtration rate.
Results indicate percentages.
Parentheses indicate 95% confidence interval.
*indicates a statistically significant association with gender (p value<0.05).

Table 5. Estimated glomerular filtration rate in patients at follow-up.

GFR (ml/min/ 1.73m^2)	Male	Female	Total
	n = 99	n = 299	n = 398
>60*	44 (35, 54)	33 (28, 39)	36 (31, 41)
30–60	51 (41, 61)	58 (53, 64)	56 (51, 61)
15–30	5 (1, 9)	8 (5, 11)	7 (5, 10)
<15	0.0 (0,0)	1 (0, 1.6)	0.5 (−.2, 1)

Abbreviation: GFR, glomerular filtration rate.
Results indicate percentage.
Percentages indicate 95% confidence interval.
*indicates a statistically significant association with gender (p value<0.05).

who lost ≥5 ml/min/1.73 m^2 of eGFR was not determined to be statistically significant (p value 0.82) (Table 5, Figure 1).

Gender and CKD Prevalence

The unadjusted odds ratio (OR) of the association between female gender and an impaired eGFR at initial assessment was 1.82 (95% CI 1.15, 2.87), with an adjusted OR of 3.19 (95% CI 1.72, 5.93, p value<0.001). Analysis was adjusted for available Framingham risk factors of age, body mass index, systolic blood pressure, diastolic blood pressure, total cholesterol, and high-density lipoprotein (HDL) cholesterol.

Estimate of population size with reduced eGFR

We performed a crude estimation of the percentage of diabetics within the Cambodian population calculated to have a reduced eGFR. The 2010 Cambodian census lists the national population at 14.1 million, 60.5% of which were between the ages of 25–64 years [17]. 2.9% of the population between the ages of 25–64 years was determined to have elevated blood glucose according to the 2010 Cambodian STEPS survey. Of those individuals, from our results we estimate 40.0% to have a reduced eGFR if this cohort is similar to other diabetics in Cambodia. This would amount to at least 98,954 adult individuals with diabetes mellitus and an abnormal eGFR, or 1.2% of the Cambodian population between ages 25–64 years.

Discussion

To our knowledge, this is the first-ever report of the prevalence of reduced eGFR from population-based screening within Cambodia. The results of this study involving about 400 rural diabetic Cambodian men and women indicate that there is a high prevalence of reduced renal function within this high-risk population. Reduced renal function was found to be more prevalent in women, and despite treatment of blood pressure and diabetes, kidney disease progression was noted in a significant proportion of individuals of both genders. Male patients had a lower prevalence of reduced renal function at entry, but a higher percentage progressed from normal kidney function to a diseased state. Very few men or women were found to be in or progress to advanced renal insufficiency. Our results estimate the percentage of the national diabetic population with advanced renal insufficiency to be 1.2%; this assessment does not include individuals with significant albuminuria and preserved eGFR as albuminuria data was not systematically collected for all patients. Hence, the true percentage of Cambodians with reduced renal function can be assumed to be significantly higher secondary to unmeasured earlier stages of CKD as diagnosed by persisting albuminuria with preserved eGFR.

There is expansive literature describing the role of gender in population access to primary care services, describing that women are more likely to access both mental health and primary care services than men [18–20]. The 2010 Cambodian STEPS survey and 2010 Cambodia Demographic and Health Survey results indicate this pattern to be similar within Cambodia. The 2010 STEPS study published results describing a higher initial inclusion of women than men secondary to responsiveness, and a higher response of women than men during each of the three steps of the evaluation. Further, the results of two large population-based screening studies among adults in Cambodia for diabetes and associated diseases also involved unequal gender responsiveness for unclear reasons [21]. The results of our study also indicate a noted predominance of women seeking screening or assistance with management of previously diagnosed chronic diseases. Though this gender predominance limits the ultimate generalizability of study results to the national Cambodian population, the value in these first estimates of kidney function warrant crude estimation of population burden of kidney disease until more exact estimates are available through studies structured to include more balanced gender inclusion.

The Cambodian STEPS survey also indicates that 2.3% of rural respondents and 5.6% of urban respondents had elevated fasting glucose or diabetes, a greater percentage of which were female [13]. There is a clear difference in burden of disease based on geography and gender; thus further studies are needed to more accurately characterize the incidence and progression of chronic kidney disease in both rural and urban settings. Notable differences between the MoPoTsyo participants and Cambodian STEPS study participants are that the STEPS study includes a wider age range, an urban population and larger sample size. Thus the extrapolation of national estimates of advanced renal insufficiency based on national STEPS survey report are rough estimates at best. Also, the differences in prevalence and progression of renal insufficiency by gender identified in this study will need to be validated with a larger cohort with more even distribution of men to women.

Data on the population prevalence of reduced renal function in southeast Asian countries are limited [2,7,11,22]. A recent study performed in northern Vietnam, involving about 8,500 adults, detected 3.1% of participants to have CKD stage 3–5 with use of the Cockcroft-Gault equation, 1.9% with use of the MDRD equation, and 3.6% when the MDRD equation was used with adjustment using the Japanese coefficient [7]. We note the wide heterogeneity of estimation depending on the GFR estimation equation [7]. In contrast, a recent publication from India detailing the first estimates from the country's renal registry revealed almost 50% of presenting cases to be CKD stage 5 [22]. This report from India emphasizes the importance of screening programs in resource-poor countries like Cambodia that lack a healthcare system that could bear the significant financial burden of universal access to maintenance renal replacement therapy; in such countries, many of the individuals who present with late-stage CKD are likely to die from the consequences of kidney disease.

As chronic diseases continue to play a larger role in early mortality within developing populations, accurate estimates of population burden of chronic diseases will help to determine the true population at risk. Slowing progression to ESRD is a major impetus for CKD detection in populations with limited ability to offer long-term renal replacement therapies such as dialysis and transplantation [3,4]. Early detection offers the possibility of implementation of treatments that can retard progression [4]. Early-stage detection has the added importance of understanding the mortality-risk of the CKD population, as CKD is associated with an increased likelihood of mortality secondary to cardiovascular disease, as well as being an independent risk factor for early mortality prior to development of ESRD [23].

The limitations of our study include its sample size, that all patients reside in rural areas of Cambodia, and that the CKD-Epi equation used to quantify renal function has not been validated for the Cambodian population. Further, women were over-represented in the cohort, and as we did not have urinalyses for all patients, we were limited in our ability to assess earlier stages of renal insufficiency. The strengths of this study are that it is the first to our knowledge to quantify kidney function estimates for a high-risk population within Cambodia.

Studies will need to be performed to assess the burden of disease in urban populations. Future studies will also be needed to explore the association between gender and chronic kidney disease both in rural and urban settings. Inclusion of kidney function in future STEPS analyses would greatly assist in enumerating the burden of disease within the country as well as within high-risk groups such as diabetics and patients with hypertension. National or region-level renal registries would also direct preventive measures for reducing the incidence and progression of CKD, and help target how and where best to implement renal replacement therapies. Ultimately, a multi-tiered approach of screening, disease treatment, and renal replacement therapy program development will be necessary to address the anticipated increase in the number of Cambodian individuals with CKD.

Author Contributions

Conceived and designed the experiments: BT JL MP. Analyzed the data: BT. Contributed reagents/materials/analysis tools: BT. Wrote the paper: BT. Critical review of manuscript: MP RM CRC JL.

References

1. Eknoyan G, Lameire N, Barsoum R, Eckardt KU, Levin A, et al. (2004) The burden of kidney disease: improving global outcomes. Kidney Int 66: 1310–1314.
2. Agarwal SK, Srivastava RK (2009) Chronic kidney disease in India: challenges and solutions. Nephron Clin Pract 111: c197–203; discussion c203.
3. Couser WG, Remuzzi G, Mendis S, Tonelli M (2011) The contribution of chronic kidney disease to the global burden of major noncommunicable diseases. Kidney Int 80: 1258–1270.
4. Jha V, Wang AY, Wang H (2012) The impact of CKD identification in large countries: the burden of illness. Nephrol Dial Transplant 27 Suppl 3: iii32–38.
5. Shan Y, Zhang Q, Liu Z, Hu X, Liu D (2010) Prevalence and risk factors associated with chronic kidney disease in adults over 40 years: a population study from Central China. Nephrology (Carlton) 15: 354–361.
6. Amos AF, McCarty DJ, Zimmet P (1997) The rising global burden of diabetes and its complications: estimates and projections to the year 2010. Diabet Med 14 Suppl 5: S1–85.
7. Ito J, Dung DT, Vuong MT, Tuyen do G, Vinh le D, et al. (2008) Impact and perspective on chronic kidney disease in an Asian developing country: a large-scale survey in North Vietnam. Nephron Clin Pract 109: c25–32.
8. Barsoum RS (2002) Overview: end-stage renal disease in the developing world. Artif Organs 26: 737–746.
9. Jha V (2009) Current status of end-stage renal disease care in South Asia. Ethn Dis 19: S1-27–32.
10. Naicker S (2009) End-stage renal disease in sub-Saharan Africa. Ethn Dis 19: S1-13–15.
11. Rajapurkar M, Dabhi M (2010) Burden of disease – prevalence and incidence of renal disease in India. Clin Nephrol 74 Suppl 1: S9–12.
12. World Health Organization – NCD Country Profiles, 2010.
13. Prevalence of Non-communicable Disease Risk Factors in Cambodia, STEPS Survey, Country Report, 2010.
14. van Pelt M (2013) Yes They Can: Peer Educators for Diabetes in Cambodia; Bloom G, editor. AbingdonOxon: Routledge. xvii, 197 p.
15. Stevens LA, Li S, Kurella Tamura M, Chen SC, Vassalotti JA, et al. (2011) Comparison of the CKD Epidemiology Collaboration (CKD-EPI) and Modification of Diet in Renal Disease (MDRD) study equations: risk factors for and complications of CKD and mortality in the Kidney Early Evaluation Program (KEEP). Am J Kidney Dis 57: S9–16.
16. Kirby T (2010) Screening for chronic kidney disease shows promise. Lancet 375: 1240–1241.
17. National Institute of Statistics, Directorate General for Health, and ICF Macro, 2011. Cambodia Demographic and Health Survey 2010. Phnom Penh, Cambodia and Calverton, Maryland, USA: National Institute of Statistics, Directorate General for Health, and ICF Macro.
18. Kapur N, Hunt I, Lunt M, McBeth J, Creed F, et al. (2005) Primary care consultation predictors in men and women: a cohort study. Br J Gen Pract 55: 108–113.
19. Moller-Leimkuhler AM (2002) Barriers to help-seeking by men: a review of sociocultural and clinical literature with particular reference to depression. J Affect Disord 71: 1–9.
20. Addis ME, Mahalik JR (2003) Men, masculinity, and the contexts of help seeking. Am Psychol 58: 5–14.
21. King H, Keuky L, Seng S, Khun T, Roglic G, et al. (2005) Diabetes and associated disorders in Cambodia: two epidemiological surveys. Lancet 366: 1633–1639.
22. Rajapurkar MM, John GT, Kirpalani AL, Abraham G, Agarwal SK, et al. (2012) What do we know about chronic kidney disease in India: first report of the Indian CKD registry. BMC Nephrol 13: 10.
23. Tonelli M, Wiebe N, Culleton B, House A, Rabbat C, et al. (2006) Chronic kidney disease and mortality risk: a systematic review. J Am Soc Nephrol 17: 2034–2047.

Determinants of Arterial Stiffness in Chronic Kidney Disease Stage 3

Natasha J. McIntyre[1], Richard J. Fluck[1], Christopher W. McIntyre[1,2], Apostolos Fakis[1], Maarten W. Taal[1]*

1 Department of Renal Medicine, Royal Derby Hospital, Derbyshire, United Kingdom, 2 Department of Vascular Medicine, University of Nottingham, Nottingham, United Kingdom

Abstract

Background: Early chronic kidney disease (CKD) is associated with increased cardiovascular (CV) risk but underlying mechanisms remain uncertain. Arterial stiffness (AS) is associated with increased CV risk in advanced CKD, but it is unclear whether AS is relevant to CV disease (CVD) in early CKD.

Study Design: Cross-sectional.

Setting and participants: 1717 patients with previous estimated glomerular filtration rate (eGFR) 59–30 mL/min/1.73 m^2; mean age 73±9y, were recruited from 32 general practices in primary care.

Outcomes: Increased arterial stiffness.

Measurements: Medical history was obtained and participants underwent clinical assessment, urine and serum biochemistry testing. Carotid to femoral pulse wave velocity (PWV) was determined as a measure of AS, using a Vicorder^{TM} device.

Results: Univariate analysis revealed significant correlations between PWV and risk factors for CVD including age ($r = 0.456$; $p<0.001$), mean arterial pressure (MAP) ($r = 0.228$; $p<0.001$), body mass index ($r = -0.122$; $p<0.001$), log urinary albumin to creatinine ratio ($r = 0.124$; $p<0.001$), Waist to Hip ratio ($r = 0.124$, $p<0.001$), eGFR ($r = -0.074$; $p = 0.002$), log high sensitivity c-reactive protein ($r = 0.066$; $p = 0.006$), HDL ($r = -0.062$; $p = 0.01$) and total cholesterol ($r = -0.057$; $p = 0.02$). PWV was higher in males (9.6 m/sec vs.10.3 m/sec; $p<0.001$), diabetics (9.8 m/sec vs. 10.3 m/sec; $p<0.001$), and those with previous CV events (CVE) (9.8 m/s vs. 10.3 m/sec; $p<0.001$). Multivariable analysis identified age, MAP and diabetes as strongest independent determinants of higher PWV (adjusted $R^2 = 0.29$). An interactive term indicated that PWV increased to a greater extent with age in males versus females. Albuminuria was a weaker determinant of PWV and eGFR did not enter the model.

Limitations: Data derived from one study visit, with absence of normal controls.

Conclusion: In this cohort, age and traditional CV risk factors were the strongest determinants of AS. Albuminuria was a relatively weak determinant of AS and eGFR was not an independent determinant. Long-term follow-up will investigate AS as an independent risk factor for CVE in this cohort.

Editor: Murielle Bochud, Lausanne University Hospital and University of Lausanne, Switzerland

Funding: This study was supported by a fellowship grant from Kidney Research UK and the British Renal Society, as well as an unrestricted educational grant from Roche Products plc. The funders had no role in study design, data collection and analysis, decision to publish, or preparation of the manuscript.

Competing Interests: As regards potential competing interests the authors would like to clarify that the support from Roche Products plc was in the form of an unrestricted educational grant. Specifically this means that Roche played no role whatever in the initiation, design or conduct of the study and have no ownership of the data. The authors are not obligated to provide Roche with any publications prior to submission and are not required to seek approval from Roche for any publications. The authors are therefore able to confirm unequivocally that the sponsorship from Roche does not alter their adherence to all the PLOS ONE policies on sharing data and materials.

* E-mail: maarten.taal1@nhs.net

Introduction

Multiple epidemiological studies attest that chronic kidney disease (CKD) is associated with increased cardiovascular risk compared to the general population, and may account for up to 50% of all deaths in this group [1]. In many studies people with early stage CKD are more likely to die from cardiovascular disease than progress to end stage kidney disease (ESKD) [2]. Hallan [3] reported that the risk of CKD progression is low until eGFR falls below 30 ml/min/1.73 m^2. In contrast even modest reductions in eGFR are incrementally associated with reduced survival [4]. The increased cardiovascular (CV) risk associated with advanced stages of CKD cannot be explained by traditional risk factors alone, but is attributable to a combination of traditional and non-traditional factors [5,6]. Arterial stiffness (AS) has been identified as one non-traditional risk factor associated with the large cardiovascular risk burden in CKD [7,8]. Arterial stiffness in CKD is proposed to provoke an increase in systolic blood pressure (SBP) and pulse pressure (PP). This in turn leads to an increase in ventricular afterload, myocyte hypertrophy and reduced coronary perfusion, resulting in systolic and diastolic dysfunction. Elevated systolic and pulse pressures may also contribute to vascular damage, further increasing CV risk [9].

Aortic pulse wave velocity (aPWV) is a measure of AS and has predicted cardiovascular morbidity and mortality in a number of populations including the healthy elderly and people with hypertension, diabetes or ESKD on haemodialysis [10,11,12,13,14]. On the other hand, data regarding the relationship between AS and CKD in earlier stages appear conflicting. Several studies have reported an increase in arterial stiffness and CV risk associated with early CKD [15,16,17] but others have not [18,19,20]. More data are therefore required regarding the relationship between AS and markers of kidney disease in early stage CKD. The aim of our study was to investigate if previously identified determinants of AS are also relevant in a population of predominantly elderly people with CKD stage 3, representing the majority affected by CKD.

Study Population and Methods

Participants and Recruitment

We studied 1741 patients with CKD stage 3 recruited from general practitioner (GP) practices. The methods have previously been described in detail and are summarised here with emphasis on the measurement of aPWV [21,22]. Participants were recruited as part of the Renal Risk in Derby (RRID) study, a prospective cohort study planned to continue for 10 years, with the aim of studying renal and CV risk factors in patients with CKD stage 3 in a primary care setting. Eligible participants were 18 years or over, met the KDOQI criteria for CKD stage 3 (eGFR of 30–59 mL/min/1.73 m^2 on 2 or more occasions at least 3 months apart), were able to give informed consent and attend their GP practice for assessments. People who had previously received a solid organ transplant or who were terminally ill (expected survival <1 year) were excluded. The RRID study is being conducted by a single Nephrology Department, but participants were recruited directly from 32 GP practices in Derbyshire, UK. Study visits were conducted at participating GP practices by the researchers. Twenty four participants were unable to have their aPWV measured due to a combination of technical failure or inability of the participant to lie at a 30 degree angle. Thus 1717 participants with aPWV readings were included in this analysis.

Data Collection

First study visits were conducted from August 2008 to March 2010. Screening and baseline visits were combined due to the large proportion of elderly participants and the logistical challenges associated with conducting study visits in multiple primary care centres. Participants were sent a medical questionnaire as well as 3 urine specimen bottles, and were asked not to eat cooked meat for at least 12 hours prior to the assessment [23]. At the assessment information on questionnaires was checked, anthropomorphic measurements and blood pressure taken, and urine analysis was performed. Blood and urine specimens were submitted for biochemical analysis to a single laboratory.

Previous diabetes was defined by having a previous clinical diagnosis according to WHO criteria [24]. Previous cardiovascular event (CVE) was defined as subject reported myocardial infarction, stroke, transient ischaemic attack, revascularisation or amputation due to peripheral vascular disease, or aortic aneurysm. Anaemia was defined as hemoglobin <11.5 g/dL for women and <13.5 g/dL for men. Obesity was defined as BMI>30 kg/m^2. Central fat distribution was defined as a waist to hip ratio (WHR) of ≥0.9 for men or ≥0.8 for women [25].

Blood pressure. Blood pressure (BP) was measured after a minimum of five minutes rest in the sitting position, using a calibrated oscillometric device, recommended by the British Hypertension Society (Digital Blood Pressure Monitor Model UA-767, A&D Instruments Ltd, Abingdon, UK). A single device was used for all readings. Measurements were taken until three readings that were within 10% of each other were obtained. BP was calculated as the mean of these three readings. Hypertension was defined as a systolic BP≥140 mmHg, diastolic BP≥90 mmHg, or current antihypertensive medication [26]. Mean arterial pressure (MAP) was calculated as 1/3 the average SBP plus 2/3 the average DBP.

Pulse wave velocity. Carotid to femoral pulse wave velocity was measured as a marker of arterial stiffness, a critical determinant of cardiovascular outcomes in CKD [7,27,28], and considered the gold standard measurement of AS [12]. Measurements were performed using a Vicorder™ device (Skidmore Medical Ltd, Bristol, UK). The Vicorder™ is small, portable, non-invasive and non-operator dependant making it well suited for use in community based studies. Readings take only 2–3 minutes to complete. Assessments were performed after at least 5 minutes of rest, according to manufacturers' instructions in the semi-prone position (at approximately 30°) to prevent venous contamination of the arterial signal. The participant had a neck-pad placed around their neck with the pressure pad over the right carotid area. A blood pressure cuff was placed around the patients' upper right thigh. The distance between the supra-sternal notch and the thigh cuff was measured using the direct method. To eliminate the potential effect of abdominal obesity on the distance measurement, an imaginary line was drawn from the supra-sternal notch to the right shoulder and the measurement to the thigh cuff was made along the side of the body. The neck-pad and thigh cuff were inflated by the Vicorder to 60 mmHg and then deflated to obtain a pressure tracing. Aortic PWV is calculated by the Vicorder by comparing carotid and femoral pressure tracings after a stable pattern is obtained. The mild discomfort caused by the inflation of a cuff placed around the neck precluded us from doing multiple readings. The intra-observer coefficient of variation for PWV measurements was 6.3%.

Skin Autofluorescence

Skin autofluorescence (AF), a measure of skin Advanced Glycation Endproduct (AGE) deposition that has been identified as a marker of cumulative metabolic stress [29,30,31], was assessed on the left forearm using an AGE Reader™ device (DiagnOptics, Groningen, Netherlands). Three readings were taken and the average calculated. It was not possible to conduct these readings on dark skin. Values are expressed in arbitrary units [22].

Albuminuria. Albuminuria was assessed by measuring the urine albumin to creatinine ratio (ACR) on three consecutive early morning urine specimens collected prior to the clinic visit and stored in a refrigerator. Microalbuminuria was defined as a mean urine ACR of >2.5 mg/mmol in males or >3.5 mg/mmol in females and overt albuminuria as >30 mg/mmol [23].

Estimation of glomerular filtration rate (eGFR). Biochemical assessments were performed by autoanalyser in a single laboratory. The creatinine assay has been standardised against an isotope dilution mass spectrometry (IDMS) method and the 4-variable MDRD equation modified for use with IDMS standardised creatinine measurement was used to estimate GFR. This study was commenced prior to publication of the

CKD-EPI formula and eGFR derived from the MDRD formula was therefore used for recruitment and baseline study assessments.

The study was approved by the Nottingham Research Ethics Committee 1 and abided by the principles of the Declaration of Helsinki. All participants provided written informed consent. The study was included on the National Institute for Health Research (NIHR) Clinical Research Portfolio (NIHR Study ID:6632) and was independently audited by QED Clinical Services in November 2009.

Statistical Analysis

Results presented are a cross sectional analysis of data from the first study visit. Continuous variables are reported as the mean and standard deviation (SD) if normally distributed or the median and inter-quartile range (IQR) if not. A t-test was used to compare two groups where variables were normally distributed and a Mann U Whitney test used if not. Pearson's test was used to assess univariate correlations with aPWV for variables with normal distribution or Spearman's test if distribution was not normal. Partial correlations were used to correct for MAP. Variables with skewed distribution (exponential) were log transformed for the correlations. SPSS version 15.0 was used for univariate analysis. $P<0.05$ was considered statistically significant.

Multivariable linear regression analysis, using the forward stepwise method, was used to identify independent determinants of arterial stiffness. $P<0.05$ was used for a variable to enter the model. The model was built using a hierarchical approach that introduced variables one-by-one on the basis of biological plausibility as well as strength of association in univariate analyses adjusted for age and diabetes. Nested models were tested using the Akaike Information Criterion (AIC). Models with a smaller AIC value were selected. An interactive term for age by gender was also tested in the final model. A scatter plot of regression residuals versus predicted values and Cook's Distance plot were used for testing the assumptions of linear regression and identifying any outliers. The adjusted R-squared value is reported as a measure of goodness-of-fit. The regression coefficients (95% Confidence Intervals) and standardised coefficients (Beta) from the final multivariable model are presented. STATA version 11.1 was used for multivariable analysis.

Results

Baseline characteristics are summarised in Table 1. Over a third of participants were obese (37%). Most (88%) had hypertension and 65% were treated with a renin angiotensin aldosterone system inhibitor (RAASi).

Mean aPWV was 9.9±2 m/sec. Aortic PWV was significantly higher in participants who were male, had diabetes, had had previous CVE, had albuminuria (microscopic or overt), were hypertensive, were not obese (as defined by BMI), had a blood pressure over 130/80 mmHg or were ≥75 years of age (Table 2). People who evidenced increased central fat distribution (central obesity), anaemia, were receiving antihypertensive medication, had CKD stage 3B or who had previously smoked also had significantly higher aPWV (Table 2). Age evidenced the strongest correlation with aPWV before and after adjusting for MAP (Table 3). Mean arterial pressure was also strongly correlated with aPWV. Other significant correlations are shown in Table 3. Adjustment for MAP produced little change in the correlations.

Multivariable analysis was performed to identify independent determinants of a higher aPWV (Table 4; adjusted $R^2=0.29$). The strongest and most significant of these were age, MAP, diabetes and BMI. Interestingly, BMI showed a negative relationship with aPWV. Other relatively weak independent determinants included serum total protein, log urine ACR and HDL cholesterol. An interactive term indicated that PWV increased to a greater extent with age in males versus females.

Table 1. Baseline characteristics.

	Females	n	Males	n	Total	n
Age (years)	73 (66–79)	1037	75 (69–80)*	680	74 (67–79)	1717
Ethnicity white	1014 (98)	1037	661 (97)	680	1675 (98)	1717
Diabetes	158 (15)	1037	129 (19)*	680	287 (17)	1717
Previous CVE	185 (18)	1037	195 (29)*	680	380 (22)	1717
Current smoker	47 (5)	1037	31 (5)	680	78 (4.5)	1717
Previous smoker	407 (39)	1037	444 (65)*	680	851 (50)	1717
BMI (kg/m^2)	29.0 (25.6–32.5)	1037	27.8 (25.7–30.5)*	680	28.4 (25.6–31.8)	1717
Systolic BP (mmHg)	133±19	1037	136±18*	680	134±18	1717
Diastolic BP (mmHg)	72±11	1037	74±11*	680	73±11	1717
MAP (mmHg)	92±12	1037	94±11*	680	93±12	1717
eGFR (mL/min/ 1.73 m^2)	54.4 (46.7–61.1)	1037	51.1 (44.1–57.6)*	680	53.3 (45.5–59.8)	1717
HDL Cholesterol (mmol/L)	1.55 (1.27–1.85)	1032	1.19 (1.00–1.45)*	676	1.40 (1.13–1.71)	1708
Total Cholesterol (mmol/L)	4.90 (4.10–5.80)	1032	4.20 (3.60–4.98)*	676	4.6 (3.9–5.5)	1708
Serum total protein (g/L)	74.2±4.8	1031	74.4±4.9	677	74.3±4.9	1708
Serum albumin (g/L)	40.5±3.0	1036	40.9±3.3*	678	40.7±3.2	1714
Corrected calcium (mmol/L)	2.39±0.10	1033	2.35±0.09*	673	2.38±0.10	1706
Phosphate (mmol/L)	1.15±0.17	1018	1.05±0.18*	667	1.11±0.18	1685
UACR (mg/mmol)	0.23 (0.00–0.90)	1035	0.63 (0.00–3.27)*	679	0.33 (0.00–1.50)	1714
CKD 3B	208 (20)	1037	194 (29)*	680	402 (23)	1717
aPWV (m/sec)	9.7±2.0	1037	10.3±2*	680	9.9±2	1717
hs CRP (mg/L)	2.23 (1.13–4.67)	1036	2.21 (1.14–4.28)	680	2.22 (1.13–4.50)	1716
Waist to Hip Ratio	0.86 (0.81–0.90)	1037	0.98 (0.94–1.02)*	680	0.91 (0.84–0.97)	1717
SAF (AU)	2.60 (2.30–3.00)	1023	2.73 (2.33–3.18)*	665	2.67 (2.30–3.07)	1688

Data are mean±SD, median (IQR) or number (%).
*$P<0.05$ versus females.
aPWV = aortic pulse wave velocity; AU = Arbitrary units.; BP = blood pressure; BMI = body mass index; CKD 3B = eGFR 30–44 mLs/min/1.73 m^2; CVE = cardiovascular event; eGFR = estimated glomerular filtration rate; HDL = high density lipo-protein; hs CRP = high sensitivity C-reactive protein; MAP = mean arterial pressure; SAF = skin autofluorescence; UACR = urine albumin to creatinine ratio.

Discussion

We have identified age as the strongest determinant of arterial stiffness in this cohort of predominantly elderly patients with CKD stage 3. Other significant independent determinants of aPWV included traditional cardiovascular risk factors such as blood pressure, diabetes, obesity and a marker of dyslipidaemia. Markers of CKD were associated with aPWV only in univariate analysis (eGFR) or were weak determinants of aPWV (albuminuria). Our

Table 2. aPWV readings in selected subgroups.

	Yes	No	P value
Male	10.3±2.0	9.7±2.0	<0.001
Diabetes	10.3±2.0	9.8±2.0	<0.001
Previous CVE	10.3±0.7	9.8±0.6	<0.001
Albuminuria*	10.3±2.0	9.8±2.0	<0.001
Hypertension‡	10.0±2.0	9.1±2.0	<0.001
BP<130/80 at baseline visit	9.2±1.7	10.3±2.1	<0.001
Obese	9.5±1.9	10.1±2.0	<0.001
Age <75 years	9.1(8.1–10.3)	10.5(9.4–11.8)	<0.001
Anaemia	10.2±1.9	9.8±2	0.003
Central Obesity	9.9±2	9.5±1.9	0.003
On antihypertensive medication	10.0±2.0	9.6±2.1	0.007
CKD stage 3B	10.1±2	9.8±2.1	0.009
Previous Smoker	10.0±2.1	9.8±1.9	0.011

Data are presented as mean ± standard deviation or median (interquartile range).
aPWV (aortic pulse wave velocity) readings expressed as m/sec.
*Microalbuminuria or greater levels of proteinuria.
CKD 3B = eGFR 30–44 mls/min/1.73 m^2; CVE = cardiovascular event;
MAP = Mean arterial pressure;
‡ = Hypertension at entry into study;
Mann U Whitney tests used where data were not normally distributed.

Table 3. Significant Correlations with aPWV.

	Total Cohort (unadjusted)		Total Cohort (adjusted for MAP)	
	r	P-value	r	P-value
Age (years)	0.456*	<0.001	0.461	<0.001
MAP (mmHg)	0.228	<0.001	-	-
Urine ACR (mg/mmol)‡	0.124	<0.001	0.111	<0.001
Waist to Hip ratio‡	0.124	<0.001	0.121	<0.001
BMI (kg/m^2)‡	−0.122	<0.001	−0.133	<0.001
Skin autofluorescence‡	0.117	<0.001	0.133	<0.001
Total Protein (g/L)	0.084	0.001	0.049	0.046
eGFR (mL/min/1.73 m^2)	−0.074*	0.002	−0.096	<0.001
hs CRP‡	0.066	0.006	0.057	0.020
HDL Cholesterol (mmol/L)‡	−0.062	0.010	−0.069	0.005
Total Cholesterol (mmol/L)‡	−0.057	0.018	−0.100	<0.001

*Spearman correlation, otherwise Pearson correlation used. For adjusted values partial correlations were used.
‡ = log transformed data. r = correlation coefficient.
ACR = albumin to creatinine ratio; aPWV = aortic pulse wave velocity; BP = blood pressure; BMI = Body Mass Index; eGFR = estimated glomerular filtration rate; IMD = Indicies of multiple deprivation; HDL = high density lipo-protein; HS CRP = High sensitivity C-reactive protein; MAP = Mean arterial pressure.

data therefore suggest that markers of kidney disease are not strong determinants of AS in early CKD and that traditional risk factors for CVD may be more important, or that mechanisms unrelated to AS mediate the association between early CKD and increased cardiovascular risk in this population.

Published data regarding the relationship between AS and CKD appear contradictory. Studies of patients receiving dialysis or with advanced CKD reported significantly increased AS compared with the general population [32,33] but results from studies that included those with earlier stages of CKD are variable. A number of studies have reported associations with reduced GFR and increased AS [15,17,34]. In a relatively small study of 102 people with a wide spectrum of CKD (stages 1–5) a clear stepwise increase corresponding to stage of CKD was reported [15]. Multivariable analysis confirmed an independent association between GFR and aPWV; however only a small number of participants (n = 45) had CKD stage 3–4 and GFR was substantially lower than in our cohort (mean eGFR of 38 mL/min/1.73 m^2). In a larger study of 2564 patients with CKD who were not receiving dialysis (almost half with diabetes, mean age 60.7 years, mean eGFR 40.7 mL/min/1.73 m^2), Townsend et al. also found an increase in aPWV with declining GFR [17]. Similarly, a population-based study of 767 people (mean age 68 years, eGFR 60.6 mL/min/1.73 m^2 and ACR 0.57 mg/mmol) targeting screening for type 2 diabetes, found that AS increased as GFR decreased in those with mild CKD (stage 2–3) [34]. In addition urinary ACR was positively associated with increased AS. On the other hand Briet et al [18] reported that AS was higher in patients with CKD than in hypertensive patients without CKD, but in the analysis of patients with CKD stage 3–5 they did not find a significant relationship between measured GFR and aPWV. Similarly, in a study of 150 patients with CKD stages 2–5D, aPWV was significantly higher in patients with CKD versus controls without CKD, but aPWV was not higher in those with more advanced CKD [20]. In another study of patients with CKD, blood pressure was the major determinant of PWV and although PWV correlated with GFR in a univariate analysis, GFR was not an independent determinant of PWV in a multivariable analysis [35]. Similarly, in 113 patients with CKD, PWV increased

Table 4. Independent Determinants of higher aPWV.

	Total Cohort Adjusted R^2 = 0.29		
	B (95% CI)	β	p value
Age (10 years)	1.09 (0.94 to 1.24)	0.49	<0.001
Gender (female)	1.46 (0.07 to 2.85)	0.35	0.04
MAP (10 mmHg)	0.43 (0.35 to 0.50)	0.24	<0.001
Diabetes Mellitus	0.61 (0.38 to 0.83)	0.11	<0.001
Body Mass Index (kg/m^2)	−0.042 (−0.058 to −0.025)	−0.11	<0.001
Total serum protein	0.025 (0.0084 to 0.042)	0.06	0.003
‡UACR (mg/mmol)	0.060 (0.0061 to 0.11)	0.05	0.03
HDL Cholesterol (mmol/L)	−0.21 (−0.42 to −0.0028)	−0.046	0.047
Interactive term age by gender (F)	−0.22 (−0.41 to −0.031)	−0.39	0.02

B = un-standardised coefficient (95% confidence intervals).
β = standardized coefficient (Beta).
F = female.
‡log-transformed data.
aPWV = aortic pulse wave velocity; HDL = high density lipo-protein; MAP = mean arterial blood pressure; UACR = urine albumin to creatinine ratio.
Independent variables that did not enter the equation were: eGFR, previous smoker status, past history of cardiovascular event, anaemia, white cell count, serum potassium, total cholesterol, skin autofluorescence, log urine protein to creatinine ratio, log high sensitivity CRP, waist to hip ratio, serum glucose. treatment with inhibitors on the renin angiotensin aldosterone system (RAASi), antihypertensive treatment.

with increasing number of components of the metabolic syndrome irrespective of GFR [36]. In one analysis of data from the Framingham Heart Study that included 181 patients with early CKD and characteristics very similar to ours (mean age 70 years, mean eGFR 51 mL/min/1.73 m^2, median urinary ACR 10 mg/g), AS was not different between those with or without CKD (defined by reduced GFR) after multivariable adjustment at baseline. In a longitudinal analysis, increased AS was not associated with increased risk of developing CKD [6]. On the other hand, higher aPWV was associated with elevated urinary albumin excretion at baseline and increased risk of developing microalbuminuria. Finally, in the Nephro Test cohort of 180 patients with CKD (mean age 59.6years, eGFR 32 mL/min/1.73 m^2) aortic PWV remained stable during 3.5 years of follow up despite a significant decline in GFR and an increase in albuminuria. Interestingly, increased carotid circumferential wall stress and pulse pressure were associated with a greater risk of progression to ESKD [19]. Taken together, published data show that arterial stiffness increases in advanced stages of CKD but that changes are more variable in early stages, probably reflecting differences in the populations studied, particularly with respect to age. Thus the lack of an independent negative association between eGFR and increased aPWV in our study as well as the weak association between urinary ACR and increased aPWV are probably attributable to the fact that our study population was predominantly elderly, the range of eGFR values was relatively small and albuminuria was present only in a small minority. These observations are nevertheless important because our study cohort is representative of the majority of people affected by early stage CKD, at least in the UK.

Previous studies have also identified age, blood pressure and the presence of diabetes as determinants of higher aPWV [6,17,20]. Our observation that aPWV increased to a greater extent with age in males versus females is consistent with data from another study that identified male gender as an independent determinant of increased aPWV in a large cohort of people with CKD [17].The increase in AS with age is proposed to be due to overproduction of abnormal collagen fibres and a loss of elastin from the extracellular matrix [9,37]. It is not clear, however, whether this is a time dependant phenomenon directly related to chronological age or if it reflects exposure to other risk factors. Hypertension has long been recognised as a major determinant of arterial stiffness due to the associated medial hypertrophy [38]. The association between diabetes and arterial stiffness may be due to accumulation of advanced glycation endproducts (AGE) that provoke structural changes in the arterial wall [22] and the generation of reactive oxygen species that deactivate nitric oxide resulting in endothelial dysfunction [39].

BMI had an inverse relationship with aPWV. This is surprising because AS has previously been associated with obesity, particularly abdominal obesity [40], and increased waist to hip ratio was associated with higher aPWV in our univariate analysis. We have previously described that BMI decreased with age in our cohort, likely reflecting a loss of muscle mass [21]. Our observation may therefore be explained by lower BMI acting as marker of increased age (the dominant determinant of aPWV) that could not be completely corrected for in the multi-variable analysis. Furthermore, we have previously shown that measures of obesity that include central fat distribution are more closely related to important risk factors in those with CKD than BMI [41].

There are a several limitations to this study. First, this analysis includes only cross-sectional data and we are therefore unable to draw any firm conclusions regarding possible causal relationships between AS and the determinants identified. However, the planned 10-year follow up of the cohort will allow us to investigate the factors that contribute to AS prospectively. Many studies have used aplanation tonometry devices (SphygmoCor^{TM} or Complior^{TM}) to measure PWV [17,19,20], but these are operator dependant, time consuming to use and not easy to transport. We therefore used the more portable Vicorder^{TM} device which is also operator independent and requires only minutes to obtain a reading. Vicorder^{TM} measurements of aPWV have been shown to be reproducible and correlate well with SphygmoCor^{TM} measurements [42] but as yet there is no agreed method for making direct comparisons between results obtained by different methods [43]. A third limitation of our study is the absence of normal controls. Finally, participants comprised only 22% of people invited to participate and may therefore not be representative of all people with CKD stage 3. We were unable for ethical reasons to obtain data on non-participants but our study population was similar to a large population of people with CKD stage 3 derived by pooling data on all patients from several GP databases, suggesting that our participants were broadly representative of patients with CKD stage 3 in primary care in the UK, though with a low proportion of people from ethnic minorities [44]. Strengths of the study include the large cohort size, robust measures of eGFR and UACR, and detailed clinical assessment of each participant. A single operator performed all assessments, eliminating inter-observer variability.

Conclusion

Age was the strongest determinant of arterial stiffness in this cohort of predominantly elderly patients with CKD stage 3. Other significant independent determinants of aPWV included traditional cardiovascular risk factors such as blood pressure, diabetes, obesity and a marker of dyslipidaemia. Markers of CKD were associated with aPWV only in univariate analysis (eGFR) or were weak determinants of aPWV (albuminuria). Long term follow-up will investigate the importance of arterial stiffness as an independent risk factor for cardiovascular events in this cohort.

Acknowledgments

Thanks go to the collaborating GP practices and their staff. In addition we gratefully acknowledge the invaluable assistance of: Mrs Diane Taal, Ms Rani Uppal, Mrs Rebecca Packington, Mrs Maureen Franklin, Mrs Sue Hodkinson, Mr Richard Turck and Mrs Paula Welch. We also thank all the participants for their time and commitment.

The results presented in this paper have not been published previously in whole or in part, except in abstract form.

Author Contributions

Conceived and designed the experiments: NJM RJF CWM AF MWT. Performed the experiments: NJM MWT. Analyzed the data: NJM AF MWT. Wrote the paper: NJM RJF CWM AF MWT.

References

1. Vanholder R, Massy Z, Argiles A, Spasovski G, Verbeke F, et al. (2005) Chronic kidney disease as cause of cardiovascular morbidity and mortality. Nephrol Dial Transplant 20: 1048–1056.
2. Keith DS, Nichols GA, Gullion CM, Brown JB, Smith DH (2004) Longitudinal follow-up and outcomes among a population with chronic kidney disease in a large managed care organization. Arch Intern Med 164: 659–663.

3. Hallan SI, Dahl K, Oien CM, Grootendorst DC, Aasberg A, et al. (2006) Screening strategies for chronic kidney disease in the general population: follow-up of cross sectional health survey. BMJ 333: 1047.
4. Go AS, Chertow GM, Fan D, McCulloch CE, Hsu CY (2004) Chronic kidney disease and the risks of death, cardiovascular events, and hospitalization. New Engl J Med 351: 1296–1305.
5. Stenvinkel P, Carrero JJ, Axelsson J, Lindholm B, Heimburger O, et al. (2008) Emerging biomarkers for evaluating cardiovascular risk in the chronic kidney disease patient: how do new pieces fit into the uremic puzzle? Clin J Am Soc Nephrol 3: 505–521.
6. Upadhyay A, Hwang SJ, Mitchell GF, Vasan RS, Vita JA, et al. (2009) Arterial stiffness in mild-to-moderate CKD. J Am Soc Nephrol 20: 2044–2053.
7. Safar ME, London GM, Plante GE (2004) Arterial stiffness and kidney function. Hypertension 43: 163–168.
8. Mitchell GF (2004) Increased aortic stiffness: an unfavorable cardiorenal connection. Hypertension 43: 151–153.
9. Chue CD, Townend JN, Steeds RP, Ferro CJ (2010) Arterial stiffness in chronic kidney disease: causes and consequences. Heart 96: 817–823.
10. Sutton-Tyrrell K, Najjar SS, Boudreau RM, Venkitachalam L, Kupelian V, et al. (2005) Elevated aortic pulse wave velocity, a marker of arterial stiffness, predicts cardiovascular events in well-functioning older adults. Circulation 111: 3384–3390.
11. Cruickshank K, Riste L, Anderson SG, Wright JS, Dunn G, et al. (2002) Aortic pulse-wave velocity and its relationship to mortality in diabetes and glucose intolerance: an integrated index of vascular function? Circulation 106: 2085–2090.
12. Laurent S, Cockcroft J, Van Bortel L, Boutouyrie P, Giannattasio C, et al. (2006) Expert consensus document on arterial stiffness: methodological issues and clinical applications. Eur Heart J 27: 2588–2605.
13. Blacher J, London GM, Safar ME, Mourad JJ (1999) Influence of age and end-stage renal disease on the stiffness of carotid wall material in hypertension. J Hypertens 17: 237–244.
14. London GM, Blacher J, Pannier B, Guerin AP, Marchais SJ, et al. (2001) Arterial wave reflections and survival in end-stage renal failure. Hypertension 38: 434–438.
15. Wang MC, Tsai WC, Chen JY, Huang JJ (2005) Stepwise increase in arterial stiffness corresponding with the stages of chronic kidney disease. Am J Kidney Dis 45: 494–501.
16. Mourad JJ, Pannier B, Blacher J, Rudnichi A, Benetos A, et al. (2001) Creatinine clearance, pulse wave velocity, carotid compliance and essential hypertension. Kidney Int 59: 1834–1841.
17. Townsend RR, Wimmer NJ, Chirinos JA, Parsa A, Weir M, et al. (2010) Aortic PWV in chronic kidney disease: a CRIC ancillary study. Am J Hypertens 23: 282–289.
18. Briet M, Bozec E, Laurent S, Fassot C, London GM, et al. (2006) Arterial stiffness and enlargement in mild-to-moderate chronic kidney disease. Kidney Int 69: 350–357.
19. Briet M, Collin C, Karras A, Laurent S, Bozec E, et al. (2011) Arterial remodeling associates with CKD progression. J Am Soc Nephrol 22: 967–974.
20. Temmar M, Liabeuf S, Renard C, Czernichow S, Esper NE, et al. (2010) Pulse wave velocity and vascular calcification at different stages of chronic kidney disease. J Hypertens 28: 163–169.
21. McIntyre NJ, Fluck RJ, McIntyre CW, Taal MW (2011) Risk Profile in Chronic Kidney Disease Stage 3: Older versus Younger Patients. Nephron Clinical Practice 119: c269–c276.
22. McIntyre NJ, Fluck RJ, McIntyre CW, Taal MW (2011) Skin Autofluorescence and the Association with Renal and Cardiovascular Risk Factors in Chronic Kidney Disease Stage 3. Clin J Am Soc Nephrol.
23. National Institute for Health and Clinical Excellence (2008) Chronic Kidney Disease: National clinical guideline for early identification and management in adults in primary and secondary care. The National Institute for Health and Clincal Excellence. www.nice.org.uk/nicemedia/pdf/CG073NICEGuideline.pdf.
24. The World Health Organisation and the International Diabetes Federation. (2006) The definition and diagnosis of diabetes mellitus and intermediate glycaemia. WHO Press.
25. Pinto-Sietsma SJ, Navis G, Janssen WM, de Zeeuw D, Gans RO, et al. (2003) A central body fat distribution is related to renal function impairment, even in lean subjects. Am J Kidney Dis 41: 733–741.
26. Chobanian AV, Bakris GL, Black HR, Cushman WC, Green LA, et al. (2003) The Seventh Report of the Joint National Committee on Prevention, Detection, Evaluation, and Treatment of High Blood Pressure: the JNC 7 report. JAMA 289: 2560–2572.
27. Blacher J, Safar ME, Guerin AP, Pannier B, Marchais SJ, et al. (2003) Aortic pulse wave velocity index and mortality in end-stage renal disease. Kidney Int 63: 1852–1860.
28. Blacher J, Guerin AP, Pannier B, Marchais SJ, Safar ME, et al. (1999) Impact of aortic stiffness on survival in end-stage renal disease. Circulation 99: 2434–2439.
29. Meerwaldt R, Graaff R, Oomen PH, Links TP, Jager JJ, et al. (2004) Simple non-invasive assessment of advanced glycation endproduct accumulation. Diabetologia 47: 1324–1330.
30. Meerwaldt R, Lutgers HL, Links TP, Graaff R, Baynes JW, et al. (2007) Skin autofluorescence is a strong predictor of cardiac mortality in diabetes. Diabetes Care 30: 107–112.
31. Hartog JW, Gross S, Oterdoom LH, van Ree RM, de Vries AP, et al. (2009) Skin-autofluorescence is an independent predictor of graft loss in renal transplant recipients. Transplantation 87: 1069–1077.
32. London GM, Marchais SJ, Safar ME, Genest AF, Guerin AP, et al. (1990) Aortic and large artery compliance in end-stage renal failure. Kidney Int 37: 137–142.
33. Shinohara K, Shoji T, Tsujimoto Y, Kimoto E, Tahara H, et al. (2004) Arterial stiffness in predialysis patients with uremia. Kidney Int 65: 936–943.
34. Hermans MM, Henry R, Dekker JM, Kooman JP, Kostense PJ, et al. (2007) Estimated glomerular filtration rate and urinary albumin excretion are independently associated with greater arterial stiffness: the Hoorn Study. J Am Soc Nephrol 18: 1942–1952.
35. Lilitkarntakul P, Dhaun N, Melville V, Blackwell S, Talwar DK, et al. (2011) Blood pressure and not uraemia is the major determinant of arterial stiffness and endothelial dysfunction in patients with chronic kidney disease and minimal co-morbidity. Atherosclerosis 216: 217–225.
36. Lilitkarntakul P, Dhaun N, Melville V, Kerr D, Webb DJ, et al. (2012) Risk factors for metabolic syndrome independently predict arterial stiffness and endothelial dysfunction in patients with chronic kidney disease and minimal comorbidity. Diabetes Care 35: 1774–1780.
37. Greenwald SE (2007) Ageing of the conduit arteries. J Pathol 211: 157–172.
38. Haider AW, Larson MG, Franklin SS, Levy D (2003) Systolic blood pressure, diastolic blood pressure, and pulse pressure as predictors of risk for congestive heart failure in the Framingham Heart Study. Ann Intern Med 138: 10–16.
39. Bucala R, Tracey KJ, Cerami A (1991) Advanced glycosylation products quench nitric oxide and mediate defective endothelium-dependent vasodilatation in experimental diabetes. J Clin Invest 87: 432–438.
40. Orr JS, Gentile CL, Davy BM, Davy KP (2008) Large artery stiffening with weight gain in humans: role of visceral fat accumulation. Hypertension 51: 1519–1524.
41. Evans PD, McIntyre NJ, Fluck RJ, McIntyre CW, Taal MW (2012) Anthropomorphic measurements that include central fat distribution are more closely related with key risk factors than BMI in CKD stage 3. PLoS One 7: e34699.
42. Hickson SS, Butlin M, Broad J, Avolio AP, Wilkinson IB, et al. (2009) Validity and repeatability of the Vicorder apparatus: a comparison with the SphygmoCor device. Hypertens Res 32: 1079–1085.
43. The Reference Values for Arterial Stiffness' Colaboration (2010) Determinants of pulse wave velocity in healthy people and in the presence of cardiovascular risk factors: 'establishing normal and reference values'. Eur Heart J 31: 2338–2350.
44. de Lusignan S, Tomson C, Harris K, van Vlymen J, Gallagher H (2010) Creatinine Fluctuation Has a Greater Effect than the Formula to Estimate Glomerular Filtration Rate on the Prevalence of Chronic Kidney Disease. Nephron Clin Pract 117: c213–c224.

23

Adrenomedullin-RAMP2 System Suppresses ER Stress-Induced Tubule Cell Death and Is Involved in Kidney Protection

Ryuichi Uetake[1], Takayuki Sakurai[1], Akiko Kamiyoshi[1], Yuka Ichikawa-Shindo[1], Hisaka Kawate[1], Yasuhiro Iesato[1], Takahiro Yoshizawa[1], Teruhide Koyama[1], Lei Yang[1], Yuichi Toriyama[1], Akihiro Yamauchi[1], Kyoko Igarashi[1], Megumu Tanaka[1], Takashige Kuwabara[2], Kiyoshi Mori[2,3], Motoko Yanagita[4], Masashi Mukoyama[2], Takayuki Shindo[1]*

1 Department of Cardiovascular Research, Shinshu University Graduate School of Medicine, Matsumoto, Japan, **2** Department of Medicine and Clinical Science, Kyoto University Graduate School of Medicine, Kyoto, Japan, **3** Medical Innovation Center, Kyoto University Graduate School of Medicine, Kyoto, Japan, **4** Department of Nephrology, Kyoto University Graduate School of Medicine, Kyoto, Japan

Abstract

Various bioactive peptides have been implicated in the homeostasis of organs and tissues. Adrenomedullin (AM) is a peptide with various bioactivities. AM-receptor, calcitonin-receptor-like receptor (CLR) associates with one of the subtypes of the accessory proteins, RAMPs. Among the RAMP subisoforms, only RAMP2 knockout mice (−/−) reproduce the phenotype of embryonic lethality of AM−/−, illustrating the importance of the AM-RAMP2-signaling system. Although AM and RAMP2 are abundantly expressed in kidney, their function there remains largely unknown. We used genetically modified mice to assess the pathophysiological functions of the AM-RAMP2 system. RAMP2+/− mice and their wild-type littermates were used in a streptozotocin (STZ)-induced renal injury model. The effect of STZ on glomeruli did not differ between the 2 types of mice. On the other hand, damage to the proximal urinary tubules was greater in RAMP2+/−. Tubular injury in RAMP2+/− was resistant to correction of blood glucose by insulin administration. We examined the effect of STZ on human renal proximal tubule epithelial cells (RPTECs), which express glucose transporter 2 (GLUT2), the glucose transporter that specifically takes up STZ. STZ activated the endoplasmic reticulum (ER) stress sensor protein kinase RNA-like endoplasmic reticulum kinase (PERK). AM suppressed PERK activation, its downstream signaling, and CCAAT/enhancer-binding homologous protein (CHOP)-induced cell death. We confirmed that the tubular damage was caused by ER stress-induced cell death using tunicamycin (TUN), which directly evokes ER stress. In RAMP2+/− kidneys, TUN caused severe injury with enhanced ER stress. In wild-type mice, TUN-induced tubular damage was reversed by AM administration. On the other hand, in RAMP2+/−, the rescue effect of exogenous AM was lost. These results indicate that the AM-RAMP2 system suppresses ER stress-induced tubule cell death, thereby exerting a protective effect on kidney. The AM-RAMP2 system thus has the potential to serve as a therapeutic target in kidney disease.

Editor: Hideharu Abe, University of Tokushima, Japan

Funding: This study was supported by the Funding Program for Next Generation World-Leading Researchers (NEXT Program) from the Cabinet Office, Government of Japan, Research Grant for Cardiovascular Disease from the National Cardiovascular Center, Research grant from the Naito Foundation, SENSHIN Medical Research Foundation,the NOVARTIS Foundation (Japan) for the Promotion of Science,Novartis Foundation for Gerontological Research, and Japan vascular disease research foundation. The funders had no role in study design, data collection and analysis, decision to publish, or preparation of the manuscript.

Competing Interests: The authors have declared that no competing interests exist.

* E-mail: tshindo@shinshu-u.ac.jp

Introduction

Epidemiological studies have shown that chronic kidney disease (CKD) is a serious risk factor for cardiovascular disease, and that there is a high incidence of death due to cardiovascular events among CKD patients [1]. At present there is no way to stop the progression of CKD, and new and more effective approaches to the treatment of CKD are greatly needed. During the progression of CKD, damage caused by uremic toxins can degrade renal function. For example, it was recently reported that the uremic toxin indoxyl sulfate induces endoplasmic reticulum (ER) stress that can aggravate CKD, particularly renal tubule injury [2]. More interestingly, it is now recognized that chronic albuminuria, a major symptom of CKD, is a detrimental factor that promotes CKD by enhancing ER stress and injuring tubule cells [3]. ER stress occurs as a result of the accumulation of unfolded proteins, which activates the unfolded protein response (UPR) [4]. Normally, the UPR works to maintain cellular homeostasis, but when the stress is excessive it can lead to cell death [5] and to disease [6,7]. For example, an exaggerated ER stress response contributes to kidney disease due to glomerular and tubular damage [8]. Thus, controlling ER stress could be an effective approach to breaking the vicious cycle of CKD progression.

Originally identified as a vasodilating peptide from human pheochromocytoma [9], AM is now known to be widely secreted in a number of organs and tissues, and to be involved in a variety of biological functions [10,11,12,13,14,15,16,17]. In the kidney, AM is distributed in the glomerulus, renal tubules, collecting ducts, and vasculature [18], where it contributes to the regulation of renal blood flow [19] and water/Na diuresis [20] and suppresses the growth of mesangial cells [21]. Blood AM levels are elevated in patients with hypertension or congestive heart failure [22,23] and in patients with renal failure, and AM is elevated in proportion to the severity of their disease [22]. Moreover, it was recently shown that the blood AM level is a sensitive marker, predictive of the long-term prognosis in CKD [24].

We previously showed that homozygotic AM knockout (KO) (AM−/−) mice die mid-gestation due to edema and hemorrhage [25]. Heterozygotic AM KO (AM+/−) mice grow to adulthood with no apparent deficits, but show accelerated damage to some organs, including the kidneys [26]. The clear importance of endogenous AM for cardiovascular and renal function suggests a therapeutic benefit may be gained from administration of the exogenous peptide. However, AM has a very short half-life in the bloodstream [27], which limits its utility for the treatment of chronic diseases requiring long-term therapy. For that reason, we have been focusing on the AM receptor system. AM is a member of the calcitonin superfamily and acts via a G protein-coupled seven transmembrane domain receptor (GPCR), calcitonin-receptor-like receptor (CLR) [28,29]. The specificity of CLR for its ligands is regulated by three receptor-activity-modifying proteins, RAMP1, RAMP2, and RAMP3. We previously showed that homozygotic RAMP2 KO (RAMP2−/−) mice die in utero and that they die from vascular abnormalities similar to those observed in AM−/− mice [30], which suggests RAMP2 is important in the cellular function of AM. In addition, we recently generated a line of endothelial cell-specific RAMP2 KO (E-RAMP2−/−) mice. Most E-RAMP2−/− mice die perinatally, and in the surviving adults we observed the spontaneous occurrence of several renal abnormalities, including polycystic kidney, hydronephrosis, and glomerular sclerosis [31]. These findings suggest that the vascular endothelial AM-RAMP2 system is involved in mediating renal homeostasis. Notably, RAMP2 is also distributed in other cell types throughout the kidney, though its significance there remains unknown.

Our aim in the present study was to further clarify the function of the AM-RAMP2 system in the kidney. For that purpose, we used adult heterozygous RAMP2 KO (RAMP2+/−) mice in a kidney injury model. Our findings indicate that the AM-RAMP2 system is a crucial regulator of ER stress in renal tubules.

Materials and Methods

Animals

Wild-type (WT) C57BL/6J mice were purchased from Charles River Laboratories Japan (Yokohama, Japan). RAMP2 KO mice were originally generated by our group [30]. Because homozygous RAMP2 KO mice die in utero, we used heterozygous RAMP2 KO male mice (RAMP2+/−) and their wild-type littermate male mice in this study. All animal handling procedures were performed in accordance with a protocol approved by the Ethics Committee of Shinshu University.

Streptozotocin (STZ) Administration Model

Four-week-old mice received a single intraperitoneal injection of 250 mg/kg body weight STZ (WAKO) dissolved in 0.9% NaCl [32]. Blood glucose levels were measured at 10:00 a.m. without fasting. Two, 4, or 12 weeks later, the mice were sacrificed and their kidneys were collected.

Tunicamycin Administration Model

Eight-week-old mice received a single intraperitoneal injection of 0.5–1.0 mg/kg body weight tunicamycin (TUN) (Sigma). TUN was initially dissolved in dimethyl sulfoxide (DMSO), which was then diluted in 150 mM dextrose solution for injection. Four days after the TUN injection, the mice were sacrificed and their kidneys were collected [33].

Adrenomedullin (AM) Administration Model

The AM-treated group received continuous subcutaneous administration of recombinant human AM dissolved in 0.9% NaCl at a delivery rate of 0.05 μg/kg/min using osmotic pumps (Alzet Model 2002). AM administration began 1 week before the TUN administration and continued to the end of the study.

Cisplatin Administration Model

Eight-week-old mice received a single intraperitoneal injection of 20 mg/kg body weight cisplatin (Sigma). Three days after the cisplatin injection, the mice were sacrificed and their kidneys were collected [34].

Cell Culture

Normal human renal proximal tubule epithelial cells (RPTECs) were purchased from Lonza. They were cultured in REGM medium (Lonza). Cells passaged up to three times were used for experimentation.

Histology

Tissues were fixed overnight in 4% paraformaldehyde, embedded in paraffin, and cut into 1.5-μm-thick sections for histological examination. The specimens were then deparaffinized for hematoxylin/eosin (H & E) staining, periodic acid-Schiff (PAS) staining, terminal deoxynucleotidyl transferase dUTP nick end labeling (TUNEL), and immunohistochemistry using anti-LC3 antibody (Cell Signaling Technology), and nuclear staining with DAPI (Life Technologies).

Transmission Electron Microscopy

Specimens were fixed in 2.5% glutaraldehyde (pH 7.2), embedded in epoxy resin (Epok) 812 (Oken Shoji Co.), cut into ultrathin sections, double-stained with uranyl acetate and lead citrate, and examined with an electron microscope.

RNA Extraction and Quantitative Real-Time RT-PCR Analysis

Total RNA was extracted from tissues using Trireagent (Molecular Research Center, Inc.), after which the RNA was treated with DNA-free (Ambion) to remove contaminating DNA and then subjected to reverse transcription using a High Capacity cDNA Reverse Transcription Kit (Applied Biosystems). Quantitative real-time RT-PCR was carried out using an Applied Biosystems 7300 real-time PCR System with SYBR green (Toyobo, Japan) or Realtime PCR Master Mix (Toyobo) and TaqMan probes (MBL). The primers and probes used are listed in Table. 1. Values were normalized to mouse GAPDH (Pre-Developed TaqMan assay reagents, Applied Biosystems).

Western Blot Analysis

Western blot analysis was carried out using protein extracts from RPTECs. The lysates were subjected to electrophoresis using TGX gel (Bio-Rad Laboratories), transferred to PVDF mem-

Table 1. Primers and probes used for quantitative real-time RT-PCR.

AM Forward	CTACCGCCAGAGCATGAACC
AM Reverse	GAAATGTGCAGGTCCCGAA
AM Probe	CCCGCAGCAATGGATGCCG
CLR Forward	AGGCGTTTACCTGCACACACT
CLR Reverse	CAGGAAGCAGAGGAAACCCC
CLR Probe	ATCGTGGTGGCTGTGTTTGCGGAG
RAMP2 Forward	GCAGCCCACCTTCTCTGATC
RAMP2 Reverse	AACGGGATGAGGCAGATGG
RAMP2 Probe	CCCAGAGGATGTGCTCCTGGCCAT
RAMP3 Forward	TGCAACGAGACAGGGATGC
RAMP3 Reverse	GCATCATGTCAGCGAAGGC
RAMP3 Probe	AGAGGCTGCCTCGCTGTGGGAA
Bax Forward	AGACACCTGAGCTGACCTTGGA
Bax Reverse	GAGACACTCGCTCAGCTTCTTG
Bcl-2 Forward	TGTGAGGACCCAATCTGGAAA
Bcl-2 Reverse	TTGCAATGAATCGGGAGTTG
BiP Forward	TCTGCCATGGTTCTCACTAAAATG
BiP Reverse	CAGTAACAATTGCATGGGTAACCT
CHOP Forward	TCCAGAAGGAAGTGCATCTTCA
CHOP Reverse	GGACTCAGCTGCCATGACT
GLUT-2 Forward	AGTACAGATGAACTGCCCACAATC
GLUT-2 Reverse	ATGGCCAGCTGATGAAAAGTG
p53 Forward	TGCATGGACGATCTGTTGCT
p53 Reverse	TGACACTCGGAGGGCTTCA
TNF-α Forward	ACGGCATGGATCTCAAAGAC
TNF-α Reverse	AGATAGCAAATCGGCTGACG
MCP-1 Forward	GCAGTTAACGCCCCACTCA
MCP-1 Reverse	CCTACTCATTGGGATCATCTTGCT
p47phox Forward	ATCCTATCTGGAGCCCCTTGA
p47phox Reverse	CACCTGCGTAGTTGGGATCC
p67phox Forward	CAGACCCAAAACCCCAGAAA
p67phox Reverse	AAAGCCAAACAATACGCGGT

branes (Bio-Rad Laboratories) and probed with anti-BiP, anti-ATF6, anti-PERK, anti-phospho-PERK (P-PERK), anti-IRE1, anti-phospho-IRE1 (P-IRE1), anti-eIF2α, anti-phospho-eIF2α (P-eIF2α), anti-ATF4, anti-CHOP (anti-ATF4 obtained from abcam, all others from Cell Signaling Technology), and anti-β-tubulin (Santa Cruz Biotechnology) antibodies. The blots were then developed using an ImageQuant LAS 4000 (GE Healthcare).

Statistical Analysis

Values are expressed as the mean ± SE. Student's t test was used to determine significant differences between two groups. One-way ANOVA followed by Fisher's PLSD was used to determine significant differences between three groups. Pearson's correlation coefficient was used to evaluate the correlation between two groups. Values of $p<0.05$ were considered significant.

Results

RAMP2+/− Mice Showed Enhanced Renal Tubular Injury in a STZ Nephropathy Model

Because RAMP2−/− mice exhibit lethal phenotypes similar to those of AM−/− mice, we hypothesized that endogenous RAMP2 is the most important in the function of AM. Heterozygous RAMP2 KO (RAMP2+/−) mice were apparently normal and fertile, though the level of RAMP2 expression in various organs, including kidney, was about half that seen in wild-type (WT) mice (Fig. 1A). To evaluate their susceptibility to renal injury, we examined RAMP2+/− mice and their WT littermates in a STZ-induced diabetic nephropathy model. Using STZ to induce hyperglycemia is a well-established method for generating experimental glomerular sclerosis. According to previous studies and the manufacturer's information, we performed a 100 mg/kg day STZ injection for 3 consecutive days or a single injection of 250 mg/kg. Because both showed similar results for the glucose level and pathological changes, we decided to use the latter protocol thereafter.

After administering 250 mg/kg STZ to mice, hyperglycemia was observed within about 1 week.?In both the control and STZ-treated groups, blood glucose levels did not differ between the WT and RAMP2+/− mice at 2 weeks (Fig. 1B). Blood pressure (BP) measured using tail cuff sphygmomanometry was not different between the 2 groups (Systolic BP: WT: 105.8±5.1, RAMP2+/−: 110.7±6.8 mmHg). After 12 weeks of STZ administration, glomeruli in both mice showed slight sclerotic changes, however, measurements of glomerular and mesangial area revealed no difference between WT and RAMP2+/− (Fig. 1C–E).

In contrast, we found urinary tubular changes to be much more prominent in STZ-treated RAMP2+/− than in WT mice. After 4 weeks of STZ administration, histological analysis showed RAMP2+/− kidneys stained poorly with H&E, suggesting interstitial edema (Fig. 2A), and in the cortical region of RAMP2+/− kidneys there was substantial degeneration of tubule cells (Fig. 2B). Some tubules were atrophic and even disappeared. No obvious inflammation, deposits, or vascular changes were found. Similar tubular damage was also confirmed in AM+/− with STZ administration, however, it was not found in RAMP2+/− without STZ administration. Using electron microscopy, the cellular membranes of tubule cells could be seen protruding into the tubule lumen in RAMP2+/− kidneys, suggesting destruction of the brush border (Fig. 2C). Taken together, these changes indicate that the proximal renal tubules of RAMP2+/− are severely damaged after STZ administration. Consistent with this finding, TUNEL assays confirmed tubule cell death to be enhanced in STZ-treated RAMP2+/− kidneys (Fig. 3A), and there was a corresponding downregulation of the anti-apoptotic factor Bcl-2 (Fig. 3B). To determine whether the tubular damage was caused by hyperglycemia, we administered insulin (glargine at a dose of 0.5–2 U daily) and STZ for 2 weeks, which normalized their blood glucose levels but did not mitigate the damage seen in RAMP2+/− kidneys (Fig. 3C). Based on these findings, we speculated that STZ acts directly to cause tubular injury, and RAMP2+/− mice were more susceptible to injury than WT mice.

Direct Renal Tubule Cell Damage Caused by STZ

We next utilized cultured human renal tubule cells (RPTECs) to evaluate the direct toxicity of STZ. STZ is a naturally occurring glucosamine-nitrosourea, and is transported into cells by the glucose transporter 2 (GLUT2) [35], which is expressed in pancreatic β cells. Notably, we found that GLUT2 is also highly expressed in renal tubule cells (Fig. 4A). When we treated

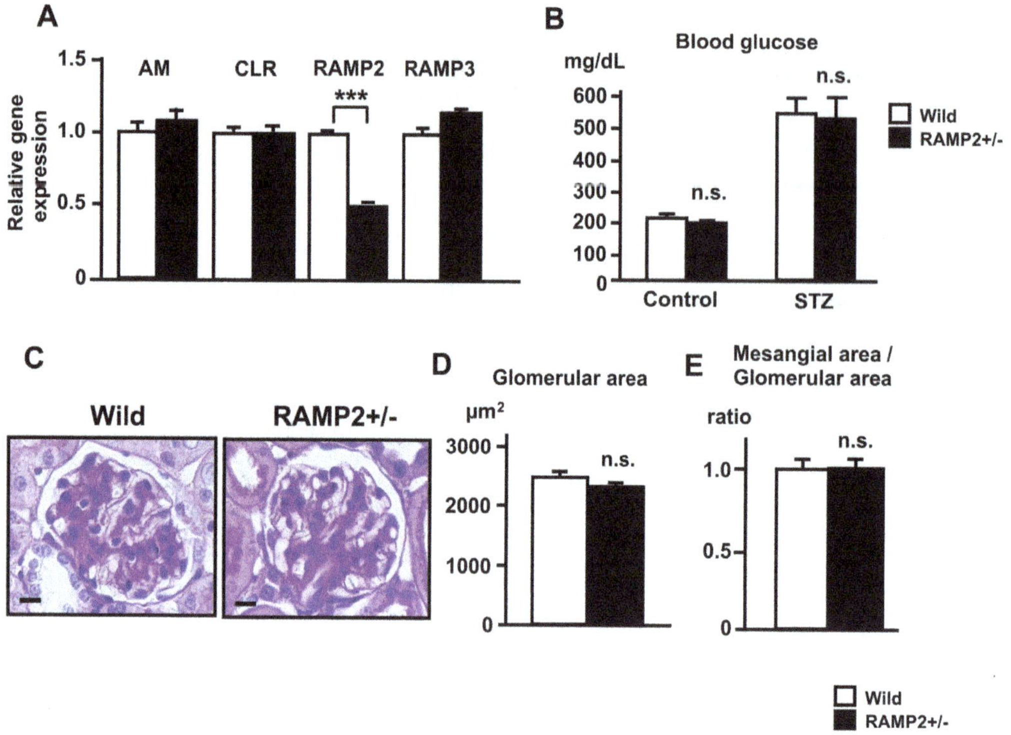

Figure 1. Blood glucose and glomerular changes in the STZ-induced diabetic nephropathy model. (A) Bar graphs showing relative gene expression determined by quantitative real-time PCR. Gene expression of RAMP2 was downregulated in RAMP2+/− kidney. (B) Effect of STZ treatment on blood glucose levels. In both the control and STZ groups, blood glucose levels did not differ between wild-type and RAMP2+/− mice 2 weeks after STZ administration. Data were obtained at 10:00 a.m. without fasting. (C-E) Comparison of glomerular lesions in wild-type and RAMP2+/− kidneys following STZ treatment. (C) PAS staining of glomeruli 12 weeks after STZ administration. Scale bars = 10 μm. (D) Glomerular area. (E) Mesangial area/glomerular area ratios. n = 5 in each group. Bars are means ± SEM. ***p<0.001. n.s. = not significant.

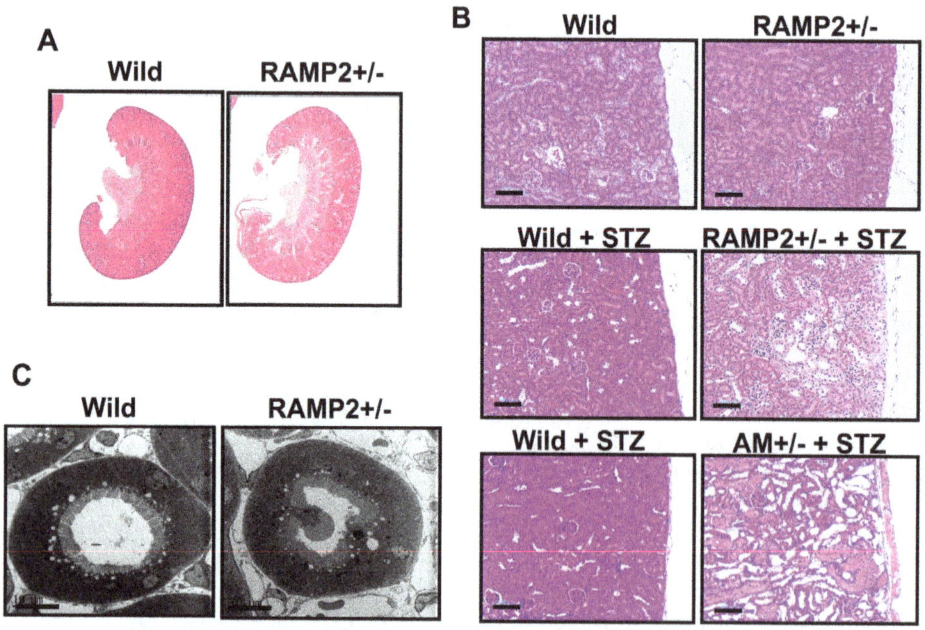

Figure 2. Renal tubular changes induced by the STZ treatment. (A) Cross-sections of kidneys collected from wild-type and RAMP2+/− mice 4 weeks after STZ administration (H & E staining). (B) Higher magnification of the renal cortex. STZ-administered RAMP2+/− and AM+/− showed substantial degeneration of tubule cells, which was not detected in RAMP2+/− without STZ administration. (C) Electron micrograph of a section of proximal tubule shows destruction of the brush border (protrusion of a tubule cellular membrane into the lumen) in a RAMP2+/− kidney. Scale bars = 100 μm (B), 10 μm (C).

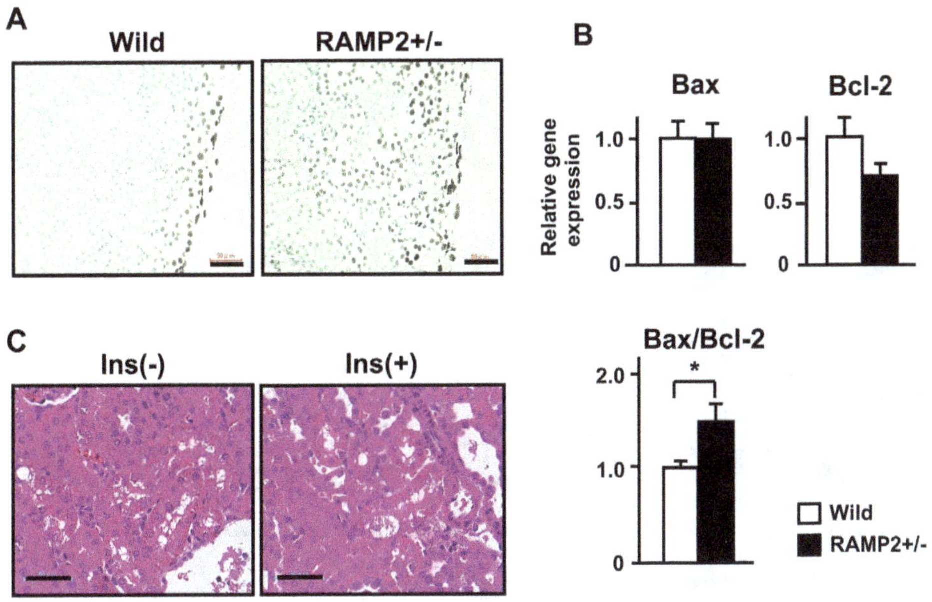

Figure 3. STZ-induced tubule cell death was enhanced in RAMP2+/− kidneys. (A) TUNEL assays of the renal cortex 4 weeks after STZ administration showed tubule cell death to be increased in RAMP2+/− kidneys. (B) Quantitative real-time PCR analysis of samples from the renal cortex. Shown are the relative gene expression levels of Bax and Bcl-2 (upper panels). Data from the wild-type control group were assigned a value of 1. Note the downregulation of Bcl-2 in RAMP2+/− kidneys indicated by the higher Bax/Bcl-2 ratio (lower panel). n = 5 in each group. Bars are means ± SEM. *$p<0.05$. (C) H&E staining of the renal cortex from RAMP2+/− kidneys 2 weeks after STZ administration, with or without insulin (Ins) treatment. Although insulin-treated RAMP2+/− mice had normal blood glucose levels, they showed the same level of tubular injury as mice not receiving insulin. Arrows indicate vacuolated proximal tubules. Scale bars = 50 μm (A), (C).

RPTECs for 4 h with STZ (10 mM) or with STZ (10 mM)+AM (0.1 μM), we found that STZ induced a 4.5-fold increase in cell death, but that AM strongly inhibited the effect (Fig. 4B, C).

STZ Induces ER Stress in Tubule Cells and the Effect is Suppressed by AM

We also found that the number of particles immunostaining positively for LC3, an autophagosome membrane protein, was greater in STZ-treated RAMP2+/− than in WT kidneys (Fig. 5A, B). Electron microscopic observation confirmed that autophagy was enhanced in STZ-treated tubule cells (Fig. 5C), which suggests that accumulation of foreign matter within tubule cells is a key contributor to STZ-induced tubule cell death.

In that context, we examined endoplasmic reticulum (ER) stress and the unfolded protein response (UPR) system, a mechanism by which foreign materials are eliminated from cells [36]. Activating transcription factor 6 (ATF6), protein kinase RNA-like endoplasmic reticulum kinase (PERK), and inositol-requiring 1 (IRE1) are three ER stress sensing proteins, whose activations are regulated by binding immunoglobulin protein (BiP). Using Western blot analysis of cultured RPTECs, we found that STZ administration directly evoked elevation of BiP and activation of PERK (elevation of phosphorylated PERK (p-PERK)), and that AM suppressed the STZ-induced elevations of BiP and p-PERK (Fig. 6A, B). We then analyzed three downstream mediators of PERK, eukaryotic initiation factor 2α (eIF2α), ATF4, and CCAAT/enhancer-binding homologous protein (CHOP), which is a critical component of the ER stress-UPR system and induces cell death [37,38]. Under basal conditions, little or no CHOP was detected in cultured RPTECs, but its expression was markedly upregulated by STZ, and this effect was significantly inhibited by AM (Fig. 6C, D). These results clearly show that STZ directly induces ER stress in renal tubule cells, and that AM suppresses the STZ-induced ER stress-UPR system and cell death.

ER Stress Causes Tubular Injury and Renal Dysfunction in RAMP2+/−

Given that AM reduces STZ-induced ER stress in RPTECs and tubule cell damage is enhanced in the STZ-treated RAMP2+/−, we hypothesized that the endogenous AM-RAMP2 system is a key regulator controlling ER stress in tubule cells *in vivo*. To test this hypothesis, we compared the effects of administering tunicamycin (TUN) to RAMP2+/− and WT mice. TUN is known to directly induce ER stress by inhibiting the synthesis of N-linked glycoproteins (N-glycans) [39] and causing cell cycle arrest at G1 phase [36]. RAMP2+/− mice administered TUN (0.5 mg/kg) exhibited slightly elevated levels of serum BUN and Cr (Fig. 7A). RAMP2+/− showed vacuolation of tubule cells (Fig. 7B) as well as upregulation of the ER stress-related factors BiP and CHOP (Fig. 7C). In contrast, TUN had little effect on WT kidneys, suggesting endogenous AM-RAMP2 signaling exerts a protective effect.

AM Reverses ER Stress-induced Tubular Injury

We next assessed the therapeutic potential of exogenous AM administration *in vivo*. Using an implanted osmotic pump, recombinant AM was continuously administered to mice beginning 1 week prior to TUN administration. At 0.05 μg/kg/min, AM administration had no significant effect on blood pressure during the study (data not shown). In wild-type mice, a higher dose of TUN (1 mg/kg) induced renal tubular injury, and it was reduced in the AM-treated group (Fig. 8A). In addition, AM administration inhibited the renal expression of the Bax and CHOP (Fig. 8B).

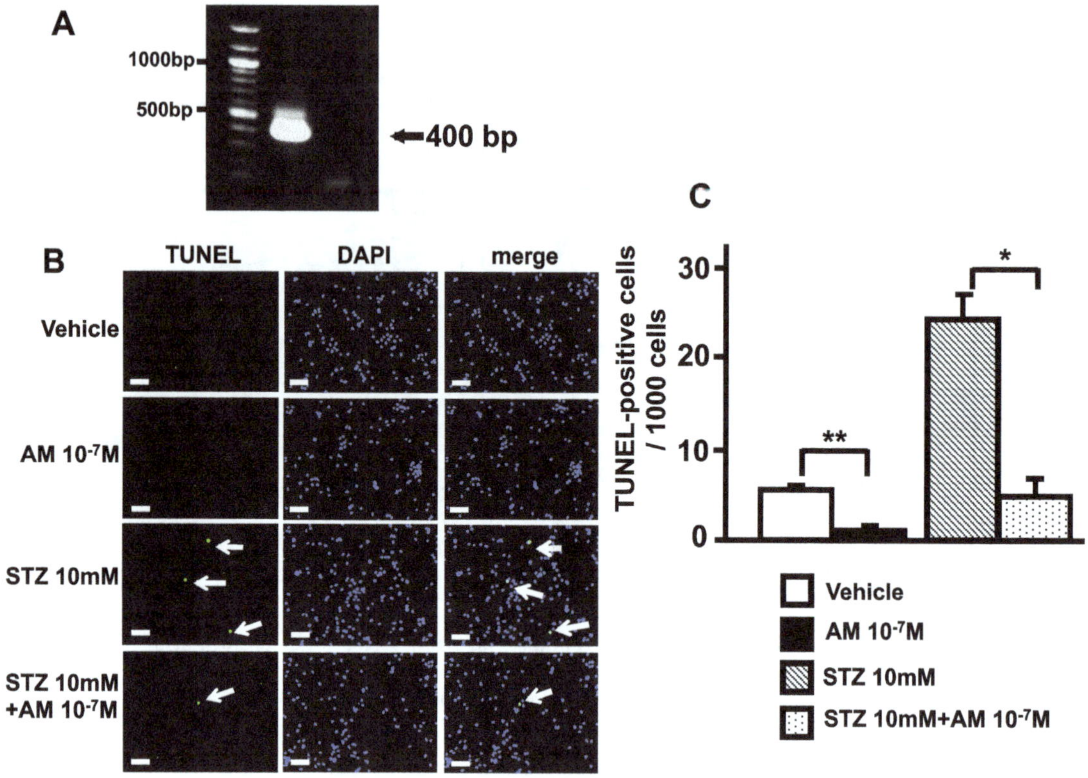

Figure 4. AM suppresses STZ-induced apoptosis among human renal tubule cells (RPTECs). (A) RT-PCR analysis showing the expression of GLUT2 in RPTECs. The arrow indicates the GLUT2 PCR product. (B) TUNEL assays of cultured RPTECs treated with vehicle, AM, STZ, or STZ+AM. Arrows show the TUNEL-positive cells. Scale bars = 100 μm. (C) Numbers of TUNEL-positive cells per 1,000 cultured cells. The experiments were repeated 3 times. Bars are means ± SEM. *p<0.05, **p<0.01.

On the other hand, in RAMP2+/−, the rescue effect of exogenous AM was lost; we could not detect the beneficial effects of AM, which was observed in wild-type mice (Fig. 8C, D). These results clearly indicate that the AM-RAMP2 system is important in the renal protection.

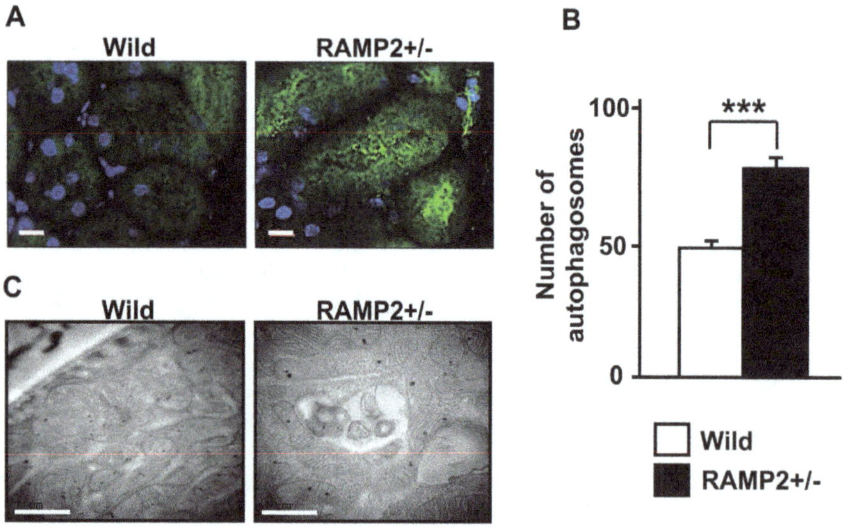

Figure 5. STZ enhances tubule cell autophagy in RAMP2+/− kidneys. (A) Fluorescent immunostaining of LC3 (green) and DAPI (blue) in proximal renal tubules 4 weeks after STZ administration to wild-type and RAMP2+/− mice. (B) Comparison of autophagosome numbers between wild-type and RAMP2+/− kidneys. Numbers of LC3-positve particles per microscope field were counted in LC3 immunostained sections. A total of 10 fields were analyzed. (C) Electron micrograph showing autophagosomes in a renal tubule cell. Bars are means ± SEM. ***p<0.001. Scale bars = 10 μm (A), 1 μm (C).

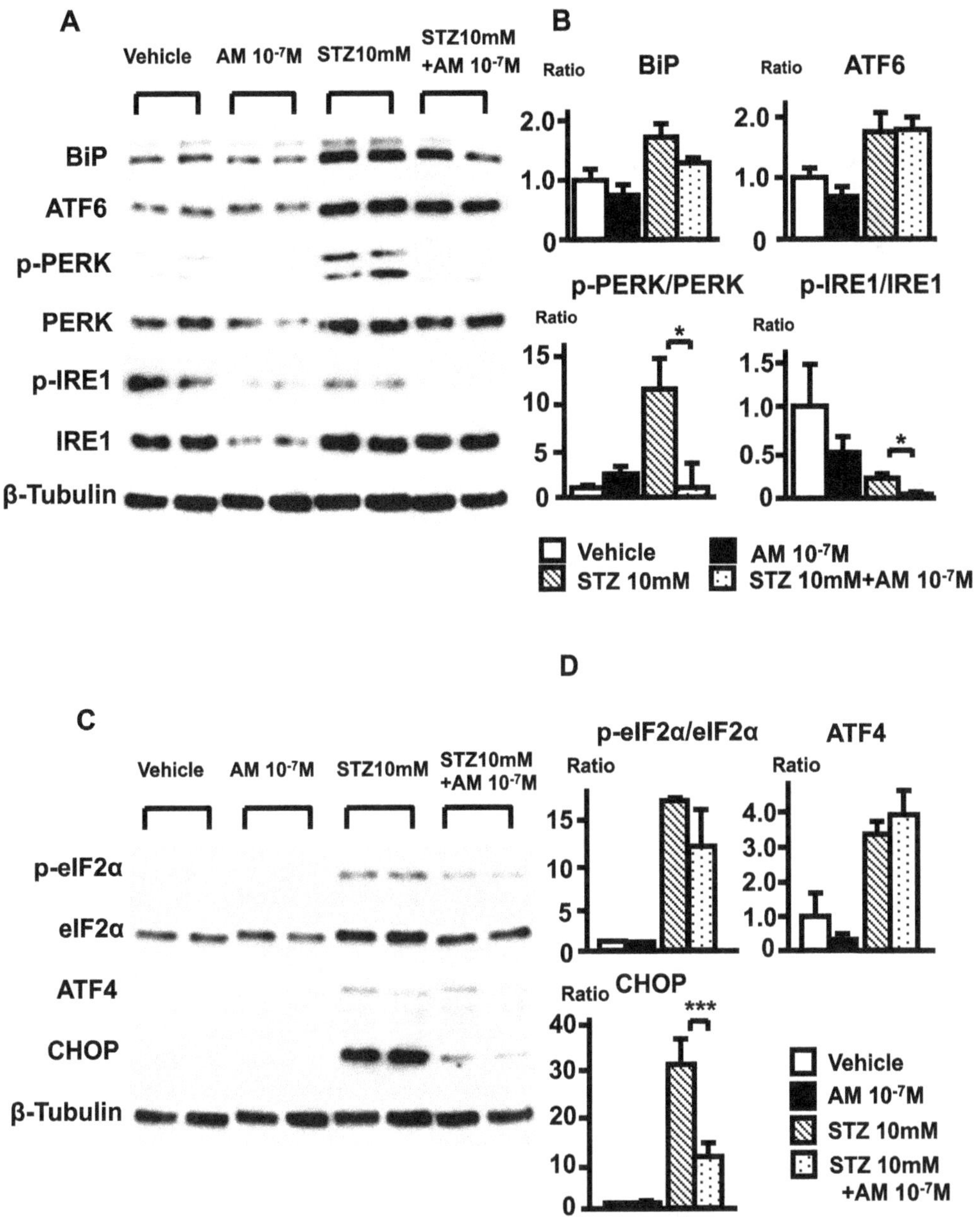

Figure 6. Western blot analysis of ER stress-related factors in STZ-treated RPTECs. (A) Western blot analysis of ER stress sensor molecules in STZ-treated RPTECs. (B) Optical densities of Western blots were quantified, and the relative expression of BiP and ATF6 and the p-PERK/PERK and p-IRE1/IRE1 ratios (PERK and IRE1 activation level) are shown. (C) Western blot analysis of the mediators downstream of PERK. (D) Quantification of the results in (C). The experiments were repeated 3 times. Data from the vehicle group were assigned a value of 1. Bars are means ± SEM. *p<0.05, ***p<0.001.

Cisplatin Induces Enhanced Tubular Injury in RAMP2+/− with Elevation of Inflammatory and Oxidative Stresses

As TUN-induced renal injury is a rather specific model, we finally evaluated the beneficial effect of the AM-RAMP2 system using a cisplatin-induced renal injury model. Cisplatin is a widely used chemotherapeutic agent. However, it is widely known to cause renal failure as a side effect. Cisplatin selectively damages proximal tubules due to its preferential accumulation within the proximal tubule cells [40]. In cisplatin-mediated nephrotoxicity, DNA injury, decreased protein synthesis, oxidative stress, and inflammation are thought to be involved [41,42]. Furthermore, cisplatin is reported to evoke ER stress and cell death [43].

Cisplatin administration (20 mg/kg) caused renal dysfunction with elevation of BUN and Cr, and the increases were slightly higher in RAMP2+/− (Fig. 9A). Cisplatin-administered RAMP2+/− showed enhanced tubular damage compared with wild-type mice (Fig. 9B). Cisplatin administration results in upregulation of cell death markers (p53 and Bax) and ER-stress markers (BiP and CHOP), as well as inflammatory markers (TNF-α and MCP-1) and oxidative stress markers (NADPH subunit, p47phox and p67phox), and again all were slightly higher in RAMP2+/−.

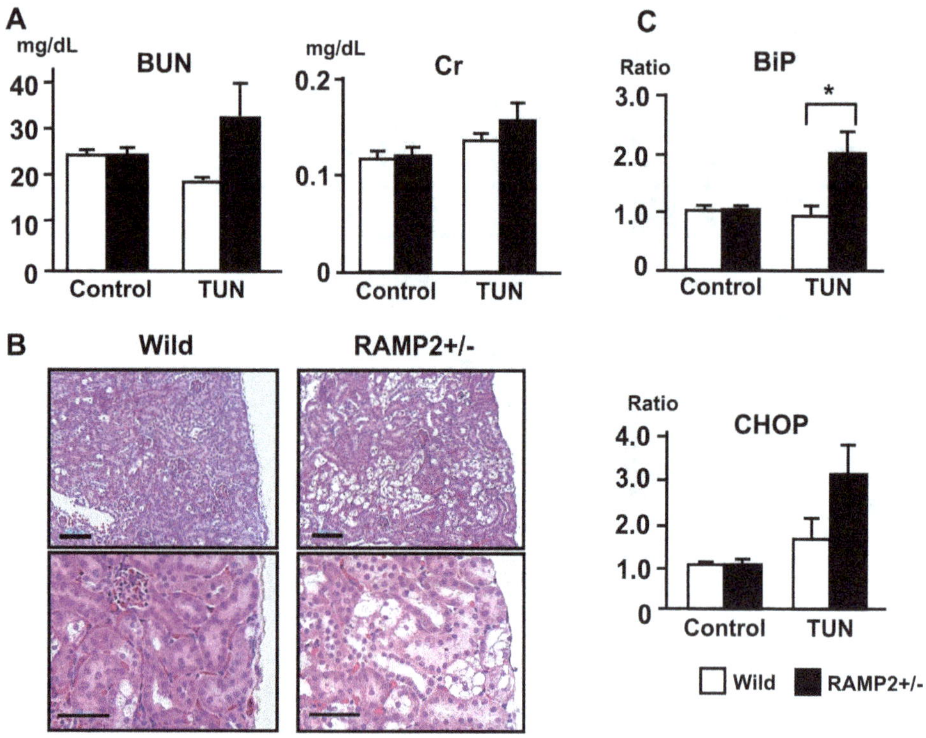

Figure 7. Tunicamycin (TUN) induces tubular injury and upregulation of ER stress-related factors in RAMP2+/− kidneys. (A) Serum BUN and creatinine (Cr) in wild-type and RAMP2+/−4 days after administration of vehicle (Control) or TUN (0.5 mg/kg). (B) H&E staining of the renal cortex in TUN-treated wild-type and RAMP2+/− kidneys. Scale bars in upper panels = 100 μm, lower panels = 50 μm. Sections from RAMP2+/− kidneys showed severe tubular injury with cell vacuolation. (C) Quantitative real-time PCR analysis of BiP and CHOP gene expression. TUN-treated RAMP2+/− kidneys showed upregulation of ER stress-related factors. Data from the wild-type control group were assigned a value of 1. n = 5 in each group. Bars are means ± SEM. $^{*}p<0.05$.

Discussion

It has been suggested that endogenous AM makes an important contribution to the maintenance of proper renal physiological function [19,20,21]. It has also been reported that AM levels are elevated in renal failure [22] and are a good predictor of who will or will not experience CKD progression [24]. Consistent with that finding, the expressions of CLR and RAMPs reportedly increase with progression of renal fibrosis in experimental models of CKD [44,45]. These reports thus implicate AM and its receptor in the development of CKD, although their precise pathophysiological significance remains unclear. In the present study, we used RAMP2 KO mice to show that endogenous AM-RAMP2 signaling exerts a protective effect on the kidney by regulating the ER stress-UPR system in the proximal renal tubules.

AM-induced effects that may work toward organ protection include the reduction of blood pressure and suppression of inflammation, oxidative stress, and fibrosis. Although we and others have shown that AM+/− mice grow to adulthood with no apparent deficits, these animals do exhibit accelerated organ damage when put under stress [13,25,46]. For example, we previously observed that ischemia/reperfusion injury is exacerbated in AM+/− kidneys [26]. Meanwhile, AM-overexpressing transgenic mice showed resistance to the injury [26]. We also found that continuous administration of angiotensin II to AM+/− mice induces severe glomerular injury with enhanced expression of TGF-β [47]. These results suggest that endogenous AM actively functions to protect the kidneys from injury.

Interestingly, RAMP2−/− phenotypes are embryonically lethal and similar to AM−/− phenotypes [25,30,48,49,50]. However, although both AM−/− and RAMP2−/− embryos exhibit abnormal vascular development, we detected no major renal deformities during embryogenesis. Recently, we developed a line of endothelial cell-specific RAMP2 KO (E-RAMP2−/−) mice. Most E-RAMP2−/− mice die perinatally; however, about 5% survive to adulthood. In the surviving E-RAMP2−/− adults, liver cirrhosis, cardiac fibrosis, and hydronephrosis all developed spontaneously. This organ damage is associated with marked fibrosis and oxidative stress and chronic inflammation. Thus, RAMP2 appears to be the critical determinant of AM function in adults, with AM-RAMP2 signaling exerting a protective effect by inhibiting inflammation and oxidative stress.

Glomerular lesions are the major pathological finding in diabetic nephropathy. From the results summarized above, we initially hypothesized that STZ-induced hyperglycemia would induce more severe glomerular lesions in RAMP2+/− than in WT kidneys. Both WT and RAMP2+/− showed similar blood glucose and BP levels, indicating that RAMP2 reduction did not have an effect on these parameters. We found, however, that RAMP2+/− mice administered STZ did not exhibit accelerated glomerular sclerosis when compared to WT mice. Instead, renal tubular injury due to ER stress was the major finding in the RAMP2+/− kidney, which suggests AM-RAMP2 exerts its protective effects by regulating the ER stress-UPR system.

The ER stress-UPR system is a stress response system initiated by accumulation of unfolded proteins [4]. Excessive accumulation

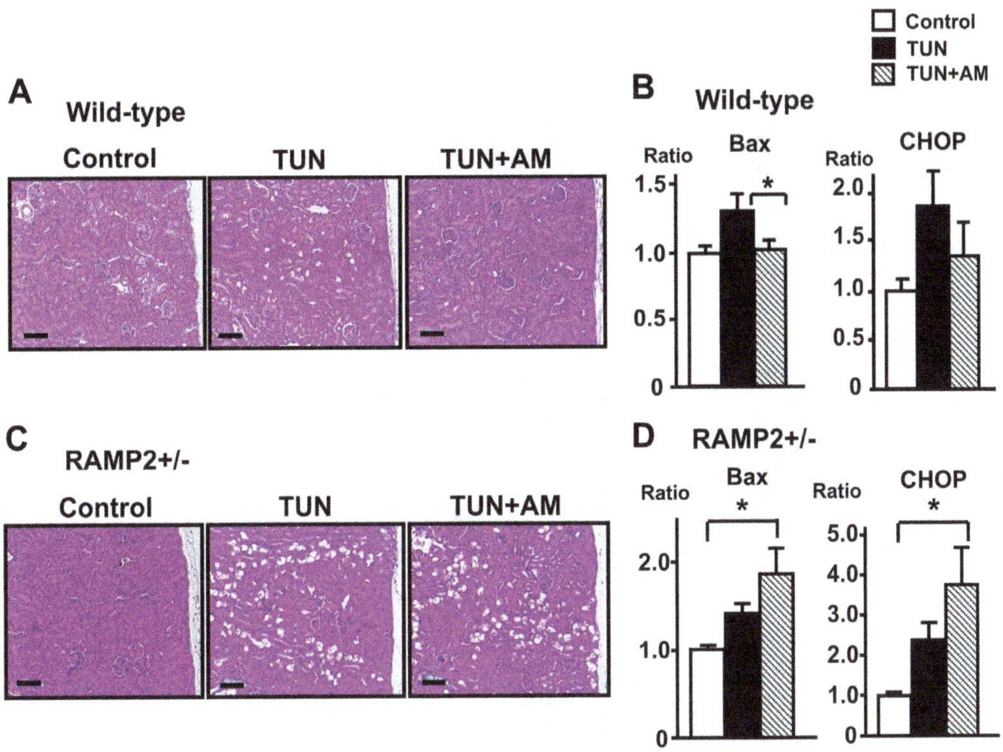

Figure 8. Exogenous AM reverses ER stress-induced tubular injury. (A) H&E staining of the renal cortex from wild-type mice treated with vehicle (Control), TUN, or TUN+AM. Samples were collected 4 days after TUN (1 mg/kg) administration. In the TUN+AM group, continuous AM administration at a rate of 0.05 μg/kg/min, beginning 1 week prior to TUN administration, reversed the TUN-induced tubular injury. (B) Quantitative real-time PCR analysis showing TUN-induced upregulation of ER stress-related factors CHOP and the apoptosis-related factor Bax, and their suppression by AM. (C, D) AM-treatment in RAMP2+/−. Even with the AM-treatment, RAMP2+/− showed enhanced tubular damage and upregulation of CHOP and Bax. (A, C) Scale bars = 100 μm. (B, D) Data from the control group were assigned a value of 1. n = 5 in each group. Bars are means ± SEM. *$p<0.05$.

of unfolded proteins disturbs cell homeostasis and can induce cell death [5]. It was recently reported, for example, that chronically elevated ER stress in pancreatic β cells induces diabetes [51], and that ER stress is increased in adipocytes in obese patients and is related to insulin resistance [52]. ER stress also appears to contribute to the pathogenesis of neurodegenerative diseases [53,54]. In an experimental model, angiotensin II administration led to upregulated expression of BiP and CHOP and induction of cardiomyocyte apoptosis [55]. In the kidney, uremic toxins and urinary proteins reportedly cause injury by inducing ER stress [2,3].

STZ injures pancreatic β cells, and the STZ administration model is often used to study hyperglycemia-induced organ damage. STZ-treated RAMP2+/− mice showed greater renal tubular injury than similarly treated WT mice. Notably, however, the tubular injury induced by STZ in RAMP2+/− kidneys was not mitigated by insulin treatment that normalized serum glucose levels. We therefore considered the renal tubular injury seen in RAMP2+/− kidneys to be a direct effect of STZ, not a secondary effect of hyperglycemia. Like other alkylating agents in the nitrosourea class, STZ is toxic to cells because it damages their DNA [56]. A glucose derivative, STZ is transported by GLUT2, which in addition to pancreatic β cells, is expressed in hepatocytes [57], small intestine epithelium [58], and renal tubules [59]. Our observation that autophagosome numbers are increased in tubule cells in STZ-treated RAMP2+/− kidneys was yet another observation highlighting the importance of the ER stress-UPR system in STZ-induced tubular injury.

In a set of *in vitro* experiments, we showed that STZ directly induces ER stress in cultured RPTECs, and that there is a corresponding upregulation of the activated form of the ER stress sensor, PERK. Interestingly, treating the cells with AM suppressed signaling downstream of PERK, in the eIF2α-ATF4-CHOP pathway, as well as CHOP-induced cell death. We then used TUN to confirm the tubular injury was caused by ER stress-induced cell death. TUN, which is commonly used to study the ER stress-UPR system, acts by inhibiting the synthesis of N-linked glycoproteins [39] and causes cell cycle arrest in G1 phase [36], which evokes ER stress. In the TUN-induced ER stress model, CHOP appeared to play a critical role by inducing cell death, which is consistent with the earlier report that CHOP KO mice are protected against TUN-induced renal tubular injury [37]. In RAMP2+/− mice, TUN administration caused tubule cell vacuolization and upregulation of the ER stress-related factors BiP and CHOP.

Our study using STZ and TUN may appear to be a rather specific situation. We chose these models because we found that these molecules clearly upregulate ER stress in renal tubular cells and RAMP2+/− are susceptible to them. Moreover, TUN is commonly used to evaluate ER stress-induced cellular and organ damage, as it directly evokes ER stress. However, drugs commonly used in clinical practice may also cause ER stress-related renal injury. Cisplatin is a major antineoplastic drug used in the treatment of solid tumors. However, it is also known to cause renal failure due to its preferential accumulation within the proximal tubule cells [42]. The mechanism of cisplatin-induced tubular

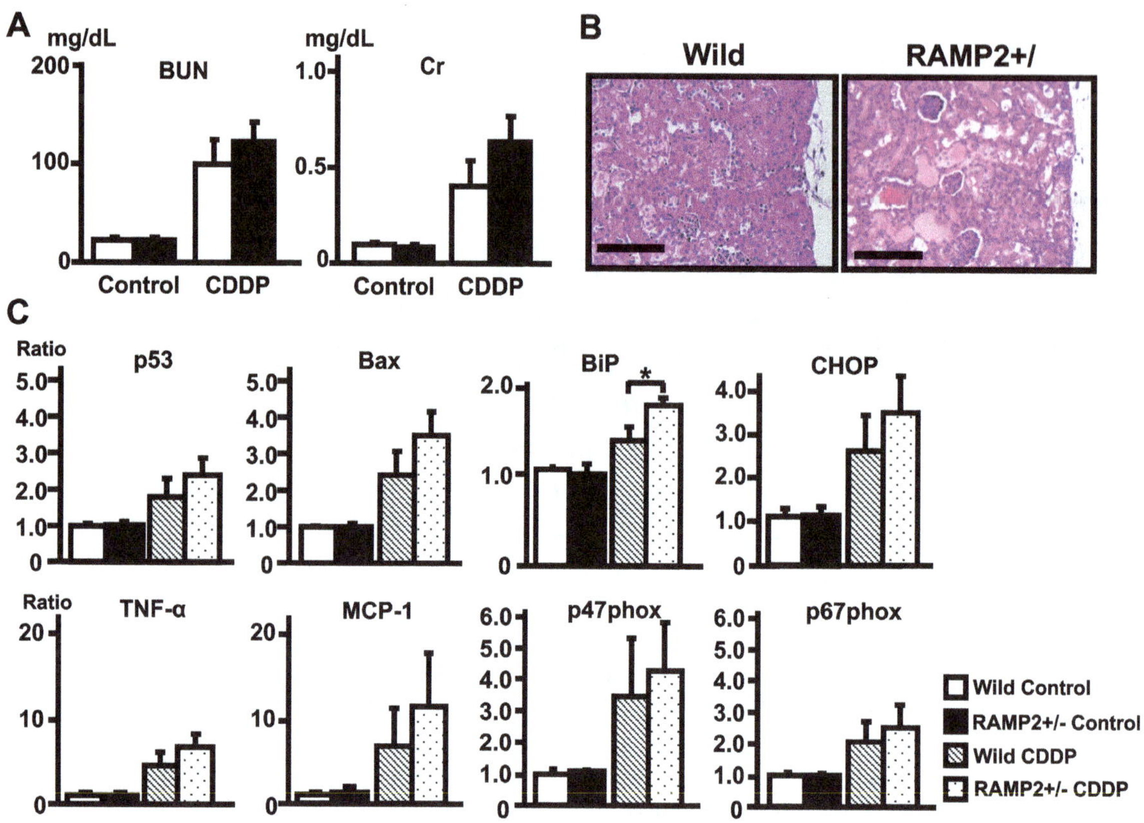

Figure 9. Cisplatin induces enhanced renal injury in RAMP2+/−. (A) Serum BUN and creatinine (Cr) in wild-type and RAMP2+/−3 days after administration of vehicle (Control) or cisplatin (CDDP) (20 mg/kg). (B) H&E staining of the renal cortex in CDDP-treated wild-type and RAMP2+/− kidneys. Scale bars = 100 μm. Sections from RAMP2+/− kidneys showed severe tubular injury. (C) Quantitative real-time PCR analysis of the indicated gene expression. Data from the wild-type control group were assigned a value of 1. n = 5 in each group. Bars are means ± SEM. *$p<0.05$.

injury is complex. Cisplatin causes a decrease in protein synthesis, as well as membrane peroxidation, mitochondrial dysfunction, and DNA injury. There is also evidence that ER stress is an important contributor to cisplatin-induced tubular damage [33]. We evaluated cisplatin-induced renal toxicity and found that RAMP2+/− kidneys showed greater tubular damage than WT kidneys. RAMP2+/− kidney showed upregulation of ER stress marker, as well as inflammatory and oxidative stress markers.

The specific signaling pathway, which directly upregulates UPR, is still largely unknown. UPR is evoked directly or indirectly through various stresses, including inflammation, toxin, oxidative stress, and other stresses. These stresses can cause the production of unfolded proteins, misfolded proteins, or simple overexpression of some proteins. As shown in the cisplatin study, inflammation and oxidative stress were enhanced in RAMP2+/−. We speculate that one explanation for the enhanced ER-stress in RAMP2+/− is the enhanced inflammation and oxidative stress, as endogenous AM has been shown to suppress excess inflammation and oxidative stress [13]. Another possibility is that RAMPs may work as chaperones, which carry some GPCRs from ER to the cell membrane [60]. RAMPs bind to other GPCRs including calcitonin receptor, parathyroid hormone receptor, and glucagon receptor, and not only AM receptor CLR, although their function with other GPCRs is largely unknown. In RAMP2+/−, reduction in the receptor trafficking of GPCRs might cause accumulation of excess GPCRs at ER, which might directly influence the enhanced ER stress.

In this study, we also analyzed whether exogenous AM treatment can protect against renal injury. In the TUN model, we found AM treatment can reduce the tubular injury in wild-type mice, however, it was not very effective in RAMP2+/− mice. This result again clearly indicates that the AM-RAMP2 system works to prevent organ damage. It has been reported that the blood AM level is elevated in patients with renal failure. Moreover, AM is elevated in proportion to the severity of the disease [22]. From the data obtained in this study, we speculate that elevation of AM in CKD functions as a compensatory mechanism against organ damage, although more intensive clinical studies are necessary in the future.

In this study, we did not find that hyperglycemia itself is involved in ER stress-evoked renal tubular injury, as the normalization of glucose levels in the STZ model could not rescue the injury. To clarify if the accumulation of metabolic abnormalities over a long period can also cause tubular injury, further studies in type II diabetic models or high fat-diet induced obese models should be conducted in the future.

Because elevated ER stress could be the cause of various diseases, chemicals that modulate ER stress are attracting attention due to their potential for clinical application. One of these compounds, 4-phenylbutyric acid (4-PBA), a non-peptide chaperone that can reduce ER stress by suppressing BiP and PERK [61], reportedly prevents the progression of diabetic nephropathy. In addition, it is anticipated that various endogenous molecules may eventually serve as new therapeutic targets. For example, nitric oxide (NO) reportedly reduces ER stress and protects against renal ischemia-reperfusion injury [62]. In the present study, we found that endogenous AM-RAMP2 signaling in renal tubule cells works to protect against renal injury by suppressing ER stress. Not surprisingly, the clinical application of AM is being much anticipated [63,64,65,66,67]. Unfortunately, AM is a peptide with a short half-life in the bloodstream, which limits its usefulness for the treatment of chronic diseases. However, we were able to mimic AM function by modulating RAMP2, which suggests RAMP2 could be a useful therapeutic alternative. Because RAMP2 is a low molecular weight protein, structural analysis and the synthesis of specific agonists or antagonists are much more realistic compared with the AM receptor CLR, which belongs to seven-transmembrane domain GPCRs. In this context, our findings provide a clear basis for the development of drugs to modulate RAMP2, and thereby, the renal effects of AM.

Supporting Information

Figure S1 Comparison of gene expression and ERK/pERK between wild-type and RAMP2+/− mice. (A) Quantitative real-time PCR analysis of VE-cadherin, p53, and TGF-β gene expression in kidney. Data from the wild-type control group were assigned a value of 1. n = 5 in each group. Bars are means ± SEM. (B) Immunohistostaining of ERK and pERK in the section of kidney. Bars = 100 μm. No change was detected between wild-type and RAMP2+/− mice.

Figure S2 Effect of STZ administration in other organs expressing GLUT2. H&E staining of intestine, pancreas, and liver sections sampled from wild-type or RAMP2+/− with or without STZ administration. STZ administration caused cell death in these organs, however, the difference was not apparent between wild-type and RAMP2+/−. Bars = 50 μm.

Figure S3 ER-stress related gene expression in STZ model. Quantitative real-time PCR analysis of BiP and CHOP after 4 weeks with STZ (250 mg/kg) administration. Data from the wild-type was assigned a value of 1. n = 5 in each group. Bars are means ± SEM. *$p<0.05$.

Figure S4 Urinary albumin level and megalin expression in STZ model. (A) Comparison of urinary albumin after 4 weeks of STZ (250 mg/kg) administration. (B) Quantitative real-time PCR analysis of megalin with or without STZ. No change was detected between wild-type and RAMP2+/− mice.

Figure S5 Proximal tubule changes in STZ administration. (A) Toluidine blue staining of renal cortex obtained from each mouse after 2 weeks of STZ (250 mg/kg) administration. Bars = 50 μm. (B) Low magnification electron micrograph of a section of proximal tubule. In RAMP2+/−, tubular atrophy, microvesicular degeneration, and protrusion of luminal side of cell membrane were prominent.

Acknowledgments

AM was kindly provided by Dr. Kangawa, Director General of the National Cardiovascular Center Research Institute, Japan.

Author Contributions

Conceived and designed the experiments: RU T. Shindo. Performed the experiments: RU T. Sakurai AK Y. Ichikawa-Shindo HK Y. Iesato TY T. Koyama LY YT AY KI MT. Analyzed the data: RU T. Shindo. Contributed reagents/materials/analysis tools: T. Kuwabara KM MY MM. Wrote the paper: RU T. Shindo.

References

1. Jaradat MI, Molitoris BA (2002) Cardiovascular disease in patients with chronic kidney disease. Semin Nephrol 22: 459–473.
2. Kawakami T, Inagi R, Wada T, Tanaka T, Fujita T, et al. (2010) Indoxyl sulfate inhibits proliferation of human proximal tubular cells via endoplasmic reticulum stress. Am J Physiol Renal Physiol 299: F568–576.
3. Ohse T, Inagi R, Tanaka T, Ota T, Miyata T, et al. (2006) Albumin induces endoplasmic reticulum stress and apoptosis in renal proximal tubular cells. Kidney Int 70: 1447–1455.
4. Bernales S, Papa FR, Walter P (2006) Intracellular signaling by the unfolded protein response. Annu Rev Cell Dev Biol 22: 487–508.
5. Szegezdi E, Logue SE, Gorman AM, Samali A (2006) Mediators of endoplasmic reticulum stress-induced apoptosis. EMBO Rep 7: 880–885.
6. Imaizumi K, Miyoshi K, Katayama T, Yoneda T, Taniguchi M, et al. (2001) The unfolded protein response and Alzheimer's disease. Biochim Biophys Acta 1536: 85–96.
7. Harding HP, Ron D (2002) Endoplasmic reticulum stress and the development of diabetes: a review. Diabetes 51 Suppl 3: S455–461.
8. Inagi R (2010) Endoplasmic reticulum stress as a progression factor for kidney injury. Curr Opin Pharmacol 10: 156–165.
9. Kitamura K, Kangawa K, Kawamoto M, Ichiki Y, Nakamura S, et al. (1993) Adrenomedullin: a novel hypotensive peptide isolated from human pheochromocytoma. Biochem Biophys Res Commun 192: 553–560.
10. Abe M, Sata M, Nishimatsu H, Nagata D, Suzuki E, et al. (2003) Adrenomedullin augments collateral development in response to acute ischemia. Biochemical and biophysical research communications 306: 10–15.
11. Kato K, Yin H, Agata J, Yoshida H, Chao L, et al. (2003) Adrenomedullin gene delivery attenuates myocardial infarction and apoptosis after ischemia and reperfusion. American journal of physiology Heart and circulatory physiology 285: H1506–1514.
12. Isumi Y, Kubo A, Katafuchi T, Kangawa K, Minamino N (1999) Adrenomedullin suppresses interleukin-1beta-induced tumor necrosis factor-alpha production in Swiss 3T3 cells. FEBS Lett 463: 110–114.
13. Shimosawa T, Shibagaki Y, Ishibashi K, Kitamura K, Kangawa K, et al. (2002) Adrenomedullin, an endogenous peptide, counteracts cardiovascular damage. Circulation 105: 106–111.
14. Nishikimi T, Matsuoka H (2005) Cardiac adrenomedullin: its role in cardiac hypertrophy and heart failure. Curr Med Chem Cardiovasc Hematol Agents 3: 231–242.
15. Petrie MC, Hillier C, Morton JJ, McMurray JJ (2000) Adrenomedullin selectively inhibits angiotensin II-induced aldosterone secretion in humans. J Hypertens 18: 61–64.
16. Samson WK, Murphy T, Schell DA (1995) A novel vasoactive peptide, adrenomedullin, inhibits pituitary adrenocorticotropin release. Endocrinology 136: 2349–2352.
17. Shimosawa T, Ogihara T, Matsui H, Asano T, Ando K, et al. (2003) Deficiency of adrenomedullin induces insulin resistance by increasing oxidative stress. Hypertension 41: 1080–1085.
18. Liu X, Zhang Z, Zhang X, Zhu H, Chen Q, et al. (2002) The localization of adrenomedullin in rat kidney tissue and its inhibitory effect on the growth of cultured rat mesangial cells. Chin Med Sci J 17: 129–133.
19. Ebara T, Miura K, Okumura M, Matsuura T, Kim S, et al. (1994) Effect of adrenomedullin on renal hemodynamics and functions in dogs. Eur J Pharmacol 263: 69–73.
20. Jougasaki M, Wei CM, Aarhus LL, Heublein DM, Sandberg SM, et al. (1995) Renal localization and actions of adrenomedullin: a natriuretic peptide. Am J Physiol 268: F657–663.
21. Parameswaran N, Nowak W, Hall CS, Sparks HV, Spielman WS (2001) Cellular and molecular actions of adrenomedullin in glomerular mesangial cells. Peptides 22: 1919–1924.
22. Ishimitsu T, Nishikimi T, Saito Y, Kitamura K, Eto T, et al. (1994) Plasma levels of adrenomedullin, a newly identified hypotensive peptide, in patients with hypertension and renal failure. J Clin Invest 94: 2158–2161.
23. Nishikimi T, Saito Y, Kitamura K, Ishimitsu T, Eto T, et al. (1995) Increased plasma levels of adrenomedullin in patients with heart failure. J Am Coll Cardiol 26: 1424–1431.
24. Kronenberg F (2009) Emerging risk factors and markers of chronic kidney disease progression. Nat Rev Nephrol 5: 677–689.
25. Shindo T, Kurihara Y, Nishimatsu H, Moriyama N, Kakoki M, et al. (2001) Vascular abnormalities and elevated blood pressure in mice lacking adrenomedullin gene. Circulation 104: 1964–1971.

26. Nishimatsu H, Hirata Y, Shindo T, Kurihara H, Kakoki M, et al. (2002) Role of endogenous adrenomedullin in the regulation of vascular tone and ischemic renal injury: studies on transgenic/knockout mice of adrenomedullin gene. Circ Res 90: 657–663.
27. Cockcroft JR, Noon JP, Gardner-Medwin J, Bennett T (1997) Haemodynamic effects of adrenomedullin in human resistance and capacitance vessels. Br J Clin Pharmacol 44: 57–60.
28. McLatchie LM, Fraser NJ, Main MJ, Wise A, Brown J, et al. (1998) RAMPs regulate the transport and ligand specificity of the calcitonin-receptor-like receptor. Nature 393: 333–339.
29. Parameswaran N, Spielman WS (2006) RAMPs: The past, present and future. Trends Biochem Sci 31: 631–638.
30. Ichikawa-Shindo Y, Sakurai T, Kamiyoshi A, Kawate H, Iinuma N, et al. (2008) The GPCR modulator protein RAMP2 is essential for angiogenesis and vascular integrity. J Clin Invest 118: 29–39.
31. Koyama T, Ochoa-Callejero L, Sakurai T, Kamiyoshi A, Ichikawa-Shindo Y, et al. (2013) Vascular endothelial adrenomedullin-RAMP2 system is essential for vascular integrity and organ homeostasis. Circulation 127: 842–853.
32. Hard GC (1985) Identification of a high-frequency model for renal carcinoma by the induction of renal tumors in the mouse with a single dose of streptozotocin. Cancer research 45: 703–708.
33. Mandic A, Hansson J, Linder S, Shoshan MC (2003) Cisplatin induces endoplasmic reticulum stress and nucleus-independent apoptotic signaling. J Biol Chem 278: 9100–9106.
34. Miyawaki Y, Ueki M, Ueno M, Asaga T, Tokuda M, et al. (2012) D-allose ameliorates cisplatin-induced nephrotoxicity in mice. The Tohoku journal of experimental medicine 228: 215–221.
35. Schnedl WJ, Ferber S, Johnson JH, Newgard CB (1994) STZ transport and cytotoxicity. Specific enhancement in GLUT2-expressing cells. Diabetes 43: 1326–1333.
36. Madhavan S, Singh AK, Maheshawari RK (2000) Tunicamycin enhances the anticellular activity of interferon by inhibiting G1/S phase progression in 3T3 cells. J Interferon Cytokine Res 20: 281–290.
37. Marciniak SJ, Yun CY, Oyadomari S, Novoa I, Zhang Y, et al. (2004) CHOP induces death by promoting protein synthesis and oxidation in the stressed endoplasmic reticulum. Genes & development 18: 3066–3077.
38. Novoa I, Zhang Y, Zeng H, Jungreis R, Harding HP, et al. (2003) Stress-induced gene expression requires programmed recovery from translational repression. EMBO J 22: 1180–1187.
39. McLawhon RW, Berry-Kravis E, Dawson G (1986) Differential regulation of multiple neuroreceptors in a somatic cell hybrid by inhibitors of glycoprotein processing. Biochem Biophys Res Commun 134: 1387–1394.
40. Yao X, Panichpisal K, Kurtzman N, Nugent K (2007) Cisplatin nephrotoxicity: a review. The American journal of the medical sciences 334: 115–124.
41. Ramesh G, Reeves WB (2002) TNF-alpha mediates chemokine and cytokine expression and renal injury in cisplatin nephrotoxicity. The Journal of clinical investigation 110: 835–842.
42. Davis CA, Nick HS, Agarwal A (2001) Manganese superoxide dismutase attenuates Cisplatin-induced renal injury: importance of superoxide. Journal of the American Society of Nephrology : JASN 12: 2683–2690.
43. Mandic A, Hansson J, Linder S, Shoshan MC (2003) Cisplatin induces endoplasmic reticulum stress and nucleus-independent apoptotic signaling. The Journal of biological chemistry 278: 9100–9106.
44. Mukoyama M, Sugawara A, Nagae T, Mori K, Murabe H, et al. (2001) Role of adrenomedullin and its receptor system in renal pathophysiology. Peptides 22: 1925–1931.
45. Nagae T, Mukoyama M, Sugawara A, Mori K, Yahata K, et al. (2000) Rat receptor-activity-modifying proteins (RAMPs) for adrenomedullin/CGRP receptor: cloning and upregulation in obstructive nephropathy. Biochem Biophys Res Commun 270: 89–93.
46. Miyamoto N, Tanaka R, Shimosawa T, Yatomi Y, Fujita T, et al. (2009) Protein kinase A-dependent suppression of reactive oxygen species in transient focal ischemia in adrenomedullin-deficient mice. Journal of cerebral blood flow and metabolism : official journal of the International Society of Cerebral Blood Flow and Metabolism 29: 1769–1779.
47. Niu P, Shindo T, Iwata H, Iimuro S, Takeda N, et al. (2004) Protective effects of endogenous adrenomedullin on cardiac hypertrophy, fibrosis, and renal damage. Circulation 109: 1789–1794.
48. Fritz-Six KL, Dunworth WP, Li M, Caron KM (2008) Adrenomedullin signaling is necessary for murine lymphatic vascular development. J Clin Invest 118: 40–50.
49. Dackor R, Fritz-Six K, Smithies O, Caron K (2007) Receptor activity-modifying proteins 2 and 3 have distinct physiological functions from embryogenesis to old age. J Biol Chem 282: 18094–18099.
50. Tsujikawa K, Yayama K, Hayashi T, Matsushita H, Yamaguchi T, et al. (2007) Hypertension and dysregulated proinflammatory cytokine production in receptor activity-modifying protein 1-deficient mice. Proceedings of the National Academy of Sciences of the United States of America 104: 16702–16707.
51. Oyadomari S, Koizumi A, Takeda K, Gotoh T, Akira S, et al. (2002) Targeted disruption of the Chop gene delays endoplasmic reticulum stress-mediated diabetes. J Clin Invest 109: 525–532.
52. Boden G, Duan X, Homko C, Molina EJ, Song W, et al. (2008) Increase in endoplasmic reticulum stress-related proteins and genes in adipose tissue of obese, insulin-resistant individuals. Diabetes 57: 2438–2444.
53. Lindholm D, Wootz H, Korhonen L (2006) ER stress and neurodegenerative diseases. Cell Death Differ 13: 385–392.
54. Rao RV, Bredesen DE (2004) Misfolded proteins, endoplasmic reticulum stress and neurodegeneration. Curr Opin Cell Biol 16: 653–662.
55. Zou XJ, Yang L, Yao SL (2012) Endoplasmic reticulum stress and C/EBP homologous protein-induced Bax translocation are involved in angiotensin II-induced apoptosis in cultured neonatal rat cardiomyocytes. Exp Biol Med (Maywood) 237: 1341–1349.
56. Szkudelski T (2001) The mechanism of alloxan and streptozotocin action in B cells of the rat pancreas. Physiological research/Academia Scientiarum Bohemoslovaca 50: 537–546.
57. Li SR, Alcolado JC, Stocks J, Baroni MG, Oelbaum RS, et al. (1991) Genetic polymorphisms at the human liver/islet glucose transporter (GLUT2) gene locus in Caucasian and West Indian subjects with type 2 (non-insulin-dependent) diabetes mellitus. Biochim Biophys Acta 1097: 293–298.
58. Bell AI, Cole JA, Busby SJ (1990) Molecular genetic analysis of an FNR-dependent anaerobically inducible Escherichia coli promoter. Mol Microbiol 4: 1753–1763.
59. Dominguez JH, Camp K, Maianu L, Garvey WT (1992) Glucose transporters of rat proximal tubule: differential expression and subcellular distribution. Am J Physiol 262: F807–812.
60. Hay DL, Poyner DR, Sexton PM (2006) GPCR modulation by RAMPs. Pharmacology & therapeutics 109: 173–197.
61. Qi W, Mu J, Luo ZF, Zeng W, Guo YH, et al. (2011) Attenuation of diabetic nephropathy in diabetes rats induced by streptozotocin by regulating the endoplasmic reticulum stress inflammatory response. Metabolism 60: 594–603.
62. Mahfoudh-Boussaid A, Zaouali MA, Hadj-Ayed K, Miled AH, Saidane-Mosbahi D, et al. (2012) Ischemic preconditioning reduces endoplasmic reticulum stress and upregulates hypoxia inducible factor-1alpha in ischemic kidney: the role of nitric oxide. J Biomed Sci 19: 7.
63. Nagaya N, Mori H, Murakami S, Kangawa K, Kitamura S (2005) Adrenomedullin: angiogenesis and gene therapy. Am J Physiol Regul Integr Comp Physiol 288: R1432–1437.
64. Iwase T, Nagaya N, Fujii T, Itoh T, Ishibashi-Ueda H, et al. (2005) Adrenomedullin enhances angiogenic potency of bone marrow transplantation in a rat model of hindlimb ischemia. Circulation 111: 356–362.
65. Hanabusa K, Nagaya N, Iwase T, Itoh T, Murakami S, et al. (2005) Adrenomedullin enhances therapeutic potency of mesenchymal stem cells after experimental stroke in rats. Stroke 36: 853–858.
66. Iimuro S, Shindo T, Moriyama N, Amaki T, Niu P, et al. (2004) Angiogenic effects of adrenomedullin in ischemia and tumor growth. Circ Res 95: 415–423.
67. Maki T, Ihara M, Fujita Y, Nambu T, Miyashita K, et al. (2011) Angiogenic and vasoprotective effects of adrenomedullin on prevention of cognitive decline after chronic cerebral hypoperfusion in mice. Stroke 42: 1122–1128.

24

The Association of Pioglitazone and Urinary Tract Disease in Type 2 Diabetic Taiwanese: Bladder Cancer and Chronic Kidney Disease

Mei-Yueh Lee[1,2,3], Pi-Jung Hsiao[2,3], Yi-Hsin Yang[5], Kun-Der Lin[2,3], Shyi-Jang Shin[2,3,4]*

1 Department of Internal Medicine, Kaohsiung Municipal Hsiao-Kang Hospital, Kaohsiung, Taiwan, **2** Division of Endocrinology and Metabolism, Department of Internal Medicine, Kaohsiung Medical University Hospital, Kaohsiung, Taiwan, **3** Graduate Institute of Medicine, Kaohsiung Medical University, Kaohsiung, Taiwan, **4** Graduate Institute of Medical Genetics, Kaohsiung Medical University, Kaohsiung, Taiwan, **5** Statistical Analysis Laboratory, Department of Clinical Research, Kaohsiung Medical University Hospital, Kaohsiung, Taiwan

Abstract

Objective: Although studies have shown an association between pioglitazone and bladder cancer, the associated factors have not been identified. The aim of this study was to investigate the factors that may link pioglitazone to bladder cancer.

Materials and Methods: In total, 34,970 study subjects were identified from the National Health Insurance Research Database in 2003 with follow-up from 2005 to 2009. The demographic characteristics of patients who had used and had never used pioglitazone, including age, sex, diabetes duration, urinary tract disease, nephropathy, bladder cancer, and cumulative dose and duration of pioglitazone therapy, were analyzed using the $\chi 2$ test. Cox proportional hazard regression models were used to determine the independent effects of pioglitazone on bladder cancer and newly developed chronic kidney disease.

Results: Among 3,497 ever users and 31,473 never users of pioglitazone, the respective incident cases of bladder cancer were 12 (0.4%) and 72 (0.2%), and for newly developed chronic kidney disease 245 (8.1%) and 663 (2.3%), respectively. Ever use of pioglitazone [1.59(1.32–1.91)], cumulative dose of pioglitazone <10,500 mg [1.69 (1.37–2.01)] and >10,500 mg [1.34 (1.04–1.73)], and duration of therapy <12 months [1.68 (1.36–2.08)] and >12 months [1.39 (1.09–1.76)] were associated with the development of chronic kidney disease.

Conclusions: There was no association of pioglitazone use with bladder cancer development, however, there was an association with an increased risk of newly developed chronic kidney disease.

Editor: Yu-Kang Tu, National Taiwan University, Taiwan

Funding: This study was funded by the Department of Internal Medicine, Kaohsiung Medical University Hospital. The funders had no role in study design, data collection and analysis, decision to publish, or preparation of the manuscript.

Competing Interests: The authors have declared that no competing interests exist.

* E-mail: sjshin@kmu.edu.tw

Introduction

Peroxisome proliferator-activated receptors (PPARs) are ligand-activated transcription factors which belong to the nuclear receptor superfamily [1]. PPARγ1 is expressed in the heart, skeletal muscles, kidneys, pancreas, and some epithelial tissues such as the urothelium and intestine. In comparison, PPARγ2 is expressed exclusively in adipose tissue and induces adipocyte differentiation as well as being involved in the control of inflammatory reactions and in glucose metabolism through enhanced insulin sensitivity [1], [2]. Since urothelial cells have PPARγ receptors, it has been suggested that a direct effect of the agonist on the urothelial receptor might be the cause of bladder carcinogenesis via these non-DNA reactive agents; further, this effect may be caused by both PPARγ and PPARα agonists via an interaction between their receptors [3]. However, some studies have reported that PPARγ agonists can also inhibit cell proliferation and induce differentiation in various cancer cell lines, such as human urothelial carcinoma [1],[4], rather than increasing cell proliferation as would be expected for a non-DNA reactive chemical's carcinogenic mode of action. Two hypotheses have been formulated regarding urothelial carcinogenesis by these agents. The first involves a direct effect of the agents on the urothelial PPARγ receptors [5]. The second suggests an indirect effect of the agents, which does not specifically target the PPARγ receptors in the urothelium but instead involves physiological or pharmacological fluid changes and the modification of renal function and the altering of fluid dynamics. This then leads to significant changes in urine composition, and in turn results in the formation of various types of urinary solids (precipitate, micro-crystals, calculi). These solids are known to be irritative and toxic to the urothelium, especially in rats, and have been observed to cause sustained regenerative proliferation and ultimately to the induction of bladder (urothelial) tumors [6]. Pioglitazone is a thiazolidinedione PPARγ ligand used in the treatment of type 2 diabetes, a disease known to increase the risk of cancer. Several studies have suggested an increased risk of bladder cancer with exposure to pioglitazone [7–9]. However, these reports have come from only Western countries, the findings have been inconsistent, and the factors related to this association were not identified. This study is the first to represent an Asian ethnic group and to analyze in detail the risk of bladder cancer with the use of pioglitazone. In this study, we aimed to investigate the possible association of pioglitazone and bladder cancer via the mechanisms in the aforementioned hypotheses.

Materials and Methods

Setting

This study use data from the National Health Insurance Research Database (NHIRD), published by the National Health Research Institute (NHI) in Taiwan, which includes data for 1,000,000 randomly selected subjects who were followed from 1998 to 2009. The NHI program was implemented in Taiwan in 1995 and offers a comprehensive, unified, and universal health insurance program to all citizens, including those who have established a registered domicile for at least 4 months in the Taiwan area. The coverage provides outpatient services, inpatient care, Chinese medicine, dental care, childbirth, physical therapy, preventive health care, home care, and rehabilitation for chronic mental illnesses. The coverage rate was 96.16% of the whole the population in 2000 rising to 99% at the end of 2004. The NHI medical claims database includes data on ambulatory care, hospital inpatient care, dental services, and prescription drugs.

Study population

The entry date of 2003 was selected because pioglitazone was first marketed in Taiwan in 2002. There were no statistically significant differences in age, sex, and average insured payroll-related amount among the enrollees. The diagnosis coding of the NHI program in Taiwan is done according to the International Classification of Diseases, 9th Revision, Clinical Modification (ICD-9-CM) diagnostic criteria. All patients with type 2 diabetes (ICD-9-CM code 250.1–250.9) were followed until the end of 2009. Data on the occurrence of bladder cancer during the study follow-up period (2005 to 2009) were obtained from the same database. Bladder cancer cases were identified according to ICD-9-CM code 188 and were confirmed by the issuance of catastrophic illness cards. After excluding individuals who died or had diabetes after the occurrence of bladder cancer, 34,970 patients with type 2 diabetes were recruited.

Variables determined before entry included age, sex, diabetes duration, newly diagnosed type 2 diabetes at entry, other diabetes medications including sulfonylurea, metformin, acarbose, meglitinides, insulin, bladder cancer, urinary tract disease (ICD-9-CM codes 590-599) and nephropathy (ICD-9-CM codes 580–589). The patients prescribed with pioglitazone before entry were defined as ever users, and those who had never used pioglitazone as never users. Dose responsive parameters including a cumulative dose of less than and more than 10,500 mg, and duration of therapy of less than and more than 12 months, were included. The cutoff criteria of a 10,500 mg dose and a 12-month duration of therapy were established in previous studies [7–9].

Statistical analysis

All data processing and statistical analyses were performed with Statistical Analysis Software (SAS), version 9.1 (SAS Institute, Cary, NC, USA). Chi-square tests were used to analyze the differences in demographic characteristics between the ever users and never users of pioglitazone, which included age, sex, diabetes duration, newly diagnosed type 2 diabetes at entry, other diabetes medications including sulfonylurea, metformin, acarbose, meglitinides, insulin, bladder cancer, urinary tract disease and nephropathy. Cox regression analysis was used to calculate hazard ratios (HRs) of bladder cancer and newly developed chronic kidney disease with pioglitazone use. The confounders of cumulative dose, duration of therapy, urinary tract disease and nephropathy were adjusted by sex, age, duration of diabetes, other diabetes medications, income (monthly income $<$NT\$20,000 and $>$NT\$20,000) and residential area. A P value of less than 0.05 was considered to be statistically significant.

Results

A total of 34,970 patients with type 2 diabetes were included, with 3,497 ever users and 31,473 never users of pioglitazone. The ever users were more likely to be aged ≥ 60 years, female, lived in Northern counties with monthly income of $<$20,000 NTD and with a diabetes duration of more than 36 months. Only 69 (2.0%) newly diagnosed type 2 diabetic patients started with pioglitazone as the initial treatment. Most of the ever users had a cumulative dose of ≦ 10,500 mg and duration therapy of ≦ 12 months, but were more likely to have been treated with sulfonylureas, metformin, acarbose, meglitinides and insulin either before, along with, or after pioglitazone. During the follow-up period, there were 84 cases of newly diagnosed bladder cancer (12 ever users and 72 never users). The incidence of nephritis (1.4% vs. 1.0%), chronic kidney disease (7.3% vs. 3.3%), newly developed chronic kidney disease (8.1% vs. 2.3%), hydronephrosis (3.6% vs. 2.5%), calculus of the kidney and ureter (2.7% vs. 1.9%), and other disorders of the urethra and urinary tract (2.4% vs. 1.4%) were higher in the ever users than in the never users (Table 1).

In the analysis of the association bladder cancer, the risk of bladder cancer increased with a cumulative dose of pioglitazone of more than 10,500 mg [HR 2.21 (95% CI 1.01–4.80), P = 0.0461], and duration of therapy of pioglitazone more than 12 months [HR 2.52 (95% CI 1.26–5.05), P = 0.0090], newly developed chronic kidney disease [HR 7.50 (95% CI 4.26–13.21), P<0.0001], and calculus of the kidney and ureter [HR 3.41 (95% CI 1.38–8.41), P = 0.0078]. After fully adjusting for sex, age, duration of diabetes, other diabetes medications, income and residential area, nephritis, chronic kidney disease, kidney infections, hydronephrosis, calculus of the lower urinary tract, calculus of the kidneys and ureter, cystitis, other disorders of the urethra and urinary tract, newly developed chronic kidney disease, hypertension and hyperlipidemia, no significant associations were found between the ever users of pioglitazone, cumulative dose and duration of therapy with the risk of bladder cancer (Table 2, Figure 1). However, there were significant associations between newly developed chronic kidney disease [HR 5.45 (95% CI 2.99–9.93), P<0.0001] and calculus of the kidney and ureter [HR 2.75 (95% CI 1.01–7.52), P = 0.484] with the risk of bladder cancer (Table 2).

With regards to the association of newly developed chronic kidney disease, there were significantly increased risks of newly developed chronic kidney disease in the pioglitazone ever users [HR 1.66 (95% CI 1.37–2.01), P<0.0001), cumulative dose of pioglitazone ≦10,500 mg [HR 1.81 (95% CI 1.46–2.25), P<0.0001] and ≥ 10,500 mg [HR 1.39 (95% CI 1.07–1.80), P = 0.0134], duration of therapy of pioglitazone ≦ 12 months [HR 1.79 (95% CI 1.44–2.24), P<0.0001] and ≥ 12 months [HR 1.46 (95% CI 1.14–1.86), P = 0.0027], hypertension [HR 4.01 (95% CI 3.47–4.63), P<0.0001], hyperlipidemia [HR 2.44 (95% CI 2.14–2.78), P<0.0001] and the diabetes medication, meglitinides [HR 4.03 (95% CI 3.27–4.96), P<0.0001]. After fully

Table 1. Demographics of the study cohort according to ever use of pioglitazone.

	Ever use of Pioglitazone N (%)	Never use of Pioglitazone N (%)	P-value
N	3,497	31,473	
Age (years)			
20–29	24 (0.7)	216 (0.7)	
30–39	47 (1.3)	423 (1.3)	
40–49	283 (8.1)	2,547 (8.1)	
50–59	836 (23.9)	7,524 (23.9)	
>60	2,307 (66.0)	20,763 (66.0)	
Sex (female)	1,835 (52.5)	16,515 (52.5)	
Income			
Unemployed	1129 (32.3)	9,167 (29.1)	<.0001
<20,000 NTD	1663 (47.6)	16,072 (51.1)	
>20,000 NTD	705 (20.2)	6,234 (19.8)	
Residence			
Metropolitan	1036 (29.6)	7,851 (24.9)	<.0001
Northern Cities	222 (6.3)	2,441 (7.8)	
Southern Cities	94 (2.7)	1,331 (4.2)	
Northern Counties	1374 (39.3)	13,420 (42.6)	
Southern Counties	763 (21.8)	6,315 (20.1)	
Nephritis	50 (1.4)	307 (1.0)	0.0112
Chronic kidney disease	256 (7.3)	1,038 (3.3)	<.0001
Infection of kidney	25 (0.7)	172 (0.5)	0.2069
Hydronephrosis	125 (3.6)	790 (2.5)	0.0002
Calculus of kidney and ureter	94 (2.7)	595 (1.9)	0.0013
Cystitis	113 (3.2)	1,059 (3.4)	0.6774
Other disorder of urethra and urinary tract	84 (2.4)	455 (1.4)	<.0001
Other diabetes medication			
Sulfonylureas	1,481 (42.4)	2,916 (9.3)	<.0001
Metformin	1,344 (38.4)	2,631 (8.4)	<.0001
Acarbose	757 (21.6)	729 (2.3)	<.0001
Meglitinides	546 (15.6)	615 (2.0)	<.0001
Insulin	2,918 (83.4)	24,770 (78.7)	<.0001
Newly diagnosed diabetes at the start of follow-up	69 (2.0)	24,796 (78.8)	<.0001
Duration of diabetes (months)			
<36	667 (19.1)	2,401 (7.6)	<.0001
>36	2,761 (79.0)	4,276 (13.6)	
Cumulative dose (mg)			
<10,500	2,313 (66.1)	N/A	
>10,500	1,184 (33.9)	N/A	
Duration of therapy (months)			
<12	2,145 (61.3)	N/A	
>12	1,352 (38.7)	N/A	
Bladder cancer	12 (0.4)	72 (0.2)	0.1761
Newly developed chronic kidney disease	245 (8.1)	663 (2.3)	<.0001

adjusting for age, sex, duration of diabetes, income and residential area, nephritis, chronic kidney disease, kidney infections, hydronephrosis, calculus of the lower urinary tract, calculus of the kidney and ureter, cystitis, other disorders of the urethra and urinary tract, and other diabetes medication including sulfonylureas, metformin, acarbose, rosiglitazone and insulin, there were significantly increased risks of newly developed chronic kidney disease with hypertension [HR 2.14 (95% CI 1.82–2.52), $P<0.0001$], hyperlipidemia [HR 1.26 (95% CI 1.09–1.45), $P=0.0020$], use of meglitinides [HR 1.68 (95% CI 1.14–2.48),

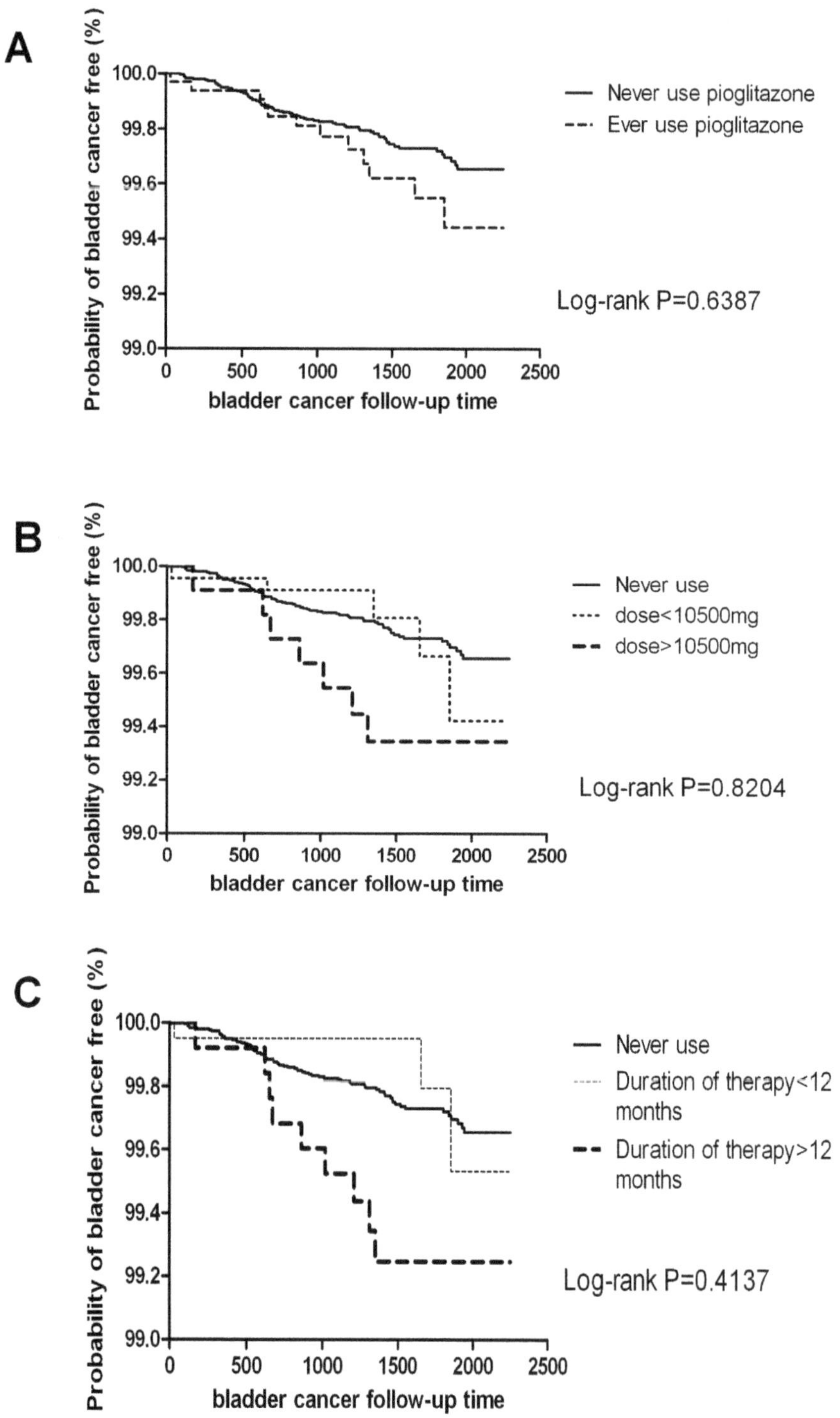

Figure 1. Disease free survival of bladder cancer. (A).never use and ever use of pioglitazone. (B).never use, cumulative dose <10500 mg and >10500 mg of pioglitazone. (C).never use, duration of therapy <12 months and >12 months of pioglitazone.

P = 0.0092], and pioglitazone ever users [HR 1.59 (95% CI 1.32–1.91), P<0.0001]. However, there were slight decreases in the adjusted hazard ratios for cumulative dose of pioglitazone ≥ 10,500 mg [HR 1.34 (95% CI 1.04–1.73), P = 0.0232] and ≦ 10,500 mg [HR 1.69 (95% CI 1.37–2.07), P<0.0001]. Decreases in the adjusted hazard ratio of newly developed chronic kidney disease were also observed with duration of therapy ≥ 12 months [HR 1.39 (95% CI 1.09–1.76), P = 0.0072] and ≦12 months [HR 1.68 (95% CI 1.36–2.08), P<0.0001]. Table 3 (see also Figure 2).

The adjusted hazard ratios in Table 2 and 3 were computed by multiple Cox regression with one of the pioglitazone usage variable at a time. Since the hazard ratios of cumulative dose and duration of therapy of pioglitazone were very similar, therefore only one set was listed in table

Table 2. Hazard ratio of bladder cancer.

Bladder Cancer	Univariate		Multivariate*	
	HR (95% CI)	*P*	HR (95% CI)	*P*
Pioglitazone use				
Never use (n = 72)	1		1	
Ever use (n = 12)	1.52 (0.83–2.80)	0.1787	1.03 (0.45–2.35)	0.9452
Cumulative dose of pioglitazone (mg)				
Never use (n = 72)	1		1	
<10,500 (n = 5)	1.03 (0.42–2.55)	0.9530	0.84 (0.30–2.35)	0.7429
>10,500 (n = 7)	2.21 (1.01–4.80)	0.0461	1.27 (0.45–3.61)	0.6540
Duration of therapy of pioglitazone (months)				
Never use (n = 72)	1		1	
<12 (n = 3)	0.67 (0.21–2.13)	0.4978	0.56 (0.16–1.95)	0.3605
>12 (n = 9)	2.52 (1.26–5.05)	0.0090	1.58 (0.62–4.02)	0.3355
Newly developed chronic kidney disease				
No	1		1	
Yes	7.50 (4.26–13.21)	<.0001	5.45 (2.99–9.93)	<.0001
Calculus of kidney and ureter				
No	1		1	
Yes	3.41 (1.78–8.41)	0.0078	2.75 (1.04–7.52)	0.0484

*Adjusted by sex, age, duration of diabetes, other diabetes medications, income (monthly income <NT$20,000; monthly income >NT$20,000), residential area, nephritis, chronic kidney disease, kidney infections, hydronephrosis, calculus of the lower urinary tract, cystitis, other disorders of the urethra and urinary tract, hypertension and hyperlipidemia. The adjusted HR of newly developed chronic kidney disease and calculus of the kidney and ureter were computed with the indicated variable of pioglitazone use.

Discussion

We observed no association of bladder cancer with the ever users, cumulative dose and therapy duration of pioglitazone, but a positive association with newly developed chronic kidney disease. Using pioglitazone and/or meglitinides as the initial treatment increased the risk of chronic kidney disease, and also for those with a history of hypertension and hyperlipidemia.

Although several studies have suggested an increased risk of bladder cancer with exposure to pioglitazone [7–9], the factors related to this association have not been identified. In the current study, we found that urinary tract diseases, such as calculus of the kidney and ureter, and chronic kidney diseases increased the risk of developing bladder cancer rather than the use of pioglitazone, for which we found no association with the development of bladder cancer in contrast to previous studies.

PPARγ and combined agonists have been shown to produce urothelial tumors in rats as well as suspected urothelial changes in monkeys and possibly in dogs [10]. These effects are either due to a direct effect on PPARγ in the urothelium or a pharmacologically based indirect mechanism in the animals leading to alterations in urine composition. A characteristic effect of PPARγ and dual agonists is the induction of an enlarged cardiac size and accumulation of body water. Physiological or pharmacological effects involving fluid changes modify renal function, alter fluid dynamics, and lead to significant changes in urine composition, which result in the formation of various types of urinary solids (precipitate, microcrystals, calculi). These these urinary solids are known to be irritative and toxic to the urothelium, especially in rats, and have been observed to lead to sustained regenerative proliferation and ultimately to the induction of bladder (urothelial) tumors [6]. This effect has been reported to be greater in male than in female rats, and greater in rats than in mice, however much less likely in primates such as humans [11]. In the current study, the associations of calculus of the kidney and ureter and bladder cancer were not related to pioglitazone. The Food and Drug Administration has accepted an increase in heart size as a determinant for a maximum tolerated dose for this class of drugs [12]. This effect has been reported to be dose-dependent and a pharmacologically-based response to these agents [13–15]. The indirect pharmacological mode of action produced by PPAR agonists is not unique to the urothelium, and indirect effects have also been seen with PPARγ agonists in the production of rat pancreatic acinar cell tumors and, to some extent, rat testicular Leydig cell neoplasms. However, these neoplasms do not appear to be relevant to humans [16]. A variety of other indirect mechanisms have been identified with other classes of chemicals operating through other modes of action. However, a direct effect on urothelial PPARγ receptors as the cause of the carcinogenic response is highly unlikely for a variety of reasons, most notably the fact that the biological effect of these agonists on the urothelium is to inhibit proliferation rather than to increase the rate of proliferation expected for a carcinogen [17].

Chronic kidney disease is a proinflammatory state [18–20], and there is now emerging evidence of an association between chronic inflammation and the risk of cancer [21]. Recently, an association between elevated albumin-to-creatinine ratio and cancer was reported in a longitudinal population-based study of older individuals [22]. Observational studies have also suggested an increased cancer risk in people with early-stage chronic kidney disease before requiring dialysis or transplantation [23]. It has been reported that for every 10-ml/min decrement in estimated glomerular filtration rate (eGFR), the risk of cancer increases by 29% (adjusted HR 1.29; 95% CI 1.10 to 1.53), with the greatest

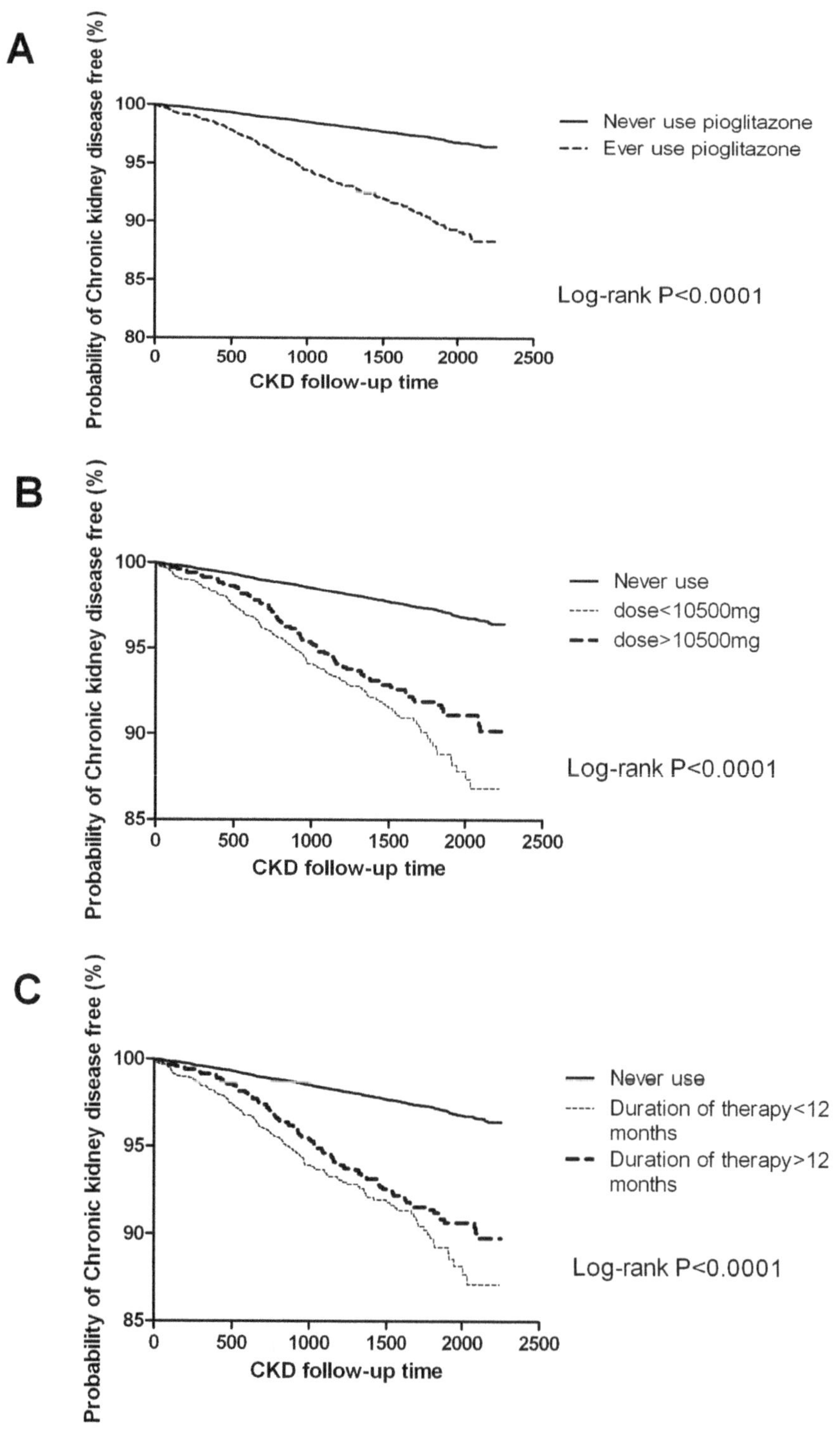

Figure 2. Disease free survival of newly developed chronic kidney disease after use of pioglitazone. (A).never use and ever use of pioglitazone. (B). never use, cumulative dose <10500 mg and >10500 mg of pioglitazone. (C). never use, duration of therapy <12 months and >12 months of pioglitazone.

risk at an eGFR ≦40 ml/min per 1.73 m2 (adjusted HR 3.01; 95% CI 1.72 to 5.27), especially in the risk for lung and urinary tract cancers but not prostate cancer in men with chronic kidney disease [24]. In the current study, chronic kidney disease was found to increase the risk of bladder cancer. Chronic kidney disease is associated with significant morbidity and premature death. Markers of inflammation such as white blood cell count have also been associated with an increased risk for cancer mortality in the general population [25–27].

Among oral antihyperglycemic agents, sulfonylureas (glyburide, gliclazide, glipizide, glibenclamide, tolbutamide, and chlorpropamide) have been reported to have increased potency as renal

Table 3. Hazard ratios of newly developed chronic kidney disease.

	Univariate		Multivariate*	
Pioglitazone use	HR (95% CI)	*P*	HR (95% CI)	*P*
Never use (n = 663)	1		1	
Ever use (n = 245)	1.66(1.37–2.01)	<.0001	1.59(1.32–1.91)	<.0001
Cumulative dose of pioglitazone (mg)				
Never use (n = 663)	1		1	
<10,500 (n = 160)	1.81(1.46–2.25)	<.0001	1.69(1.37–2.07)	<.0001
>10,500 (n = 85)	1.39(1.07–1.80)	0.0134	1.34(1.04–1.73)	0.0232
Duration of therapy of pioglitazone (months)				
Never use (n = 663)				
<12 (n = 144)	1.79(1.44–2.24)	<.0001	1.68(1.36–2.08)	<.0001
>12 (n = 101)	1.46(1.14–1.86)	0.0027	1.39(1.09–1.76)	0.0072
Hypertension				
No	1		1	
Yes	4.01(3.47–4.63)	<.0001	2.14(1.82–2.52)	<.0001
Hyperlipidemia				
No	1		1	
Yes	2.44(2.14–2.78)	<.0001	1.26(1.09–1.45)	0.0020
Other diabetes medication				
Meglitinides				
No	1		1	
Yes	4.03 (3.27–4.96)	<.0001	1.68 (1.14–2.48)	0.0092

*Adjusted by age, sex, diabetes duration, income (monthly income <NT$20,000; monthly income >NT$20,000) residential area, nephritis, chronic kidney disease, kidney infections, hydronephrosis, calculus of the lower urinary tract, calculus of the kidney and ureter, cystitis, other disorders of the urethra and urinary tract, other diabetes medication including sulfonylureas, metformin, acarbose, rosiglitazone and insulin. The adjusted HR of hypertension, hyperlipidemia and other diabetes medication were computed with the indicated variable of pioglitazone use.

function decreases, and are contraindicated in patients with severe renal failure [28]. Similarly, α-glucosidase inhibitors (acarbose and miglitol) are also contraindicated in patients with renal failure, whereas the non-sulfonylurea insulin secretagogues repaglinide and nateglinide can be used in patients with renal failure without dose adjustments [29]. In the absence of contraindications, metformin is preferred over other agents due to equal potency and a low risk of hypoglycemia, and also as it causes less weight gain compared with insulin secretagogues. In obese patients, metformin has shown strong clinical evidence of reduced microvascular and macrovascular outcomes [30]. Metformin is contraindicated in patients with renal failure because of the associated risk of lactic acidosis [31]. In the presence of contraindications or intolerance to metformin or when metformin alone does not result in optimal control, thiazolidinediones should be used [30]. Although the metabolism of thiazolidinediones is unaffected by renal failure, they must be used with caution in this context because of their volume retaining effect with a risk of heart failure [32]. Therefore, in chronic renal failure, the oral agents that can be used include the insulin secretagogues repaglinide and nateglinide and the thiazolidinediones (rosiglitazone and pioglitazone), although they should be used with caution. Insulin can also be used safely in patients with renal failure [30]. However, in the current study, we found that pioglitazone, repaglinide and nateglinide increased the risk of developing chronic kidney disease.

Cardiovascular complications and mortality have been reported to be increased in patients with chronic kidney disease independent of traditional risk factors such as diabetes, hypertension, and dyslipidemia [33–35]. Post hoc analysis from the PROspective pioglitAzone Clinical Trial In macroVascular Events (PROactive) investigated the relationship between chronic kidney disease and the incidence of cardiovascular disease in patients with diabetes and documented macrovascular disease, as well as the effects of pioglitazone treatment on recurrent cardiovascular disease, and found that pioglitazone was more effective than placebo in reducing the rate of both primary and secondary composite end points in the patients with chronic kidney disease. There was a nonsignificant 25% risk reduction for pioglitazone relative to the placebo for the primary end point (95% CI 0.55 to 1.03) and a significant 34% relative risk reduction for the secondary end point (95% CI 0.45 to 0.98). The yearly declines in GFR (0.9 ml/min per 1.73 m2 with placebo and 1.8 ml/min per 1.73 m2 with pioglitazone) in one study [36] were considerably lower than the decline of 3 to 4 ml/min per 1.73 m2 observed in patients with diabetes in previous studies [37],[38], and were more in the range of the GFR decrease found in an aging healthy population (1 ml/min per 1.73 m2/year) [39]. In the current study, the use of pioglitazone was found to increase the risk of chronic kidney disease.

There are several strengths to this study. It is a prospective follow-up study of a very large cohort of diabetic and cancer patients with a high likelihood of the correct diagnosis of cancer and diabetes by use of the computerized data files for each individual from the NHIRD. Nevertheless, there are some limitations including the lack of actual measurements for confounders such as biochemical data, obesity, tobacco smoking, occupational exposure, lifestyle and diet. Instead of tobacco smoking history, we thus analyzed the association of bladder cancer, calculus of the kidney and ureter, and newly developed chronic kidney disease with pioglitazone separately by gender, however no significant differences were found. We also included the residential area and income as confounders instead of occupational exposure, lifestyle and diet, and used hyperlipidemia for obesity. In addition, the relationship between the duration of therapy and cumulative dose of pioglitazone with the possibility of renoprotection cannot be proven further due to the short historical use of pioglitazone in Taiwan. Further studies are warranted to elucidate this relationship.

In summary, there was no significant increases in the incidence of bladder cancer in the ever users of pioglitazone, therapy duration and cumulative dose of pioglitazone. However, pioglitazone use increased the risk of developing chronic kidney disease,

Acknowledgments

The authors thank the Statistical Analysis Laboratory, Department of Internal Medicine, Kaohsiung Medical University Hospital for providing access to the NHIRD database, and Yu-Ting Hwang for their contribution during data analysis.

Author Contributions

Conceived and designed the experiments: SJS MYL. Performed the experiments: MYL KDL. Analyzed the data: MYL SJS PJH YHY. Contributed reagents/materials/analysis tools: MYL KDL YHY. Wrote the paper: MYL.

References

1. Tachibana K, Yamasaki D, Ishimoto K, Doi T (2008) The role of PPARs in cancer. PPAR Res 2008:102737.
2. Berger J, Moller DE (2002) The mechanisms of action of PPARs. Annu Rev Med 53:409–435.
3. Varley CL, Southgate J (2008) Effects of PPAR agonists on proliferation and differentiation in human urothelium. Exp Toxicol Pathol 60:435–441.
4. Varley CL, Bacon EJ, Holder JC, Southgate J (2009) FOXA1 and IRF-1 intermediary transcriptional regulators of PPARgamma-induced urothelial cytodifferentiation. Cell Death Differ 16:103–114.
5. Varley CL, Stahlschmidt J, Smith B, Stower M, Southgate J (2004) Activation of peroxisome proliferators-activated receptor-c reverses squamous metaplasia and induces transitional differentiation in normal human urothelial cells. Am J Pathol 164:1789–1798.
6. IARC Working Group (1999) Consensus Report. IARC Sci Publ 147:1–32.
7. Neumann A, Weill A, Ricordeau P, Fagot JP, Alla F, et al (2012) Pioglitazone and risk of bladder cancer among diabetic patients in France: a population-based cohort study. Diabetologia 55:1953–1962.
8. Lewis JD, Ferrara A, Peng T, Hedderson M, Bilker WB, et al (2011) Risk of bladder cancer among diabetic patients treated with pioglitazone: interim report of a longitudinal cohort study. Diabetes Care 34:916–922.
9. Piccinni C, Motola D, Marchesini G, Poluzzi E (2011) Assessing the association of pioglitazone use and bladder cancer through drug adverse event reporting. Diabetes Care 34:1369–71.
10. Takayama S, Sieber SM, Adamson RH, Thorgeirsson UP, Dalgard DW, et al (1998) Long-term feeding of sodium saccharin to nonhuman primates: Implications for urinary tract cancer. J Natl Cancer Inst 90:19–25.
11. Cohen SM (1995) Role of urinary physiology and chemistry in bladder carcinogenesis. Food Chem Toxicol 33:715–730.
12. El-Hage J (2005) Peroxisome proliferation-activated receptor agonists: Carcinogenicity findings and regulatory recommendations. International Atherosclerosis Society Symposium on PPAR, Monte Carlo.
13. Cohen SM (1998) Urinary bladder carcinogenesis. Toxicol Pathol 26:121–127.
14. Cohen SM (1999) Calcium phosphate-containing urinary precipitate in rat urinary bladder carcinogenesis. IARC Sci Publ 147:175–189.
15. IARC Working Group (1999) Consensus Report. IARC Sci Publ 147:1–32.
16. Klaunig JD, Babich MA, Baetcke KP, Cook JC, Corton JC, et al (2003) PPARγ agonist-induced rodent tumors: Modes of action and human relevance. Crit Rev Toxicol 33:655–780.
17. Varley CL, Stahlschmidt J, Lee W, Holder J, Dibble C, et al (2003) Role of PPARγ and EGFR signalling in the urothelial terminal differentiation programme. J Cell Sci 117:2029–2036.
18. Keller CR, Odden MC, Fried LF, Newman AB, Angleman S, et al (2007) Kidney function and markers of inflammation in elderly persons without chronic kidney disease: The health, aging, and body composition study. Kidney Int 71:239–244.
19. Tonelli M, Sacks F, Pfeffer M, Jhangri GS, Curhan G (2005) Cholesterol and Recurrent Events (CARE) Trial Investigators: Biomarkers of inflammation and progression of chronic kidney disease. Kidney Int 68:237–245.
20. de Vinuesa SG, Goicoechea M, Kanter J, Puerta M, Cachofeiro V, et al (2006) Insulin resistance, inflammatory biomarkers, and adipokines in patients with chronic kidney disease: Effects of angiotensin II blockade. J Am Soc Nephrol 17 [Suppl 3]:S206–S212.
21. Coussens LM, Werb Z (2002) Inflammation and cancer. Nature 420:860–867.
22. Jorgensen L, Heuch I, Jenssen T, Jacobsen BK (2008) Association of albuminuria and cancer incidence. J Am Soc Nephrol 19:992–998.
23. Cengiz K (2002) Increased incidence of neoplasia in chronic renal failure (20-year experience). Int Urol Nephrol 33:121–126.
24. Wong G, Hayen A, Chapman JR, Webster AC, Wang JJ, et al (2009) Association of CKD and cancer risk in older people. J Am Soc Nephrol. 6:1341–1350.
25. Grimm RH Jr, Neaton JD, Ludwig W (1985) Prognostic importance of the white blood cell count for coronary, cancer, and all-cause mortality. JAMA 254:1932–1937.
26. Friedman GD, Fireman BH (1991) The leukocyte count and cancer mortality. Am J Epidemiol 133:376–380.
27. Shankar A, Wang JJ, Rochtchina E, Yu MC, Kefford R, et al (2006) Association between circulating white blood cell count and cancer mortality: A population-based cohort study. Arch Intern Med 166:188–194.
28. Krepinsky J, Ingram AJ, Clase CM (2000) Prolonged sulfonylurea- induced hypoglycemia in diabetic patients with endstage renal disease. Am J Kidney Dis 35:500–505.
29. Schumacher S, Abbasi I, Weise D, Hatorp V, Sattler K, et al (2001) Single- and multiple-dose pharmacokinetics of repaglinide in patients with type 2 diabetes and renal impairment. Eur J Clin Pharmacol 57:147–152.
30. Yale JF (2005) Oral antihyperglycemic agents and renal disease: new agents, new concepts. J Am Soc Nephrol. 16 Suppl 1:S7–10.
31. Gan SC, Barr J, Arieff AI, Pearl RG (1992) Biguanide-associated lactic acidosis. Case report and review of the literature. Arch Intern Med 152:2333–2336.
32. Chapelsky MC, Thompson-Culkin K, Miller AK, Sack M, Blum R, et al.(2003) Pharmacokinetics of rosiglitazone in patients with varying degrees of renal insufficiency. J Clin Pharmacol 43:252–259.
33. Fried LF, Shlipak MG, Crump C, Bleyer AJ, Gottdiener JS, et al (2003) Renal insufficiency as a predictor of cardiovascular outcomes and mortality in elderly individuals. J Am Coll Cardiol 41:1364–1372.
34. Shlipak MG, Simon JA, Grady D, Lin F, Wenger NK, et al (2001) Heart and Estrogen/progestin Replacement Study (HERS) Investigators: Renal insufficiency and cardiovascular events in postmenopausal women with coronary heart disease. J Am Coll Cardiol 38:705–711.
35. Mann JF, Gerstein HC, Pogue J, Bosch J, Yusuf S (2001) Renal insufficiency as a predictor of cardiovascular outcomes and the impact of ramipril: The HOPE randomized trial. Ann Intern Med 134:629–636.
36. Schneider CA, Ferrannini E, Defronzo R, Schernthaner G, Yates J, et al (2008) Effect of pioglitazone on cardiovascular outcome in diabetes and chronic kidney disease. J Am Soc Nephrol 19:182–187.
37. Fox CS, Larson MG, Leip EP, Meigs JB, Wilson PW, et al (2005) Glycemic status and development of kidney disease: The Framingham Heart Study. Diabetes Care 28:2436–2440.
38. Perkins BA, Nelson RG, Ostrander BE, Blouch KL, Krolewski AS, et al (2005) Detection of renal function decline in patients with diabetes and normal or elevated GFR by serial measurements of serum cystatin C concentration: results of a 4-year follow-up study. J Am Soc Nephrol 16:1404–1412.
39. Davies DF, Shock NW (1950) Age changes in glomerular filtration rate, effective renal plasma flow, and tubular excretory capacity in adult males. J Clin Invest 29:496–507.

Allopurinol is an Independent Determinant of Improved Arterial Stiffness in Chronic Kidney Disease

Khai P. Ng[1], Stephanie J. Stringer[1,2], Mark D. Jesky[1,2], Punit Yadav[1,2], Rajbir Athwal[1], Mary Dutton[1], Charles J. Ferro[1,2], Paul Cockwell[1,2]*

1 Department of Renal Medicine, Queen Elizabeth Hospital Birmingham, Birmingham, United Kingdom, **2** School of Immunity and Infection, University of Birmingham, Birmingham, United Kingdom

Abstract

Background: Arterial stiffness is increased in patients with CKD and is a powerful predictor of cardiovascular morbidity and mortality. Use of the xanthine oxidase inhibitor allopurinol has been shown to improve endothelial function, reduce left ventricular hypertrophy and possibly improve cardiovascular outcome. We explored the relationship between use of allopurinol and arterial stiffness in patients with chronic kidney disease (CKD).

Methods: Cross-sectional observational study of 422 patients with CKD with evidence of, or at high risk of, renal disease progression. Arterial stiffness was determined by carotid-femoral pulse wave velocity (PWV).

Results: The mean age was 63±16 years, median estimated glomerular filtration rate was 25 (interquartile range: 19–31) ml/min/1.73 m^2 and mean PWV was 10.2±2.4 m/s. Seventy-seven patients (18%) were receiving regular allopurinol, 61% at a dose of 100 mg/day (range: 50–400 mg/day). Patients receiving allopurinol had significantly lower peripheral pulse pressure, central pulse pressure, central systolic blood pressure, serum uric acid level tissue advanced glycation end product levels but comparable high-sensitivity C-reactive protein levels. Use of allopurinol was associated with lower PWV. After adjusting for age, gender, ethnicity, tissue advanced glycation end product level, peripheral pulse pressure, smoking pack years, presence of diabetes mellitus and use of angiotensin converting enzyme inhibitor or angiotensin II receptor blocker, the use of allopurinol remained a significant independent determinant of PWV (mean difference: −0.63 m/s; 95% CI, −0.09 to −1.17 m/s, p = 0.02).

Conclusion: In patients with CKD, use of allopurinol is independently associated with lower arterial stiffness. This study provides further justification for a large definitive randomised controlled trial examining the therapeutic potential of allopurinol to reduce cardiovascular risk in people with CKD.

Editor: Jose Vina, University of Valencia, Spain

Funding: The study is supported by JABBS foundation (Birmingham, United Kingdom) (URL: http://opencharities.org/charities/1128402), University Hospital Birmingham Charities (URL: http://qehb.org/) and the British Renal Society (URL: http://www.britishrenal.org/). CJF is supported through a National Institute for Health Research Fellowship (URL: http://www.nihrtcc.nhs.uk/). The funders had no role in study design, data collection and analysis, decision to publish, or preparation of the manuscript.

Competing Interests: The authors have read the journal's policy and have the following conflicts: PC has received an honorarium for a lecture and research funding for investigator led studies from the Binding Site. CJF has received lecture fees and advisory board fees from Genzyme Corp. The other authors have declared no competing interests exist. This does not alter their adherence to PLOS ONE policies on sharing data and materials.

* E-mail: paul.cockwell@uhb.nhs.uk

Introduction

Asymptomatic hyperuricaemia is associated with increased cardiovascular (CV) and all-cause mortality in the general population [1–6] and in patients with chronic kidney disease (CKD) [7–12]. Use of the xanthine oxidase inhibitor allopurinol in patients with CKD is associated with improvements in surrogate markers for CV disease (CVD) including endothelial function [13,14] and left ventricular hypertrophy [14]. Furthermore, allopurinol use is associated with a slower progression of renal dysfunction [15] and a reduction in CV events [15,16] in CKD cohorts.

Arterial stiffness is increased in patients with CKD and is a powerful predictor of mortality in this patient group [17–19]. Arterial stiffness is associated with endothelial dysfunction and increased left ventricular mass and is thought to be a key initiating factor contributing to the elevated CV risk observed in patients with CKD [17]. Carotid-femoral pulse wave velocity (PWV) is considered to be the current 'gold-standard' measurement of arterial stiffness [20]. Although allopurinol has been shown to improve endothelial function, lower central aortic pressure and regress left ventricular hypertrophy in patients with CKD, its effects on PWV remain unclear [14]. We therefore examined the relationship between allopurinol use and carotid-femoral PWV in patients with CKD recruited into the Renal Impairment In Secondary Care (RIISC) cohort study.

Methods

Ethics Statement

The study was approved by the South Birmingham Local Research Ethics committee (reference: 10/H1207/6) and all participants gave informed and written consent. The study was conducted in accordance with the Declaration of Helsinki. (Clinical Trials Registration Number: NCT01722383; Date of Registration: November 11, 2012)

Study Design and Participants

The RIISC study is a prospective, observational cohort study of patients with CKD with evidence of, or at high risk of, renal disease progression. The inclusion and exclusion criteria have previously been reported in detail [21]. In brief, patients were included if they had stage 3 CKD with a declining estimated glomerular filtration rate (eGFR) of ≥5 ml/min/year or ≥10 ml/min/5years or a urine albumin creatinine ratio (uACR) ≥70 mg/mmol on three consecutive occasions, or stage 4/5 CKD. GFR was estimated (eGFR) using the four-variable Modification of Diet in Renal Disease (MDRD) equation with serum creatinine recalibrated to be traceable to an isotope derived mass spectroscopy method [22]. Patients with established renal failure receiving dialysis treatment and patients receiving immunosuppressive medication were excluded from the study. From October 2010 to November 2012, 437 out-patients under regular follow-up were recruited from renal clinics at two large teaching hospitals in the United Kingdom.

Baseline measurements

Baseline clinical information on participants' demographics, renal diagnosis, diagnosis of diabetes mellitus (DM), CV history, past medication history, family history, concomitant medication, smoking and alcohol consumption history were recorded. Presence of CVD was defined by history or other evidence of angina, previous myocardial infarction, previous stroke or transient ischaemic attack, peripheral vascular disease, a previous revascularisation procedure or heart failure. Presence of DM was defined as receiving treatment for DM or a confirmed clinical diagnosis of diet-controlled DM. Smoking history and pack years were determined by participant self-reporting. An allopurinol user was defined as a participant who was receiving any dosage of allopurinol on recruitment. We contacted the primary care physician of all allopurinol users to obtain further details on the reason for prescription, presence of side effect related to allopurinol in the initial 3 months of treatment and start date of allopurinol to determine the duration of exposure.

Peripheral blood pressure (BP) was measured in the dominant arm using a British Hypertension Society approved automated oscillometric sphygmomanometer (BPM-100, BpTRU™), which obtained a series of six BP readings at 1-minute intervals after 5 minutes of rest [23]. Mean peripheral BP was derived from the average of the 2nd to 6th BP readings. Carotid-femoral PWV was measured non-invasively using the Vicorder system (Skidmore Medical, Bristol, UK) as previously described [24]. This is an operator independent and highly reproducible technique with low within-subject variation [24]. After 5 minutes of lying supine, PWV measurements were obtained in duplicate; the mean of the measurements was used in data analyses. Central pressure waveforms were derived and analysed using pulse wave analysis as previously described [25]. The central pressure waveform was analysed to determine the augmentation index (AIx) and central aortic pressures. AIx represents the difference between the second and first peaks of the central pressure waveform in systole, expressed as a percentage of the pulse pressure. Given the known effects of heart rate, AIx was corrected to a heart rate of 75 beats per minute (AIx_{75}) [26].

Routine laboratory testing included blood haematological (Beckman Coulter Haematology Analyzer) and biochemical profiles and urinary albumin creatinine ratios (ACR) (Roche Hitachi 702 Analyser). Additional samples were centrifuged and serum was aliquoted and stored at −80°C and subsequently batch analysed for high sensitivity C-reactive protein (hsCRP) using a commercially available assay (SpaPlus assay, Binding Site). Tissue advanced glycation end product (AGE) level was determined by skin autofluorescence (SAF) using a validated AGE Reader™ (DiagnOptics BV, Groningen, The Netherlands).

Statistical Analysis

Statistical analysis was performed using SPSS version 19.0 (SPSS Inc, Chicago, IL). Numerical values are expressed as mean ± standard deviation for parametric data or median (interquartile range) for non-parametric data. Normality of the distribution of data was assessed by visual inspection of histogram and normal probability plot [27]. Non-parametric variables were log transformed prior to analysis to achieve normal distribution. If normal distribution was not achieved after transformation, non-parametric tests were used. Parametric continuous data were compared using student t-tests and non-parametric using Mann-Whitney tests. Pearson or Spearman's bivariate correlation analysis was used to examine the relationship between parametric and non-parametric numerical variables, respectively. Correlation coefficient factors were expressed as 'r' for Pearson correlation analyses and 'rho' for Spearman's analysis. Categorical data were compared by χ^2 tests. As age is strongly correlated with arterial stiffness, we divided the studied population into 4 age quartiles. Two-way analysis of variance (ANOVA) was performed to examine the interaction between age and the use of allopurinol as well as their individual effect on PWV. In addition, multiple linear regression was performed to explore the relationship between PWV and independent variables. Missing data was excluded by cases pairwise during analyses. Statistical significance is defined as a two-tailed p value <0.05.

Results

Baseline characteristics

Four hundred and thirty-seven patients were recruited; of whom 14 did not have PWV measured for technical reasons and were therefore excluded from the study. One patient who was receiving febuxostat was excluded. Therefore 422 patients were included in the analyses. The numbers of individuals at each stage of study are detailed in Figure 1. The baseline demographic and biochemical characteristics of the study population are shown in Table 1. The mean age was 63±16 years with 60% of male gender and 71% of white ethnicity. Use of antihypertensive agents was common and 67% were receiving either an angiotensin converting enzyme inhibitor (ACEI) or angiotensin II receptor blocker (ARB). A small number (5%) were on both an ACEI and an ARB. There was a high prevalence of hyperuricaemia; 84% had a serum uric acid concentration greater than 360 μmol/L. The frequencies of different stages of CKD were: stage 1, 0.2%; stage 2, 1%; stage 3a, 5.3%; stage 3b, 23.1%; stage 4, 61.7%; stage 5, 8.7%. Seventy-seven patients (18%) were receiving regular allopurinol, 61% as a

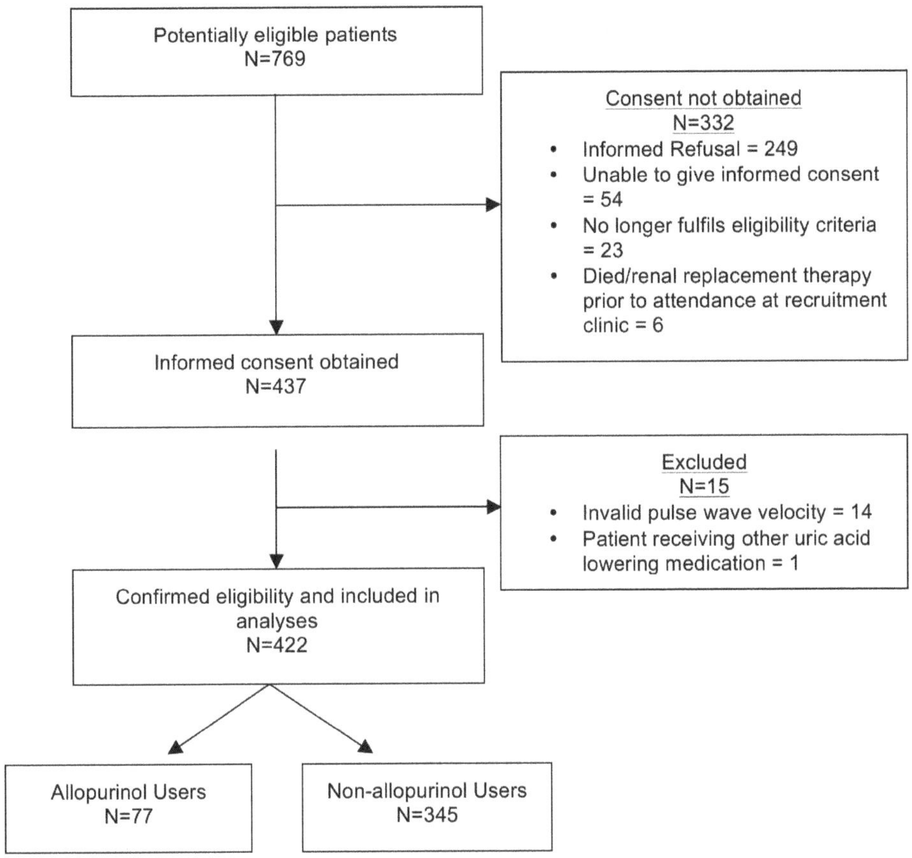

Figure 1. Flow diagram of the participants included in the study.

dose of 100 mg/day (range: 50–400 mg/day). Haemodynamic parameters are presented in Table 2.

Use of allopurinol

The demographic, clinical and biochemical characteristics of the cohort and a comparison between allopurinol users and non-allopurinol users is shown in Table 1. There was a significantly higher proportion of patients of male gender and white ethnicity and a significantly lower proportion of patients who were current smokers among allopurinol users. Allopurinol users had a higher body mass index (BMI) than non-allopurinol users. There was no significant difference in age, prevalence of DM, prevalence of CVD, percentage of ex-smokers, smoking pack years, total number of antihypertensive agents used and use of ACEI/ARB between the groups. Allopurinol users had significantly lower serum uric acid concentrations and lower SAF level compared to non-allopurinol users. Other biochemical variables, including kidney function, albuminuria, lipid and bone profiles and hsCRP levels were not different between the groups. Allopurinol users had significantly lower peripheral and central pulse pressures (PP), central systolic BP (SBP) and PWV (Table 2). There were no differences in heart rate, peripheral SBP, AIx and AIx_{75} between allopurinol and non-allopurinol users.

Among the 77 allopurinol users, details regarding allopurinol prescription were available from their primary care physician on 59 patients. Ninety four per cent were commenced on allopurinol for gout and 6% for asymptomatic hyperuricaemia. Side effects were reported in 12% during the first 3 months of allopurinol treatment: 3 had acute gout, 2 had a skin rash, 1 had diarrhoea and 1 complained of increased thirst. The mean duration of allopurinol use at recruitment was 74 months (SD: 54 months).

Use of allopurinol and pulse wave velocity

Univariate correlations with PWV are shown in Table 3. Although BMI positively correlated with serum uric acid level ($r = 0.178$, $p<0.001$), there was no significant correlation between BMI and PWV. Uric acid levels, kidney function and hsCRP also did not correlate with PWV. In participants who were not receiving ACEI/ARB (n = 141), there was no correlation between uric acid and PWV ($p = 0.66$). Six per cent of participants were receiving a thiazide, use of this drug did not correlate with levels of uric acid ($p = 0.58$) or PWV ($p = 0.66$).

Pulse wave velocity positively correlated with increasing age, white ethnicity, SAF, peripheral and central SBP and PP. Ex-smokers and smoking pack years had a significant positive correlation with PWV whilst current smoking did not. Use of allopurinol (mean difference: −0.8 m/s; 95% CI, −0.2 to −1.4 m/s, $p = 0.006$), use of ACEI/ARB and Afro-Caribbean ethnicity were also associated with lower PWV. Neither the dose of allopurinol or duration of use of allopurinol had a significant correlation with PWV. Fifty-one per cent (n = 39) of the allopurinol users had a uric acid level below 416 μmol/L. Among allopurinol users, there was no difference in PWV between those with a uric acid below or above this threshold ($p = 0.92$).

Two-way ANOVA was used to explore the impact of age and use of allopurinol on PWV. Participants were divided into quartiles of age (19–50, 51–65, 66–76 and 77–92 years). Pulse wave velocity increased with age and was significantly lower in

Table 1. Baseline demographic, clinical and biochemical characteristic of all participants and according to the usage of allopurinol.

	All participants (n = 422)	Allopurinol user (n = 77)	Non-allopurinol user (n = 345)	P Value	Number missing data (%)
Age (years)	63±16	62±15	64±17	0.31	0
Male	225 (60%)	59 (77%)	196 (57%)	**0.001**	0
Ethnicity				**0.006**	1 (0.2)
White	301 (71%)	67 (87%)	234 (67%)		
Asian	64 (15%)	4 (5%)	60 (17%)		
Afro-Caribbean	40 (10%)	3 (4%)	37 (11%)		
Body Mass Index (kg/m^2)	29.8±6.8	31.8±6.4	29.3±6.8	**0.003**	9 (2)
Presence of Diabetes Mellitus	152 (36%)	24 (31%)	128 (37%)	0.33	0
Presence of CVD	142 (34%)	21 (27%)	121 (35%)	0.19	0
Current smoker	58(14%)	4 (5%)	54 (16%)	**0.02**	0
Ex-smoker	174 (41%)	35 (46%)	139 (40%)	0.41	0
Smoking pack years *§§	2 (0–22)	0 (0–15)	2 (0–24)	0.25	13 (3)
Number of antihypertensive agents	2.4±1.3	2.5±1.0	2.4±1.4	0.49	6 (1)
Use of ACEI/ARB	281 (67%)	55 (71%)	227 (66%)	0.32	0
Use of thiazide	24 (6%)	1 (1%)	23 (7%)	0.10	0
Use of Antiplatelet agents	166 (39%)	37 (48%)	129 (37%)	0.08	0
Use of Statin	247 (59%)	46 (60%)	201 (58%)	0.81	0
Duration of allopurinol exposure	-	74±54	-	-	18 (23)
Serum creatinine*§ (μmol/L)	213 (169–263)	216 (174–270)	212 (167–263)	0.77	6 (1)
eGFR*§ (ml/min/1.73 m^2)	25 (19–31)	26 (21–33)	24 (19–31)	0.24	6 (1)
Urine ACR*§ (mg/mmol)	35.0 (6.9–163.1)	40.1 (7.4–134.3)	33.8 (6.7–166.7)	0.70	45 (11)
Serum uric acid (μmol/L)	479±121	431±123	489±117	**<0.001**	8 (2)
Cholesterol (mmol/L)	4.6±1.2	4.5±1.1	4.7±1.2	0.33	5 (1)
Corrected calcium (mmol/L)	2.26±0.14	2.25±0.14	2.26±0.14	0.82	10 (2)
Phosphate*§ (mmol/L)	1.13 (0.99–1.28)	1.10 (1.00–1.23)	1.13 (0.98–1.30)	0.50	7 (1)
hsCRP*§ (mg/L)	3.280 (1.228–9.332)	3.678 (1.215–9.246)	3.203 (1.257–9.332)	0.92	103 (24)
SAF (a.u.)	3.0±0.8	2.8±0.7	3.1±0.8	**0.02**	60 (14)

*Data are presented as frequency (percentage), mean ± standard deviation or *median (interquartile range).*
Parametric data was analysed using unpaired two-tailed t-test or Pearson's χ^2 unless otherwise specified.
§Log-transformed prior to analyses.
§§Analysed using Mann-Whiteney U test.
Abbreviations: ACR = albumin creatinine ratio; bpm = beats per minutes; CVD = cardiovascular disease; ACEI = angiotensin converting enzyme inhibitor; ARB = Angiotensin II receptor blocker; eGFR = estimate glomerular filtration rate, hsCRP = high sensitivity C-reactive protein; SAF = skin autofluorescence.

Table 2. Haemodynamic parameters of all participants and according to the usage of allopurinol.

	All participants (n = 422)	Allopurinol user (n = 77)	Non-allopurinol user (n = 345)	P Value	Number missing data (%)
Peripheral SBP (mmHg)	129±20	126±22	129±20	0.19	14 (3)
Peripheral DBP (mmHg)	76±13	76±12	75±13	0.59	14(3)
Peripheral PP (mmHg)	71±18	67±18	72±17	**0.02**	16 (4)
Central SBP (mmHg)	141±20	136±22	142±20	**0.02**	16 (4)
Central PP (mmHg)	65±18	61±18	66±17	**0.02**	16 (4)
AIx (%)	21±9	20±9	21±9	0.45	12 (3)
AIx_{75} (%)	21±9	20±8	21±9	0.35	12 (3)
Heart Rate (bpm)	69±13	68±15	69±15	0.42	8 (2)
PWV (m/s)	10.2±2.4	9.5±2.3	10.3±2.4	**0.006**	0

Abbreviations: AIx: augmentation index; AIx_{75} = augmentation index adjusted to heart rate of 75 bpm; bpm = beats per minute; DBP = diastolic blood pressure; SBP = systolic blood pressure; PP = pulse pressure; PWV = pulse wave velocity.

Table 3. Univariate analyses with pulse wave velocity (PWV) as the dependent outcome variable.

	Correlation coefficient	P value
Demographics		
Age (years)	0.534	**<0.001**
Gender (Male)	0.088	0.07
Ethnicity		
White	0.105	**0.03**
Asian	0.014	0.77
Afro-Caribbean	−0.105	**0.03**
Body Mass Index (kg/m²)	−0.057	0.25
Presence of diabetes mellitus	0.082	0.09
Presence of cardiovascular disease	0.044	0.37
Current smoker	0.021	0.67
Ex-smoker	0.198	**<0.001**
Smoking Pack Years**	0.244	**<0.001**
Haemodynamics		
BpTRU Peripheral SBP (mmHg)	0.320	**<0.001**
BpTRU Peripheral DBP (mmHg)	−0.061	0.21
Peripheral PP (mmHg)	0.454	**<0.001**
Central SBP (mmHg)	0.440	**<0.001**
Central PP (mmHg)	0.442	**<0.001**
AIx (%)	0.024	0.63
AIx_{75} (%)	0.023	0.64
Biochemical markers		
Serum creatinine* (μmol/L)	0.039	0.43
eGFR (ml/min/1.73 m²)*	−0.078	0.11
Urine ACR (mg/mmol)*	−0.042	0.40
Serum uric acid (μmol/L)	−0.035	0.48
Cholesterol (mmol/L)	−0.080	0.11
Corrected calcium (mmol/L)	−0.001	0.98
Phosphate (mmol/L)*	0.019	0.71
hsCRP (mg/L)*	0.062	0.27
SAF (a.u.)	0.253	**<0.001**
Medications		
Use of allopurinol	−0.135	**0.006**
Dose of allopurinol (mg)	−0.185	0.11
Duration of allopurinol exposure (months)	−0.019	0.89
Use of ACEI/ARB	−0.163	**0.001**
Use of thiazide	0.021	0.66

Abbreviations: ACEI = angiotensin converting enzyme inhibitor; ACR = albumin creatinine ratio; AIx: augmentation index; AIx_{75} = augmentation index adjusted to heart rate of 75 bpm; ARB = angiotensin II receptor blocker; SBP = systolic blood pressure; DBP = diastolic blood pressure; PP = pulse pressure; SAF = skin autofluorescence.
Parametric data was analysed using Pearson correlation unless otherwise specified.
**Natural Log transformed prior to analyses.*
***Non-parametric data was analysed using Spearman's bivariate correlation analysis.*

non-allopurinol users (Figure 2). There was no interaction between age and use of allopurinol (p = 0.27). There were significant main effects for both age and use of allopurinol, with age having a large effect size (partial eta squared = 0.201, p<0.001) and use of allopurinol having a small albeit significant effect size (partial eta squared = 0.011, p = 0.03).

A linear regression model was created with PWV as the dependent variable. Variables which correlated with PWV at a p value <0.1 were included in a standard regression model. As there was strong co-linearity among the BP measures, peripheral PP was selected from these parameters for incorporation in the regression model as it had the strongest correlation (r = 0.45, p<0.001) with PWV. Similarly, smoking pack years was selected to adjust for the relationship between smoking history and PWV in the regression model. Preliminary analyses were performed to ensure no violation of the assumptions of normality, linearity and multi-collinearity. Factors entered into the model were age, gender, ethnicity, smoking pack years, diagnosis of DM, SAF level, peripheral PP, use of ACEI/ARB and use of allopurinol. Age, peripheral PP and use of allopurinol were significant independent determinants of PWV (Table 4). In the regression model, the use of allopurinol was associated with a mean reduction of PWV of 0.63 m/s (95% CI, −0.09 to −1.17 m/s, p = 0.02). The model explained 35% of the variance in PWV. Substituting peripheral SBP, central SBP or central PP, for peripheral PP and substituting smoking pack years for current or previous smoking status made no appreciable difference to the model.

Discussion

This observational study in a prospectively recruited CKD cohort suggests that the use of allopurinol was associated with reduced arterial stiffness as measured by carotid-femoral PWV, the current gold-standard measurement of arterial stiffness [20]; this association was independent of age and BP. Arterial stiffness, which is a hallmark of CKD, is a well-recognised, powerful prognostic marker of CV morbidity and mortality in both the general and CKD population [17–19]. Increased arterial stiffness results in higher systolic pressures, greater pressure fluctuations and leads to ventricular-arterial uncoupling, myocardial hypertrophy and fibrosis. Alterations in the extracellular matrix and endothelial dysfunction promoted by chronic inflammation, increase oxidative stress and accumulation of advanced glycation end products, vascular calcification, and activation of renin-angiotensin-aldosterone system (RAAS) have been postulated to contribute to increased arterial stiffness [17,28].

Allopurinol, a xanthine oxidase inhibitor, is commonly prescribed for patients with gout as a uric acid lowering agent. During the catalytic reaction that produces uric acid, xanthine oxidase generates reactive oxidative species, which may contribute to the development of endothelial dysfunction, hypertension and vascular damage [29]. Accumulating evidence from interventional studies indicates that allopurinol improves endothelial dysfunction [14,30], lowers left ventricular mass [14], and may slow progression of CKD and lower CV risk [15]. The results of this current study suggest that some of the beneficial effect of allopurinol may occur through reducing arterial stiffness.

Even among allopurinol users there was a high prevalence of hyperuricaemia. Although several large observational studies have reported a strong association between hyperuricaemia and CV morbidity or mortality, the evidence for hyperuricaemia as a risk factor or risk marker of CVD is conflicting [31–39]. Despite a significant association between allopurinol use and PWV, we found no significant direct association between serum uric acid levels and PWV. In a small group of patients with chronic heart failure, George et al demonstrated that the mechanism of improvement in endothelial function with allopurinol was

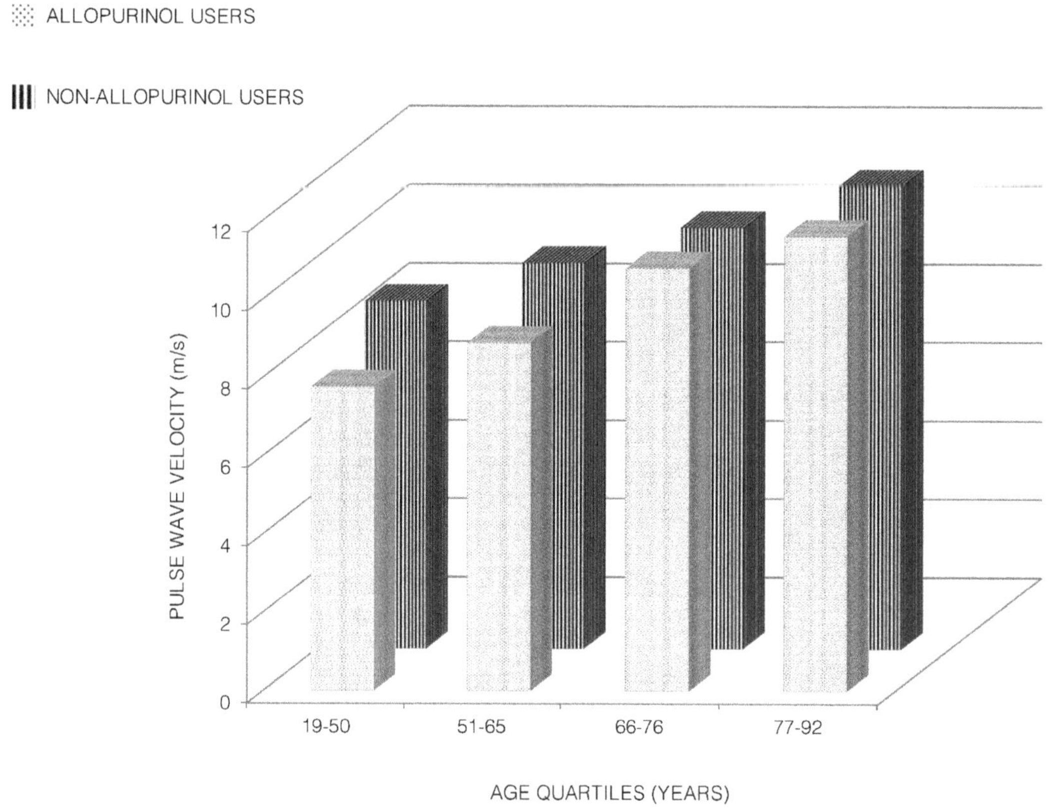

Figure 2. Differences in pulse wave velocity according to use of allopurinol and age quartiles.

attributable to reduced oxidative stress and not to uric acid reduction [30]. CKD is known to be associated with increased oxidative stress and acute-phase inflammation, which may both contribute to increased CV risk [40]. We found no significant difference in the levels of hsCRP between allopurinol users and non-allopurinol users, suggesting that inflammation was not a prominent mechanism in this association. Advanced glycation end product (AGE) has a bi-directional relationship with oxidative stress, including studies showing that increased oxidative stress is associated with formation and accumulation of AGE [41–45]. Level of tissue AGE as measured by SAF, which positively correlated with arterial stiffness, was found to be significantly lower in the allopurinol users when compared to non-allopurinol users, indicating that this biological pathway may be relevant to the link between allopurinol use and PWV described here.

Table 4. Multiple regression with pulse wave velocity as the dependent outcome variable.

	Mean change of PWV	95% CI		P value
		Lower bound	Upper bound	
Age (/5 years)	**0.306**	**0.225**	**0.387**	**<0.001**
Gender (male)	0.423	−0.009	0.856	0.06
White ethnicity	0.252	−0.296	0.800	0.4
Afro-caribbean ethnicity	0.552	−0.245	1.350	0.2
Smoking pack years	0.005	−0.006	0.015	0.4
Presence of diabetes mellitus	0.163	−0.261	0.586	0.5
SAF (/1 a.u.)	−0.258	−0.559	0.043	0.09
Peripheral PP (/5 mmHg)	**0.186**	**−0.0121**	**0.251**	**<0.001**
Use of ACEI/ARB	−0.136	−0.579	0.307	0.5
Use of allopurinol	**−0.633**	**−1.174**	**−0.092**	**0.02**

Adjusted R^2 for model = 0.348, $p<0.001$.

Abbreviations: ACEI = angiotensin converting enzyme inhibitor; ARB = angiotensin II receptor blocker; CI = confidence interval; PP = pulse pressure, PWV = pulse wave velocity; SAF = skin autofluorescence.

As arterial stiffness and BP are closely related, it is possible that the effect of allopurinol on arterial stiffness may be mediated through improved BP. A recent meta-analysis showed that allopurinol is associated with a small but significant reduction in BP [46]. Several hypotheses have been postulated to explain this apparent association. The antioxidant effect of allopurinol was considered to play a major role in improving endothelial function and blood pressure regulation [46]. Nonetheless, there was no clear consensus to-date with regards to the effects of oral antioxidant on arterial blood pressure. While some demonstrated blood pressure lowering effect of antioxidant vitamins [47,48], others did not [49–52] and one study showed paradoxical blunting of exercise training-induced improvement in endothelial function with antioxidant administration [53]. In addition to its antioxidant property, there is emerging evidence that allopurinol can block the deleterious cardiovascular effect of angiotensin II [54–56]. In this current study we found a significant difference in both peripheral and central BP between allopurinol users and non-allopurinol users, despite a comparable prevalence of ACEI/ARB use and total numbers of anti-hypertensive agents between groups. However, after adjustment in a multivariate analysis, the use of allopurinol remained significantly associated with arterial stiffness. This suggests a distinct direct effect of allopurinol on vascular stiffness that is independent of BP and the use of ACEI/ARB. This observation is supported by an RCT of 66 patients with mild to moderate hypertension which reported a favourable effect of allopurinol on aortic compliance, independent of ACEI or thiazide-based antihypertensive therapy [57].

Limitations

There were a number of limitations in this study. Due to the observational, cross-sectional nature of the study and non-randomised use of allopurinol, the association between allopurinol use and lower arterial stiffness reported here does not prove causality.

Although there were unequal distributions of gender, race, BMI, current smoking status and differences in serum uric acid between the groups, these are unlikely to have resulted in bias. Male gender was associated with higher PWV, however despite a higher proportion of males amongst allopurinol users, use of allopurinol remained associated with a lower PWV. In addition, people of Afro-Caribbean ethnicity had a lower PWV; most of the Afro-Caribbean participants were non-allopurinol users. The unequal distribution of gender and race between the groups was therefore unlikely to have resulted in bias against non-allopurinol use. As the number of non-white participants was small, we were unable to confidently examine the influence of allopurinol in different ethnic groups; this should be an area for future study. Although there were differences in BMI and serum uric acid level between the groups, these parameters did not have a significant bivariate association with PWV; hence, they were unlikely to confound the findings. Smoking history is known to have significant influence on arterial stiffness and there was a higher proportion of current smokers in the allopurinol non-user group. In addition, the comparatively lower peripheral and central pressures in the allopurinol user group might have contributed to lower PWV as BP is a strong determinant of arterial stiffness. However, after adjusted for haemodynamic parameters and smoking history in the regression model, use of allopurinol remained associated with lower PWV.

Although all available confounding variables were included in this study, there may be other potential unknown confounders as the biology of vascular disease in CKD is complex. The measurement of hsCRP was performed only at single time-point rather than the two time-points two weeks apart recommended by the American Heart Association [58]. We did not have measurements of endothelial dysfunction, which is closely linked to arterial stiffness and CKD [17]. Finally, encouraging results have been reported on an effect of allopurinol in improving renal function in patients with asymptomatic hyperuricaemia [59] or delaying disease progression in patients with CKD [15,60]. However, due to the cross-sectional nature of the data we were unable to examine this relationship.

Conclusion

In summary, the data shown here suggests that allopurinol is independently associated with lower arterial stiffness in patients with progressive CKD. This adds to accumulating evidence of the favourable effect of allopurinol on cardiovascular outcomes in a well-defined CKD cohort and indicates one mechanism by which this may occur. This study provides further justification for a large definitive RCT examining the therapeutic potential of allopurinol to reduce cardiovascular risk in people with CKD.

Acknowledgments

The authors would like to acknowledge the support of the staff in the renal outpatients department at University Hospital Birmingham, the research and development department at University Hospital Birmingham and the remainder of the recruiting RIISC study team.

Author Contributions

Conceived and designed the experiments: SJS MD CJF PC. Performed the experiments: KPN SJS MDJ PY RA MD. Analyzed the data: KPN CJF PC. Wrote the paper: KPN CJF PC.

References

1. Perlstein TS, Gumieniak O, Williams GH, Sparrow D, Vokonas PS, et al. (2006) Uric acid and the development of hypertension: the normative aging study. Hypertension 48: 1031–1036.
2. Erdogan D, Gullu H, Caliskan M, Yildirim E, Bilgi M, et al. (2005) Relationship of serum uric acid to measures of endothelial function and atherosclerosis in healthy adults. International journal of clinical practice 59: 1276–1282.
3. Freedman DS, Williamson DF, Gunter EW, Byers T (1995) Relation of serum uric acid to mortality and ischemic heart disease. The NHANES I Epidemiologic Follow-up Study. American journal of epidemiology 141: 637–644.
4. Fang J, Alderman MH (2000) Serum uric acid and cardiovascular mortality the NHANES I epidemiologic follow-up study, 1971–1992. National Health and Nutrition Examination Survey. JAMA : the journal of the American Medical Association 283: 2404–2410.
5. Strasak A, Ruttmann E, Brant L, Kelleher C, Klenk J, et al. (2008) Serum uric acid and risk of cardiovascular mortality: a prospective long-term study of 83,683 Austrian men. Clinical chemistry 54: 273–284.
6. Strasak AM, Kelleher CC, Brant LJ, Rapp K, Ruttmann E, et al. (2008) Serum uric acid is an independent predictor for all major forms of cardiovascular death in 28,613 elderly women: a prospective 21-year follow-up study. International journal of cardiology 125: 232–239.
7. Edwards NL (2008) The role of hyperuricemia and gout in kidney and cardiovascular disease. Cleveland Clinic journal of medicine 75 Suppl 5: S13–16.
8. Chonchol M, Shlipak MG, Katz R, Sarnak MJ, Newman AB, et al. (2007) Relationship of uric acid with progression of kidney disease. American journal of kidney diseases : the official journal of the National Kidney Foundation 50: 239–247.
9. Madero M, Sarnak MJ, Wang X, Greene T, Beck GJ, et al. (2009) Uric acid and long-term outcomes in CKD. American journal of kidney diseases : the official journal of the National Kidney Foundation 53: 796–803.
10. Iseki K, Ikemiya Y, Inoue T, Iseki C, Kinjo K, et al. (2004) Significance of hyperuricemia as a risk factor for developing ESRD in a screened cohort. American journal of kidney diseases : the official journal of the National Kidney Foundation 44: 642–650.

11. Syrjanen J, Mustonen J, Pasternack A (2000) Hypertriglyceridaemia and hyperuricaemia are risk factors for progression of IgA nephropathy. Nephrology, dialysis, transplantation : official publication of the European Dialysis and Transplant Association - European Renal Association 15: 34–42.
12. Li YL, Wang L, Li J, Huang Y, Yuan WM (2011) [The correlation between uric acid and the incidence and prognosis of kidney diseases: a systematic review and meta-analysis of cohort studies]. Zhonghua nei ke za zhi [Chinese journal of internal medicine] 50: 555–561.
13. Yelken B, Caliskan Y, Gorgulu N, Altun I, Yilmaz A, et al. (2012) Reduction of uric acid levels with allopurinol treatment improves endothelial function in patients with chronic kidney disease. Clinical nephrology 77: 275–282.
14. Kao MP, Ang DS, Gandy SJ, Nadir MA, Houston JG, et al. (2011) Allopurinol benefits left ventricular mass and endothelial dysfunction in chronic kidney disease. Journal of the American Society of Nephrology : JASN 22: 1382–1389.
15. Goicoechea M, de Vinuesa SG, Verdalles U, Ruiz-Caro C, Ampuero J, et al. (2010) Effect of allopurinol in chronic kidney disease progression and cardiovascular risk. Clinical journal of the American Society of Nephrology : CJASN 5: 1388–1393.
16. Wei L, Mackenzie IS, Chen Y, Struthers AD, MacDonald TM (2011) Impact of allopurinol use on urate concentration and cardiovascular outcome. British journal of clinical pharmacology 71: 600–607.
17. Chue CD, Townend JN, Steeds RP, Ferro CJ (2010) Arterial stiffness in chronic kidney disease: causes and consequences. Heart 96: 817–823.
18. Vlachopoulos C, Aznaouridis K, Stefanadis C (2010) Prediction of cardiovascular events and all-cause mortality with arterial stiffness: a systematic review and meta-analysis. Journal of the American College of Cardiology 55: 1318–1327.
19. Blacher J, Guerin AP, Pannier B, Marchais SJ, Safar ME, et al. (1999) Impact of aortic stiffness on survival in end-stage renal disease. Circulation 99: 2434–2439.
20. Laurent S, Cockcroft J, Van Bortel L, Boutouyrie P, Giannattasio C, et al. (2006) Expert consensus document on arterial stiffness: methodological issues and clinical applications. European heart journal 27: 2588–2605.
21. Stringer S, Sharma P, Dutton M, Jesky M, Ng K, et al. (2013) The natural history of, and risk factors for, progressive Chronic Kidney Disease (CKD): the Renal Impairment in Secondary care (RIISC) study; rationale and protocol. BMC nephrology 14: 95.
22. Levey AS, Bosch JP, Lewis JB, Greene T, Rogers N, et al. (1999) A more accurate method to estimate glomerular filtration rate from serum creatinine: a new prediction equation. Modification of Diet in Renal Disease Study Group. Annals of internal medicine 130: 461–470.
23. Wright JM, Mattu GS, Perry Jr TL, Gelferc ME, Strange KD, et al. (2001) Validation of a new algorithm for the BPM-100 electronic oscillometric office blood pressure monitor. Blood pressure monitoring 6: 161–165.
24. Hickson SS, Butlin M, Broad J, Avolio AP, Wilkinson IB, et al. (2009) Validity and repeatability of the Vicorder apparatus: a comparison with the SphygmoCor device. Hypertension research : official journal of the Japanese Society of Hypertension 32: 1079–1085.
25. Pucci G, Cheriyan J, Hubsch A, Hickson SS, Gajendragadkar PR, et al. (2013) Evaluation of the Vicorder, a novel cuff-based device for the noninvasive estimation of central blood pressure. Journal of hypertension 31: 77–85.
26. Wilkinson IB, MacCallum H, Flint L, Cockcroft JR, Newby DE, et al. (2000) The influence of heart rate on augmentation index and central arterial pressure in humans. The Journal of physiology 525 Pt 1: 263–270.
27. Altman D (1999) Practical statistics for medical research. London: Chapman & Hall.
28. Kals J, Kampus P, Kals M, Zilmer K, Kullisaar T, et al. (2006) Impact of oxidative stress on arterial elasticity in patients with atherosclerosis. American journal of hypertension 19: 902–908.
29. Touyz RM (2004) Reactive oxygen species, vascular oxidative stress, and redox signaling in hypertension: what is the clinical significance? Hypertension 44: 248–252.
30. George J, Carr E, Davies J, Belch JJ, Struthers A (2006) High-dose allopurinol improves endothelial function by profoundly reducing vascular oxidative stress and not by lowering uric acid. Circulation 114: 2508–2516.
31. Culleton BF, Larson MG, Kannel WB, Levy D (1999) Serum uric acid and risk for cardiovascular disease and death: the Framingham Heart Study. Annals of internal medicine 131: 7–13.
32. Alderman MH, Cohen H, Madhavan S, Kivlighn S (1999) Serum uric acid and cardiovascular events in successfully treated hypertensive patients. Hypertension 34: 144–150.
33. Liese AD, Hense HW, Lowel H, Doring A, Tietze M, et al. (1999) Association of serum uric acid with all-cause and cardiovascular disease mortality and incident myocardial infarction in the MONICA Augsburg cohort. World Health Organization Monitoring Trends and Determinants in Cardiovascular Diseases. Epidemiology 10: 391–397.
34. Bos MJ, Koudstaal PJ, Hofman A, Witteman JC, Breteler MM (2006) Uric acid is a risk factor for myocardial infarction and stroke: the Rotterdam study. Stroke; a journal of cerebral circulation 37: 1503–1507.
35. Moriarity JT, Folsom AR, Iribarren C, Nieto FJ, Rosamond WD (2000) Serum uric acid and risk of coronary heart disease: Atherosclerosis Risk in Communities (ARIC) Study. Annals of epidemiology 10: 136–143.
36. Hozawa A, Folsom AR, Ibrahim H, Nieto FJ, Rosamond WD, et al. (2006) Serum uric acid and risk of ischemic stroke: the ARIC Study. Atherosclerosis 187: 401–407.
37. Niskanen LK, Laaksonen DE, Nyyssonen K, Alfthan G, Lakka HM, et al. (2004) Uric acid level as a risk factor for cardiovascular and all-cause mortality in middle-aged men: a prospective cohort study. Archives of internal medicine 164: 1546–1551.
38. Krishnan E, Baker JF, Furst DE, Schumacher HR (2006) Gout and the risk of acute myocardial infarction. Arthritis and rheumatism 54: 2688–2696.
39. Verdecchia P, Schillaci G, Reboldi G, Santeusanio F, Porcellati C, et al. (2000) Relation between serum uric acid and risk of cardiovascular disease in essential hypertension. The PIUMA study. Hypertension 36: 1072–1078.
40. Oberg BP, McMenamin E, Lucas FL, McMonagle E, Morrow J, et al. (2004) Increased prevalence of oxidant stress and inflammation in patients with moderate to severe chronic kidney disease. Kidney international 65: 1009–1016.
41. Schmidt AM, Hori O, Brett J, Yan SD, Wautier JL, et al. (1994) Cellular receptors for advanced glycation end products. Implications for induction of oxidant stress and cellular dysfunction in the pathogenesis of vascular lesions. Arteriosclerosis and thrombosis : a journal of vascular biology/American Heart Association 14: 1521–1528.
42. Mulder DJ, de Boer JF, Graaff R, de Vries R, Annema W, et al. (2011) Skin autofluorescence is inversely related to HDL anti-oxidative capacity in type 2 diabetes mellitus. Atherosclerosis 218: 102–106.
43. Mulder DJ, van Haelst PL, Gross S, de Leeuw K, Bijzet J, et al. (2008) Skin autofluorescence is elevated in patients with stable coronary artery disease and is associated with serum levels of neopterin and the soluble receptor for advanced glycation end products. Atherosclerosis 197: 217–223.
44. Yan SD, Schmidt AM, Anderson GM, Zhang J, Brett J, et al. (1994) Enhanced cellular oxidant stress by the interaction of advanced glycation end products with their receptors/binding proteins. The Journal of biological chemistry 269: 9889–9897.
45. Yamagishi S, Maeda S, Matsui T, Ueda S, Fukami K, et al. (2012) Role of advanced glycation end products (AGEs) and oxidative stress in vascular complications in diabetes. Biochimica et biophysica acta 1820: 663–671.
46. Agarwal V, Hans N, Messerli FH (2012) Effect of Allopurinol on Blood Pressure: A Systematic Review and Meta-Analysis. The Journal of Clinical Hypertension: no–no.
47. Schutte AE, Huisman HW, Oosthuizen W, van Rooyen JM, Jerling JC (2004) Cardiovascular effects of oral Supplementation of vitamin C, E and folic acid in young healthy males. International journal for vitamin and nutrition research Internationale Zeitschrift fur Vitamin- und Ernahrungsforschung Journal international de vitaminologie et de nutrition 74: 285–293.
48. Galley HF, Thornton J, Howdle PD, Walker BE, Webster NR (1997) Combination oral antioxidant supplementation reduces blood pressure. Clinical science 92: 361–365.
49. Miller ER, 3rd, Appel LJ, Levander OA, Levine DM (1997) The effect of antioxidant vitamin supplementation on traditional cardiovascular risk factors. Journal of cardiovascular risk 4: 19–24.
50. Zureik M, Galan P, Bertrais S, Mennen L, Czernichow S, et al. (2004) Effects of long-term daily low-dose supplementation with antioxidant vitamins and minerals on structure and function of large arteries. Arteriosclerosis, thrombosis, and vascular biology 24: 1485–1491.
51. Eskurza I, Monahan KD, Robinson JA, Seals DR (2004) Ascorbic acid does not affect large elastic artery compliance or central blood pressure in young and older men. American journal of physiology Heart and circulatory physiology 286: H1528–1534.
52. Mottram P, Shige H, Nestel P (1999) Vitamin E improves arterial compliance in middle-aged men and women. Atherosclerosis 145: 399–404.
53. Wray DW, Uberoi A, Lawrenson L, Bailey DM, Richardson RS (2009) Oral antioxidants and cardiovascular health in the exercise-trained and untrained elderly: a radically different outcome. Clinical science 116: 433–441.
54. Jia N, Dong P, Ye Y, Qian C, Dai Q (2012) Allopurinol attenuates oxidative stress and cardiac fibrosis in angiotensin II-induced cardiac diastolic dysfunction. Cardiovascular therapeutics 30: 117–123.
55. Ercan ZS, Ilhan M, Oguz A, Turker RK (1992) Superoxide dismutase and allopurinol prevent the pressor effects of angiotensin II and histamine in the guinea-pig isolated perfused lung exposed to hypoxia. General pharmacology 23: 1149–1151.
56. Kasal DA, Neves MF, Oigman W, Mandarim-de-Lacerda CA (2008) Allopurinol attenuates L-NAME induced cardiomyopathy comparable to blockade of angiotensin receptor. Histology and histopathology 23: 1241–1248.
57. Kostka-Jeziorny K, Uruski P, Tykarski A (2011) Effect of allopurinol on blood pressure and aortic compliance in hypertensive patients. Blood pressure 20: 104–110.
58. Pearson TA, Mensah GA, Alexander RW, Anderson JL, Cannon RO, 3rd, et al. (2003) Markers of inflammation and cardiovascular disease: application to clinical and public health practice: A statement for healthcare professionals from the Centers for Disease Control and Prevention and the American Heart Association. Circulation 107: 499–511.
59. Kanbay M, Ozkara A, Selcoki Y, Isik B, Turgut F, et al. (2007) Effect of treatment of hyperuricemia with allopurinol on blood pressure, creatinine clearence, and proteinuria in patients with normal renal functions. International urology and nephrology 39: 1227–1233.
60. Siu Y-P, Leung K-T, Tong MK-H, Kwan T-H (2006) Use of Allopurinol in Slowing the Progression of Renal Disease Through Its Ability to Lower Serum Uric Acid Level. american journal of kidney diseases 47: 51–59.

Permissions

All chapters in this book were first published in PLOS ONE, by The Public Library of Science; hereby published with permission under the Creative Commons Attribution License or equivalent. Every chapter published in this book has been scrutinized by our experts. Their significance has been extensively debated. The topics covered herein carry significant findings which will fuel the growth of the discipline. They may even be implemented as practical applications or may be referred to as a beginning point for another development.

The contributors of this book come from diverse backgrounds, making this book a truly international effort. This book will bring forth new frontiers with its revolutionizing research information and detailed analysis of the nascent developments around the world.

We would like to thank all the contributing authors for lending their expertise to make the book truly unique. They have played a crucial role in the development of this book. Without their invaluable contributions this book wouldn't have been possible. They have made vital efforts to compile up to date information on the varied aspects of this subject to make this book a valuable addition to the collection of many professionals and students.

This book was conceptualized with the vision of imparting up-to-date information and advanced data in this field. To ensure the same, a matchless editorial board was set up. Every individual on the board went through rigorous rounds of assessment to prove their worth. After which they invested a large part of their time researching and compiling the most relevant data for our readers.

The editorial board has been involved in producing this book since its inception. They have spent rigorous hours researching and exploring the diverse topics which have resulted in the successful publishing of this book. They have passed on their knowledge of decades through this book. To expedite this challenging task, the publisher supported the team at every step. A small team of assistant editors was also appointed to further simplify the editing procedure and attain best results for the readers.

Apart from the editorial board, the designing team has also invested a significant amount of their time in understanding the subject and creating the most relevant covers. They scrutinized every image to scout for the most suitable representation of the subject and create an appropriate cover for the book.

The publishing team has been an ardent support to the editorial, designing and production team. Their endless efforts to recruit the best for this project, has resulted in the accomplishment of this book. They are a veteran in the field of academics and their pool of knowledge is as vast as their experience in printing. Their expertise and guidance has proved useful at every step. Their uncompromising quality standards have made this book an exceptional effort. Their encouragement from time to time has been an inspiration for everyone.

The publisher and the editorial board hope that this book will prove to be a valuable piece of knowledge for researchers, students, practitioners and scholars across the globe.

List of Contributors

Martin J. Raftery
Department of Renal Medicine, Barts Health NHS Trust, London, United Kingdom

Muhammad M. Yaqoob, Gavin Dreyer
Department of Renal Medicine, Barts Health NHS Trust, London, United Kingdom
Department of Translational Medicine and Therapeutics, Queen Mary University of London, London, United Kingdom

Rupert M. Pearse
Department of Critical Care Medicine, Barts Health NHS Trust, London, United Kingdom,

Steven M. Harwood
Department of Translational Medicine and Therapeutics, Queen Mary University of London, London, United Kingdom,

Arthur T. Tucker
Ernest Cooke Microvascular Unit, Barts Health NHS Trust, London, United Kingdom

Nathalie Neirynck, Sunny Eloot, Griet Glorieux, Raymond Vanholder
Nephrology Section, Department of Internal Medicine, Ghent University Hospital, Gent, Belgium

Daniela V. Barreto, Fellype C. Barreto, Sophie Liabeuf
INSERM U-1088, Amiens, France
Clinical Research Centre, Division of Clinical Pharmacology, Amiens University Hospital, Amiens, France and the Jules Verne University of Picardy, Amiens, France

Ziad A. Massy
INSERM U-1088, Amiens, France
Clinical Research Centre, Division of Clinical Pharmacology, Amiens University Hospital, Amiens, France and the Jules Verne University of Picardy, Amiens, France
Division of Nephrology, Amiens University Hospital, Amiens, France

Aurélie Lenglet
INSERM U-1088, Amiens, France
Division of Nephrology, Amiens University Hospital, Amiens, France

Horst D. Lemke
EXcor Lab GmbH, Obernburg, Germany

Aurore Halkovich, Anne-Marie Dupuy
Laboratoire de Biochimie, CHRU de Montpellier, Montpellier, France

Marion Morena
Laboratoire de Biochimie, CHRU de Montpellier, Montpellier, France
Institut de Recherche et de Formation en Dialyse, Montpellier, France
UMR 204, Nutripass, UniversitéMontpellier I, Montpellier, France

Anne-Sophie Bargnoux, Jean-Paul Cristol
Laboratoire de Biochimie, CHRU de Montpellier, Montpellier, France
UMR 204, Nutripass, UniversitéMontpellier I, Montpellier, France

Bernard Canaud
Institut de Recherche et de Formation en Dialyse, Montpellier, France
UMR 204, Nutripass, UniversitéMontpellier I, Montpellier, France
Service de Néphrologie-Hémodialyse et Soins Intensifs, CHRU de Montpellier, Montpellier, France

Kada Klouche
UMR 204, Nutripass, UniversitéMontpellier I, Montpellier, France
V6 Service de Re´animation Me´tabolique, CHRU de Montpellier, Montpellier, France

Isabelle Jaussent
INSERM, U1061 and UniversitéMontpellier I, Montpellier, France

Leila Chenine, Héléne Leray-Moragues
Service de Néphrologie-He´modialyse et Soins Intensifs, CHRU de Montpellier, Montpellier, France

Héléne Vernhet
Service de Radiologie, CHRU de Montpellier, Montpellier, France

Arianne van Koppen, Jaap A. Joles, Bas W. M. van Balkom, Rachel H. Giles, Marianne C. Verhaar
Department of Nephrology and Hypertension, University Medical Center Utrecht, Utrecht, the Netherlands

Sai Kiang Lim
Institute of Medical Biology, A*STAR, Singapore, Republic of Singapore

Dominique de Kleijn
Department of Experimental Cardiology, University Medical Center Utrecht, Utrecht, the Netherlands

Melissa S. Nolan, Kristy O. Murray
Department of Pediatrics, Baylor College of Medicine, Houston, Texas, United States of America

Amber S. Podoll, Katherine M. Akers, Kevin W. Finkel
Department of Internal Medicine, Medical School, University of Texas Health Science Center at Houston, Houston, Texas, United States of America

Anne M. Hause
Department of Epidemiology, School of Public Health, University of Texas Health Science Center at Houston, Houston, Texas, United States of America

Darren A. Yuen, Kim A. Connelly andrew Advani, Christine Liao, Michael A. Kuliszewski, Judy Trogadis, Kerri Thai, Suzanne L. Advani, Howard Leong-Poi, Philip A. Marsden, Richard E. Gilbert
Keenan Research Centre of the Li Ka Shing Knowledge Institute, St. Michael's Hospital, Department of Medicine, University of Toronto, Toronto, Ontario, Canada,

Yuan Zhang, Darren J. Kelly
Department of Medicine, St. Vincent's Hospital, University of Melbourne, Melbourne, Victoria, Australia,

Armand Keating
Department of Medicine, Princess Margaret Hospital, University of Toronto, Toronto, Ontario, Canada,

Duncan J. Stewart
Ottawa Health Research Institute, University of Ottawa, Ottawa, Ontario, Canada

Michael Rudnicki, Hannes Neuwirt, Susie-Jane Noppert, Johannes Leierer, Judith Sunzenauer, Susanne Eder, Gert Mayer
Medical University Innsbruck, Deptartment of Internal Medicine IV - Nephrology and Hypertension, Innsbruck, Austria,

Kathrin Eller, Alexander R. Rosenkranz
Medical University Innsbruck, Deptartment of Internal Medicine IV - Nephrology and Hypertension, Innsbruck, Austria
Medical University of Graz, Deptartment of Internal Medicine, Clinical Division of Nephrology and Hemodialysis, Graz, Austria

Paul Perco, Bernd Mayer
Emergentec Biodevelopment GmbH, Vienna, Austria,

Carlamaria Zoja
Mario Negri Institute for Pharmacological Research, Centro Anna Maria Astori, Science and Technology Park Kilometro Rosso, Bergamo, Italy

Gerhard A. Müller
Georg-August-University Göttingen, Department of Medicine, Nephrology and Rheumatology, Göttingen, Germany

Colin D. Chue, William E. Moody, Nicola C. Edwards
School of Clinical and Experimental Medicine, College of Medical and Dental Sciences, University of Birmingham, Birmingham, United Kingdom
Department of Cardiology, Queen Elizabeth Hospital Birmingham, Birmingham, United Kingdom

Richard P. Steeds, Jonathan N. Townend
Department of Cardiology, Queen Elizabeth Hospital Birmingham, Birmingham, United Kingdom

Nadezhda A. Wall
School of Immunity and Infection, College of Medical and Dental Sciences, University of Birmingham, Birmingham, United Kingdom

Nicola J. Crabtree
Department of Endocrinology, Birmingham Children's Hospital, Birmingham, United Kingdom

Daniel Zehnder
Clinical Sciences Research Institute, University of Warwick, Coventry, United Kingdom,

Charles J. Ferro
Department of Nephrology, Queen Elizabeth Hospital Birmingham, Birmingham, United Kingdom

Wen-Hsien, Lee Po-Chao Hsu
Division of Cardiology, Department of Internal Medicine, Kaohsiung Medical University Hospital, Kaohsiung Medical University, Kaohsiung, Taiwan

Ho-Ming Su
Division of Cardiology, Department of Internal Medicine, Kaohsiung Medical University Hospital, Kaohsiung Medical University, Kaohsiung, Taiwan,
Department of Internal Medicine, Kaohsiung Municipal Hsiao-Kang Hospital, Kaohsiung Medical University, Kaohsiung, Taiwan
Faculty of Medicine, College of Medicine, Kaohsiung Medical University, Kaohsiung, Taiwan

Tsung-Hsien Lin, Chee-Siong Lee, Wen-Chol Voon, Wen-Ter Lai, Sheng-Hsiung Sheu
Division of Cardiology, Department of Internal Medicine, Kaohsiung Medical University Hospital, Kaohsiung Medical University, Kaohsiung, Taiwan
Faculty of Medicine, College of Medicine, Kaohsiung Medical University, Kaohsiung, Taiwan

Szu-Chia Chen
Division of Nephrology, Department of Internal Medicine, Kaohsiung Medical University Hospital, Kaohsiung Medical University, Kaohsiung, Taiwan
Department of Internal Medicine, Kaohsiung Municipal Hsiao-Kang Hospital, Kaohsiung Medical University, Kaohsiung, Taiwan
Faculty of Medicine, College of Medicine, Kaohsiung Medical University, Kaohsiung, Taiwan

Chiung-Chi Peng
Graduate Institute of Clinical Medicine, College of Medicine, Taipei Medical University, Taipei, Taiwan
Department of Physical Therapy, Graduate Institute of Rehabilitation Science, China Medical University, Taichung, Taiwan
Graduate Institute of Rehabilitation Science, China Medical University, Taichung, Taiwan

Kuan-Chou Chen
Department of Urology, School of Medicine, College of Medicine, Taipei Medical University, Taipei, Taiwan,
Department of Urology, Shuang Ho Hospital, Taipei Medical University, Zhonghe, Taipei, Taiwan,

Chiu-Lan Hsieh
Graduate Institute of Biotechnology, National Changhua University of Education, 1, Changhua City, Taiwan

Robert Y. Peng
Research Institute of Biotechnology, Hungkuang University, Shalu County, Taichung, Taiwan

Ling-I Chen
Division of Nephrology, Department of Internal Medicine, Kaohsiung Medical University Hospital, Kaohsiung, Taiwan

Jinn-Yuh Guh, Mei-Chuan Kuo, Shang-Jyh Hwang, Hung-Chun Chen
Division of Nephrology, Department of Internal Medicine, Kaohsiung Medical University Hospital, Kaohsiung, Taiwan
Faculty of Renal Care, College of Medicine, Kaohsiung Medical University, Kaohsiung, Taiwan

Tzu-Hui Chen
Department of Nursing, Kaohsiung Medical University Hospital, Kaohsiung, Taiwan

Kwan-Dun Wu, Yung-Ming Chen
Department of Internal Medicine, National Taiwan University Hospital, Taipei, Taiwan

Fabrizio Veglia, Isabella Squellerio, Monica De Metrio, Mara Rubino, Benedetta Porro, Marco Moltrasio, Giancarlo Marenzi
Centro Cardiologico Monzino, I.R.C.C.S, Milan, Italy

Viviana Cavalca
Centro Cardiologico Monzino, I.R.C.C.S, Milan, Italy
Dipartimento di Scienze Cliniche e di Comunitá, Universitá degli Studi di Milano, Milan, Italy

Elena Tremoli
Dipartimento di Scienze Farmacologiche e Biomolecolari, Universita` degli Studi di Milano, Milan, Italy

Martin H. de Borst, Ferdau L. Nauta, Gozewijn D. Laverman, Ron T. Gansevoort, Gerjan Navis
Division of Nephrology, Department of Internal Medicine, University Medical Center Groningen and University of Groningen, Groningen, the Netherlands

Liffert Vogt
Department of Nephrology, Academic Medical Center, Amsterdam, the Netherlands

David M. Charytan, Alexander M. Helfand, Angeles Cinelli
Renal Division, Department of Medicine, Brigham and Women's Hospital, Boston, Massachusetts, United States of America

Raghu Kalluri, Elisabeth M. Zeisberg Brian A. MacDonald
Division of Matrix Biology, Department of Medicine, Beth Israel Deaconess Medical Center, Boston, Massachusetts, United States of America

Marie Frimodt-Møller, Anne-Lise Kamper
Departments of Nephrology, Rigshospitalet, University of Copenhagen, Copenhagen, Denmark,

Svend Strandgaard, Arne Høj Nielsen
Herlev Hospital, Copenhagen, Denmark,

Svend Kreiner
Department of Biostatistics, University of Copenhagen, Copenhagen, Denmark

Andréia M. Menezes, Jorge Torelly Jr, Lúcia Real, Julia Poeta
Faculdade de Medicina, Universidade Federal do Rio Grande do Sul, Porto Alegre, Rio Grande do Sul, Brazil

Eduardo Sprinz
Faculdade de Medicina, Universidade Federal do Rio Grande do Sul, Porto Alegre, Rio Grande do Sul, Brazil
Hospital de Clı´nicas de Porto Alegre, Porto Alegre, Rio Grande do Sul, Brazil

Mônica Bay
Hospital de Clínicas de Porto Alegre, Porto Alegre, Rio Grande do Sul, Brazil

Chih-Kang Chiang, Yung-Ming Chen, Ming-Shiou Wu, Kwan-Dun Wu
Renal Division, Department of Medicine, National Taiwan University Hospital, Taipei, Taiwan,

Tzong- Shinn Chu
Renal Division, Department of Medicine, National Taiwan University Hospital, Taipei, Taiwan
Department of Internal Medicine, National Taiwan University Hospital Chu-Tung Branch, Hsin-Chu County, Taiwan

Fan-Chi Chang
Renal Division, Department of Medicine, National Taiwan University Hospital, Taipei, Taiwan
Department of Internal Medicine, National Taiwan University Hospital Chu-Tung Branch, Hsin-Chu County, Taiwan
Graduate Institutes of Physiology, College of Medicine, National Taiwan University, Taipei, Taiwan

Shuei-Liong Lin
Renal Division, Department of Medicine, National Taiwan University Hospital, Taipei, Taiwan
Graduate Institutes of Physiology, College of Medicine, National Taiwan University, Taipei, Taiwan

Tai-Shuan Lai
Renal Division, Department of Medicine, National Taiwan University Hospital, Taipei, Taiwan
Department of Internal Medicine, National Taiwan University Hospital Bei-Hu Branch, Taipei, Taiwan

Massimiliano Fedecostante, Francesco Spannella, Emma Espinosa, Paolo Dessí-Fulgheri, Riccardo Sarzani
Internal Medicine and Geriatrics and ''Hypertension Excellence Centre'' of the European Society of Hypertension, Department of Clinical and Molecular Sciences, University ''Politecnica delle Marche'', Italian National Research Centre on Aging ''U. Sestilli'', IRCCS-INRCA, Ancona, Italy

Giovanna Cola
Cardiology Clinic, Department of Cardiovascular Sciences, University ''Politecnica delle Marche'', ''Ospedali Riuniti'', Ancona, Italy

Melissa E. Stauffer
SCRIBCO, Effort, Pennsylvania, United States of America

Tao Fan
Merck & Co., Inc., Whitehouse Station, New Jersey, United States of America

Ju-Ae Kim
Integrated Metabolomics Research Group, Seoul Center, Korea Basic Science Institute, Seoul, Korea
Department of Chemistry, Sungkyunkwan University, Suwon, Korea

Yong-Kook Kwon, Geum-Sook Hwang
Integrated Metabolomics Research Group, Seoul Center, Korea Basic Science Institute, Seoul, Korea
Graduate School of Analytical Science and Technology, Chungnam University, Daejeon, Korea

Do Hyun Ryu
Department of Chemistry, Sungkyunkwan University, Suwon, Korea

Tae-Hwan Kwon, Hyo-Jung Choi
Department of Biochemistry and Cell Biology, School of Medicine, Kyungpook National University, Taegu, Korea

Bernadette Thomas, Rajnish Mehrotra
Division of Nephrology, Department of Medicine, University of Washington, Seattle, Washington, United States of America

Maurits van Pelt
MoPoTsyo Patient Information Centre, Phnom Penh, Cambodia

Cassianne Robinson-Cohen
Kidney Research Institute, University of Washington, Seattle, Washington, United States of America

James Lo Gerfo
Department of Medicine, University of Washington, Seattle, Washington, United States of America

Natasha J. McIntyre, Richard J. Fluck, Apostolos Fakis, Maarten W. Taal
Department of Renal Medicine, Royal Derby Hospital, Derbyshire, United Kingdom

Christopher W. McIntyre
Department of Renal Medicine, Royal Derby Hospital, Derbyshire, United Kingdom,
Department of Vascular Medicine, University of Nottingham, Nottingham, United Kingdom

Ryuichi Uetake, Takayuki Sakurai, Akiko Kamiyoshi, Yuka Ichikawa-Shindo, Hisaka Kawate, Yasuhiro Iesato, Takahiro Yoshizawa, Teruhide Koyama, Lei Yang, Yuichi Toriyama, Akihiro Yamauchi, Kyoko Igarashi, Megumu Tanaka, Takayuki Shindo
Department of Cardiovascular Research, Shinshu University Graduate School of Medicine, Matsumoto, Japan

Takashige Kuwabara, Masashi Mukoyama
Department of Medicine and Clinical Science, Kyoto University Graduate School of Medicine, Kyoto, Japan

Kiyoshi Mori
Department of Medicine and Clinical Science, Kyoto University Graduate School of Medicine, Kyoto, Japan
Medical Innovation Center, Kyoto University Graduate School of Medicine, Kyoto, Japan

Motoko Yanagita
Department of Nephrology, Kyoto University Graduate School of Medicine, Kyoto, Japan

Mei-Yueh Lee
Department of Internal Medicine, Kaohsiung Municipal Hsiao-Kang Hospital, Kaohsiung, Taiwan
Division of Endocrinology and Metabolism, Department of Internal Medicine, Kaohsiung Medical University Hospital, Kaohsiung, Taiwan
Graduate Institute of Medicine, Kaohsiung Medical University, Kaohsiung, Taiwan

Pi-Jung Hsiao, Kun-Der Lin
Division of Endocrinology and Metabolism, Department of Internal Medicine, Kaohsiung Medical University Hospital, Kaohsiung, Taiwan
Graduate Institute of Medicine, Kaohsiung Medical University, Kaohsiung, Taiwan

Shyi-Jang Shin
Division of Endocrinology and Metabolism, Department of Internal Medicine, Kaohsiung Medical University Hospital, Kaohsiung, Taiwan
Graduate Institute of Medicine, Kaohsiung Medical University, Kaohsiung, Taiwan
Graduate Institute of Medical Genetics, Kaohsiung Medical University, Kaohsiung, Taiwan

Yi-Hsin Yang
Statistical Analysis Laboratory, Department of Clinical Research, Kaohsiung Medical University Hospital, Kaohsiung, Taiwan

Rajbir Athwal, Mary Dutton, Khai P. Ng
Department of Renal Medicine, Queen Elizabeth Hospital Birmingham, Birmingham, United Kingdom,

Stephanie J. Stringer, Mark D. Jesky, Punit Yadav, Charles J. Ferro, Paul Cockwell
Department of Renal Medicine, Queen Elizabeth Hospital Birmingham, Birmingham, United Kingdom,
School of Immunity and Infection, University of Birmingham, Birmingham, United Kingdom

Index

www.ingramcontent.com/pod-product-compliance
Lightning Source LLC
LaVergne TN
LVHW060559210926
848485LV00005B/1341